Non-Neoplastic Hematologic Disorders

Lubomir Sokol • Ling Zhang
Editors

Non-Neoplastic Hematologic Disorders

A Quick Review of Modern Diagnostic and Therapeutic Approaches

Springer

Editors
Lubomir Sokol
Department of Malignant Hematology
Moffitt Cancer Center
Tampa, FL, USA

Ling Zhang
Department of Hematopathology
Moffitt Cancer Center
Tampa, FL, USA

ISBN 978-3-031-62372-1 ISBN 978-3-031-62373-8 (eBook)
https://doi.org/10.1007/978-3-031-62373-8

This Springer imprint is published by the registered company Springer Nature Switzerland AG
The registered company address is: Gewerbestrasse 11, 6330 Cham, Switzerland

Preface

Nonmalignant hematology, also known in the literature as classical or benign hematology, comprises a large group of hereditary and acquired blood diseases such as anemias, bleeding and clotting disorders, hemoglobinopathies, and other disorders of blood, bone marrow, and blood vessels. This topic is very important since general hematology/oncology specialists receive up to 40% of consults related to nonmalignant hematology. In the past decades, the progress in diagnosis and therapy in the field of nonmalignant blood diseases was rather slower and in the shadow of discoveries made in malignant hematology. However, more recently, the major progress in development of novel therapeutic agents including recombinant coagulation factors, direct oral anticoagulants, monoclonal antibodies for patients with microangiopathies, and gene therapy for genetic diseases such as sickle cell disease and beta-thalassemia highlights the evolving landscape of modern treatment options. Furthermore, the advent of advanced cellular, molecular, and genomic diagnostic technologies resulted in the discovery of somatic and germline mutations in many hematologic disorders and led to the development of more effective therapeutic strategies with improved patient outcomes. Mastering both routine and advanced diagnostic and therapeutic approaches in classical hematology is not only crucial for providing excellent personalized patient care but also essential for the ongoing professional development of clinical hematology fellows. This pocket-sized compendium with over 50 chapters is designed to be a practical guide in clinical settings, providing quick reference and essential algorithms for the diagnosis and management of nonmalignant hematologic disorders. The electronic version of this book also includes relevant board exam-like questions following each chapter. We have aimed to assemble a diverse team of contributors, who bring their wealth of knowledge and clinical experience. We hope that this pocketbook will serve as a valuable up-to-date resource for practicing hematologists, oncologists, hematopathologists, laboratory scientists, clinical fellows, residents, medical students, and allied health professionals, guiding them in the diagnosis and management of nonmalignant hematologic disorders. Thank you for joining us on this exciting journey through the fascinating world of discoveries and innovations in nonmalignant hematology.

Tampa, FL, USA

Lubomir Sokol
Ling Zhang

Contents

Contributors

Yasmin Abaza Department of Medicine, Hematology Oncology Division, Feinberg School of Medicine, Northwestern University, Chicago, IL, USA

Ziad Abuhelwa Department of Hematology/Oncology, Moffitt Cancer Center, University of South Florida, Tampa, FL, USA

Hassan Abushukair Department of Medicine, Jordan University of Science and Technology, Irbid, Jordan

Barina Aqil Department of Pathology, Feinberg School of Medicine, Northwestern University, Chicago, IL, USA

Ahmed Arfa Department of Pathology, Medical College of Georgia, Augusta University, Augusta, GA, USA

Department of Hematopathology, Moffitt Cancer Center & Research Institute, University of South Florida, Tampa, FL, USA

Sabarish Ayyappan Division of Hematology–Oncology, University of Iowa Hospitals and Clinics, Iowa City, IA, USA

Department of Internal Medicine, University of Iowa, Carver College of Medicine, Iowa City, IA, USA

Abida Babu Department of Hematology Oncology, H Lee Moffitt Cancer Center, University of South Florida, Tampa, FL, USA

Somedeb Ball, MD Division of Hematology and Oncology, Vanderbilt University School of Medicine, Nashville, TN, USA

Mark Ballow Department of Pediatrics, Allergy and Immunology Division, University of South Florida at Johns Hopkins All Children's Hospital, St. Petersburg, FL, USA

Sudeepthi Bandikatla Moffitt Cancer Center, Tampa, FL, USA

Kaaron Benson Department of Pathology, H. Lee Moffitt Cancer Center, Tampa, FL, USA

Mishi Bhushan Department of Pathology, University of Alabama Birmingham, Birmingham, AL, USA

Amalia Bonano-Rios Memorial Cancer Institute at Memorial Healthcare System, Pembroke Pines, FL, USA

Aaron B. Boothby University of Washington, Seattle, WA, USA

Sanjay Bridgelall USF/Moffitt Cancer Center, Tampa, FL, USA

Lugen Chen Department of Pathology, Tampa General Hospital, Tampa, FL, USA

Jinjun Cheng Department of Pathology and Laboratory Medicine, Children's National Hospital, Washington, DC, USA

Shivani M. Dalal Memorial Cancer Institute at Memorial Healthcare System, Pembroke Pines, FL, USA

Nyein Thaw Dar Memorial Health Care, Memorial Cancer Institute, Hollywood, FL, USA

Jerel David Hematology Oncology Fellow, Moffitt Cancer Center/University of South Florida, Tampa, FL, USA

Yehuda Deutsch Department of Malignant Hematology and Cellular TherapyMemorial Healthcare System, Moffitt Cancer Center, Pembroke Pines, FL, USA

Jaime Roman Diaz Department of Blood and Marrow Transplant and Cellular Immunotherapy, H. Lee Moffitt Cancer Center and Research Institute, Tampa, FL, USA

Mohammad Ammad Ud Din Department of Hematology/Oncology, H Lee Moffitt Cancer Center and Research Institute, Tampa, FL, USA

Dimitrios Drekolias Moffitt Cancer Center, University of South Florida, Tampa, FL, USA

Alexandra Dreyzin Center for Cancer and Blood Disorders, Children's National Hospital, Washington, DC, USA

Jennifer Eatrides H. Lee Moffitt Cancer Center and Research Institute, Tampa, FL, USA

Department of Oncologic Sciences, Morsani College of Medicine, University of South Florida, Tampa, FL, USA

Department of Satellite and Community Oncology, H. Lee Moffitt Cancer Center and Research Institute, Tampa, FL, USA

Department of Malignant Hematology, H. Lee Moffitt Cancer Center and Research Institute, Tampa, FL, USA

Kleber Y. Fertrin Fred Hutchinson Cancer Center, Seattle, WA, USA

Juehua Gao Department of Pathology, Feinberg School of Medicine, Northwestern University, Chicago, IL, USA

Franco C. Garcia Department of Satellite and Community Oncology, H. Lee Moffitt Cancer Center and Research Institute, Tampa, FL, USA

Curtis Gravenmier Department of Hematopathology and Laboratory Medicine, Moffitt Cancer Center, Tampa, FL, USA

Udhayvir Singh Grewal Division of Hematology–Oncology, University of Iowa Hospitals and Clinics, Iowa City, IA, USA

Caroline K. Hana Department of Hematology and Medical Oncology, Memorial Healthcare System, Hollywood, FL, USA

Memorial Healthcare System, Pembroke Pines, FL, USA

Wissam Hanayneh Our Lady of Lourdes- JD Moncus Cancer Center, Lafayette, LA, USA

Guy Handley H. Lee Moffitt Cancer Center and Research Institute, Tampa, FL, USA

Department of Medicine, Division of Infectious Disease and International Medicine, Morsani College of Medicine, University of South Florida, Tampa, FL, USA

Jesse J. Hubbard Moffitt Cancer Center, Tampa, FL, USA

Atif Hussein Department Hematology and Oncology, Memorial Cancer Institute, Miami, FL, USA

Memorial Healthcare System, Pembroke Pines, FL, USA

Atif M. Hussein Department of Hematology and Medical Oncology, Memorial Healthcare System, Hollywood, FL, USA

Stanislav Ivanov Department Hematology and Oncology, Memorial Cancer Institute, Miami, FL, USA

Ajay B. Iyer Department of Internal Medicine, HCA Healthcare, Sarasota, FL, USA

Michael Jaglal Department of Hematology and Oncology, Moffitt Cancer Center, Tampa, FL, USA

Moffitt Cancer Center, University of South Florida, Tampa, FL, USA

Akriti G. Jain H. Lee Moffitt Cancer and Research Center, Tampa, FL, USA

Akriti Jain Department of Hematology/Oncology, Moffitt Cancer Center, University of South Florida, Tampa, FL, USA

Jesse M. Jaso Department of Hematopathology, University of Texas Southwestern Medical Center, Dallas, TX, USA

Yulan Jin Department of Pathology, H.Lee Moffitt Cancer Center and Research Institute, University of South Florida, Tampa, FL, USA

Aryanna Jordan Department of Malignant Hematology, H. Lee Moffitt Cancer Center and Research Institute, Tampa, FL, USA

Loveleen C. Kang Department of Pathology and Laboratory Medicine, James A. Haley, Veterans' Hospital, Tampa, FL, USA

James A Haley VA, Tampa, FL, USA

Syeda Saba Kareem Department of Malignant Hematology, Moffitt Cancer Center, Tampa, FL, USA

Sushmita Khadka Moffitt Cancer Center, Tampa, FL, USA

Robert Killeen Moffitt Cancer Center, Tampa, FL, USA

Julie Li Department of Pathology, Moffitt Cancer Center, Tampa, FL, USA

Hien D. Liu Department of Blood and Marrow Transplant and Cellular Immunotherapy, H. Lee Moffitt Cancer Center and Research Institute, Tampa, FL, USA

Chuanyi M. Lu Department of Laboratory Medicine, University of California San Francisco & San Francisco VA Health Care System, San Francisco, CA, USA

Fernando Vargas Madueno Memorial Cancer Institute at Memorial Healthcare System, Pembroke Pines, FL, USA

Mariola Vazquez Martinez Department of Blood and Marrow Transplant and Cellular Immunotherapy, H. Lee Moffitt Cancer Center and Research Institute, Tampa, FL, USA

Manuel Martinez-Rio Memorial Health Care, Memorial Cancer Institute, Hollywood, FL, USA

Ruoyu Miao Moffitt Cancer Center, University of South Florida, Tampa, FL, USA

Meri Muminovic Memorial Cancer Institute at Memorial Healthcare System, Pembroke Pines, FL, USA

Olger Nano Memorial Cancer Institute at Memorial Healthcare System, Pembroke Pines, FL, USA

Mandy O'Leary USF/Moffitt Cancer Center, Tampa, FL, USA

Oluwatobi Ozoya Department of Infectious Diseases, H. Lee Moffitt Cancer Center and Research Institute, Tampa, FL, USA

Nagehan Pakasticali Department of Pathology, University of South Florida, Tampa, FL, USA

Nikolaos Papadantonakis Department of Hematology and Medical Oncology, Winship Cancer Institute of Emory University, Atlanta, GA, USA

Parth C. Patel, DO, MS Division of Hematology and Oncology, Vanderbilt University School of Medicine, Nashville, TN, USA

Deniz Peker Department of Pathology and Laboratory Medicine, Winship Cancer Institute of Emory University, Emory University School of Medicine, Atlanta, GA, USA

Jerrin Joy Pullukkara Department of Internal Medicine, University of South Florida, Tampa, FL, USA

Prerna Rastogi Department of Pathology, University of Iowa, Carver College of Medicine, Iowa City, IA, USA

Tauseef Ur Rehman Memorial Healthcare System, Pembroke Pines, FL, USA

Clark R. Robinson University of Texas Southwestern Medical Center, Dallas, TX, USA

Kai J. Rogers Department of Pathology, University of Iowa, Carver College of Medicine, Iowa City, IA, USA

Ashley M. Rose Department of Hematology and Oncology, H. Lee Moffitt Cancer Center and Research Institute, Tampa, FL, USA

Department of Hematology and Oncology, University of South Florida, Tampa, FL, USA

Elizabeth Rubin Memorial Healthcare System, Pembroke Pines, FL, USA

Aditi Saha Department of Internal Medicine, USF Health Morsani College of Medicine, University of South Florida, Tampa, FL, USA

David Sallman Department of Malignant Hematology, Moffitt Cancer Center, Tampa, FL, USA

Ramon Sandin Department of Hematopathology, H. Lee Moffitt Cancer Center and Research Institute, Tampa, FL, USA

José D. Sandoval-Sus Department of Malignant Hematology and Cellular Therapy, Moffitt Cancer Center at Memorial Healthcare System, Pembroke Pines, FL, USA

Department of Hematology/Oncology, Moffitt Cancer Center/University of South Florida, Tampa, FL, USA

Natasha M. Savage Department of Pathology, Medical College of Georgia, Augusta University, Augusta, GA, USA

Olga Sazanova Department of Pathology, University of Iowa, Carver College of Medicine, Iowa City, IA, USA

Brian D. Schlick Tennessee Oncology, Nashville, TN, USA

Department of Internal Medicine, USF Health, Moffitt Cancer Center, Tampa, FL, USA

Zaker Schwabkey Division of Hematology and Hematologic Malignancies, Huntsman Cancer Institute at University of Utah, Salt Lake City, UT, USA

Joseph Schwartz Department of Pathology/Hematopathology and Laboratory Medicine, H. Lee Moffitt Cancer Center and Research Institute, Tampa, FL, USA

Savan S. Shah Moffitt Cancer Center, Tampa, FL, USA

Khine Swe Shan Memorial Health Care, Memorial Cancer Institute, Hollywood, FL, USA

Avani M. Singh Department of Hematology & Oncology, University of South Florida/Moffitt Cancer Center, Tampa, FL, USA

Nirupama Singh Division of Laboratory Medicine, Department of Pathology, University of Alabama at Birmingham, Birmingham, AL, USA

Lubomir Sokol Department of Malignant Hematology, H. Lee Moffitt Cancer Center and Research Institute, Tampa, FL, USA

Moffitt Cancer Center, Tampa, FL, USA

Caroline Stanek Department of Pathology, University of Alabama at Birmingham, Birmingham, AL, USA

Shrinjaya Thapa H. Lee Moffitt Cancer and Research Center, Tampa, FL, USA

Pankit Vachhani Division of Hematology/Oncology, Department of Medicine, University of Alabama at Birmingham, Birmingham, AL, USA

Ana Paula Velez Department of Infectious Diseases, H. Lee Moffitt Cancer Center and Research Institute, Tampa, FL, USA

Nathan Visweshwar Department of Hematology and Oncology, University of South Florida, Tampa, FL, USA

Hematology/Oncology, University of South Florida, Tampa, FL, USA

Michel Vulfovich Memorial Cancer Institute at Memorial Healthcare System, Pembroke Pines, FL, USA

Anthony Wood Department of Internal Medicine, USF Health Morsani College of Medicine, University of South Florida, Tampa, FL, USA

Yu Yang Department of Pathology, Immunology and Laboratory Medicine, University of Florida College of Medicine, Gainesville, FL, USA

Ling Zhang Department of Hematopathology, H. Lee Moffitt Cancer Center and Research Institute, Tampa, FL, USA

Yumeng Zhang Department of Malignant Hematology, H. Lee Moffitt Cancer Center and Research Institute, Tampa, FL, USA

Department of Malignant Hematology, Moffitt Cancer Center, Tampa, FL, USA

Part I

Benign Disorders of White Blood Cells

Benign Neutrophilic Disorders

1

Yumeng Zhang and Ling Zhang

Introduction

Neutrophils are the most common type of white blood cells (WBC) in the human body, comprising up to approximately 70% of circulating leukocytes. These cells play a crucial role in innate immunity in response to infections, injuries, and other threats to the body's well-being. Neutrophils kill microorganisms via complex activities, e.g., migration to tissue; phagocytosis; release of primary, secondary, and tertiary granules; and neutrophilic extracellular traps' effect. While neutrophils play an essential role in the immune response, their activity can also contribute to tissue damage and inflammation, particularly in chronic inflammatory disease.

The normal range of the WBC count in adults is from 4.0 to 11.0×10^9 cells/L, of which 60% to 70% are mature neutrophils. An absolute neutrophil count (ANC) is between 2.5 and 7.0×10^9 neutrophils/L in adults. ANC includes both mature neutrophils

Y. Zhang
Department of Malignant Hematology, H. Lee Moffitt Cancer Center and Research Institute, Tampa, FL, USA
e-mail: Yumeng.zhang@moffitt.org

L. Zhang (✉)
Department of Hematopathology, H. Lee Moffitt Cancer Center and Research Institute, Tampa, FL, USA
e-mail: Ling.Zhang@moffitt.org

L. Sokol, L. Zhang (eds.), *Non-Neoplastic Hematologic Disorders*,
https://doi.org/10.1007/978-3-031-62373-8_1

and band neutrophils. The normal range of ANC varies based on age, ethnicity, and underlying medical conditions. For instance, people of African descent have been found to have lower-normal neutrophil counts compared to Caucasians [1]. The normal ANC is lower in infants ($1.2–8.5 \times 10^9$/L) and gradually increases with age to reach the adult range ($1.8–8 \times 10^9$/L).

Neutrophilia is the most common type of leukocytosis and is defined as an increase in the ANC to more than 7.7×10^9 neutrophils/L, e.g., +/− 2 SD (standard deviations) above the mean. Neutropenia is characterized by a decrease in the ANC to less than 2 standard deviations below the mean, which is typically less than 1.5×10^9/L and further separated with mild (ANC ≥ 1.0 and $< 1.6 \times 10^9$/L), moderate (ANC ≥ 0.5 and $< 1.0 \times 10^9$/L), severe (ANC $<0.5 \times 10^9$/L), or agranulocytosis (ANC $<0.2 \times 10^9$/L).

Pathogenesis

Mature neutrophils are produced in the bone marrow from myeloid progenitor cells. In response to infections or other stimuli, cytokines and various transcription and growth factors increase neutrophil production, proliferation, and release from the bone marrow.

Neutrophilic/neutropenic disorders can occur via four main mechanisms: (1) changes in neutrophil production or maturation in the bone marrow (caused by factors such as drugs, infections, or nutritional deficiencies); (2) intrinsic defect of the neutrophils; (3) redistribution of circulating neutrophils to the spleen or vascular endothelium (known as *margination*); or (4) immune destruction caused by a drug reaction or autoimmunity [2].

Diagnosis

Neutrophilia

Both good clinical history and laboratory investigation are necessary to help with the differential diagnosis of neutrophilic disorders. Attention must be paid to the history of active or prior history of infection or inflammation; malignancies; trends of complete blood count (CBC) result; recent physical or emotional distress; cigarette smoking; recent medication use; family history of neutrophilia; surgical or functional asplenia; and other conditions associated with neutrophilia (refer to Table 1.1). For the diagnostic algorithm for neutrophilia, see Fig. 1.1a.

Physical examination is performed to collect vital signs (e.g., fever, tachycardia) and identify organomegaly, musculoskeletal deformity, and cutaneous lesion.

Laboratory evaluation includes CBC with manual differential. A peripheral blood smear is reviewed to assess neutrophil morphology, left shift, circulating blasts, and exclusion of factitious neutrophilia caused by platelet clumping. Left-shifted granulocytosis, toxic granulation, and Dölhe bodies suggest infection or an inflammatory state (Fig. 1.2). Dysplastic neutrophilia may be caused by chronic myeloid neoplasm with neutrophilia based on the 5th edition of WHO classification, previously called atypical chronic myeloid leukemia. Liver and renal function tests, coagulation profile, inflammatory markers such as erythrocyte sedimentation rate (ESR), C-reactive protein (CPR), lactate dehydrogenase, and ferritin are ordered for patients with a critical illness. Imaging study is optional, based on clinical suspicion and specific etiology. If an infection is suspected, blood culture, urine culture/urinalysis, sputum culture, cerebrospinal fluid analysis, stool culture, and *Clostridiodes difficile* testing will be selectively ordered. Bone marrow aspirate and biopsy are optional only if clinically indicated to exclude disseminated fungal infection and hematological or non-hematological malignancy.

In a patient with a clinical suspicion for leukocyte adhesion deficiency (LAD), molecular testing (*ITGB2*, *SLC35C1*, or *FERMT3* gene mutation) is performed for LAD types I, II, and III, respectively [3]. In addition, flow cytometry is performed to detect reduced CD18 and reduced CD11b expression on neutrophils for LAD type I and reduced CD15 expression on neutrophils for LAD type II.

Table 1.1 Major differential diagnosis for neutrophilia

Category	Subcategory	Mechanisms	Treatment
Inherited			
Inherited causes	Leukocyte adhesion deficiency type I, II, III	*ITGB2*, *SLC35C1*, *FERMT3* gene mutation	Optional ustekinumab, a monoclonal antibody
Down syndrome	None	Trisomy 21, *GATA1* gene mutation	NA
Cryopyrin-associated periodic syndrome	None	Cold agglutination	NA
Acquired			
Infection	Bacterial, viral, fungal, and parasitic	Reactive	Control infection
Acute and chronic inflammation	Rheumatoid arthritis, systemic lupus erythematosus, adult-onset Still's disease, vasculitis, myositis, chronic hepatitis, inflammatory bowel disease, granulomatous disease, etc.	Reactive	Disease-specific treatment
Hematological and nonhematological malignancies	MPN, MDS/MPN, MM, CNL, BM metastases from solid tumor	*e.g., CSF3R* mutation for CNL	Chemotherapy, immunotherapy, or clinical trials

(continued)

Table 1.1 (continued)

Category	Subcategory	Mechanisms	Treatment
Medications	(a) G-CSF or GM-CSF, ATRA (b) glucocorticoids, plerixafor; (c) catecholamines, lithium; (d) others	(a) Direct stimulation of bone marrow myelopoiesis; (b) release of granulocytes from the bone marrow into circulation; (c) De-margination of neutrophils within the vasculature; (d) allergic or inflammation reactions to many drugs can cause neutrophilia	NA
Asplenia or hyposplenia	Sickle-cell disease, trauma	Auto-splenectomy, post-splenectomy	Treating underlying disease, if any
Physical or emotional stress	Cigarette smoking, obesity, pregnancy-associated conditions, vigorous exercise	Transient response to environmental stimulant, compartmental shift	No treatment
Tissue damage	Surgery, trauma, burns	In response to tissue repair	Treating underlying disease
Endocrine causes	Thyroid storm, hypercortisolism	Response to hormonal stimulation	Treating underlying disease

ATRA all-trans-retinoic acid, *BM* bone marrow, *CNL* chronic neutrophilic leukemia, *G-CSF, CM-CSF* recombinant granulocyte, and granulocyte-macrophage colony-stimulating factors, *MDS* myelodysplastic syndromes/neoplasms, *MPN* myeloproliferative neoplasms, *NA* not applicable

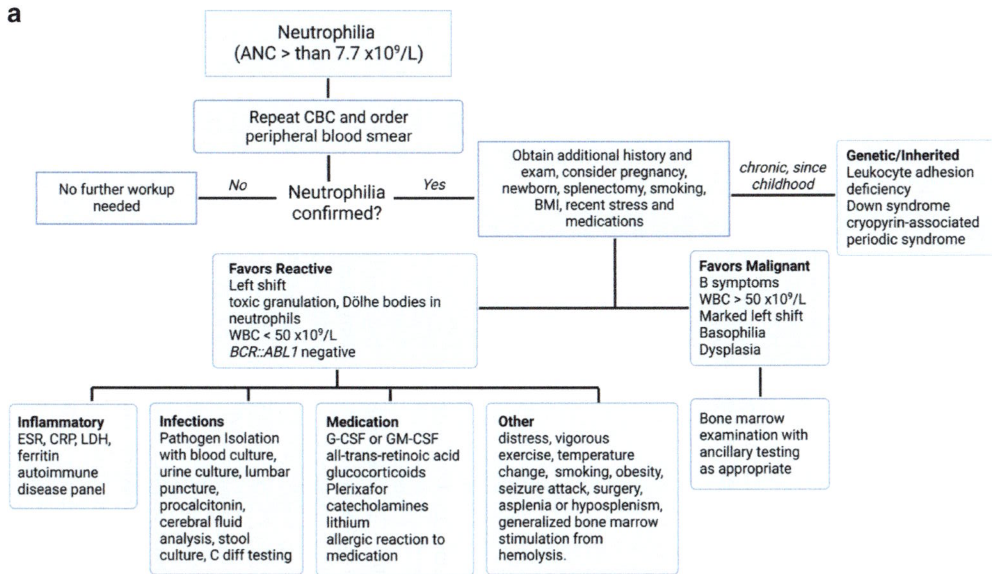

Fig. 1.1 (**a**) Diagnostic Algorithm of Neutrophilia. *ANC* absolute neutrophil count, *ANA* antinuclear antibody, *BMI* body-mass index *C diff Clostridioides difficile*, *CRP* C-reactive protein, *ESR* erythrocyte sedimentation rate, *G-CSF* Granulocyte colony-stimulating factor, *GM-CSF* Granulocyte-macrophage colony-stimulating factor, *LDH* Lactate dehydrogenase, *WBC* white blood cells. (**b**) Diagnostic Algorithm of Neutropenia. *ANA* antinuclear antibody, *CMV* Cytomegalovirus, *EBV* Epstein-Barr Virus, *flu* influenza, *HIV* human immunodeficiency virus, *RA* rheumatoid arthritis, *SLE* Systemic lupus erythematosus, white blood cells

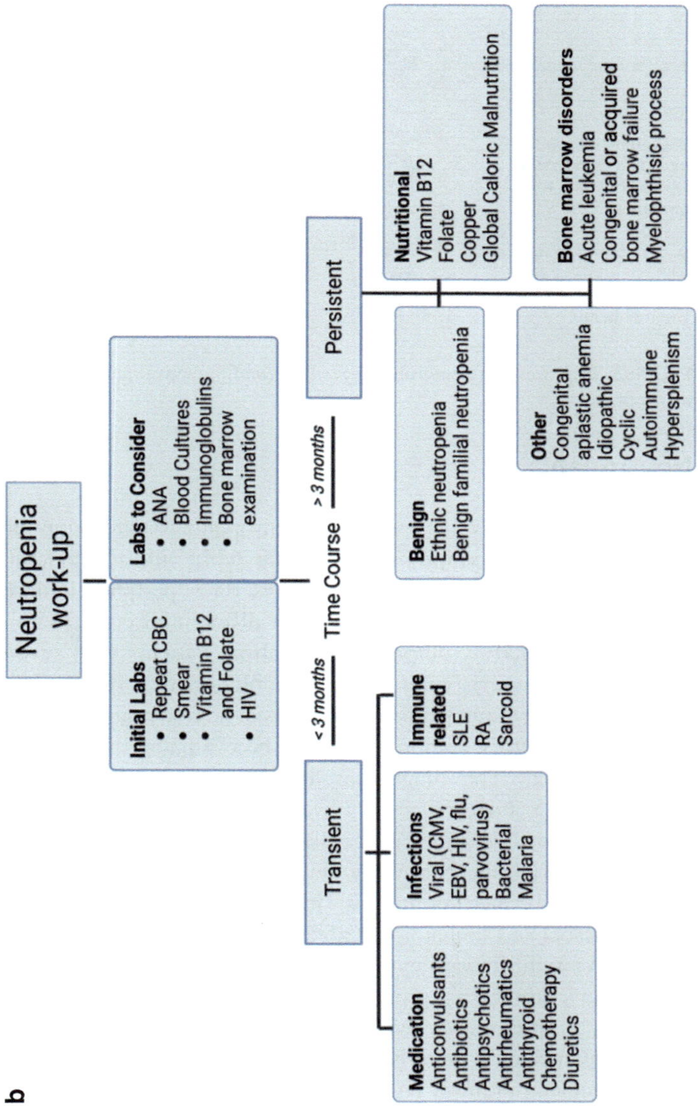

Fig. 1.1 (continued)

1–4: Normal neutrophils;

3–8: reactive neutrophils including cytoplasmic Dohle body and toxic Granules;

9–12: dysplastic neutrophils with pseudo-Pelger changes or abnormal Segmentation.

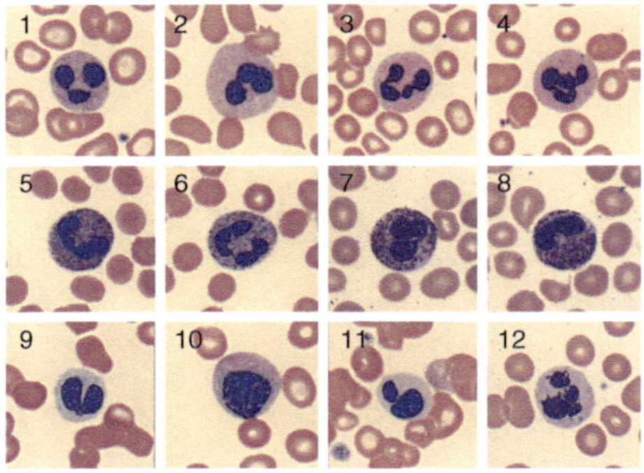

Fig. 1.2 Representative morphology of normal, reactive and dysplastic neutrophils

Neutropenia

It is critical to assess the severity of neutropenia to determine further evaluation. Asymptomatic patients with mild-to-moderate neutropenia and no worrisome findings on a peripheral blood smear should have a repeat CBC with differential count within 2 weeks, followed by outpatient evaluation. Patients with severe neutropenia or worrisome findings on a blood smear (e.g., leukemic blasts, schistocytes) or signs of sepsis, hemodynamical instability, or respiratory compromise must be evaluated immediately or hospitalized. The diagnostic algorithm for neutropenia is depicted in Fig. 1.1b.

Minimal considerations in the diagnostic evaluation of neutropenia include (1) the chronicity, degree, and duration of neutropenia; (2) associated symptoms (infections); (3) comorbidities; and (4) associated hematologic abnormalities (e.g., isolated neutropenia vs multilineage cytopenias) [4]. History should include the patient's ethnic background, family, and dietary and medication lists [5]. Laboratory evaluation beyond CBC and peripheral blood smears should be targeted based on the differential diagnosis. Antinuclear antibody (ANA) and rheumatoid factors are good diagnostic screening tests for systemic rheumatologic diseases. All patients with neutropenia should be tested for HIV. A bone marrow examination is indicated for neutropenia with unknown etiology.

Other diagnostic tests in bone marrow in the right clinical context include flow cytometry, chromosomal analysis, and targeted gene sequencing for hematological malignancies. Other tests are selective, e.g., chromosome instability test for Fanconi syndrome and *ELANE* mutations for congenital or cyclical neutropenia [6].

Differential Diagnosis

Neutrophilia

There are three main types of benign neutrophilia: factitious, primary, and secondary.

Factitious neutrophilia: an artificially increased number of neutrophils caused by laboratory errors or manipulation of the blood sample. Examples of factitious neutrophilia include inadequately anticoagulated samples resulting in platelet clumping in an automated cell counter or precipitated cryoglobulin particles in mixed cryoglobulinemia. A repeat blood sample with adequate anticoagulation and peripheral blood smear examination can solve this problem.

Primary neutrophilia: caused by increased neutrophil production in the bone marrow from dysregulated neutrophil production. This type of neutrophilia is relatively rare and often associated with other hematological disorders [2].

1. Neutrophilia can often be seen with a myeloid neoplasm, in particular, myeloproliferative neoplasms (MPN), such as chronic myelogenous leukemia, chronic neutrophilic leukemia, and the proliferative phase of primary myelofibrosis.
2. Genetic/inherited neutrophilia: It is a rare condition caused by an inherited genetic mutation that increases the number of neutrophils. It is generally diagnosed in neonates and children, though sometimes discovered in adulthood. Leukocyte adhesion deficiency (LAD) is a rare but life-threatening example that affects the ability of neutrophils to adhere to blood vessel walls and migrate to sites of infection or injury. It can be characterized by leukocytosis, recurrent infection, and delayed umbilical cord separation.

3. Neutrophil counts can be variable among healthy individuals (normal variation). Repeated CBCs and evaluation of siblings' or parents' blood count might also be helpful since the neutrophil count is influenced by genetics.

Secondary neutrophilia: occurs in response to an external factor, such as an infection, autoimmune disorder, or certain medications. This type of neutrophilia is much more common than primary neutrophilia.

1. Infections: Bacterial and viral infections are common causes of neutrophilia. Left shift (e.g., increased percentage of neutrophil band forms), toxic granulation, and Döhle bodies on peripheral smears suggest bacterial infection.
2. Autoimmune disorders/inflammatory conditions: They can result in neutrophilia caused by the release of cytokines, which stimulate the bone marrow to produce more neutrophils.
3. Nonhematological neoplasms: Neutrophilia is not uncommonly seen in solid tumors, e.g., lung cancer. Proposed mechanisms include paraneoplastic leukemoid reaction, infections, nonspecific tumor-related inflammation, high-dose corticosteroids as therapy, or tumor metastases to bone marrow.
4. Medications: A number of medications can induce neutrophilia by different pathways.
5. Other causes include physical or emotional distress, vigorous exercise, temperature change, cigarette smoking, seizure attack, overweight, surgery, hyposplenism or asplenia, and generalized bone marrow response to hemolysis.

Neutropenia

The differential diagnosis for neutropenia includes both benign and malignant conditions. In some cases, neutropenia can be a temporary condition that resolves on its own or with treatment. Examples of benign conditions that can cause neutropenia include viral infections, such as influenza or hepatitis, as well as certain medications, such as chemotherapy or antibiotics [7]. Other benign causes of neutropenia include pregnancy, alcohol abuse, and vitamin deficiencies [4].

By contrast, neutropenia can also be a sign of more serious conditions, such as benign or malignant bone marrow disorders or autoimmune diseases. Examples of bone marrow disorders that cause neutropenia include myelodysplastic syndromes/neoplasms, aplastic anemia, leukemias, and paroxysmal nocturnal hemoglobinuria. Autoimmune diseases that lead to neutropenia include lupus, rheumatoid arthritis, and Felty syndrome (Table 1.2). Differential diagnosis is essential to identify the underlying cause and determines the appropriate treatment approach.

It is important to examine neutrophilia with other abnormal WBC conditions (Table 1.3) to identify the potential etiology.

Table 1.2 Major differential diagnosis for congenital and acquired neutropenia

Category	History clues	Mechanism	Treatment
Congenital			
Constitutional/ ethnic neutropenia	Linked to ethnic group such as Mediterranean and African descents; mild, chronic in nature; no history of recurrent infection	Polymorphisms in the *DARC* gene	Observation
Benign familial neutropenia	Not linked to ethnic group but hereditary		Observation
Severe congenital neutropenia	Agranulocytosis: recurrent, severe infections that begin during infancy	Inherited mutations, e.g., the primary granule protein gene neutrophil elastase (*ELANE*), the mitochondrial gene *HAX1* in several neutrophil-specific genes.	Periodic G-CSF therapy. Curative therapy is allogeneic hematopoietic stem cell transplant

(continued)

Table 1.2 (continued)

Category	History clues	Mechanism	Treatment
Cyclic neutropenia	Episodes of self-limited neutropenia, mild to severe, onset of every 2 to 5 weeks; during their neutrophil nadir, patient could develop infections or oral ulcers	Autosomal dominant syndrome, e.g., mutations in *ELANE*	G-CSF at lower dose to target ANC > 500/mm^2
Others congenital syndrome	Primary immunodeficiency	SDS, Fanconi anemia, DKC, CHS, myelokathesis, Griscelli syndrome II, and cartilage-hair hypoplasia	
Acquired			
Infection-associated			
Sepsis	Fever, hypotension, tachycardia	Any bacteria, but most notably, *Brucella*, rickettsial, and mycobacterial	
Postinfection	After acute viral infection	Varicella, measles, rubella, influenza, hepatitis, EBV, or HIV	Often recover or improve within one to 2 weeks

(continued)

Table 1.2 (continued)

Category	History clues	Mechanism	Treatment
Drug-induced			
Agranulocytosis	Medication changes: e.g., TMP-SMX, dapsone, chloramphenicol, quinine, ibuprofen, sulfasalazine, clozapine	Varies based on drugs, e.g., toxic metabolites from clozapine	Discontinuation of the drug. G-CSF can be considered but benefits are unproven.
Mild neutropenia	Medication changes: e.g., thiazide, acetazolamide, ethosuximide, valproate, macrolides, vancomycin		Discontinuation of drug
Autoimmune			
Primary autoimmune	Occurs during first year of life; moderate to severe neutropenia complicated by serious infection	Autoantibodies directed at specific neutrophil antigens, e.g., FcγIIIb, CD177, CD11a, and CD11b	
Secondary autoimmune	History of systemic autoimmune diseases; changes based on the severity of underlying disorder; usually mild		

(continued)

Table 1.2 (continued)

Category	History clues	Mechanism	Treatment
Felty syndrome	Rheumatoid arthritis, splenomegaly	Polyclonal or oligoclonal LGL	Treatment of RA with methotrexate, corticosteroid, or TNF-a blocking antibodies
Malignancy			
Acute leukemia	Weight loss, fever/chills, fatigue	Bone marrow infiltration of malignant cells	Treat primary causes
Myelodysplasia	Weight loss, fever/chills, fatigue	Bone marrow infiltration of malignant cells	Treat primary causes
Large granular lymphocytic leukemia	Rheumatoid arthritis, splenomegaly, severe neutropenia	Clonal LGL, TCR gene rearrangement, *STAT3 or STAT5bB* mutation	If severe, treat with methotrexate, cyclosporine, or cyclophosphamide.
Myeloma, lymphoma	Weight loss, fever/chills, fatigue, bone pain, lymphadenopathy	Bone marrow infiltration of malignant cells	Treat primary causes
Myelophthisic processes	History of cancer	Bone marrow infiltration of malignant cells	Treat primary causes
Dietary			
Vitamin B12, folate deficiency	Low BMI, macrocytosis, and pancytopenia	Ineffective hematopoiesis	Nutrition supplement
Copper deficiency	Neurologic symptoms	Inhibition of differential and self-renewal of hematopoietic progenitor cells	Copper supplement
Global caloric malnutrition	Anorexia nervosa	Multifactorial	Nutritional supplement

(continued)

Table 1.2 (continued)

Category	History clues	Mechanism	Treatment
Hypersplenism	Splenomegaly	Portal hypertension induces congestive hypersplenism and results in increased sequestration of circulating blood cells	G-CSF is contraindicated given risk of splenic rupture

BMI body-mass index, *CHS* Chediak-Higashi syndrome, *DARC* Duffy Antigen Receptor Complex, *DKC* dyskeratosis congenita, *EBV* Epstein–Barr virus, *G-CSF* Granulocyte colony-stimulating factor, *LGL* large granular lymphocytic leukemia, *RA* rheumatoid arthritis, *SDS* Schwachman-Diamond syndrome

Table 1.3 Samples of combined neutrophilia with other situations

Situation	Potentially associated disease
Neutrophilia with monocytosis	Infections (bacterial endocarditis, brucellosis, varicella-zoster, tuberculosis, malaria, typhoid fever, syphilis, trypanosomiasis), inflammatory conditions (sarcoidosis, inflammatory bowel disease), medications (corticosteroid, GM-CSF), asplenia, pregnancy, and malignancies
Neutrophilia with eosinophilia and basophilia	Allergic conditions, parasitic infections, malignancies (e.g., MPN, systemic mastocytosis), and inflammatory processes (e.g., sarcoidosis, inflammatory bowel disease)
Neutrophilia with microangiopathic hemolytic anemia	Thrombotic thrombocytopenic purpura, disseminated intravascular coagulation, and related disorders
Leukoerythroblastosis and neutrophilia	Myelophthisic process (e.g., primary myelofibrosis, tumor metastases to the bone marrow, vasculitis, or fungal infection)
Neutrophilia and thrombocytosis or thrombocytopenia	Various infections, inflammatory conditions, and malignancies

Prognosis

The prognosis of neutrophilia depends on the underlying cause of the condition. In most cases in general medical practice, neutrophilia is a transient condition that resolves on its own or with the treatment of the underlying cause. If neutrophilia is caused by cancer or a chronic inflammatory condition, the prognosis may be more guarded. Neutrophilia, in certain circumstances, can be associated with an increased risk of adverse health events. For example, leukemoid reaction can be associated with hypercoagulability; untreated severe infection can lead to multiorgan failure, thrombosis, or hemorrhage. LAD can be associated with severe mental impairment, failure to thrive, and severe infections.

The prognosis of neutropenia also depends on the underlying etiology as well as the degree of severity. The outcome of congenital neutropenia is variable, e.g., familial cyclic neutropenia is usually benign. Dietary neutropenia can be collected after nutritional supplement therapy with a good prognosis. Neutropenia secondary to cytotoxic chemotherapy could be transient and recovered after stopping cytoreductive therapy and administration of G-CSF.

Treatment

The treatment and management of benign neutrophilia depend on its underlying cause and specific underlying pathologies (Table 1.1).

1. Leukemoid reaction: WBC count is increased to 50×10^9/L composed of mostly neutrophils. Treatment is based on the etiology and causes. Hyperleukocytosis, defined as a WBC count above 100×10^9/L, can lead to increased blood viscosity and tumor lysis syndrome if caused by an underlying malignancy. To prevent hypercoagulability-associated complications, initiating aggressive hydration, treatment of underlying malignancies +/− hydroxyurea should be considered in symptomatic patients.
2. LAD: Hematopoietic stem cell transplantation is the only corrective treatment for the severe phenotype.

The management of neutropenia depends on the underlying pathology. Some pathologies, such as familial neutropenia and most cyclic neutropenias, do not require treatment. The decision for treatment should be made based on infectious complications from neutropenia and is usually deferred until infections are cleared. Neutropenia secondary to T-LGL leukemia responds to monotherapy with low-dose methotrexate, cyclophosphamide, or cyclosporine A [8]. Rituximab can be used for autoimmune neutropenia, even though it is considered a cytotoxic T-cell-mediated process [9]. For other disease-specific treatments, please see Table 1.2.

G-CSF is recommended for recurrent or severe infections, mucosal erosions, or skin infections for patients with neutropenia. We usually use the minimal dose and frequency of G-CSF to maintain ANC > 0.25–0.3 × 10^9/L.

Promising Clinical Study

Ustekinumab, a monoclonal antibody to the p40 subunit common to IL-12 and IL-23, can treat refractory LAD in mild and moderate phenotypes [10]. Gene therapy has been studied in preclinical studies (ClinicalTrials.gov Identifier: NCT03366142).

Caveats

- Reactive neutrophilia accounts for most of the neutrophilic cases. Repeat CBC with differential and peripheral blood smear review is the first step to evaluate for neutrophilia.
- The urgency of the evaluation on neutropenia depends on the degree and chronicity of the neutropenia. Severe neutropenia (ANC <0.5 × 10^9/L), blasts or schistocytes on the blood smear, signs of sepsis, hemodynamical instability, or respiratory compromise need immediate evaluation or hospitalization.
- *CSF3R* mutation status helps differentiate between chronic neutrophilic leukemia and sustained reactive neutrophilia. Sustained leukocytosis with granulocytosis with basophilia or eosinophilia warrants a fluorescence in situ hybridization test or polymerase chain reaction test for *BCR::ABL1* fusion products.

Board Questions

1. Neutrophilia

   A 36-year-old female is referred for evaluation of leukocytosis for 2 months. Her lab showed WBC count of 19.1×10^9 cells/L. The differential showed 70% neutrophils. She smokes occasionally and works in a stressful job. She is on birth control pills, levothyroxine for hypothyroidism, loratadine for seasonal allergies, and lithium for bipolar disorder. She is slightly obese, with BMI of 30.1 kg/M^2. On exam, she had no fever, lymphadenopathy, or splenomegaly. What is the most likely etiology for her neutrophilia?

   A. Obesity
   B. Smoking
   C. Levothyroxine
   D. Lithium
   E. Stress

   Correct Answer: D

   This patient could have several etiologies that could explain leukocytosis; however, the use of lithium is the most compelling. Lithium has been widely reported to cause neutrophilia and carries no clinical sequalae. Her minimal smoking, slight obesity, and stressful job should not lead her to have neutrophils over 13.3×10^9/L.

2. Neutropenia

   Which of the following drugs does not cause neutropenia?

   A. Beta-lactam antibiotics
   B. Antithyroid drugs
   C. Ticlopidine
   D. Clozapine
   E. Epinephrine

The correct Answer is E. Antithyroid medication, clozapine, and ticlopidine can potentially cause severe neutropenia or agranulocytosis. Beta-lactam causes immune-mediated neutrophil destruction. Clozapine leads to oxidant-mediated damage to white blood cells. Toxic and reactive metabolite of ticlopidine can cause neutropenia. Catecholamines, such as epinephrine, can cause neutrophilia.

References

1. Azab B, Camacho-Rivera M, Taioli E. Average values and racial differences of neutrophil lymphocyte ratio among a nationally representative sample of United States subjects. PLoS One. 2014;9:e112361.
2. George TI. Malignant or benign leukocytosis. Hematology Am Soc Hematol Educ Program. 2012;2012:475–84.
3. Roos D, van Leeuwen K, Madkaikar M, Kambli PM, Gupta M, Mathews V, Rawat A, Kuhns DB, Holland SM, de Boer M, Kanegane H, Parvaneh N, Lorenz M, Schwarz K, Klein C, Sherkat R, Jafari M, Wolach B, den Dunnen JT, Kuijpers TW, Koker MY. Hematologically important mutations: leukocyte adhesion deficiency (second update). Blood Cells Mol Dis. 2023;99:102726.
4. Solomou EE, Salamaliki C, Lagadinou M. How to make the right diagnosis in neutropenia. Clin Hematol Int. 2021;3:41–6.
5. Haddy TB, Rana SR, Castro O. Benign ethnic neutropenia: what is a normal absolute neutrophil count? J Lab Clin Med. 1999;133:15–22.
6. Horwitz MS, Corey SJ, Grimes HL, Tidwell T. ELANE mutations in cyclic and severe congenital neutropenia: genetics and pathophysiology. Hematol Oncol Clin North Am. 2013;27(19-41):vii.
7. Curtis BR. Drug-induced immune neutropenia/agranulocytosis. Immunohematology. 2014;30:95–101.
8. Pontikoglou C, Kalpadakis C, Papadaki HA. Pathophysiologic mechanisms and management of neutropenia associated with large granular lymphocytic leukemia. Expert Rev Hematol. 2011;4:317–28.
9. Martin J, Audrain M, Durant C, Rimbert M, Fromont P, Hamidou M. Autoimmune neutropenia. Rev Med Interne. 2011;32:26–32.
10. Moutsopoulos NM, Zerbe CS, Wild T, Dutzan N, Brenchley L, DiPasquale G, Uzel G, Axelrod KC, Lisco A, Notarangelo LD, Hajishengallis G, Notarangelo LD, Holland SM. Interleukin-12 and interleukin-23 blockade in leukocyte adhesion deficiency type 1. N Engl J Med. 2017;376:1141–6.

Benign Eosinophil Disorders

2

Chuanyi M. Lu

Introduction

Eosinophils are a type of specialized myeloid cells (eosinophilic granulocytes) found in peripheral blood, which originate from multipotent hematopoietic stem cells and play a crucial rule in host innate defense [1]. In healthy subjects, the eosinophil count in peripheral blood ranges from 0.05 to 0.5×10^9/L (50–500 cells per μL). *Eosinophilia* is defined as a blood eosinophil count greater than 0.5×10^9/L, which can be further divided into mild (0.5–1.5×10^9/L), moderate (1.5–5.0×10^9/L), and severe eosinophilia ($>5.0 \times 10^9$/L) [2–4]. The definition of eosinophilia also includes relative eosinophilia (>6% in white blood cell differential counts). The term *hypereosinophilia* (HE) is defined as marked blood eosinophilia ($\geq 1.5 \times 10^9$/L) that is documented on at least two occasions with a minimum "time interval" of 2 weeks (Fig. 2.1). For patients with certain myeloid leukemias (such as chronic myeloid leukemia and some variants of acute myeloid leukemia), HE is defined as persistent blood eosinophilia

C. M. Lu (✉)
Department of Laboratory Medicine, University of California San Francisco & San Francisco VA Health Care System, San Francisco, CA, USA
e-mail: chuanyi.lu@ucsf.edu

L. Sokol, L. Zhang (eds.), *Non-Neoplastic Hematologic Disorders*, https://doi.org/10.1007/978-3-031-62373-8_2

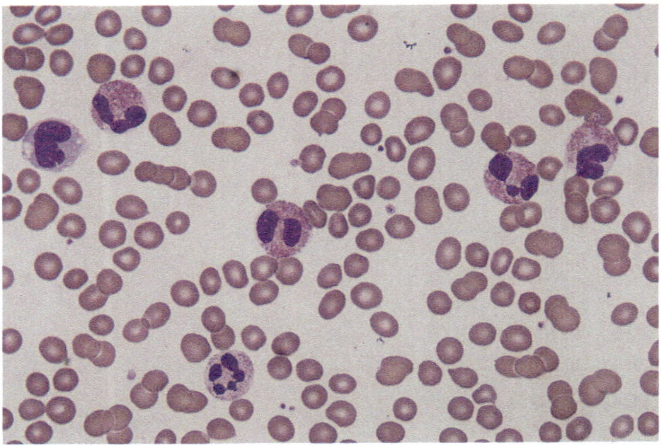

Fig. 2.1 Peripheral blood smear from an adult male shows marked eosinophilia (absolute eosinophil count, 6.83×10^9/L). The white cells include 4 eosinophils, 1 segmented neutrophil, and 1 monocyte (Wright stain, ×1000)

$\geq 1.5 \times 10^9$/L and $\geq$ 10% eosinophils in peripheral blood differential counts.

Mature eosinophils are present in normal bone marrow aspirates, ranging between <1% and 6% in differential counts. Eosinophils are also found in the healthy thymus, spleen, lymph nodes, uterus, and the entire gastrointestinal tract distal to the esophagus, but the physiological counts of eosinophils in these organs vary. The term *tissue HE* has also been proposed, though the defining criteria remain to be accepted [4].

Mild blood eosinophilia is seen among 4 to 10% of individuals in the primary care setting, whereas HE is much less common and seen in ~0.3% of the patient population [1, 5, 6]. HE can be transient, episodic, or persistent (chronic). The etiology of HE is diverse and can be grouped under three categories, primary (neoplastic or clonal), secondary (reactive), and idiopathic (Table 2.1) [3]. In this chapter, we focus on secondary and idiopathic HE and aim to distinguish them from their neoplastic counterparts.

Table 2.1 Common causes of hypereosinophilia [3]

• Secondary HE (reactive, HE_R)[a]	
Non-neoplastic conditions	– Allergy and hypersensitivity (e.g., asthma) – Drug reactions (allergic or toxic) – Parasitic infections (e.g., helminthiasis) – Scabies and other infestations – Collagen vascular disorders (autoimmune) – Skin diseases (e.g., atopic dermatitis) – Chronic inflammatory disorders (e.g., IBD) – Metabolic condition (e.g., adrenal insufficiency) – Chronic graft-versus-host disease – Eosinophilic myalgia syndrome – Lymphoid variant HE/HES
Neoplastic conditions (paraneoplastic)	– Solid tumors – T-cell lymphoma/leukemia – Hodgkin lymphoma – B-cell ALL with t(5;14)/IL3-IgH – Langerhans cell histiocytosis
• Primary HE (neoplastic, HE_N)[b]	– Chronic eosinophilic leukemia (CEL)-NOS – Myeloid/lymphoid neoplasms with eosinophilia and tyrosine kinase gene fusions (*PDGFRA*, *PDGFRB*, *FGFR1*, *JAK2*, *FLT3*, *ABL1*) – MPN with eosinophilia (e.g., CML and JAK2 V617F+ MPN) – AML with inv(16) or t(16;16)/*CBFB-MYH11* – MDS with eosinophilia – MDS/MPN with eosinophilia – ASM with eosinophilia
• Idiopathic HE (HE_{US})	Defined as HE that lasts ≥6 months and without an underlying reactive or neoplastic cause
• Familial HE (HE_{FA})	Rare inherited condition with an autosomal dominant inheritance; pathogenesis unknown; benign clinical course

ALL acute lymphoblastic leukemia, *AML* acute myeloid leukemia, *ASM* aggressive systemic mastocytosis, *CML* chronic myeloid leukemia, *HE* hypereosinophilia (absolute eosinophil count in blood >1.5 × 109/L on 2 occasions that are at least 2 weeks apart), *HEUS* HE of undetermined significance, *MDS* myelodysplastic syndrome, *MPN* myeloproliferative neoplasm, *MDS/MPN* myelodysplastic/myeloproliferative overlap neoplasm, *NOS* not otherwise specified

[a] HE is triggered by eosinopoietic cytokines in most cases

[b] Eosinophils are clonal cells (neoplastic eosinophils)

Secondary HE (reactive, HE_R) is caused by an underlying condition of nonneoplastic or paraneoplastic origin, in which the eosinophils themselves are benign.

Primary HE (neoplastic/clonal, HE_N), by contrast, is caused by clonal stem cell disorders of myeloid or lymphoid origin, in which the eosinophils belong to the malignant clone and eosinophilia could be the initial manifestation of disease.

If neither secondary nor primary etiology can be identified and no organ dysfunction is detected, the HE is then considered idiopathic (also referred to as HE of undetermined significance, HE_{US}). Of note, the WHO Classification [7, 8] specified that HE must persist for ≥6 months to classify a case as idiopathic HE.

In addition to these three categories, a rare hereditary (familial, HE_{FA}) variant of HE with autosomal-dominant inheritance has been reported. The hereditary form of HE typically has a benign clinical course with only rare reports of associated organ dysfunction [3, 4].

Hypereosinophilic syndrome (HES) applies to organ damage that can be attributed to the eosinophilic infiltrate. Therefore, the terms of HE and HES are different and should not be used interchangeably. Like HE, HES can be divided into variant types based on the underlying etiology: primary (neoplastic) HES, secondary (reactive) HES, and idiopathic HES (with unknown etiology) [3, 4]. If tissue HE is present and causing organ damage but criteria for blood HE are not fulfilled, the term *tissue/organ-restricted HES* could be used. In addition, a so-called lymphocyte-variant of HE/HES (LV-HE/HES) is also recognized, which is a hypereosinophilic condition resulting from excess production of eosinophilic cytokines secreted by immunophenotypically aberrant T cells [3, 4, 9].

Many organ systems may be affected in HES. The most common tissues/organs affected by HE are skin (40–70%), lungs (25–40%), and gastrointestinal tract (15–35%), followed by heart (5–20%) and nervous system (5–20%) [10]. The most critical organ that may be affected is the heart, as cardiac involvement can be life-threatening. HES involving cardiac damage may manifest as myocardial infarction, heart failure, thromboembolism, or rarely, endomyocardial fibrosis, restrictive cardiomyopathy, or valvular insufficiency [11].

Secondary HE/HES is most common (45–50%), including cases with eosinophilic disease restricted to a single organ system (eg, skin, lungs, intestines, etc.), followed by 10% to 20% primary HE/HES (myeloid or lymphoid), 15% to 25% LV-HE/HES, 5% to 10% idiopathic HE/HES, and rare familial HE.

Pathogenesis

Reactive eosinophilia is induced by eosinophilic cytokines, such as interleukin (IL)-5, IL-3, or granulocyte-macrophage colony-stimulating factor (GM-CSF). These eosinophilic cytokines are primarily produced by activated T cells, mast cells, and stromal cells. *IGH::IL3* rearrangement not only causes B-cell acute lymphoblastic leukemia but is also a rare cause of reactive eosinophilia due to overproduction of IL-3. Other cytokines and chemokines, such as transforming growth factors, platelet-derived growth factors (PDGF), and CC/CXC ligands, can modulate eosinophil function [1].

Primary (neoplastic) eosinophilia can be associated with various hematolymphoid neoplasms and is typically caused by rearrangements in certain oncogenic target genes, including *PDGFRA*, *PDGFRB*, *FGFR1*, *JAK2*, *ABL1*, and *ETV6*. These neoplasms are grouped under "myeloid/lymphoid neoplasms with eosinophilia and tyrosine kinase gene fusions." [3] Underlying clonal genetic or molecular alterations (e.g., acquired somatic variants) might be also attributable to CEL. The *CBFB::MYH11* rearrangement leads to a subtype of acute myeloid leukemia (AML) that is characterized by eosinophilia.

Eosinophils produce, store, and release a large quantity of biologically active substances, including cytotoxic proteins, lipid mediators, chemotactic proteins (chemokines), and cytokines (many have cytotoxic properties, such as eosinophil-derived cationic protein, major basic proteins, peroxidase, and neurotoxin) [1]. Under various physiologic conditions and pathologies, eosinophils migrate into certain target organs and, once activated, release their products in affected tissue sites, thereby promoting local inflammation, tissue remodeling, and sometimes tissue damage. In a subset of these patients, tissue fibrosis and/or thrombosis with end-organ damage develops, resulting in the diagnosis of HES.

Diagnosis

The first step in HE tests is to identify the possible etiology to trigger a secondary (reactive) eosinophilia, followed by an exclusion of primary, paraneoplastic HE and LV-HE (Table 2.1) [3, 4]. Detailed history (allergy, travel, medications, food, domestic pets, etc.), physical examination, and clinical evaluation are essential. In all patients with HE, routine laboratory examinations should be performed, including complete blood count (CBC) with differential counts, serum chemistry (including a basal serum tryptase level), inflammation markers (including fibrinogen and CRP), autoantibodies, serum IgE, and vitamin B12. Diagnostic imaging (X-ray, computed tomography, magnetic resonance imaging, and/or positron emission tomography, if indicated) and additional laboratory testing (e.g., parasitology and allergy testing, flow cytometry, serology, etc.) are often needed. A diagnostic algorithm is proposed as a guide for HE workup (Fig. 2.2).

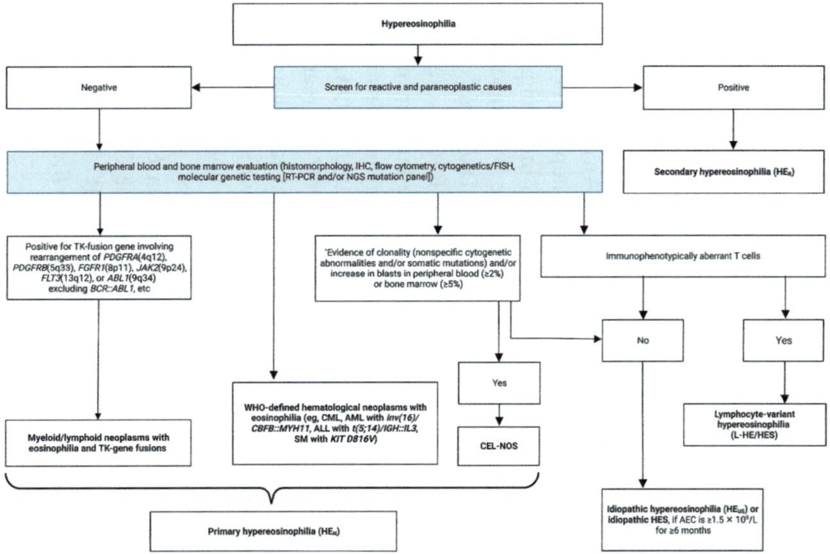

Fig. 2.2 Diagnostic algorithm for patients with hypereosinophilia (AEC >1.5 × 10^9/L for ≥4 weeks). *Nonspecific cytogenetic abnormalities include +8, +15, −7, del(5q), i(17q), complex karyotype, and nonspecific somatic mutations include mutations in *ASXL1, TET2, EZH2, DNMT3A,* or *STAT5B,* etc. ALL, acute lymphoblastic leukemia; AML, acute myeloid leukemi; CEL-NOS, chronic eosinophilic leukemia, not otherwise specified; CML, chronic myeloid leukemia, *Bcr::Abl1*-positive; IHC, immunohistochemistry; NGS, next-generation sequencing; RT-PCR, reverse transcription polymerase chain reaction; SM, systemic mastocytosis; TK, tyrosine kinase

Differential Diagnosis

The most important differential diagnosis is secondary (reactive)-vs-primary (clonal) HE. Features suggestive of primary HE include constitutional symptoms (e.g., fever, weight loss, fatigue, cough, dyspnea, etc.); persistent and worsening eosinophilia that is refractory to steroids; leukocytosis (neutrophilia, monocytosis, and/or basophilia); the presence of both mature and immature and/or dysplastic cells in peripheral blood; anemia; abnormal platelet count (thrombocytopenia or thrombocytosis); and/or increase in serum vitamin B12 (e.g., >1000 pg/mL) or tryptase (e.g., >20 ng/mL), among other abnormal laboratory findings. When primary HE is suspected, bone marrow aspiration and core biopsy should always be offered to the patient. An abnormal bone marrow is considered a strong indicator of eosinophilic neoplasm and should be one of the major considerations in distinguishing patients with primary (clonal) HE from those with reactive or idiopathic hypereosinophilic disorder [3, 12]. Diagnosis of neoplastic eosinophilia should follow the current WHO Classifications.

Routine cytogenetic analysis, if an adequate number of metaphases are obtained for analysis, can detect translocations involving 5q31-33 (*PDGFRB*), 8p11 (*FGFR1*), and 9p24.1 (*JAK2*), as well as t(12;13)/*ETV6-FLT3,* but not 4q12 (*PDGFRA*) rearrangement. The *FIP1L1-PDGFRA* is typically associated with a cryptic 4q12 deletion (e.g., ~800 kb interstitial deletion) which can be detected by FISH and/or RT-PCR [3]. Of note, cytogenetically cryptic *PDGFRB* rearrangement has also been reported, especially with variant partner genes other than *ETV6* [13]. The t(9;12)/*ETV::ABL1* is usually cryptic on routine G-banded chromosome analysis [14]; therefore, FISH and/or RT-PCR should be ordered if clinically indicated [3]. FISH for *CBFB::MHY11* would help diagnosis of AML with eosinophilia.

Next-generation sequencing (NGS)–based targeted mutation panel has become available and used in studying eosinophilic myeloid neoplasms [3, 15]. Somatic mutations are significantly more frequent in *FGFR1*-rearranged cases than other gene rearrangements. Performing an NGS myeloid panel should be considered for HE cases if a secondary cause is excluded, the karyotype is normal or of no diagnostic significance (e.g., -Y in elders), and the HE is considered as a result of a myeloid neoplasm or to be idiopathic. The utilities of an NGS myeloid panel in an HE diagnostic workup include detecting rare activating mutation(s) in a TK (e.g., *PDGFRA*) that can be targeted by TKI and predicting outcome in "idiopathic" HES (e.g., if mutation is detected, the outcome would be closer to that of CEL-NOS) [3]. Rare activating mutations have been identified in *PDGFRA* and *STAT5B* [16]. In addition, detection of myeloid neoplasm-associated mutation(s) helps differentiate truly idiopathic HE vs CEL-NOS.

Treatment

The clinical treatment of HE and HES depends on disease etiology and subtypes. However, even in the absence of a known cause, HES must be promptly treated to reduce potential morbidity that can result from organ damage [3, 17].

For patients with mild eosinophilia (AEC $<1.5 \times 10^9$/L) and without symptoms or evidence of organ dysfunction, a watch-and-wait approach with close follow-up may be undertaken, especially if the eosinophil count fluctuates.

The reactive form of HE (HE_R) is best managed by treating and (if possible) eradicating the underlying disease or pathology. When eradication is not possible, symptomatic therapy may be sufficient to control problems related to eosinophilia and eosinophil activation. Organ damage can often be prevented by administration of corticosteroids (e.g., prednisone) and/or other anti-inflammatory drugs. For patients with severe eosinophilic granulomatosis and polyangiitis, additional drugs such as cyclophosphamide may be required. Anti-IL-5 and anti-IL-5 receptor antibodies (e.g., mepolizumab, reslizumab, benralizumab) have been shown to be effective in patients with organ-restricted eosinophilic inflammatory disorders involving respiratory or digestive system [2, 17].

Corticosteroids are the first line of treatment for patients with LV-HE/HES or idiopathic HE/HES, and allogeneic hematopoietic stem cell transplant (allo-HSCT) may be pursued for the latter. About 10% to 20% of patients with LV-HE/HES eventually progress to overt T-cell lymphoma; following up with patients with LV-HE/HES is therefore recommended. Alternatively, corticosteroid-sparing agents should be considered to avoid side effects of long-term corticosteroid therapy.

Patients with primary (neoplastic) HE and HES_N are not responding to corticosteroids or other anti-inflammatory agents. For patients with HE and rearrangement of *PDGFRA* or *PDGFRB*, with or without organ dysfunction, imatinib is the treatment of choice [2, 3, 17]. Note that patients with certain rare *PDGFRA* mutations (e.g., T674I, D842V, or tandem S601P and L629P) are typically resistant to imatinib.

For patients with HE and *FGFR1* rearrangement, intensive chemotherapy is the treatment of choice [2, 17, 18]. Variable short-term responses to midostaurin (a multitarget kinase inhibitor) and ponatinib have been reported. Allo-HSCT is the only option to achieve long-term remission or cure, but recently pemigatinib, a highly selective inhibitor of FGFR, showed promising results in a clinical trial. Additionally, in one study, 78% of cases with *FGFR1* rearrangement have a *RUNX1* mutation, suggesting *RUNX1* could be a novel therapeutic target [19].

Patients with *PCM1-JAK2* may respond to ruxolitinib (a JAK2 inhibitor), but the response is usually short-term with relapse within 1 to 2 years [18]. Allo-HSCT should be explored early for eligible patients, because the utility of ruxolitinib is in disease cytoreduction and as a bridge to transplant.

Patients diagnosed with CEL-NOS are typically treated with hydroxyurea or interferon-α. Allo-HSCT should be explored for eligible patients. Empiric imatinib treatment and investigational clinical trials may be pursued.

Patients diagnosed with HE and AML or ALL/LBL (T- or B-cell type) often require high-dose chemotherapy in addition to selective tyrosine kinase inhibitor.

Prognosis

Prognosis of eosinophil disorders varies significantly, depending on the underlying etiology and diagnostic classification.

Board Questions

56-year-old female presented with generalized body itching and dysphagia for the past 2 months. She denied any weight loss, diarrhea, and abdominal pain, and she is recently not on any medication. On physical examination, diffuse skin rash was found in her arms and lower extremities. Laboratory study revealed hemoglobin of 140 g/L, WBC of 9.1 × 10^9/L, and absolute eosinophil count increased to 4. 5 × 10^9/L. Which of the following studies should be done as the first approach?

A. Order *PDGFRA/PDGFRB/FGFR1* FISH panel
B. Perform Bone marrow biopsy
C. Obtain medical history of allergy, autoimmune, or infection
D. Biopsy of skin lesions
E. Perform flow cytometry to detect abnormal T-cell population

Answer C: There is a broad spectrum of differential diagnoses for a patient who suffered from diffuse skin rash and hypereosinophilia. Obtaining medical history is the initial step to identify potential etiology that could lead to a reactive eosinophilia before performing any invasive procedure, e.g., bone marrow biopsy (B) and skin biopsy (D). Flow cytometry T-cell panel can be pursued either on peripheral blood or skin biopsy sample to exclude cutaneous T-cell lymphoma with eosinophilia or T-cell-variant hypereosinophilia (E) if clinically indicated. FISH study for *PDGFRA/PDGFRB/FGFR1* is ordered when clinically suspicious for myeloid/lymphoid neoplasm with eosinophilia.

References

1. Valent P, Degenfeld-Schonburg L, Sadovnik I, et al. Eosinophils and eosinophil-associated disorders: immunological, clinical, and molecular complexity. Semin Immunopathol. 2021;43:423–38.
2. Shomali W, Gotlib J. World Health Organization–defined eosinophilic disorders: 2019 update on diagnosis, risk stratification, and management. Am J Hematol. 2019;94:1149–67.
3. Mattis DM, Wang S, Lu CM. Contemporary classification, and diagnostic evaluation of hypereosinophilia: an ACLPS critical review. Am J Clin Pathol. 2020;154:305–18.

4. Valent P, Klion AD, Roufosse F, et al. Proposed refined diagnostic criteria and classification of eosinophil disorders and related syndromes. Allergy. 2023;78:47–59.
5. Anderson CL, Siersma VD, Hasselbalch HC, et al. Eosinophilia in routine blood samples and the subsequent risk of hematological malignancies and death. Am J Hematol. 2013;88:843–7.
6. Schulte C, Krebs B, Jelinek T, et al. Diagnostic significance of blood eosinophilia in returning travelers. Clin Infect Dis. 2002;34:407–11.
7. Swerdlow SH, Campo E, Harris NL, et al., editors. WHO classification of tumours of haematopoietic and lymphoid tissues. Revised 4th ed. Lyon: IARC; 2017.
8. Khoury JD, Solary E, Abla O, et al. The 5th edition of the World Health Organization classification of haematolymphoid tumours: myeloid and histiocytic/dendritic neoplasms. Leukemia. 2022;36:1703–19.
9. Shi M, Rech KL, Otteson GE, et al. Prevalence and spectrum of T-cell lymphoproliferative disorders in patients with Hypereosinophilia: a reference laboratory experience. Ann Diagn Pathol. 2020;44:151412.
10. Ogbogu PU, Bochner BS, Butterfield JH, et al. Hypereosinophilic syndrome: a multicenter, retrospective analysis of clinical characteristics and response to therapy. J Allergy Clin Immunol. 2009;124:1319–25.
11. Cheung CC, Constantine M, Ahmadi A, et al. Eosinophilic myocarditis. Am J Med Sci. 2017;354:486–92.
12. Wang SA, Hasserjian RP, Tam W, et al. Bone marrow morphology is a strong discriminator between chronic eosinophilic leukemia, not otherwise specified and reactive idiopathic hypereosinophilic syndrome. Haematologica. 2017;102:1352–60.
13. Jawhar M, Naumann N, Knut M, et al. Cytogenetically cryptic ZMYM2-FLT3 and DIAPH1-PDGFRB gene fusions in myeloid neoplasms with eosinophilia. Leukemia. 2017;31:2271–3.
14. Cessna MH, Paulraj P, Hilton B, et al. Chronic myelomonocytic leukemia with ETV6-ABL1 rearrangement and SMC1A mutation. Cancer Genet. 2019;238:31–6.
15. Wang SA, Tam W, Tsai AG, et al. Targeted next-generation sequencing identifies a subset of idiopathic hypereosinophilic syndrome with features similar to chronic eosinophilic leukemia, not otherwise specified. Mod Pathol. 2016;29:854–64.
16. Cross NCP, Hoade Y, Tapper WJ, et al. Recurrent activating STAT5B N642H mutation in myeloid neoplasms with eosinophilia. Leukemia. 2019;33:415–25.
17. Stella S, Massimino M, Manzella L, et al. Molecular pathogenesis and treatment perspectives for hypereosinophilia and hypereosinophilic syndromes. Int J Mol Sci. 2021;22(2):486.
18. Reiter A, Gotlib J. Myeloid neoplasms with eosinophilia. Blood. 2017;129:704–14.
19. Strati P, Tang G, Duose DY. Myeloid/lymphoid neoplasms with FGFR1 rearrangement. Leuk Lymphoma. 2018;59:1672–6.

Benign Monocytic Disorders

3

Barina Aqil, Yasmin Abaza,
and Juehua Gao

Introduction

Monocytes normally comprise between 2% and 8% of the peripheral blood leukocytes with absolute monocyte count between 0.2 and 0.8 × 10^9/L, although it has been proposed that absolute counts as low as 0.5 × 10^9/L should qualify as clonal monocytosis if there is an associated clonal genetic abnormality. Monocytes belong to the mononuclear phagocyte system, spend only a short time in the marrow, and after circulating for 20 to 40 hours, leave the blood to enter solid tissues where they differentiate into macrophages (histiocytes) and survive for months or even years.

The monocyte precursors in the marrow are monoblasts and promonocytes. Mature monocytes average 12 μm to 15 μm in diameter and possess a large central oval or indented nucleus with clumped chromatin. They contain abundant cytoplasm pale blue or gray abundant cytoplasm and many fine purple-red granules

B. Aqil (✉) · J. Gao
Department of Pathology, Feinberg School of Medicine, Northwestern University, Chicago, IL, USA
e-mail: barina.aqil@northwestern.edu

Y. Abaza
Department of Medicine, Hematology Oncology Division, Feinberg School of Medicine, Northwestern University, Chicago, IL, USA

L. Sokol, L. Zhang (eds.), *Non-Neoplastic Hematologic Disorders*,
https://doi.org/10.1007/978-3-031-62373-8_3

and vacuoles (Fig. 3.1). The granules contain enzymes that are positive for a cytochemical nonspecific esterase stain (α-naphthyl butyrate esterase) (Fig. 3.2).

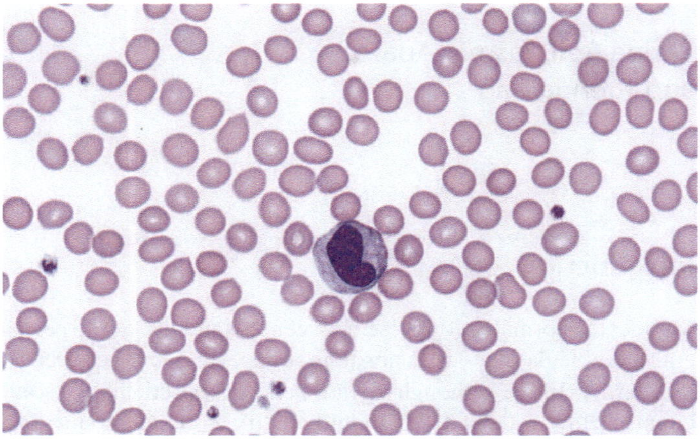

Fig. 3.1 Peripheral blood smear shows monocytes with a central oval/indented nucleus, clumped chromatin and abundant pale blue/gray cytoplasm with fine purple-red granules (Wright-Giemsa stain, magnification 1000×)

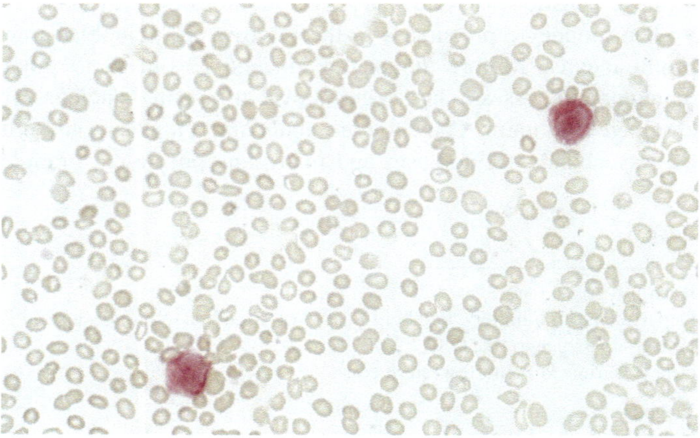

Fig. 3.2 Monocytes show staining with alpha-napthyl butyrate esterase stain (ANBE stain, magnification 600×)

By flow cytometry immunophenotyping, normal monocytes are commonly positive for CD14, CD4 (dim), CD11b, CD11c, CD18, CD64 (bright), CD36 (bright), CD33, CD13, HLA-DR, CD38, and CD45, and negative for CD34 and CD117 (Fig. 3.3). By immunohistochemical staining, CD68, CD163, and lysozyme are additional monocytic markers.

Human monocytes mature in the bone marrow and are subsequently released into circulation. They can be divided into three subsets based on microarray, flow cytometry, and cytokine production. $CD14^{+}$ classical monocytes (CM) ($CD14^{++}CD16^{-}$) subsequently give rise to nonclassical monocytes (N-CM) ($CD14^{dim+}CD16^{++}$) through an intermediate step of $CD14^{++}CD16^{+}$ monocytes (IM). CM in humans can also be distinguished from the other two subsets via expression of CD36, CCR2, and CD64. CM produce the highest level of G-CSF, IL10, CCL2, and IL6, while N-CM secrete a higher level of TNF-α and IL-1β, and IM produce all these kinds of cytokines but in low levels [1–4].

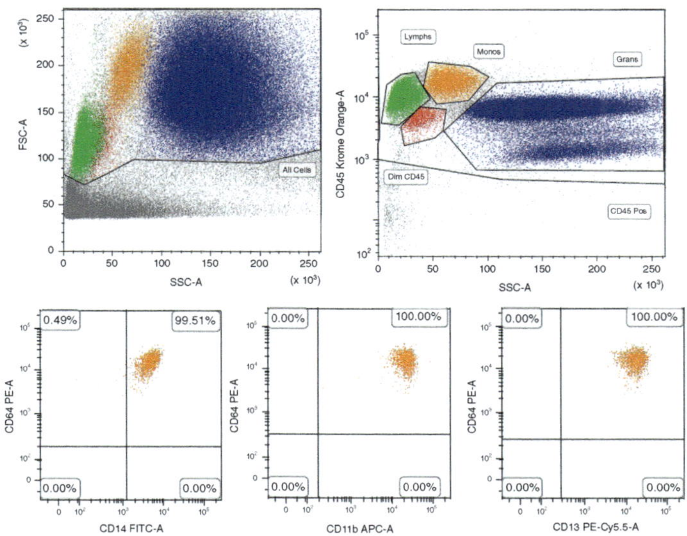

Fig. 3.3 Flow cytometry identified monocytes which are bright $CD45^{+}$, $CD64^{+}$, $CD14^{+}$, $CD11b^{+}$ and $CD13^{+}$

The functions of CM, N-CM, and IM are slightly different, but together they play critical roles in transmigration to tissue, antigen processing, phagocytosis, and antiviral response [5, 6].

Pathogenesis

The pathogenesis of monocytosis is complex and involves the regulation of monocyte production, differentiation, and turnover. Monocytosis is a result of disturbed balance between production and removal, which can occur in multiple ways, including increased production triggered by cytokines, such as GM-CSF and IL-3, or clonal proliferation caused by gene mutations. Decreased removal from blood circulation or blockage of apoptosis can also cause accumulation of monocytes in blood. Monocytopenia can be caused by decreased production (e.g., bone marrow injury), immunosuppression, or increased monocyte destruction.

Diagnosis

There are multiple non-neoplastic causes of monocytosis (Table 3.1). Reactive monocytosis can be transient and reversible. The most cost-effective evaluation is to repeat the complete blood count and differential once the presumed etiology has resolved. In cases of persistent monocytosis, a more comprehensive evaluation of reactive causes and, sometimes, additional laboratory investigation to exclude clonal proliferation may be undertaken. The evaluation starts with a thorough history and physical examination, including consideration of recent travel and exposures to illness to assess for infectious disease. Associated symptoms may also suggest a chronic systemic disorder and trigger appropriate laboratory testing for inflammatory or autoimmune conditions.

Acquired monocytopenia can occur in a variety of clinical settings (Table 3.2). Monocytopenia is also a characteristic feature of hairy-cell leukemia. Clinically, hairy-cell leukemia often presents

Table 3.1 Common non-neoplastic causes of monocytosis and monocytopenia

Main cause	Subcategory
Infection	Bacteria: tuberculosis, brucellosis, syphilis, subacute bacterial endocarditis
	Viruses: cytomegalovirus, parvovirus, Epstein-Barr virus, varicella-zoster
	Parasites: malaria, leishmaniasis, rickettsial infection (e.g., Rocky Mountain spotted fever)
Immune-mediated/ inflammatory disorders	Collagen vascular diseases: SLE, rheumatoid arthritis, polyarteritis nodosa, temporal arteritis, sarcoidosis
	GI and liver disorders: Crohn's disease, UC, regional enteritis, autoimmune hepatitis, primary biliary cirrhosis
	Immune-mediated hemolytic anemia, thrombocytopenia
Hematological disorders	Hemolytic anemia
	Congenital neutropenias: cyclic neutropenia, Wiskott-Aldrich syndrome, idiopathic thrombocytopenic purpura
	Chronic neutropenia
Medications/alcohol	GM-CSF, phenytoin, phenobarbital, valproic acid, carbamazepine, olanzapine, corticosteroid
Cardiovascular disease	Acute myocardial infarction, CAD
Medications	Chlorpromazine, ampicillin
Acute stress or trauma	Thermal injury, severe trauma, marathon running

CAD coronary artery disease, *GI* Gastrointestinal, *GM-CSF* granulocyte-macrophage colony-stimulating factor, *SLE* systemic lupus erythematosus, *UC* ulcerative colitis

among elderly patients with pancytopenia, circulating lymphocytes with hairy projections, splenomegaly, and marrow fibrosis.

The laboratory testing of monocytic disorders often starts with complete blood count with differential cell count demonstrating absolute monocytosis with monocytes accounting for more than 10% of the white blood cell (WBC) differential. Peripheral blood smear review is often used to confirm monocytosis and evaluate the morphology of the monocytes. Identification of dysplastic granulocytes, circulating blasts/promonocytes, and associated

Table 3.2 Common etiology of acquired monocytopenia

Main cause	Subcategory
Congenital	Germline *GATA2* deficiency/MonoMAC, Kostmann's syndrome, Shwachman-Diamond syndrome, cyclic neutropenia
Infection	HIV, sepsis
Autoimmune	SLE, rheumatoid arthritis
Bone marrow failure	Aplastic anemia
Medications	Glucocorticoid administration, radiation therapy
Others	Gaucher disease, decreased monocyte superoxide production, chemotaxis, microbial killing, hemodialysis

HIV human immunodeficiency virus, *MonoMAC* monocytopenia and mycobacterial infection, *SLE* systemic lupus erythematosus

hematologic abnormalities, such as anemia, thrombocytopenia, or eosinophilia, may suggest a clonal etiology. These findings may prompt a bone marrow biopsy and further evaluation. Findings of toxic changes in granulocytes and monocytes, intracellular microorganism, or evidence of hemolysis may suggest reactive causes. A repeat complete blood count and differential in 3 to 6 months are suggested to monitor resolution.

Flow cytometric immunophenotyping may aid in the differential of reactive vs clonal proliferation. Aberrant CD56 and CD7 expression, downregulation of CD14 and HLA-DR–aberrant monocyte repartition, and increased $CD34^+$ or $CD117^+$ blasts are observed in clonal monocytic proliferation. In chronic myelomonocytic leukemia (CMML), there is expansion of the CM ($CD14^+CD16^-$) fraction as opposed to N-CM ($CD14^{dim+}CD16^{++}$) or IM ($CD14^{++}CD16^+$) seen in sepsis, HIV, chronic kidney disease, inflammatory bowel disease, diabetes, obesity, atherosclerotic cardiovascular disease, and other reactive conditions [7]. If a clonal process is suspected, a bone marrow biopsy with additional fluorescence in situ hybridization, chromosome, and molecular studies are required for more definitive evaluation. The presence of clonal cytogenetic abnormalities such as trisomy 8, −7/del(7q), −5/del(5q) or detection of mutations commonly associated with myeloid neoplasms by next-generation sequence study (*TET2*,

SRSF2, *ASXL1*, *RUNX1*, *SETBP1*, *CBL*, *EZH2*, *KRAS*, *NRAS*) supports a diagnosis of myeloid neoplasm or clonal monocytosis.

Differential Diagnosis

Monocytosis is also commonly seen in myeloproliferative neoplasms, myelodysplastic/myeloproliferative neoplasms (e.g., CMML), and acute myeloid leukemia (AML) with monocytic differentiation. A representative list of myeloid neoplasms with monocytosis can be found in Table 3.3. In the recently published International Consensus Classification of Myeloid Neoplasms and Acute Leukemias [8], a new entity of "clonal monocytosis of undetermined significance" (CMUS) is added. CMUS is defined by persistent monocytosis (monocytes >10% and > 0.5×10^9/L of the WBCs) and the presence of myeloid neoplasm-associated mutations (variant allele frequency of ≥2%) without meeting CMML

Table 3.3 Myeloid neoplasms with monocytosis

Category	Names of diseases
Preneoplastic status	CMUS
	CCMUS
MPN	CML with increased monocytes
MDS/MPN	CMML
	MDS/MPN MPN, including JMML
M/LN-TK	Mainly including myeloid/lymphoid neoplasms with eosinophilia and *PDGFRB* rearrangement
AML	AML with inv(16)/*CBFB::MYH11*, AML with *KMT2A* rearrangement, AML with t(6;9)/*DEK::NUP214*, AML with *NPM1* mutation, acute myelomonocytic leukemia, acute monocytic leukemia, AML–myelodysplasia related

AML acute myeloid leukemia, *CCMUS* clonal cytopenia and monocytosis of undetermined significance, *CML* chronic myeloid leukemia, *CMML* chronic myelomonocytic leukemia, *CMUS* clonal monocytosis of undetermined significance, *JMML* juvenile myelomonocytic leukemia, *M/LN-TK* myeloid and lymphoid neoplasms with eosinophilia and tyrosine kinase gene rearrangement, *MDS/MPN* myelodysplastic/myeloproliferative neoplasms, *MPN* myeloproliferative neoplasms criteria or other hematopoietic neoplasms on bone marrow examination (Table 3.3). If there is cytopenia, then the nomenclature is clonal cytopenia and monocytosis of undetermined significance (CCMUS). The mutations that can be seen with CMUS or CCMUS are *SRSF2*, *TET2*, *ASXL1*, *SETBP1*, *NRAS/KRAS*, *RUNX1*, *CBL*, and *EZH2* [7]. These provisional entities are used when the available clinical, laboratory, and morphologic features are not sufficient to definitively diagnose CMML or another myeloid neoplasm. CMUS and CCMUS diagnoses are intended to further investigations and monitoring among individuals with monocytosis and myeloid neoplasm-associated mutations to determine if the elevated monocyte count is part of a benign process or represents the early stages of a myeloid neoplasm. Another major differential diagnosis of reactive monocytosis is CMML. Bone marrow examination shows hypercellularity, variable dyspoiesis, and monocytosis, but does not meet the morphological and molecular criteria for AML defined by the International Consensus Classification or WHO classification [8, 9]. A more detailed differential and subclassification of myeloid neoplasms with monocytosis is beyond the scope of the chapter; however, myeloid neoplasms can have a spectrum of presentation, and the differential from reactive monocytosis is not always straightforward. The distinction should be made based on peripheral blood, bone marrow morphology, ancillary studies (particularly molecular findings), as well as appropriate clinicopathologic correlation.

Compared to monocytosis, monocytopenia is relatively uncommon and frequently associated with other cytopenias (anemia and leukopenia). In the pediatric and young-adult group, monocytopenia can be observed as part of congenital disorders, such as Kostmann's syndrome, Shwachman-Diamond syndrome, or cyclic neutropenia and may warrant genetic consultation. Monocytopenia is also a main feature of germline *GATA2* deficiency, which is associated with a range of phenotypes, including monocytopenia, dendritic cell, B- and NK-lymphoid deficiency, and mycobacterial infection, lymphedema, and predisposition to myelodysplastic syndrome/AML. Monocytopenia is a characteristic finding of hairy-cell leukemia. Diagnosis of hairy-cell leukemia relies on immunophenotyping for clonal B-cells expressing CD11c, CD25, CD103, ANEXIN 1, and TRAP.

Prognosis

The prognosis of monocytosis and monocytopenia depends on the underlying etiology. Reactive monocytosis is usually self-limited and may occur in the recovery phase from an acute viral infection or during bone marrow regeneration after insults, such as chemotherapy or drugs. Chronic infections (such as tuberculosis, chronic fungal infections, brucellosis, and subacute bacterial endocarditis) and autoimmune/ inflammatory disorders (such as systemic lupus erythematosus and sarcoidosis) are among the most common benign causes of persistent monocytosis that need to be ruled out during initial investigation. Persistent monocytosis (absolute peripheral blood monocytosis $\geq 1 \times 10^9/L$ and monocytes $\geq 10\%$ of WBC differential for >3 consecutive months) may be caused by reactive or malignant causes and typically needs further investigation. Prognosis of patients with benign persistent monocytosis is favorable and dependent on underlying etiology.

Treatment

In general, reactive monocytosis or monocytopenia is often reversible with treatment of the offending etiology. Reactive monocytosis has also been reported with solid tumors as a paraneoplastic process and attributed to either increased mobilization of monocytes from bone marrow or increased monopoiesis [10]. Once reactive causes for sustained monocytosis are ruled out, primary bone marrow disorders, including clonal myeloid neoplasms, need to be considered. Treatment and prognosis of malignant monocytosis, such as CMML or AML, vary significantly based on the disease subtype and molecular characteristics. Please refer to the WHO classification of hematolymphoid neoplasms and NCCN guidelines.

Promising Clinical Studies

NA.

Caveats

- Monocytosis or monocytopenia is a result of disturbed balance between the production and consumption.
- Persistent peripheral blood monocytosis with immature/abnormal morphology, circulating blasts, and granulocytic dysplasia may prompt bone marrow examination for further evaluation.
- Expanded CM subset (>94% of circulating monocytes) is one of the supporting criteria for diagnosis of CMML according to 5th Edition of the WHO classification [8].
- NGS myeloid mutation panel including *TET2*, *SRSF2*, *ASXL1*, and *SETBP1* would be useful to distinguish between benign and clonal monocytosis.

Board Questions

1. The diagnostic criteria for CMUS include which of the following?

   A. Persistent monocytosis, monocytes $>2.0 \times 10^9$/L and > 10% of the WBCs
   B. Presence of dysplasia
   C. Hypercellular marrow with monocytosis and atypical megakaryocytes
   D. Myeloid-associated gene mutation (VAF >2%)
   E. Increased blasts

Answer: D. According to International Consensus Classification (ICC), CMUS is defined as persistent monocytosis $>= 0.5 \times 10^9$/uL and 10% of the WBCs after excluding reactive condition, presence of myeloid-associated gene mutations (> = 2% VAF), without overt dysplasia or increased blasts, lacking definite evidence of a myeloid or other hematopoietic neoplasm.

2. Which of the following lymphoma is associated with monocytopenia?

   A. Hepatosplenic T-cell lymphoma
   B. Hairy-cell leukemia
   C. Splenic marginal-zone lymphoma
   D. Chronic lymphocytic leukemia/small lymphocytic lymphoma
   E. Mantle-cell lymphoma

Answer: B. Of the listed malignant lymphoid neoplasms, hairy cell leukemia often accompanies with monocytopenia.

References

1. Wong KL, Tai JJ-Y, Wong WC, Han H, Sem X, Yeap WH, et al. Gene expression profiling reveals the defining features of the classical, intermediate, and nonclassical human monocyte subsets. Blood. 2011;118:e16–31. PMID: 21653326.
2. Weber C, Belge KU, von Hundelshausen P, Draude G, Steppich B, Mack M, et al. Differential chemokine receptor expression and function in human monocyte subpopulations. J Leukoc Biol. 2000;67:699–704. PMID: 10811011.
3. Boyette LB, Macedo C, Hadi K, Elinoff BD, Walters JT, Ramaswami B, et al. Phenotype, function, and differentiation potential of human monocyte subsets. PLoS ONE. 2017;12:e0176460. PMID: 28445506.
4. Dutertre CA, Amraoui S, DeRosa A, Jourdain JP, Vimeux L, Goguet M, et al. Pivotal role of M-DC8+ monocytes from viremic HIV-infected patients in TNFα overproduction in response to microbial products. Blood. 2012;120:2259–68. PMID: 22802339.
5. Wong KL, Yeap WH, Tai JJY, Ong SM, Dang TM, Wong SC. The three human monocyte subsets: implications for health and disease. Immunol Res. 2012;53:41–57. PMID: 22430559.
6. Heine GH, Ortiz A, Massy ZA, Lindholm B, Wiecek A, Martínez-Castelao A, et al. Monocyte subpopulations and cardiovascular risk in chronic kidney disease. Nat Rev Nephrol. 2012;8:362. PMID: 22410492.
7. Selimoglu-Buet D, Wagenr-Ballon O, Saada V, et al. Characteristic repartition of monocyte subsets as a diagnostic signature of chronic myelomonocytic leukemia. Blood. 2015;125(23):3618–26. PMID: 25852055.
8. Arber DA, Orazi A, Hasserjian RP, et al. International Consensus Classification of Myeloid Neoplasms and Acute Leukemias: integrating

morphologic, clinical, and genomic data. Blood. 2022;140(11):1200–28. PMID: 35767897.
9. Khoury JD, Germing U, Kikkeri N, et al. Chronic myelomonocytic leukemia. 5th ed. International Agency for research on cancer, World Health Organization; 2022.
10. Kiss M, Caro AA, Raes G, et al. Systemic reprogramming of monocytes in cancer. Front Oncol. 2020;10:1399. PMID: 33042791.

Benign Basophil and Mast Cell Disorders

4

Parth C. Patel and Somedeb Ball

Basophils

Introduction

Basophils are a type of granulocyte in the peripheral blood. They are so named because their granules stain with basic dyes. Basophils play an important role in allergic late-phase reactions and atopic disease and may bridge innate and adaptive immunity by driving T helper 2 (Th2) cell differentiation and IgE class switching in response to both antigenic and nonantigenic inputs. The normal range for basophils in the peripheral blood is only 0.5% to 1% of the total white blood cell count. Basophils are similar in size to neutrophils (10–14 μm across) with a 2- to 3-lobed or reniform nucleus that is usually obscured by coarse, basophilic (blue-black), or purple-red granules. These granules are often unevenly distributed and at times appear as a washed-out pattern

P. C. Patel · S. Ball (✉)
Division of Hematology and Oncology, Vanderbilt University School of Medicine, Nashville, TN, USA
e-mail: parth.c.patel@vumc.org; somedeb.ball@vumc.org

L. Sokol, L. Zhang (eds.), *Non-Neoplastic Hematologic Disorders*,
https://doi.org/10.1007/978-3-031-62373-8_4

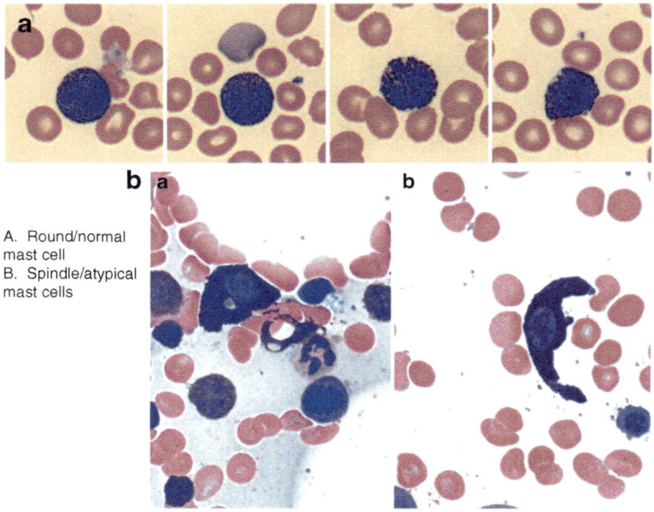

Fig. 4.1 (**a**) Normal Basophils in Peripheral Blood Smear (Cellavision). (**b**) Mast Cells (Bone Marrow, Wright-Giemsa Stain, ×1000)

(Fig. 4.1a) [1]. An increase in absolute basophils (usually greater than 0.2×10^9/L) is referred to as basophilia, which can be associated with reactive and neoplastic processes. We focus on reactive basophilia and distinguish it from its neoplastic counterpart.

Pathophysiology

Basophils differentiate from an eosinophil/basophil progenitor in bone marrow. The major cytokine that stimulates basophil production is IL-3. Additional cytokines involved in basophil growth and differentiation include IL-5, GM-CSF, TGF-β, and nerve growth factor. Basophils express surface IL-3 α chain (CD123) and eotaxin receptor (CCR3), which are critical to their function. Important effectors secreted by basophils following activation include histamine (found in granules), leukotriene (LTC_4), and the cytokines IL-4 and IL-13, which result in an increased vascular permeability and production of cell adhesion molecules by endothelium, thereby promoting leukocyte extravasation at sites of inflammation. Histamine and LTC_4 cause vasodilation and bronchoconstriction, which are critical to the pathophysiology of anaphylaxis and asthma. Moreover, IL-4 induces eotaxin synthesis by stromal cells, contributing to the recruitment of tissue eosinophils in allergic-disease states, while IL-13 is known to induce an asthmatic phenotype in mice (bronchial eosinophilia, mucus hypersecretion, subepithelial fibrosis, and hyperresponsiveness to methacholine challenge) [2].

Basophil activation can occur by at least two pathways: one antigenic and another nonantigenic. IgE receptor crosslinking in the presence of an antigen activates basophils via phosphatidylinositol 3-kinase and calcium-dependent signal-transduction pathways. In the absence of a specific antigen, basophils may be activated by co-stimulation with IL-3 and C5a, suggesting basophils also have a more general role in inflammation. IL-4 and IL-13 promote Th2 cell differentiation and IgE class switching. In normal physiology, this type of immune response is useful to eliminate certain infections (e.g., helminths) and enhance wound healing. However, this response may alternatively foster allergic disease [2, 3].

Diagnosis

Basophilia is diagnosed through a complete blood count (CBC) with a differential showing increased basophils in the peripheral blood. It is good practice to repeat the CBC after 2 to 3 weeks and request a manual slide review if basophilia persists, because spurious basophilia can result from misinterpreting atypical lymphocytes or degranulated neutrophils by automated hematology analyzers. Additionally, bone marrow biopsy with ancillary studies is only needed to exclude underlying myeloid and lymphoid neoplasms that could be associated with paraneoplastic basophilia or neoplastic proliferation of basophilic cells, e.g., accelerated phase of chronic myeloid leukemia, and rarely acute basophilic leukemia [4, 5].

Basopenia is difficult to define and study since basophils are infrequent in peripheral blood under normal conditions. It has been reported following severe allergic reactions (presumably caused by basophil tissue extravasation at the involved site). Corticosteroids appear to lower the basophil count [5].

Differential Diagnosis

It is important to differentiate reactive basophilia from neoplastic causes of basophilia because the management and prognosis will differ. Some conditions associated with basophilia are summarized in Table 4.1 and Fig. 4.2a.

Treatment

Treatment, if necessary, will depend on the underlying condition. For example, if basophilia is associated with severe atopic asthma, the patient may benefit from a leukotriene receptor antagonist such as montelukast.

Treatment for malignant basophilia is based on the treatment guidelines for the specific myeloid or lymphoid neoplasms, consisting of cytoreductive therapy (e.g., hydroxyurea), targeted therapy (e.g., tyrosine kinase inhibitors), allogeneic hematopoietic transplant, or chimeric antigen receptor T-cell therapy.

- A study found that basophilia may be associated with certain genetic mutations, such as a mutation in the *JAK2* gene [8] that may be suitable for targeted therapy
- Studies are in progress to determine whether a basophil activation test may be used to diagnose food allergies in children without risks associated with giving the triggering antigen (NCT05309772).

Board Question
Which of these hematologic malignancies is most likely associated with basophilia?

Table 4.1 Differential diagnoses of basophilia [5–7]

Reactive disorders	Clinical	Laboratory/molecular	Note
Reactive			
Viral or bacterial infections	Fevers, chills, pain, symptoms specific to infection type	CBC, blood cultures, suspected infection-specific cultures	Can resolve with resolution of infection
Autoimmune conditions	Variable finding per condition	CBC, ANA panel, RF, disease-specific antibodies	
Allergic reactions	Rhinitis, rashes, pruritis, nasal congestion, shortness of breath, conjunctivitis	CBC, CMP, patch testing, lung-function tests if considering asthma, immunoglobulin levels	
Tobacco use	Tobacco use history	CBC with increase in basophils, usually mild Resolution with cessation	
Neoplastic disorders			
Myeloproliferative neoplasms	Fatigue, weight loss, splenomegaly, aquagenic pruritis (seen in PV), leukostatic symptoms	NGS, flow cytometry, cytogenetics, FISH, karyotyping Bone marrow biopsy	CML: basophilia most common abnormality, associated with *BCR::ABL1* fusion. Other mutations include *JAK2*, *MPL*, *CALR*

(continued)

Table 4.1 (continued)

Reactive disorders	Clinical	Laboratory/molecular	Note
AML	Fatigue, infections, bleeding	NGS, flow cytometry, cytogenetics, FISH, karyotyping Bone marrow biopsy with >20% myeloid blasts Cytopenia Peripheral blasts	Associated with t(6;9)(p23;q34.1); *DEK::NUP214* For CML myeloblastic crisis looking for *BCR::ABL1* and additional cytogenetic aberrations
Basophilic leukemia	Pruritis, urticarial rash, fatigue, flushing, nausea, diarrhea	Cytopenia Peripheral blasts Bone marrow biopsy with increase in basophils, basophilic blasts >20% for acute, <20% for chronic NGS, flow cytometry, cytogenetics, FISH, karyotyping	Rare, not well-defined *MYB::GATA1* fusion gene
Acute promyelocytic leukemia with basophilic differentiation (PMID: 32185069)	Fatigue, infections, bleeding	NGS, flow cytometry, cytogenetics, FISH, karyotyping Peripheral blast/promyelocytes, Auer rods	Not well-studied t(15;17)/*PML::RARA* rearrangement

AML acute myeloid leukemia, *ANA* antinuclear antibody, *CBC* complete blood count, *CML* chronic myeloid leukemia, *CMP* comprehensive metabolic panel, *FISH* Fluorescence in situ hybridization, *NGS* next-generation sequencing, *RF* Rheumatoid factor, *PV* polycythemia vera

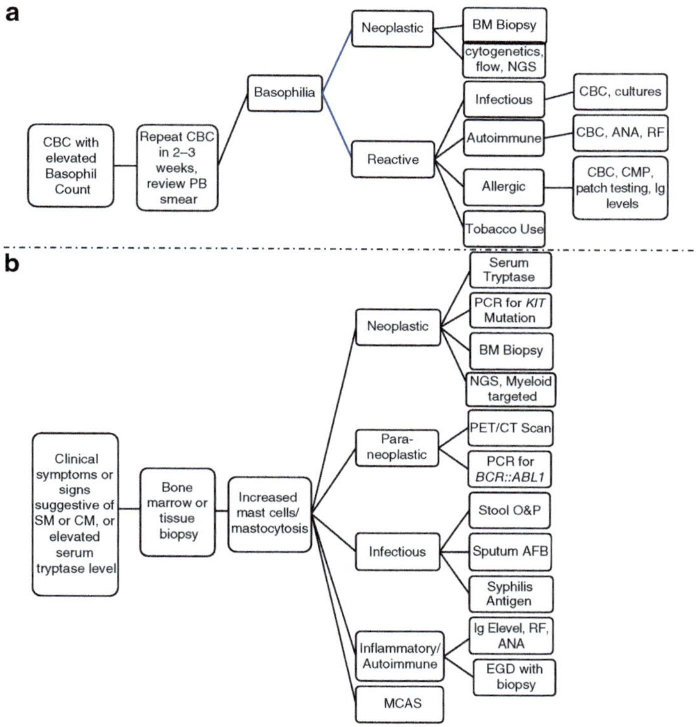

Fig. 4.2 Diagnostic Algorithms of Basophilia and Mastocytosis. AFB Acid fast bacilli, ANA antinuclear antigen, CBC complete blood count, CM cutaneous mastocytosis, CMP comprehensive metabolic profile, Ig immunoglobulin, MCAS mast cell activation syndrome, NGS next generation sequencing, O&P ova and parasites, PET/CT position Emission Tomography/Computed Tomography, PCR polymerase chain reaction, RF rheumatoid factor, SM systemic mastocytosis

a. Acute promyelocytic leukemia
b. Indolent systemic mastocytosis
c. Myeloproliferative neoplasm
d. Myelodysplastic syndrome

Answer: c. Myeloproliferative neoplasms, especially chronic myeloid leukemia.

Mast Cells

Introduction

Mast cells are singly scattered throughout loose connective tissue and are especially abundant in the skin, lungs, and gastrointestinal mucosa. They are important mediators of allergic reactions and have several functions which overlap basophils, although the two cell types are distinct. Mast cells also play a variety of regenerative and protective roles in the human body. They are morphologically characterized by numerous cytoplasmic granules (metachromatic in Wright stain, eosinophilic on H&E) which partially obscure the nucleus, like basophils. However, mast cells are larger (15–30 μm across) and have a nonsegmented nucleus. Normal mast cells are round-to-oval and scattered, whereas neoplastic mast cells aggregates (Fig. 4.1b) [9]. Abnormal proliferation of mast cells can be primary, derived from a mutant hematopoietic stem cell, or secondary to infection, allergy/anaphylaxis, inflammatory conditions, medications, or paraneoplastic syndromes. Mast cells can also be increased in idiopathic disorders, such as mast cell activation syndrome [10].

Pathophysiology

Mast cells arise from pluripotent stem cells (CD34+) in bone marrow and spleen. Stem cell factor is an important growth factor for mast cell development. Surface receptor for stem cell factor is receptor tyrosine kinase kit (CD117), produced from gene *KIT*, and it is expressed in hematopoietic stem cells. Unlike other myeloid cells, mast cells continue to retain kit throughout their life cycle. Interaction with various cytokines and tissue factors determines the differentiation and migration of mast cells to different tissues.

Mucosal mast cells are commonly associated with Th2 cell-mediated inflammation [11].

Diagnosis

It is important to separate reactive or paraneoplastic mastocytosis from the neoplastic process. A careful inquiry of current and past medical clinical history, performing an adequate physical examination, and ordering appropriate laboratory tests, imaging study, and tissue-biopsy procedures would be helpful for an accurate diagnosis. Clinically, patients with high mast cell burden may have history of skin rash, diarrhea, allergy, asthma, or anaphylaxis. Rarely, mastocytosis could indicate a primary malignancy, such as systemic mastocytosis (SM). In these cases, patients may have low blood counts, fatigue, infection, or bleeding. Patients with SM can also have hepatosplenomegaly or bone disease. Imaging study can be used to assess systemic involvement and staging for SM.

Workup should include CBC, CMP, immunoglobulin E level, rheumatoid factor, stool for ova–parasite–cyst, and serum tryptase level. Additionally, a polymerase chain reaction test for *KIT* mutation should be done if SM is suspected. A point mutation in the - *KIT* gene at codon 816 is detected in the majority (>90%) of patients with SM. Presence of any activating *KIT* mutation has been accepted as a minor diagnostic criterion for SM in the new WHO classification [12]. Rarely, mast cells could be found in peripheral blood smear examination (mast cell leukemia). Usually, biopsy of relevant organ or tissue (e.g., skin, gastric tissue, or bone marrow) based on symptoms and signs could yield the finding of high mast cell burden. Multifocal dense mast cell infiltrates (≥15 mast cells in aggregates) and atypical *spindle-shaped* morphology could suggest a neoplastic process like SM (refer to the 5th edition of WHO diagnostic criteria for SM) (12). Targeted DNA sequencing could identify non-*KIT* mutations (*TET2*, *SRSF2*, *ASXL1*, *RUNX1*, and *JAK2*) relevant for associated myeloid neoplasms (SM-AMN).

Differential Diagnosis

Differential diagnoses for mastocytosis are summarized in Table 4.2 and Fig. 4.2b [10].

Table 4.2 Differential diagnoses for mastocytosis

Disorders	Clinical findings	Laboratory/ molecular	Note
Infections			
Parasites, tuberculosis, syphilis	Fever, pruritus, cough, hemoptysis, genital lesions, hepatosplenomegaly	Stool examination for ova–parasite–cyst Sputum for acid fast bacilli Rapid antigen test for syphilis	Reversible mastocytosis, resolves with resolution of infection
Inflammatory/autoimmune			
Allergic rhinitis, asthma, urticaria, eosinophilic esophagitis RA, scleroderma	Allergic symptoms, dyspnea with seasonal variation, dysphagia, joint pain, and swelling	Serum IgE level Serology for Rheumatoid factor, antinuclear antibodies Esophago-gastro-duodenoscopy with biopsy	Can resolve with improvement in underlying condition
Neoplastic			
Cutaneous mastocytosis SM MCS	Allergic symptoms, diarrhea, skin rash, bone pain, ascites, hepatosplenomegaly, cytopenias	Serum tryptase level PCR for *KIT* mutation Bone marrow aspiration and biopsy Myeloid-targeted DNA sequencing (for SM-AMN)	Mastocytosis may improve with local and systemic therapies as applicable. Systemic therapy may include KIT inhibitors
Paraneoplastic			

(continued)

Table 4.2 (continued)

Disorders	Clinical findings	Laboratory/ molecular	Note
Melanoma Seminoma Hodgkin's lymphoma CML	Variable based on underlying malignancy	CT scan PET scan PCR for *BCR;ABL* transcript	
Idiopathic MCAS			Omalizumab may be effective

CML chronic myeloid leukemia, *MCAS* mast cell activation syndrome, *MCS* mast cell sarcoma, *RA* Rheumatoid arthritis, *SM* systemic mastocytosis, *SM-AMN* SM associated myeloid neoplasm

Prognosis

Prognosis depends on etiology for increased mast cell burden. Mastocytosis associated with allergic conditions should improve after the allergy is controlled. Similarly, high mast cell burden secondary to infections should also resolve once infection subsides. If mastocytosis is neoplastic, prognosis varies based on extent and severity of SM. For example, a patient with indolent SM has a survival similar to the age-matched general population, whereas presence of aggressive SM (defined by organ damage caused by mast cell infiltration) leads to a shortened median survival of about 3 years. The factors useful in assessing prognosis in SM include extent of anemia, thrombocytopenia, serum tryptase, alkaline phosphatase, and beta-2 microglobulin levels, and presence of AMN-related mutations.

Treatment

Treatment of mastocytosis depends on underlying etiologies. Allergic diseases with mastocytosis can be managed with a combination of topical and inhalational steroids or anti-IgE monoclonal antibodies (e.g., omalizumab). Autoimmune disease like RA requires treatment with disease-modifying antirheumatoid drugs (e.g., methotrexate).

KIT tyrosine kinase inhibitors (e.g., midostaurin and avapritinib) can be useful in treating advanced SM [13]. Other recommended regimens for patients with aggressive SM include cladribine and peginterferon-alfa (with or without prednisone).

For patients with SM-AMN, clinicians should first assess which component (SM or AMN) needs immediate treatment. Accordingly, a KIT-targeted therapy or AMN-directed treatment (e.g., hypomethylating agent for myelodysplastic syndrome as AMN) can be chosen.

Promising Clinical Studies

- Avapritinib, a selective KIT inhibitor, was found to be safe and effective in patients with advanced SM in the phase I trial (EXPLORER) [13].
- In a study of 55 patients with mast cell disorders, omalizumab therapy was effective in controlling mast cell-mediated symptoms in cutaneous mastocytosis, SM, and MCAS [14].

Board Question

A 55-year-old female showed up to an outside clinic because of chronic skin rash, irritation, intermittent diarrhea, and unintended weight loss. On physical examination, there were diffuse reddish-brown skin macules over the patient's upper chest, back, and thighs. Additional laboratory investigation revealed leukocytosis (white blood cell count of 11×10^9/L) and elevated serum tryptase level (121 ng/ml). A bone marrow biopsy showed atypical or spindle-shaped mast cells in big aggregates that stained positive for CD117, mast cell tryptase, CD2 (subset), and CD25. There was no overt dysplasia, no increased blasts or eosinophils, or any other evidence of abnormalities in the bone marrow examination.

Which of the following genetic aberrations is most likely to be found in this patient?

a. *BCR::ABL1* translocation
b. *CSF3R* T618I mutation

c. *KMT2A* rearrangement
d. *JAK2* V617F mutation
e. *KIT* D816V mutation

Answer: e. The patient's clinical and bone marrow findings are most consistent with systemic mastocytosis. *KIT* D816V mutation is commonly present in systemic mastocytosis. *BCR:ABL1* translocation is found in chronic myeloid leukemia. *CSF3R* T618I mutation is more associated with chronic neutrophilic leukemia. KMT2A/MLL gene rearrangement is often seen with AML, ALL, or other myeloid/lymphoid neoplasm, but not diagnostic for systemic mastocytosis. Keep in mind, it is not uncommon to have associated hematologic/myeloid neoplasm with SM (SM-AMN).

References

1. Sticco KL, Pandya NK, Lynch DT. Basophilia. StatPearls; 2022.
2. Siracusa MC, Kim BS, Spergel JM, Artis D. Basophils and allergic inflammation. J Allergy Clin Immunol. 2013;132(4):789–801; quiz 788. https://doi.org/10.1016/j.jaci.2013.07.046.
3. Redrup AC, Howard BP, MacGlashan DW Jr, Kagey-Sobotka A, Lichtenstein LM, Schroeder JT, et al. J Immunol. 1998;160(4):1957–64.
4. Grattan CE, Dawn G, Gibbs S, Francis DM. Blood basophil numbers in chronic ordinary urticaria and healthy controls: diurnal variation, influence of loratadine and prednisolone and relationship to disease activity. Clin Exp Allergy. 2003;33(3):337–41. https://doi.org/10.1046/j.1365-2222.2003.01589.x.
5. Feriel J, Depasse F, Genevieve F. How I investigate basophilia in daily practice. Int J Lab Hematol. 2020;42(3):237–45. https://doi.org/10.1111/ijlh.13146.
6. May ME, Waddell CC. Basophils in peripheral blood and bone marrow. A retrospective review. Am J Med. 1984;76(3):509–11. https://doi.org/10.1016/0002-9343(84)90671-5.
7. Smith CJ, Kluck LA, Ruan GJ, et al. Leukocytosis and tobacco use: an observational study of asymptomatic leukocytosis. Am J Med. 2021;134(1):e31–5. https://doi.org/10.1016/j.amjmed.2020.06.014.
8. Pieri L, Bogani C, Guglielmelli P, et al. The JAK2V617 mutation induces constitutive activation and agonist hypersensitivity in basophils from patients with polycythemia vera. Haematologica. 2009;94(11):1537–45. https://doi.org/10.3324/haematol.2009.007047.

9. Krystel-Whittemore M, Dileepan KN, Wood JG. Mast cell: a multi-functional master cell. Front Immunol. 2015;6:620. https://doi.org/10.3389/fimmu.2015.00620.
10. Theoharides TC, Valent P, Akin C. Mast cells, mastocytosis, and related disorders. N Engl J Med. 2015;373(2):163–72. https://doi.org/10.1056/NEJMc1510021.
11. Dahlin JS, Hallgren J. Mast cell progenitors: origin, development and migration to tissues. Mol Immunol. 2015;63(1):9–17. https://doi.org/10.1016/j.molimm.2014.01.018.
12. Khoury JD, Solary E, Abla O, et al. The 5th edition of the World Health Organization classification of haematolymphoid tumours: myeloid and histiocytic/dendritic neoplasms. Leukemia. 2022;36(7):1703–19. https://doi.org/10.1038/s41375-022-01613-1.
13. DeAngelo DJ, Radia DH, George TI, et al. Safety and efficacy of avapritinib in advanced systemic mastocytosis: the phase 1 EXPLORER trial. Nat Med. 2021;27(12):2183–91. https://doi.org/10.1038/s41591-021-01538-9.
14. Lemal R, Fouquet G, Terriou L, et al. Omalizumab therapy for mast cell-mediator symptoms in patients with ISM, CM, MMAS, and MCAS. J Allergy Clin Immunol Pract. 2019;7(7):2387–2395 e3. https://doi.org/10.1016/j.jaip.2019.03.039.

Benign Lymphocytic Disorders

5

Anthony Wood, Ling Zhang, and Lubomir Sokol

Introduction

Lymphocytes are a class of white blood cells (WBCs) comprised of mature T-cells, B-cells, and natural killer (NK) cells that are important in the maintenance of both adaptive and innate immune responses. The normal absolute lymphocyte count (ALC) for a healthy adult ranges from 1×10^9/L to 4.0×10^9/L. Lymphocytosis is present when the ALC exceeds 5×10^9/L, whereas an ALC of less than 1.0×10^9/L is termed lymphopenia. A normal lymphocyte count is variable for pediatric patients based on the child's age and is usually higher among infants and very young children. An ALC of 6×10^9/L for children and that of 9×10^9/L for infants

A. Wood
Department of Internal Medicine, USF Health Morsani College of Medicine, University of South Florida, Tampa, FL, USA

L. Zhang
Department of Hematopathology, H. Lee Moffitt Cancer Center and Research Institute, Tampa, FL, USA
e-mail: ling.zhang@moffitt.org

L. Sokol (✉)
Department of Malignant Hematology, H. Lee Moffitt Cancer Center and Research Institute, Tampa, FL, USA
e-mail: lubomir.sokol@moffitt.org

L. Sokol, L. Zhang (eds.), *Non-Neoplastic Hematologic Disorders*, https://doi.org/10.1007/978-3-031-62373-8_5

are considered absolute lymphocytosis, whereas an ALC less than 2×10^9/L is considered lymphocytopenia for children aged 6 and younger [1].

Lymphocytosis can be broadly divided into reactive and malignant categories. Reactive lymphocytosis refers to an increase of activated lymphocytes in response to triggers such as infections, autoimmune diseases, medications, transplantation, endocrine disorders, tobacco use, and stress (e.g., trauma, extreme exercise, stroke, or seizure). Malignant lymphocytosis is a clonal proliferation of neoplastic lymphocytes.

Lymphocytopenia is usually identified in adults as a laboratory finding during a regular annual checkup or follow-up for other malignancy. It is often associated with congenital or acquired immunocompromised status or post-cytotoxic therapy.

This chapter will describe a practical approach for these conditions from the perspective of a consulting hematologist.

Pathogenesis

Given varied factors are applied, the underlying mechanism leading to lymphocyte depletion or proliferation is more complicated. Reactive lymphocytosis is often secondary to an immune system response to infection or due to autoimmune process, resulting in increased lymphocyte production, decreased lymphocyte clearance, and/or release of preexisting lymphocytes into circulation from secondary lymphoid compartments. The reactive lymphocytosis is usually self-limited after elimination of antigenic stimulants. However, in autoimmune diseases, presence of unrecognized "self-antigens" could cause a sustained activation and proliferation of self-reactive T-cells and B-cells secondary to cell-mediated and humoral immune responses, leading to long-standing lymphocytosis until the "error" signals have been blocked. Under different situations, release of certain cytokines, chemokines, and growth factors (e.g., IL-6, IL-10, TNF alpha) could suppress lymphogenesis. Additionally, lymphocyte trafficking to lymphoid organs or tissues, inflammation-induced cell death, release of co-inhibitory humoral factors, and administration of glucocorticoids will result in lymphocytopenia.

Diagnosis

It is important to correctly identify lymphocytosis as reactive or malignant so that the proper clinical approach with appropriate laboratory tests can be taken. The difficulty in this task lies in the fact that reactive and malignant lymphocytosis can have similar clinical features, e.g., B-symptoms (including fevers, night sweats, fatigue, and weight loss), lymphadenopathy, and sometimes splenomegaly. A thorough understanding of the patient's history and a physical exam focused on various domains of the differential diagnosis can provide contextual clues to help come to an accurate conclusion. Family history, travel, vaccination, infection, autoimmunity, medications, herbal supplements, nicotine use, diets, animal exposures, and toxins are useful diagnostic

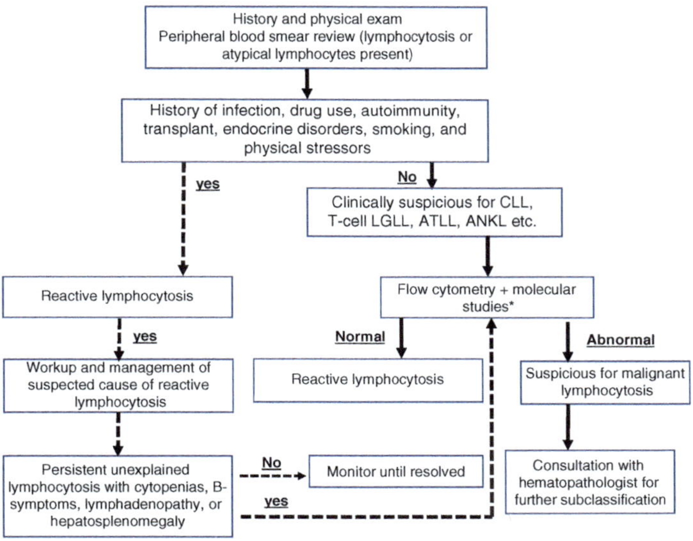

CLL: chronic lymphocytic leukemia, MCL: mantle cell lymphoma, T-cell LGLL: T-large granular lymphocytic leukemia, ATLL: adult T-cell lymphoma/leukemia, ANKL: aggressive NK cell leukemia.
*Molecular studies: TCR or BCR gene rearrangement clonality tests, NGS

Fig. 5.1 Diagnostic algorithm of clinical lymphocytosis

clues. A diagnostic algorithm for lymphocytosis is displayed in Fig. 5.1.

Patients who have lymphocytopenia often show unusual or recurrent infections, or slow wound healing. Obtaining clinical history of congenital or familial disease, immunodeficiency (e.g., HIV status, prior chemoradiation, immunosuppressive therapy, or transplantation) is a key step for patients with lymphocytopenia.

Peripheral Blood Smear Review

A peripheral blood smear is essential to evaluate morphology of lymphocytosis [2]. Reactive processes are characterized by polymorphous lymphocytes, including activated forms that are intermediate in size and have a moderate amount of cytoplasm which adhere to neighboring red blood cells. In contrast, malignant lymphocytic processes are often monotonous, with limited variation between individual cells. However, there is no morphologic gold standard to separate malignant lymphocytes from reactive lymphocytes, as neoplastic lymphocytes may be indistinguishable from normal lymphocytic counterparts (e.g., T-large granular lymphocytes). Moreover, a malignant process such as leukemia or lymphoma may be associated with reactive lymphocytosis (e.g., Sezary cells in a background of increased T-LGLs). Despite so, additional morphologic clues might be useful to help identify certain pathologies (Table 5.1, Fig. 5.2).

Flow Cytometry

Flow cytometry is usually performed for diagnosis and staging of clonal lymphoproliferative disorders, to monitor residual disease or quantitate immunodeficient T- or B-cell status.

A flow cytometry panel for lymphocytosis typically includes T- and B-cell markers, such as CD3, CD4, CD5, CD7, CD8, CD10, CD25, CD30, CD19, CD20, CD23, CD200, FMC-7, and surface kappa and lambda light chains. In general, the observation of polyclonal B-cells and intact T-cell antigen expression without aberrancy or increased immature forms excludes lymphoid malignancy.

Table 5.1 Morphologic features for common peripheral lymphocytosis, benign or malignant

Morphology	Benign examples	Neoplastic examples	Additional studies
Small, round nuclei, condensed chromatin	Naive B/T lymphocytes	CLL/SLL, monoclonal B lymphocytosis, or MCL	FCM/FISH
Small, cleaved nuclei	Reactive T-cells (e.g., pertussis)	Follicular lymphoma	FCM, microbiology
Large granular lymphocytes	Infectious mononucleosis or other viral infection or T-LGL proliferation secondary to malignancy or treatment	T/NK-LGLL, or aggressive NK-cell leukemia	FCM, TCR gene clonality test, EBV titer, virology
"Flower-cells"	–	ATLL	HTLV-1/2 serology test
"Cerebriform nuclei"	–	CTCL/Sezary syndrome	FCM, TCR gene clonality test
Cytoplasmic villous projections	Reactive small T-cells (occasional)	SMZL (polar villous), HCL, or HCL-v (circumferential villous)	FCM, TRAP, molecular study (BRAF mutation)
Enlarged lymphocytes with prominent nucleoli	Immunoblasts (occasional)	T-PLL, atypical CLL (e.g., TP53 mutation), MCL, or HCL-v	FCM, FISH, molecular study
Plasmacytoid	Reactive plasmacytoid lymphocytes, immunoblasts, or reactive plasma cells (occasional)	MZL, MM, plasma cell leukemia, or LPL (infrequent)	FCM

(continued)

Table 5.1 (continued)

Morphology	Benign examples	Neoplastic examples	Additional studies
Large, bizarre looking	–	Burkitt lymphoma, DLBCL, pleomorphic MCL, PTCL, or ALCL	FCM, FISH
Blastoid	–	MCL blastoid variant, or T- or B-ALL	FCM, FISH

ALCL anaplastic large cell lymphoma, *ALL* acute lymphoblastic leukemia, *ATLL* adult T-cell leukemia/lymphoma, *CLL* chronic lymphocytic leukemia, *CMV* cytomegalovirus, *CTCL* cutaneous T-cell lymphoma, *DLBCL* diffuse large B-cell lymphoma, *EBV* Epstein-Barr virus, *FCM* flow cytometry, *FISH* fluorescence in situ hybridization, *HCL-v* hairy cell leukemia variant, now namely splenic B-cell lymphoma/leukemia with prominent nucleoli, *HTLV-1* human T-lymphotropic virus 1, *LPL* lymphoplasmacytic lymphoma, *MCL* mantle cell lymphoma, *MM* multiple myeloma, *MZL* marginal zone lymphoma, *PCR* polymerase chain reaction, *PLL* prolymphocytic leukemia, *PTCL* peripheral T-cell lymphoma, *SMZL* splenic marginal zone lymphoma, *T/NK-LGLL* T/NK-cell large granular lymphocytic leukemia, *TRAP* tartrate-resistant acid phosphatase

However, a neoplasm may be hidden due to the marker combination used; low event number; interpretation errors; or inappropriate sampling, processing, or gating strategies. Monoclonal kappa or lambda light chain expression supports a clonal B-cell lymphocytosis diagnosis. Conversely, a lack of surface light chain restriction does not exclude B-cell lymphoma/leukemia, as chronic lymphocytic leukemia/small lymphocytic lymphoma (CLL/SLL) often shows diminished surface light chain expression, but demonstrates cytoplasmic kappa or lambda light chain clonality. Diminished light chain expression is also not uncommon in diffuse large B-cell lymphoma. The diagnosis of T-cell lymphoproliferative disorders is more complex, as the loss of certain surface antigens (e.g., CD7 or CD26) is not necessarily malignant. Identifying abnormal coexpression of bright CD25 (e.g., adult T-cell leukemia/lymphoma [ATLL]), CD10 (e.g., angioimmunoblastic T-cell lymphoma), or CD30 (e.g., anaplastic large cell lymphoma and mycosis fungoides

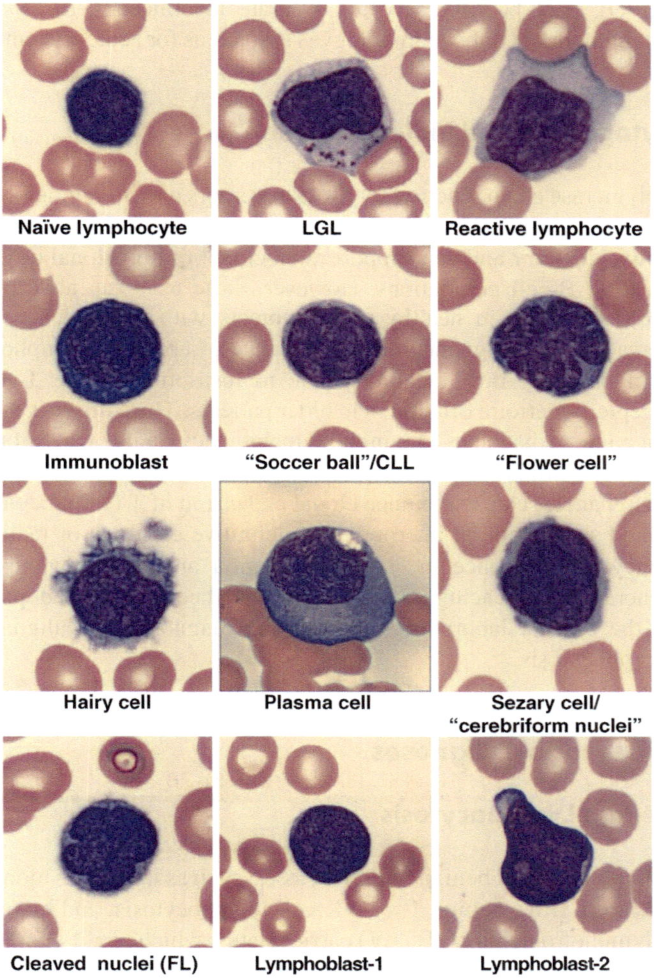

Fig. 5.2 Morphologic variation of reactive vs neoplastic lymphoid cells

with large cell transformation) might be helpful for diagnosis. In addition to routine T- or B-cell markers, an expanded flow cytometry panel, including cytoplasmic CD3, cytoplasmic light chains, terminal deoxynucleotidyl transferase (TdT), and myeloperoxidase

(MPO), may be necessary for accurate identification of B- or T-lymphoblasts if the morphology is suspicious for acute leukemia.

Cytogenetic and Molecular Tests

Polymerase chain reaction for T-cell receptors and immunoglobulin gene rearrangement clonality tests complement the results of flow cytometry and can support monoclonal or polyclonal origin of T- or B-cell populations. However, these tests can also give positive results in healthy older subjects with no evidence of hematologic malignancy or with absence of abnormal lymphoid population on flow cytometry due to restriction of the T-cell receptor repertoire often seen in older patients. Thus, this test cannot confirm diagnosis of lymphoid malignancy on its own. Strong antigenic stimulation with viruses, autoimmune diseases, and malignancies can also induce clonal expansion of T-lymphocytes, which should not be interpreted as definitive evidence of malignancy. Fluorescence in situ hybridization and emerging next-generation sequencing (NGS) studies have been recently adopted in the clinical laboratories for refining diagnosis of malignant lymphocytosis.

Differential Diagnoses

Benign Lymphocytosis

There are several benign lymphocytoses, such as infectious mononucleosis (IM), benign T- or NK-cell lymphocytosis, and human T-lymphotropic virus (HTLV) carrier status, which could mimic a malignant lymphocytosis and require special clinical attention (Table 5.2).

IM is a common infectious syndrome that manifests with fever, pharyngitis, lymphadenopathy, lymphocytosis, and splenomegaly. It is most frequently seen in adolescents and young adults and is classically associated with EBV infection [3]. However, CMV, acute HIV, human herpesvirus 6 (HHV-6), and toxoplasmosis,

Table 5.2 The etiology and diagnostic features of common reactive lymphocytosis

Category	Etiology	Phenotype and unique features	Laboratory tests
Viral infections			
Infectious mononucleosis	EBV; DDx includes CMV, acute toxoplasmosis, HHV-6, and acute HIV infection	T-cell immunophenotype	Mono-spot (+), HIV RNA/Ab (−), group A streptococcal infection (−)
T-LGL/NK-cell expansion	Age ≥ 60, EBV, CMV, HIV, HBV, HCV, VZV, HTLV-1, HIV, connective tissue diseases, malignancies, posttransplantation, dasatinib, aplastic anemia, PNH, MDS, PRCA, celiac disease, ITP, or HLH	T-LGL immunophenotype	TCR gene rearrangement +/−, age-appropriate cancer screening, viral, autoimmune, and malignancy workup as indicated
HTLV-1-positive carrier	Endemic to southern Japan, the Caribbean, Central/South America, tropical Africa, and northern Iran	T-cell immunophenotype or flower cells on PBS	HTLV-1 serology (+)
HIV and Diffuse Infiltrative Lymphocyte Syndrome (DILS)	Poorly controlled HIV; DDx includes connective tissue disease and IgG4-related disease	CD8+ T-cell immunophenotype	CD4 count (low), HIV VL (high), ANA, RF, anti-Ro/La, serum Ig with IgG subclasses (−), tissue biopsy
Varicella	Virus	–	Fluid PCR (+)
Measles	Virus	–	Serology: IgM (+), fluid PCR (+)
Mumps	Virus	–	Serology: IgM (+), fluid PCR (+)

(continued)

Table 5.2 (continued)

Category	Etiology	Phenotype and unique features	Laboratory tests
Hepatitis viruses	Virus	–	HAV: IgM (+), HBV: HbsAg and PCR (+), HCV: Ab and PCR (+)
Adenovirus	Virus	–	Fluid PCR (+)
Bacterial infections			
Bordetella pertussis	Bacteria	Small, mature lymphocytes with significantly cleaved nuclei	Sputum culture/PCR and serology (+)
Bartonella henselae	Bacteria	–	Clinical dx; serology (+)
Typhoid	Endemic to areas of poor sanitation in Asia, Africa, Latin America, and the Caribbean	–	Blood and stool cultures (+)
Brucellosis	Unpasteurized milk products, exposure to animal fluids, endemic to the Mediterranean basin, Middle East, Asia, Africa, Latin America, and the Caribbean	–	Body fluid cultures, serial serology, PCR (+)
Parasitic infections	Various kinds		Gross examination
Toxoplasmosis	Contaminated water and undercooked meat	–	Serology: IgM (+)

Rheumatology/ autoimmunity			
Sarcoidosis	–	–	Clinicopathologic diagnosis with noncaseating granulomas, hypercalcemia, ACE (high)
Rheumatoid arthritis	–	–	Clinical diagnosis, RF/anti-CCP (+), ESR/CRP (high).
Ulcerative colitis	–	–	Clinicopathologic diagnosis
Crohn's disease	–	–	Clinicopathologic diagnosis
Thymoma	–	–	Clinicopathologic diagnosis
Medications/toxins			
DRESS	Common medications include anticonvulsants, antibiotics, or allopurinol	–	Clinicopathologic diagnosis
Nicotine use	–	Both a monoclonal and polyclonal B-cell immunophenotype	Diagnosis of exclusion

(continued)

Table 5.2 (continued)

Category	Etiology	Phenotype and unique features	Laboratory tests
Others			
Physiologic stressors	Heart attacks, strokes, seizures, physical trauma, or pain	–	Diagnosis of exclusion
Hyperthyroidism	Thyroid nodule, Graves disease, thyroiditis, or exogenous thyroid hormone use	–	TSH (high or low) and free T4/total T3 (high)
Postsplenectomy	Postsplenectomy	–	–

ab antibody, *ACE* angiotensin-converting enzyme, *anti-CCP* anti-cyclic citrullinated peptide, *ATLL* adult T-cell leukemia/lymphoma, *ANA* antinuclear antibody, *CD* cluster of differentiation, *CMV* cytomegalovirus, *CRP* C-reactive protein, *DDx* differential diagnosis, *DIP* distal interphalangeal joint, *DRESS* drug rash with eosinophilia and systemic symptoms, *EBV* Epstein-Barr virus, *ESR* erythrocyte sedimentation rate, *HAV* hepatitis A virus, *HBV* hepatitis B virus, *HbsAg* hepatitis B surface antigen, *HCV* hepatitis C virus, *HHV-6* human herpesvirus 6, *HIV* human immunodeficiency virus, *HLH* hemophagocytic lymphohistiocytosis, *HTLV-1* human T-cell lymphotropic virus 1; *Ig* immunoglobulin, *ITP* immune thrombocytopenia, *MDS* myelodysplastic syndrome, *NK* natural killer, *PBS* peripheral blood smear, *PCR* polymerase chain reaction, *PNH* paroxysmal nocturnal hemoglobinuria, *PRCA* pure red cell aplasia, *RF* rheumatoid factor, *RNA* ribonucleic acid, *TCR* T-cell receptor, *T-LGL* T-cell large granular lymphocyte, *TSH* thyroid stimulating hormone, *VL* viral load, *VZV* varicella-zoster virus

among other disorders, can lead to an IM-like presentation. A positive monospot-heterophile antibody test is diagnostic of IM. EBV/CMV serology and HIV RNA/antibody analyses should be ordered for patients who are negative for heterophile antibody.

Expansion of T-/NK-LGLs can be associated with both reactive and malignant processes. It is important to exclude transiently increased T-/NK-LGLs secondary to viral infections or autoimmune disease with elevated antinuclear antibody and rheumatoid factor. T-/NK-LGL leukemia is usually associated with sustained elevation of LGLs, autoimmune diseases, unexplainable cytopenias, and splenomegaly. STAT-3 or STAT-5b gain-of-function mutations usually confirm diagnosis of T/NK-LGL leukemia [4].

HTLV-1 is a retrovirus endemic to southern Japan, the Caribbean, Central/South America, tropical Africa, and northern Iran. The majority of infected subjects are asymptomatic, but a minority of HTLV-1-infected patients show development of ATLL [5]. Therefore, positive HTLV-1 serology must be interpreted in the proper clinical context. "*Flower cells*" are frequently seen on the peripheral blood smear of both asymptomatic carriers and those with ATLL.

Relative lymphocytosis refers to the scenario in which the percentage of WBCs consisting of lymphocytes exceeds 40%, but with absolute lymphocyte count <5000 cells/uL.

Malignant Lymphocytosis

Diagnosing malignant lymphocytosis, though uncommon, is critical for treatment decision and requires a comprehensive clinical and laboratory investigation. The common clinical and diagnostic features for performing differential diagnosis are included in Table 5.3.

Table 5.3 The clinical, immunophenotypic, and diagnostic features of malignant lymphocytosis

Condition	Immunophenotype	Diagnosis/characteristics	Key cytogenetic/ Molecular findings
Mature B-cell neoplasms			
CLL	CD5+, CD10−, CD19+, CD20 dim+, CD23+, CD43+/−, sIg dim+, cyclin D1−	ALC ≥5 × 10^9/L for 3 months; associated with AIHA and hypogammaglobulinemia	
SLL	Same as CLL	ALC <5 × 10^9/L with LAD and/or splenomegaly	
MBL	CLL or non-CLL phenotype	Monoclonal B-cell count <5 × 10^9/L without meeting diagnostic criteria for CLL or SLL	
FL	CD5−, CD10+, CD19+, CD20+, CD23+/−, CD43−, BCL2+, BCL6+, cyclin D1−	Indolent course, waxing and waning LAD over time	t(14;18)::*BCL2-IgH**
MCL	CD5+, CD10−, CD19+, CD20 bright+, CD23−, CD43+, BCL6−, sIgM bright+, cyclin D1+	Both indolent and aggressive leukemic type variants	t(11;14)/ *CCDN1::IgH*
MZL	CD5−, CD10−, CD19+, CD20 bright+, CD23+/−, CD43+/−, sIgM bright+, cyclin D1−	Splenic MZL most likely to present with lymphocytosis	

HCL/HC-v	HCLc: CD5−, CD10−, CD11c+, CD20 bright+, CD22+, CD25+, CD103+, CD123+, cyclin D1+, annexin A1+ HCLv: CD25−, CD123−, annexin A1−	HCLc: Splenomegaly and monocytopenia HCLv: Severe leukocytosis with atypical lymphocytosis	*BRAF* V600E mutation
LPL/WM	CD5+/−. CD10−, CD19+, CD20+, CD22+, CD23−, CD25+, CD27+, CD103−, CD138−, sIgM+, FMC7+	IgM monoclonal protein and > 10% BM involvement of plasmacytoid lymphocytes; eccentric nucleus with clumped chromatin and paranuclear hof (clearing)	*MYD88* L265P mutation
Mature T-cell neoplasms			
SZ	CD2+, CD3+, CD4+, CD5+, CD7−, CD8−/(rarely +), CD26−, CD30+/−	Sezary syndrome; ≥1000/μL circulating Sezary cells OR ≥ 1000/μL CD4+/CD26− or CD4+/CD7− cells OR ≥ 40% CD4+/CD7− cells OR ≥ 30% CD4+/CD26− cells	
ATLL	CD2+, CD3 low+, CD4+, CD5+, CD8−/(rarely +), CD25+, CD26−, CD29+, CD45RO+, TCR αβ+, HLA-DR+	Positive HTLV-1 serology; endemic to southern Japan, the Caribbean, Central/South America, tropical Africa, and northern Iran	HTLV1/2 positive
T- or NK-LGLL	T-LGLs: CD3+, CD4− (rarely +), CD5 dim+/-, CD7 dim+/-, CD8+, CD16+, CD28−, CD45A+, CD56+/−, CD57+, CD62L−, TCRαβ+, TIA+, granzyme B+, or granzyme M+. NK-LGLLs: surface CD3-, Cd2+, CD7+, CD4-, CD8-/+, CD16+, CD56+, CD57-/+, TCR αβ−, TCRγδ−	Increased T-/NK-cell LGL clonal populations (generally >2000 cells/μL) for greater than 6 months in appropriate clinical context; less than 2000 but >=500 cells/μL could occur in certain clinical setting	*STAT3* mutations identified in 30–40% of cases

(continued)

Table 5.3 (continued)

Condition	Immunophenotype	Diagnosis/characteristics	Key cytogenetic/ Molecular findings
T-PLL	CD1a−, CD2+, CD3+, CD4+/−, CD5+, CD7+, CD8+/−, CD52+, TCR αβ+, TdT−	Diagnosis per minor/major TPLL-ISG criteria; usually clinically aggressive	Inv(14) or t(X;14)
Others			
ALL	B or T-cell markers along with markers of immaturity (TdT, CD10, CD34, CD123, HLA-DR) and aberrant myeloid expression (CD13, CD33); always MPO-unless mixed lymphoid/myeloid lineage	>20% lymphoblasts on bone marrow biopsy; can present critically ill with leukostasis, coagulopathy, and sepsis.	Ph+ (*BCR-ABL1* p190), Ph-like or Ph-
ANKL	CD2+, cCD3ε+, sCD3−, CD4−, CD7+, CD8+/−, CD11b +/−, CD16+, CD56+, CD57+/−, TCR αβ−, TCRγδ−, germline TCR and Ig, EBV-EBER+, CXCR1+, CCR5+; extranodal NKCL, see above but CD16−	Appropriate immunophenotype in a patient with an aggressive clinical course; can be associated with HLH	

*t(14;18) can be identified in some healthy individuals

ALC absolute lymphocyte count, *AIHA* autoimmune hemolytic anemia, *ALL* acute lymphoblastic leukemia, *ANKL* aggressive natural killer cell leukemia, *ATLL* adult T-cell leukemia/lymphoma, *BM* bone marrow, *CD* cluster of differentiation, *CLL* chronic lymphocytic leukemia, *CLPD-NK* chronic lymphoproliferative disorder of natural killer cells, *FL* follicular lymphoma, *HCLc* classic hairy cell leukemia, *HCLv* hairy cell leukemia variant, *Ig* immunoglobulin, *HLH* hemophagocytic lymphohistiocytosis, *HTLV-1* human T-cell lymphotropic virus 1, *LAD* lymphadenopathy, *LPL* lymphoplasmacytic lymphoma, *MBL* monoclonal B-cell lymphocytosis, *MCL* mantle cell lymphoma, *MZL* marginal zone lymphoma,, *PLL* prolymphocytic leukemia, *SLL* small lymphocytic lymphoma, *SZ* Sezary syndrome, *TdT* terminal deoxynucleotidyl transferase, *T-LGLL* T-cell large granular lymphocyte leukemia, *TPLL-ISG* T-prolymphocytic leukemia - International Study Grup, *WM* Waldenström macroglobulinemia

Table 5.4 The etiology and diagnostic features of common reactive lymphocytopenia

Category	Etiology
Infections	
	HIV, Hepatitis, Flu, COVID, tuberculosis, malaria, sepsis
Treatment-related	Cytoreduction (chemotherapy and/or radiation) Corticosteroid Certain antibiotics Hematopoietic stem cell transplant
Nutritional	Alcoholism Poor nutrition situation
Autoimmune disorder	SLE, Rheumatoid arthritis, Sjogren's syndrome
Inherited disorder	Ataxia-telangiectasia DiGeorge syndrome Common variable immunodeficiency SCID Wiskott-Aldrich syndrome
Hematologic malignancy associated	cHL AA Leukemia MDS

AA aplastic anemia, *cHL* classic Hodgkin lymphoma, *CMV* cytomegalovirus, *EBV* Epstein-Barr virus, *HIV* human immunodeficiency virus, *MDS* myelodysplastic neoplasms, *SLE* systemic lupus erythematosus, *SCID* Severe combined immunodeficiency

Lymphocytopenia

Differential diagnosis of lymphocytopenia usually depends on the underlying diseases [6]. The common etiology for lymphocytopenia is summarized in Table 5.4.

Prognosis

Benign lymphocytosis usually has a good clinical outcome with or without treatment. In contrast, malignant lymphocytosis is usually associated with worse outcomes; however, outcomes are also dependent on its disease nature, molecular profile, stage, and response to treatment. Lymphocytopenia patients have higher risk of infection. Outcome is also related to underlying condition and response to therapy.

Treatment

Treatment of reactive lymphocytosis depends upon etiology. Chemoradiation, immunotherapy, autologous hematopoietic stem cell transplant, or chimeric antigen receptor T-cell therapy are usually used for treatment of malignant lymphocytosis. For patients with mild lymphocytopenia without overt underlying disease, no treatment is needed as it may resolve on its own. Management of underlying diseases, e.g., HIV and SLE, leading to lymphocytopenia, will improve lymphocyte count. Severe depletion of B-cells with modern anti-CD19 or anti-CD20-directed immunotherapy can result in prolonged severe lymphocytopenia, hypogammaglobulinemia, and recurrent bacterial infections, which may need supplementation with IVIG. Several chemotherapy agents such as fludarabine, bendamustine, or anti-CD52 monoclonal antibodies can also lead to severe T cell lymphocytopenia, which will require antiviral antibiotic prophylaxis until T-cell recovery.

Promising Clinical Studies

There are a number of clinical trials and novel therapeutic strategies tailored for the variety of malignant lymphocytoses, which are beyond the scope of this book chapter.

Caveats

- Reactive lymphocytosis often results from infections, autoimmune diseases, adverse medication reactions, transplantation, endocrine disorders, smoking, and physical stressors.
- It is important to distinguish between reactive lymphocytosis and a neoplastic lymphocytosis. However, cytologic examination of a peripheral blood smear might not be helpful in certain settings. Flow cytometry should be ordered for all cases of unexplained, persistent lymphocytosis to assess for malignancy. Atypical circulating lymphocytes in HTLV1/2 carriers warrants clinical follow-up.
- Proliferations of T-cell large granular lymphocytes (LGLs) and natural killer (NK) cells can be natural phenomena among aging adults or may be related to an underlying medical condition. Persistent elevations of T-LGLs or NKs with associated cytopenias and splenomegaly should prompt consideration for a malignant hematologic process.
- Lymphocytopenia is usually a consequence of cytoreduction therapy or is associated with familial or acquired immunodeficiency.

Review Questions

Question 1.

38-year-old female who has a long history of SLE visited her primary care physician and was found to have splenomegaly on physical exam. CT scan imaging studies of chest, abdomen, and pelvis revealed spleen measuring 13 cm, normal size of liver, and no lymphadenopathy. CBC/Diff. test showed Hb of 11.2 g/dL, and WBC of 3.5×10^9/L. Absolute neutrophil count (ANC) was 1.0×10^9/L and absolute lymphocyte count (ALC) of 2.3×10^9/L. Peripheral blood smear reveals many mature lymphocytes with abundant cytoplasm and azurophilic granules. Flow cytometry performed on the peripheral blood revealed a population of T-cells (50% of gated lymphocytes), expressing CD3+, CD8+, CD5dim+, CD7+, CD57+, and TCR alpha-beta+. TCR gene beta was clonally rearranged per PCR study. Which of the following conditions is most probably associated with the patient's current clinical presentation?

A. Chronic lymphocytic leukemia
B. T-cell large granular lymphocytic (T-LGL) proliferation
C. Adult T cell leukemia/lymphoma
D. Felty's syndrome
E. EBV infection

Answer B. The patient has a history of autoimmune disorder that often accompanies T-cell expansion, especially T-LGL proliferation that may eventually progress into T-LGL leukemia. Flow cytometry test should be repeated in 6 months to confirm persistence of LGLs. Immunophenotype of lymphocytic population was of T cell lineage, thus the patient does not have B-CLL. The immunophenotype of ATLL is usually CD3+/CD4+/CD25+ which is different from immunophenotype of LGLs. Although viral infections such as EBV could result in reactive lymphocytosis, it is a transient process and usually does not result in persistent peripheral blood cytopenias. The patient did not demonstrate any typical symptoms of acute or chronic EBV infection. Felty's syndrome is associated with splenomegaly, neutropenia and rheumatoid arthritis.

Question 2.
A 70-years-old, otherwise healthy, male presented to his local hospital with cough, fever, and shortness of breath for approximately 7 days. Chest X-ray showed ill-defined opacities in both lungs. A laboratory study showed WBCs of 3.2×10^9/L, composed of 73% of neutrophils, 17% of monocytes, 8% lymphocytes, 1% eosinophils, and 0% basophils. Results of respiratory viral panel are pending. What would be the most probable cause of infection and lymphopenia?

A. Bacterial sepsis
B. CMV infection
C. Pulmonary embolism

D. Epstein-Barr virus infection
E. COVID19 infection

Answer: E. COVID19 infection can often be accompanied with lymphopenia. Infection leading to inflammatory cytokine storm (elevated TNF-alpha and IL-6, etc.) is likely a key factor behind the observed lymphopenia. EBV and CMV infections are often associated with infectious mononucleosis-like picture with reactive lymphocytosis. Pulmonary embolism usually does not manifest with characteristic symptoms of viral respiratory infection. Bacterial sepsis is often associated with neutrophilia.

References

1. Mims M. Lymphocytosis, lymphocytopenia, hypergammaglobulinemia, and hypogammaglobulinemia. In: Hoffman R, Benz EJ, Silberstein LE, Heslop HE, Weitz JI, Anastasi J, Salama ME, Abutalilb SA, editors. Elsevier; 2018. p. 682–90.
2. George T. Diagnostic approach to lymphocytosis. Hematologist. 2015;12:6.
3. Luzuriaga K, Sullivan JL. Infectious mononucleosis. N Engl J Med. 2010;362(21):1993–2000. https://doi.org/10.1056/NEJMcp1001116. PMID: 20505178.
4. Barilà G, Calabretto G, Teramo A, Vicenzetto C, Gasparini VR, Semenzato G, Zambello R. T cell large granular lymphocyte leukemia and chronic NK lymphocytosis. Best Pract Res Clin Haematol. 2019;32(3):207–16.
5. Durer C, Babiker HM. Adult T cell leukemia. Treasure Island: StatPearls Publishing; 2020; 2021 Jan–. PMID: 32644394.
6. Guo E, Zhang Z, Prajapati M, et al. Academic editor lymphopenia caused by virus infections and the mechanisms beyond. Viruses. 2021;13(9):1876. PMID: 34578457.

Primary and Secondary Immunodeficiency

6

Curtis Gravenmier and Mark Ballow

Introduction

Immunodeficiency refers to a defect in the immune system that leads to increased susceptibility to infection, heightened risk of malignancy, and/or impaired wound healing. It is frequently accompanied by autoimmunity or auto-inflammation caused by compromised immune regulation.

Primary immunodeficiencies (PID) may be idiopathic or arise from a specific genetic lesion as with common variable immunodeficiency, for which a monogenic cause has thus far been identified among up to 30% of patients. The International Union of Immunology Societies classifies PID based on the clinical phenotype (Table 6.1). To date, there are a total of 485 specific inborn errors of immunity and studying these has enabled profound advances in molecular medicine and human biology [1].

C. Gravenmier (✉)
Department of Hematopathology and Laboratory Medicine, Moffitt Cancer Center, Tampa, FL, USA

M. Ballow
Department of Pediatrics, Allergy and Immunology Division, University of South Florida at Johns Hopkins All Children's Hospital, St. Petersburg, FL, USA
e-mail: mballow@usf.edu

L. Sokol, L. Zhang (eds.), *Non-Neoplastic Hematologic Disorders*, https://doi.org/10.1007/978-3-031-62373-8_6

Table 6.1 IUIS Classification of human inborn errors of immunity (2022)

Main category	Subtypes	Examples
1. Immunodeficiencies affecting cellular and humoral immunity	a. Severe combined immunodeficiencies (CD3 T-cell lymphopenia) b. Combined immunodeficiencies less profound than SCID	JAK3 deficiency IL7R deficiency RAG1/2 deficiency
2. CID with associated or syndromic features	–	Wiskott-Aldrich syndrome Ataxia-telangiectasia Nijmegen breakage syndrome Bloom syndrome
3. Predominantly antibody deficiencies	a. Hypogammaglobulinemia b. Other antibody deficiencies	X-linked agammaglobulinemia Selective IgA deficiency
4. Diseases of immune dysregulation	a. HLH and EBV susceptibility b. Syndromes with autoimmunity	Familial HLH syndromes ALPS
5. Congenital defects of phagocyte number, function, or both	a. Neutropenia b. Functional phagocyte defects	Shwachman-Diamond syndrome CGD
6. Defects of intrinsic and innate immunity	a. Predisposition to viral infection b. Predisposition to bacterial, fungal, and parasitic infections	Congenital asplenia XIAP deficiency (*XLP2*) Mendelian susceptibility to mycobacterial disease
7. Auto-inflammatory disorders	–	Familial Mediterranean Fever Mevalonate kinase deficiency
8. Complement deficiencies	a. Disseminated Neisserial infections b. SLE-like syndrome with infection by encapsulated organisms c. Atypical hemolytic uremic syndrome	Terminal complement deficiencies (C6-C9) C1q deficiency Factor H deficiency

Table 6.1 (continued)

Main category	Subtypes	Examples
9. Bone marrow failure	–	FA, DKC
10. Phenocopies of PID	a. Associated with somatic mutations b. Associated with autoantibodies	ALPS-sFAS, RALD Pulmonary alveolar proteinosis

ALPS autoimmune lymphoproliferative syndrome, *ALPS-sFAS* ALPS with somatic FAS mutation, *CGD* chronic granulomatous disease, *CID* combined immunodeficiency, *DKC* dyskeratosis congenita, *EBV* Epstein-Barr virus, *FA* Fanconi anemia, *HLH* hemophagocytic lymphohistiocytosis, *IUIS* International Union of Immunology Societies, *PID* primary immunodeficiency, *RALD* RAS-associated autoimmune leukoproliferative disease, *SCID* severe combined immunodeficiency, *SLE* systemic lupus erythematosus

Individual PID are often very rare. However, in aggregate, PID occur at surprisingly high incidence and appear to be increasing with time.

Secondary immunodeficiencies (SID), by contrast, are acquired disorders which abound in the healthcare arena and are frequently overlooked even though many are iatrogenic. Both PID and SID often manifest with hematological abnormalities such as cytopenia or a lymphoproliferative disorder. In other respects, the clinical diversity of PID and SID is staggering. This chapter focuses on select PID and SID deemed of interest to hematology and oncology practice.

Pathogenesis

The pathogenesis of many PID and SID has been investigated. Tables 6.2 and 6.3 present several notable PID and SID and organize them by etiopathogenesis. Genes listed are the most affected; however, pathological variants of other genes may give rise to the same condition.

Table 6.2 Primary immunodeficiency [2–5]

Condition and mechanism	Key features
Combined immunodeficiency	
RAG1/2 deficiency *RAG1* or *RAG2* (AR) Failure of V(D)J recombination	B- and T-cell lymphocytopenia; NK cells preserved. Adverse reactions to live-attenuated vaccines. Immune cytopenias. Delayed diagnosis of combined immunodeficiency is increasingly attributed to hypomorphic RAG1/2 deficiency
Combined immunodeficiency with associated or syndromic features	
Wiskott-Aldrich syndrome *WAS* (XL) Disrupted actin remodeling	Microthrombocytopenia, eczema, immune cytopenias
Predominantly antibody deficiencies	
Activation-induced cytidine deaminase deficiency *AICDA* (AR or AD) Inability to perform antibody class switching and somatic hypermutation	Hyperimmunoglobulin M and lymphoid hyperplasia (e.g., enlarged tonsils and lymph nodes), immune cytopenias
Common variable immunodeficiency *NFKB1* (AD) B-cells fail to differentiate into plasma cells	Hypogammaglobulinemia, increased bacterial infections, immune cytopenias (especially ITP)
Diseases associated with EBV susceptibility	
X-linked lymphoproliferative disease *SH2DIA* (XL) Disrupted NK cell, cytotoxic T-cell, and antigen presenting cell interactions	Fulminant infectious mononucleosis or HLH triggered by EBV. Increased risk of extranodal B-cell lymphoma, often near ileocecal valve

Table 6.2 (continued)

Condition and mechanism	Key features
Familial HLH syndromes	
Chediak-Higashi syndrome *LYST* (AR) Disrupted intracellular vesicle trafficking	Granulocytes and large granular lymphocytes contain giant azurophilic granules. Recurrent bacterial infections and high susceptibility to EBV and HLH. Oculocutaneous albinism. Platelet storage pool disorder
Hermansky-Pudlak syndrome *HPS1* (AR) Disrupted intracellular vesicle trafficking	Variable neutropenia, oculocutaneous albinism, platelet storage pool disorder. Increased HLH risk, though much less frequent and milder than Chediak-Higashi syndrome
Syndromes with autoimmunity	
Autoimmune lymphoproliferative syndrome *TNFRSF6* or *FAS* (AD or AR) *Ineffective* Fas-mediated apoptosis of autoreactive lymphocytes	Lymphadenopathy, splenomegaly, severe immune cytopenias. Patients have a relatively high percentage of CD4-/CD8- T-cells in peripheral blood Importantly, ALPS can also arise from somatic gene variants, in which case it would be an acquired disorder
Congenital defects of phagocytes	
WHIM syndrome *CXCR4* (AD) Mature neutrophils are retained in bone marrow	Warts are HPV-related. Peripheral blood shows neutropenia and lymphopenia
Neutrophil elastase deficiency *ELA2* (AD) Abnormal elastase protein negatively impacts neutrophil lifespan	Severe congenital neutropenia. Note: Some *ELA2* variants cause intermittent or cyclic neutropenia. Bacterial and fungal skin, mucosal, or lung infections
Leukocyte adhesion deficiency (type I) *ITGB2* (AR) Neutrophils cannot adhere to endothelium or transmigrate into infected tissues	Peripheral blood neutrophilia. Skin and mucosal bacterial infection (without purulence). Severe periodontitis and tooth loss. Impaired wound healing. Delayed umbilical cord separation

(continued)

Table 6.2 (continued)

Condition and mechanism	Key features
Complement deficiency	
Factor H deficiency *CFH* (AR) Unchecked complement activation via the alternative pathway	Atypical hemolytic uremic syndrome, C3 glomerulopathy, recurrent meningococcal infections

AD autosomal dominant, *ALPS* autoimmune lymphoproliferative syndrome, *AR* autosomal recessive, *EBV* Epstein-Barr virus, *HLH* hemophagocytic lymphohistiocytosis, *HPV* human papillomavirus, *ITP* immune thrombocytopenia purpura, *NK* natural killer, *WHIM* warts, hypogammaglobulinemia, infections, myelokathexis, *XL* X-linked

Table 6.3 Secondary immunodeficiency [6, 7]

Condition and mechanism	Key features
Infections	
HIV Viral destruction of CD4+ T helper cells	Patients are rendered susceptible to numerous opportunistic pathogens when CD4+ T-cells drop below 200/μL
Medications	
Glucocorticoids Inhibition of pro-inflammatory gene expression programs	Lymphopenia and repressed cytokine production. Dose-dependent increased risk of serious bacterial infections and *Pneumocystis jirovecii* pneumonia
Methotrexate Inhibits dihydrofolate reductase and thymidylate synthetase, blocking both purine and thymidine syntheses	Low-dose MTX for rheumatological conditions is associated with modestly increased risk of infection. High-dose MTX for hematological malignancies may cause mucositis and myelosuppression leading to severe acute bacterial infection
Mycophenolate Inhibits inosine 5-monophosphate dehydrogenase and depletes guanosine	Increased susceptibility to a variety of viral, fungal, and bacterial infections but especially CMV and BK virus

Table 6.3 (continued)

Condition and mechanism	Key features
Tacrolimus Inhibits calcineurin, a phosphatase that initiates transcription of IL-2 after T-cell activation	Increased susceptibility to a variety of viral and bacterial infections, notably BK virus. Interestingly, calcineurin inhibitors have antifungal activity
Rituximab Anti-CD20 depletes B cells and impairs antibody response	Relatively high risk of HBV reactivation in affected patients. *Pneumocystis jirovecii* pneumonia and progressive multifocal leukoencephalopathy caused by JC virus may also be increased
Eculizumab Anti-C5 inhibits terminal complement activation	Increased risk of meningococcal infection
Alkylating chemotherapies Methylates guanine bases in DNA and may also generate interstrand crosslinks	Dose-related myelosuppression with infectious risk driven by neutropenia
Hematologic malignancies	
CLL/SLL and multiple myeloma Multifaceted suppression of antibody production and cellular immunity (TGF-β may play a key role)	Pneumonia caused by encapsulated bacteria is a major cause of mortality in both CLL and multiple myeloma. Herpes zoster reactivation is also increased
Syndromes	
VEXAS syndrome Somatic mutations of *UBA1*, an X-linked gene that encodes the E1 ubiquitin activating enzyme	The *UBA1* mutation is restricted to myeloid cells, which display vacuoles. Patients have inflammatory disease that is refractory to treatment and develop progressive cytopenias with high risk of MDS. Severe bacterial infections have been reported
Protein-losing states	
Nephrotic syndrome Urinary loss of serum immunoglobulins leading to hypogammaglobulinemia	Proteinuria, hypoalbuminemia, hyperlipidemia, lipiduria, and anasarca. Increased risk of infection, especially with encapsulated bacteria such as *Streptococcus pneumonia*

CLL/SLL chronic lymphocytic leukemia/small lymphocytic lymphoma, *CMV* cytomegalovirus, *HBV* hepatitis B virus, *HIV* human immunodeficiency virus, *MDS* myelodysplastic syndrome, *MTX* methotrexate, *VEXAS* vacuoles, E1 enzyme, X-linked, autoinflammatory, somatic

Diagnosis

A thorough history and physical examination are critical for diagnosis. Laboratory assessment of the immune system is complex. A good launching point is to obtain a complete blood count with differential, peripheral blood smear, comprehensive metabolic profile, urinalysis, and serum immunoglobulin concentrations (IgG, IgA, IgM, and IgE). If an antibody defect is suspected, it may be useful to measure specific antibody levels after booster vaccination. Hypogammaglobulinemia with a deficient vaccine response and no obvious SID should prompt concern for PID. Flow cytometry can be used to quantitate lymphocyte subsets and demonstrate functional or nonfunctional protein expression patterns. Complement deficiencies are screened for using CH50 (total hemolytic complement), AH50 (alternative hemolytic complement), and mannose-binding lectin tests, which measure the functional concentrations of the classical, alternative, and lectin complement pathways, respectively. Other important tests assess T-cell proliferation in response to mitogens, natural killer cell function, neutrophil function, and cytokine release. Bone marrow biopsy should be performed for cases with unexplained cytopenia or clinical suspicion for a concomitant hematologic malignancy. Finally, the definitive diagnosis of many PID requires next-generation sequencing. Targeted next-generation sequencing panels geared toward the clinical presentation are typically performed first; then, if negative, whole-exome sequencing may be pursued [8].

Differential Diagnosis

PID are uncommon, remarkably heterogeneous, and difficult to diagnose without specialized knowledge and laboratory resources. A history of intravenous antibiotics for infection, failure to thrive, or a family history of immunodeficiency suggests PID. Other features concerning for PID include nonhealing wounds, unexplained or immune cytopenia, persistent nonneoplastic lymphadenopathy or splenomegaly, hemophagocytic lymphohistiocytosis, and early-onset lymphoma.

The differential diagnosis of PID is chiefly guided by two things: (1) the clinical phenotype and (2) which pathogens are responsible for recurrent infection. The diagnosis is then pinpointed using molecular genetics. The International Union of Immunological Societies updated its classification of inborn errors of immunity in 2022 and divided PID into nine broad clinical phenotypes (Table 6.1) [1]. Each phenotype can be traced to an etiologically related group of gene mutations. The pathogen(s) responsible for recurrent infection also provide diagnostic clues. For instance, recurrent sinopulmonary infections with encapsulated bacteria (e.g., *Streptococcus pneumoniae* or *Haemophilus influenzae*) and recurrent enteroviral meningitis are associated with antibody deficiency. *Pneumocystis jirovecii* pneumonia, persistent oral or cutaneous candidiasis, gastrointestinal cytomegalovirus (CMV), and atypical mycobacterial infections are associated with T-cell deficiency. Recurrent infections with catalase-positive bacteria (e.g., *Staphylococcus aureus*) may indicate phagocyte dysfunction, while recurrent or invasive *Neisseria meningitidis* occurs with terminal complement deficiency.

SID often results from medications, diabetes mellitus, HIV, protein-losing states (nephrotic syndrome, severe burns, malnutrition, enteropathy), or malignancy. An underlying condition should be sought in cases of recurrent infection, especially among adults. It is also important to consider nonimmunological reasons for recurrent infection. For example, abnormal anatomy, such as bronchial obstruction by tumor, can lead to recurrent pneumonia, despite there being no immunological defect.

Prognosis

The prognosis of an immunodeficiency depends on the specific diagnosis and is variable. In general, newborn screening for severe combined immunodeficiencies using T-cell excision circles allows timely recognition and treatment of many patients, such that long-term survival after hematopoietic stem cell transplant (HSCT) exceeds 90% for patients with a sibling match. In the past, these conditions were uniformly fatal.

Treatment

Treatment of PID is based on a practice parameter published jointly by the American Academy of Allergy, Asthma, and Immunology and the American College of Allergy, Asthma, and Immunology [8]. For SID, it is important to identify and address the process responsible for acquired immunodeficiency.

Prophylactic Antimicrobial Therapy

Once immunodeficiency is established, management begins with efforts to prevent serious infection. This includes prophylactic antimicrobial therapy with agents such as trimethoprim-sulfamethoxazole (bacteria, *Pneumocystis jirovecii*); azithromycin (bacteria, *Mycoplasma* spp.); triazole antifungals; acyclovir (herpes simplex virus, varicella zoster virus); and/or valganciclovir (CMV), depending on the type of PID or SID. Vaccinations should be reviewed and appropriately updated to cover problematic organisms. For example, adults with sickle cell disease benefit from vaccines against encapsulated bacteria, including *Haemophilus influenzae* type b; *Streptococcus pneumoniae*; and *Neisseria meningitidis* serogroups A, C, W, and Y, as well as serogroup B. In cases of severely impaired T-cell function, blood products must be irradiated to prevent transfusion-associated graft-vs-host disease and leukoreduced to prevent CMV transmission. Live-attenuated vaccines are contraindicated in this group.

Immunoglobulin Therapy

Lifelong IgG replacement is the mainstay of treatment for patients with primary antibody deficiency and a significant component of therapy for patients with combined immunodeficiency. Some patients with secondary antibody deficiency also benefit. An initial dose of 400 to 600 mg/kg/month can be administered intravenously or subcutaneously to obtain a trough level between 600 and 800 mg/dL after 3 months; higher concentrations are desirable in some instances. The recommended intravenous infusion rate is 0.5 to 1 mg/kg/min and can be gradually increased to 8 mg/kg/min after several hours (refer to the instructions for each product). Subcutaneous IgG may be administered at home using a similar dose that is divided into several infusions per week, or weekly/biweekly injections, and offers improved quality of life. Intravenous administration is preferred for higher doses and situations where subcutaneous administration proves difficult (e.g., noncompliance, bleeding diathesis). Once a therapeutic steady state is achieved, the IgG trough, complete blood count, and liver/renal function tests should be measured 1 to 2 times annually.

Approximately 1/3 of patients developed mild systemic reactions (e.g., headache, chills, myalgia, tachycardia) after intravenous IgG within 72 hours. Severe adverse events are rare, but include anaphylaxis, aseptic meningitis, renal tubular injury, thromboembolic events, and hemolysis that should be managed accordingly. Anaphylaxis may occur among patients who lack IgA. It is recommended to use a product with less than 25 μg/mL IgA or to prescribe subcutaneous immunoglobulin for these individuals. Thromboembolic events may occur because of activated factor XI in the replacement product. For patients at high risk for thrombosis, it is advisable to consider a slower infusion rate, prophylaxis with aspirin or low molecular-weight heparin, and/or prehydration [9].

HSCT

Many types of severe combined immunodeficiency (SCID) and primary bone marrow failure are ultimately managed using HSCT. The ideal donor is a human leukocyte antigen–identical sibling. A haploidentical parent or matched-unrelated donor can be used with modestly decreased survival and higher risk of graft-vs-host disease. Of note, only a few types of SCID, including hypomorphic RAG1/2 deficiency, are capable of graft rejection and require bone marrow conditioning. Pretransplant conditioning is always required in non-SCID immunodeficiency. However, radiation and genotoxic drugs are avoided to the extent possible among patients with DNA-repair defects. Severe congenital neutropenia frequently responds to granulocyte colony-stimulating factor therapy and may not need transplantation.

Promising Clinical Studies

"JSP191 Antibody Targeting Conditioning in SCID Patients" is a phase 1/2 study to evaluate the safety and efficacy of anti-CD117 antibodies as the sole conditioning agent for patients with SCID undergoing bone marrow transplant [10].

Caveats

- A comprehensive clinical investigation and laboratory testing is needed for diagnosis and subclassification of PID or SID.
- It is necessary to obtain baseline immunoglobulin levels and pertinent serological tests before immunoglobulin replacement since therapy will invalidate these assays.
- Always consider autoimmune lymphoproliferative syndrome among patients with Evans syndrome (autoimmune destruction of at least two hematologic cell types). The prevalence of autoimmune lymphoproliferative syndrome among children with Evans syndrome nears 50%.
- Patients with PID are generally at high risk for developing malignancy or autoimmune disease and should be closely followed by a specialist.

Review Questions

1. What is the most frequent hematological manifestation of common variable immunodeficiency?

A. Immune thrombocytopenia
B. Autoimmune hemolytic anemia
C. Autoimmune neutropenia
D. Lymphocytosis

Answer: A. Immune thrombocytopenia is the most common clinical presentation for patients who have common variable immunodeficiency.

2. A young child with history of recurrent fungal infections presents with fever and malaise. Testing reveals *Aspergillus* lung infection. A flow cytometric dihydrorhodamine (DHR) respiratory burst assay shows no significant change in DHR fluorescence after neutrophil activation, and a nitroblue tetrazolium (NBT) test results in a yellow color. What is the most likely diagnosis?

A. Leukocyte adhesion deficiency
B. Neutrophil elastase deficiency
C. Chronic granulomatous disease (CGD)
D. Myeloperoxidase deficiency

Answer: C. Normally, the white blood cells turn blue when NBT is added. For the patients who have CGD, the sample does not change color when NBT is added because their white blood cells lack the substance needed to kill bacteria. No fluorescence changes in DHR respiratory burst assay after neutrophil activation also supports the diagnosis of CGD.

References

1. Bousfiha A, Moundir A, Tangye SG, et al. The 2022 update of IUIS phenotypical classification for human inborn errors of immunity. J Clin Immunol. 2022;42(7):1508–20.
2. Cunningham-Rundles C, Ponda PP. Molecular defects in T-and B-cell primary immunodeficiency diseases. Nat Rev Immunol. 2005;5(11):880–92.

3. Spoor J, Farajifard H, Rezaei N. Congenital neutropenia, and primary immunodeficiency diseases. Crit Rev Oncol Hematol. 2019;133:149–62.
4. Hanna S, Etzioni A. Leukocyte adhesion deficiencies. Ann NY Acad Sci. 2012;1250(1):50–5.
5. Wen L, Atkinson JP, Giclas PC. Clinical and laboratory evaluation of complement deficiency. J Allergy Clin Immunol. 2004;113(4):585–93.
6. Patel SY, Carbone J, Jolles S. The expanding field of secondary antibody deficiency: causes, diagnosis, and management. Front Immunol. 2019;10:33.
7. Allison AC. Immunosuppressive drugs: the first 50 years and a glance forward. Immunopharmacology. 2000;47(2–3):63–83.
8. Bonilla FA, Khan DA, Ballas ZK, et al. Practice parameter for the diagnosis and management of primary immunodeficiency. J Allergy Clin Immunol. 2015;136(5):1186–205.
9. Sriaroon P, Ballow M. Immunoglobulin replacement therapy for primary immunodeficiency. Immunol Allergy Clin North Am. 2015;35(4):713–30.
10. Agarwal R, Dvorak CC, Kwon HS, et al. Non-genotoxic anti-CD117 antibody conditioning results in successful hematopoietic stem cell engraftment in patients with severe combined immunodeficiency. Blood. 2019;134:800.

Benign Histiocytic and Dendritic Cell Disorders

7

Aditi Saha, Ling Zhang, and Lubomir Sokol

Introduction

Histiocytes and dendritic cells (DCs) play critical roles in tissue homeostasis and immunity. DCs are derivative of the hematopoietic stem cell lineage, whereas *histiocyte* is a morphological term that is used to delineate tissue macrophages and sometimes encompasses both macrophages and DCs. Morphologically, we can easily distinguish between DCs (stellate in shape, with numerous cytoplastic projections) and macrophages (large, containing abundant foamy cytoplasm, with engulfed dusty granules). Mature DCs appear to have a larger surface area than the immature forms because of their longer cytoplasmic projections.

DCs and macrophages have separate functions. The primary function of DCs is antigen presentation, whereas macrophages eliminate foreign bodies and pathogens and perform phagocyto-

A. Saha
Department of Internal Medicine, USF Health Morsani College of Medicine, University of South Florida, Tampa, FL, USA

L. Zhang
Department of Hematopathology, H. Lee Moffitt Cancer Center and Research Institute, Tampa, FL, USA

L. Sokol (✉)
Department of Malignant Hematology, H. Lee Moffitt Cancer Center and Research Institute, Tampa, FL, USA
e-mail: Lubomir.Sokol@moffitt.org

L. Sokol, L. Zhang (eds.), *Non-Neoplastic Hematologic Disorders*,
https://doi.org/10.1007/978-3-031-62373-8_7

sis. Reactive histiocytic or dendritic proliferation is often noted in response to a variety of antigen stimulations, especially in the lymph nodes, and is much more common than malignant proliferation. In this chapter, we will review common benign histiocytic and DC disorders, with a focus on diagnosis and treatment recommendations for hemophagocytic lymphohistiocytosis (HLH).

Pathogenesis

Reactive proliferation of histiocytes and dendritic cells is secondary to a variety of antigen stimulation triggering release of cytokines, such as granulocyte-macrophage colony-stimulating factor (GM-CSF), interleukin 3 and 4, and others. Activated histiocytes further differentiate into subtypes or present antigens to T-cells and stimulate B-cells in the lymph nodes, the spleen, and other lymphoid tissues, where DCs interact with T-cells and lead to antigen-specific T-cell responses. DC signaling via CD40L, IL-12, TNFR, NF-κB, and other proteins is complex but crucial for immune capacity. Clonal expansion may happen with long-standing reactive processes. An acquired *BRAF*-V600E mutation and mutations in MAPK pathway have been proven to be important for neoplastic evolution.

Diagnosis

Because of their differing underlying mechanisms, different benign histiocytic disorders show unique natural histories, histomorphologies, and clinical outcomes. Clinical courses can range from indolent to life-threatening, such as with HLH, which require aggressive treatment strategies. In Table 7.1, we list several representative histiocytic and DC disorders and summarize their clinical presentations, associated disorders, and diagnoses. Castleman disease and storage disorders are discussed in other chapters of this book.

Benign histiocytic/DC disorders could be asymptomatic and identified incidentally or manifest with lymphadenopathy. Their proliferation is often associated with infections, autoimmune diseases, or neoplasms. A skin or lymph node (LN) biopsy is necessary for micromorphological assessment, along with ancillary tests. CD163, CD68, and CD4 markers are useful for identi-

Table 7.1 List of benign histiocytic disorders with their clinical presentations and diagnoses [1]

Disorder	Clinical presentation and associated diseases	Diagnosis
Sinus histiocytosis	Young adults usually present with massive LAD; associated with autoimmune disorders	LN biopsy shows variable number of normal-appearing histiocytes, CD68 (+), cytokeratin (−), S100 (−), and mucin (−) stains
Whipple disease	Common in middle-aged population. Presents with fever, abdominal pain, diarrhea, weight loss, LAD, and arthralgia; associated with *Tropheryma whipplei*	Duodenal or proximal small bowel biopsy shows increased macrophages; intracellular bacteria are PAS-positive; Diagnosis is confirmed by PCR for *T. whipplei*
Reactive histiocytosis following prosthetic arthroplasty	Presents with arthralgia and regional LAD	PAS-positive cytoplasmic granules with small particles of foreign bodies can be seen in cells; presence of foreign bodies with iron, cobalt chromium, titanium, or polyethylene segments can be confirmed with energy-dispersive x-ray microanalysis and plasma mass spectrometry, if needed
Silicone LAD	Associated with silicone-containing medical implants; presents with regional LAD	LN biopsy shows histiocytes with non-polarizing silicone particles inside vacuoles, confirmed by energy-dispersive x-ray, confocal laser Raman microprobe spectroscopy, or Fourier transform infrared spectroscopy, if needed
Crystal storing histiocytosis	Presents with regional LAD; associated with B-cell LPD, plasma cell neoplasms, autoimmune disorders, and drugs e.g., clofazimine	LN biopsy shows histiocytes with cytoplasmic crystals

(continued)

Table 7.1 (continued)

Disorder	Clinical presentation and associated diseases	Diagnosis
Dermatopathic LAD	Localized or generalized LAD; associated with certain skin disorders, including psoriasis, eczema, exfoliative dermatitis, neurodermatitis, and MF	LN biopsy shows paracortical expansion with interdigitating DCs (S100+) and LCs (S100+, CD1a+, Langerin+). Flow cytometry or PCR shows involvement with T-cell lymphoma if history is positive for CTCL/MF
Plasmacytoid dendritic cell proliferation	Presents with LAD; associated with Castleman disease, histiocytic necrotizing disease, granulomatous adenitis, CMML, AML, and MDS	LN biopsy reveals pDCs positive for CD4, TCL1, TCF4, BDCA2/CD303, and CD123
Langerhans cell hyperplasia	Associated with mycosis fungoides; presents with skin manifestation or adjacent LAD only	CD1a-, S100-, Langerin-positive cells

AML acute myeloid leukemia, *CMML* chronic myelomonocytic leukemia, *MF* Mycosis Fungoides, *DCs* dendritic cells, *LAD* lymphadenopathy, *LC* Langerhans cells, *LN* lymph node, *LPD* lymphoproliferative disorder, *MDS* myelodysplastic neoplasms, *PAS* Periodic acid–Schiff, *pDCs* plasmacytoid dendritic cells, *PCR* polymerase chain reaction

fication of histiocytes, and CD123, CD4, TCL1, BDCA2/CD303, and TCF4 markers can identify plasmacytoid DCs. Molecular studies, such as targeted mutation panels, are useful to assess underlying or associated neoplasms.

Differential Diagnoses

It is critical to differentiate reactive histiocytosis or DC proliferation from their malignant counterparts. Several histiocytic and dendric lesions previously considered reactive are now recognized as clonal processes based on their molecular fingerprinting, such as Rosai-Dorfman disease. Table 7.2 reviews several common malignancies that could lead to diagnostic dilemmas.

Table 7.2 Malignant counterparts of benign histiocytic/dendritic cell disorders

Disease	Clinical presentation	Diagnosis	Treatment
LCH/ Langerhans cell sarcoma	Usually presents with skin lesions, lytic bone lesions, or lymphadenopathy; may involve lung, CNS, or pituitary gland	Biopsy with IHC stains positive for CD1a and CD207 (langerin); may be positive for S100. Cyclin D1/BCL1 positivity distinguishes neoplastic processes from reactive processes. Around 40% of patients have *BRAF* V600E mutation	*For BRAF V600E-positive patients*: vemurafenib/dabrafenib *For MAP kinase pathway mutation-positive patients*: cobimetinib/trametinib *For patients without specific mutations*: cytarabine, cladribine, or combination with methotrexate
Indeterminate DC tumor	Skin involvement, rarely with organ or LN involvement	Biopsy with IHC stains positive for S100, CD1a, and CD68; but negative for Langerin, distinguishing it from LCH. CD163, CD21, CD23, CD30, and MPO stains are negative.	Surgical excision of isolated lesions; psoralen; ultraviolet A therapy
Interdigitating DC sarcoma	Common in adult men; presents with painless localized LAD; most common extranodal sites are liver, lung, spleen, BM, and GI tract	Biopsy with IHC stains positive for S-100, vimentin, HLA-DR, and weak variable expression of CD68; negative for CD1a and langerin	*For localized disease*: surgery or radiation *For metastatic disease*: combination chemotherapy regimen like CHOP/ABVD/ICE
Juvenile xanthogranuloma	More common in infants and young children; most commonly presents with cutaneous lesions; rarely involves oral cavity and orbit	Biopsy with IHC stains positive for CD68, XIIIa, vimentin, and CD4; negative for CD1a and S-100	*For localized skin lesions*: surgical excision *For non-cutaneous disease*: chemotherapy/immunotherapy

(continued)

Table 7.2 (continued)

Disease	Clinical presentation	Diagnosis	Treatment
ECD	Most commonly involves long bones (symmetrical); can involve orbits, CNS, lung, and vasculature	Biopsy shows foamy histiocytes giant cells. IHC stains positive for CD68, CD163, factor XIIIa; negative for CD1a and Langerin. Around 50% of patients have *BRAF* V600E mutation	*For BRAF V600E-positive patients*: vemurafenib/dabrafenib *For MAP kinase pathway–mutation-positive patients*: cobimetinib/trametinib *For patients without specific mutations*: cladribine or pegylated interferon alpha. Targeted therapy can be used for specific mutations like *ALK* fusions, CSF1R, etc.
RDD	Presents with LAD; most common extranodal involved sites are skin, soft tissue, upper respiratory tract, and bone	Neoplastic cells positive for S100, CD68, CD163, OCT2, and Cyclin D1/BCL1; negative for CD1a and Langerin. NGS can show MAPK pathway mutation(s)	*For MAP kinase pathway–mutation-positive patients*: cobimetinib/trametinib *For patients with no specific mutation*: cladribine/cytarabine/methotrexate Targeted therapy can be used for specific mutations like *ALK* fusions, CSF1R, etc.
ALK-positive histiocytosis	Common in infants and young children; involves liver, lung, skin, bone marrow, spleen, or kidney	Neoplastic cells positive for ALK, CD68, CD163, and variable S100; negative for CD1a, Langerin, and *BRAF* V600E. NGS/Genomic study may show *KIF5B::ALK* gene fusion or *COL1A2::ALK* fusion. Other ALK partners: *CLTC, TPM3, TFG, EML4, DCTN1*, and *TRIM33*.	ALK inhibitors, including crizotinib

Histiocytic sarcoma	Adults present with unifocal or multifocal extranodal site involvement, such as GI tract, skin, and soft tissue	HS cells positive for CD68, lysozymes, PU1, CD31, CD4, and CD163; negative for specific T-cell, B-cell, Langerhans cell, or myeloid cell markers	*For patients with localized disease*: surgery or radiation *For patients with multifocal disease*: Combination chemotherapy regimen like CHOP/ABVD/ICE
MPDCP	Associated with myeloid neoplasms, such as AML, CMML, or MDS; presenting symptoms are related to underlying associated disorders	MPDCP cells are positive for CD123, HLA-DR, CD4, BDCA2/CD303, and CD304/neuropilin-1, CD2AP, SPIB; usually negative for CD56, CD34, CD117, and TdT but aberrant expression of CD34, CD56 and TdT could occur. NGS may detect *RUNX1* mutation in AML or mutations involving RAS pathway in CMML patients	Treatment for associated myeloid disease
BDPCN	Adults present with skin lesions; may be associated with cytopenia, LAD or splenomegaly	BPDCN cells are positive for CD4, CD56, CD123, BDCA2/CD303, TCF4, TCL1, CD2AP, and SPIB; negative for CD19, CD20, CD79a, CD3, CD5, CD117, lysozyme, CD13, and CD16	Anti-CD123 antibody/tagraxofusp, combination chemotherapy

LCH Langerhans cell histiocytosis, ABVD adriamycin, bleomycin, vinblastine, dacarbazine, *ALK* anaplastic lymphoma kinase, *AML* acute myeloid leukemia, *BM* bone marrow, *BPDCN* blastic plasmacytoid dendritic cell neoplasm, *CHOP* cyclophosphamide, doxorubicin, vincristine, prednisone, *CMML* Chronic myelomonocytic leukemia, *CNS* central nervous system, *DC* dendritic cell, *ECD* Erdheim-Chester disease, *RDD* Rosai-Dorfman disease, *HS* histiocytic sarcoma, *GI* gastrointestinal, *ICE* ifosfamide, carboplatin, and etoposide, *IHC* immunohistochemistry, *LAD* lymphadenopathy, *MDS* Myelodysplastic syndrome, *MPDCP* mature plasmacytoid dendritic cell proliferation, *RDD* Rosai-Dorfman disease

Treatment

No treatment is needed for most benign histiocytic or dendritic cell proliferation besides HLH, which is an emergent issue and is discussed in detail later in the chapter. Treatment for the associated disorders might be necessary in accordance with the underlying disorder's treatment guidelines.

Prognosis

Benign histiocytic/dendritic proliferations, beside HLH, have favorable clinical outcomes.

Caveats

1. Reactive histiocytosis or DC proliferation is more common than their neoplastic counterparts; however, it is critical to differentiate between benign and neoplastic histiocytosis and DC neoplasms.
2. Recent studies have shown clonal evidence for some histiocytic or dendritic cell proliferations that were previously considered benign, such as Rosai-Dorfman disease or Erdheim-Chester disease
3. NGS of targeted *BRAF*/*MAPK* pathway genes has been utilized for differential diagnosis of benign vs clonal histiocytic and DC proliferations.
4. Uniform expression of *CCND1* is more commonly associated with malignant histiocytosis than benign or reactive histiocytic and DC proliferations.

Hemophagocytic Lymphohistiocytosis

Introduction

Hemophagocytic lymphohistiocytosis (HLH) is a fatal disorder characterized by uncontrolled activation of the immune system, resulting in excessive production of cytokines and pathological inflammation. It was first recognized in children; HLH is rare in adults, but an increasing incidence rate has been noted. About 40% of total HLH cases are observed in adults, and for this population, the median age of diagnosis is 49 years.

HLH may be primary (familial) or secondary (acquired). Familial HLH predominates in children and young adults. It is postulated that genetic defects in cytotoxic T lymphocytes and natural killer (NK) cells lead to abnormal activation and persistence of the inflammatory response. The most common mutations are in *PRF1* (perforin), *UNC13D* (Munc 13-4), *STX11* (Syntaxin 11), and *STXBP2* (Munc 18-2). Familial HLH is also associated with Griscelli syndrome, Chediak-Higashi syndrome, Hermansky-Pudlak syndrome, and X-linked lymphoproliferative disorder.

Acquired HLH more often occurs in adults secondary to infection, malignancy, or an autoimmune disorder. Epstein-Barr virus (EBV), cytomegalovirus (CMV), human immunodeficiency virus (HIV), mycobacterial infection, *Rickettsia* infection, leishmaniasis histoplasmosis, and SARS CoV-2 virus are the most common infections triggering HLH. Extranodal NK/T-cell lymphoma, primary cutaneous gamma/delta T-cell lymphoma, and subacutaneous panniculitis-like T-cell lymphoma have well-known associations with HLH. HLH may also occur after stem cell transplantation. When HLH is associated with autoimmune diseases, it is referred to as *macrophage activation syndrome* (MAS). Fever, cytopenias, and organomegaly are the most common presentations of HLH. Laboratory findings include high ferritin, high triglycerides (TG), low fibrinogen, and elevated soluble interleukin-2 receptor alpha (sIL-2R) levels.

Diagnosis

Diagnosis of HLH depends on clinical, laboratory, molecular, and pathological findings. The HLH-2004 clinical trial enrollment criteria were eventually adopted as the diagnostic criteria for HLH (Table 7.3). Fever is the most common presenting symptom. Diagnostic evaluation includes laboratory assessment with

Table 7.3 Diagnostic criteria for HLH

1. A molecular diagnosis consistent with HLH
OR
2. Five out of eight following criteria fulfilled:
A. Fever
B. Splenomegaly
C. Cytopenia affecting at least two of three hematopoietic lineages
Hemoglobin <9 g/dL
Platelet $<1.0 \times 10^{11}$/L
Neutrophil $<1 \times 10^{3}$/mL
D. Hypertriglyceridemia (fasting ≥265 mg/dL) and/or hypofibrinogenemia (≤150 mg/dL)
E. Low or absent NK cell activity
F. Ferritin ≥500 mcg/mL
G. Elevated soluble CD25 (soluble IL-2 receptor alpha) of ≥2400 U/mL
H. Hemophagocytosis in bone marrow, spleen, liver, or lymph node

HLH hemophagocytic lymphohistiocytosis, *IL-2* interleukin 2, *NK* natural killer cells

complete blood count (CBC) with differential, serum ferritin, fibrinogen, lipid panel, complete metabolic panel (CMP), lactate dehydrogenase (LDH), and bone marrow biopsy. MRI of the brain and lumbar puncture are recommended if CNS involvement is suspected. The bone marrow aspirate usually reveals hemophagocytosis (phagocytosis of hematopoietic cells by activated macrophages), though this alone is not sufficient to establish a diagnosis of HLH. The probability of HLH can be predicted using the H-Score [2]. A score of ≤90 correlates with low probability (<1%) of HLH, and a score ≥ 250 correlates with high probability (>99%). Patients considered as having high clinical suspicion for HLH should be evaluated promptly, as it can be fatal if untreated.

Treatment

The main objective in treating HLH is to manage inflammation and address the underlying condition. Familial HLH is commonly treated with hematopoietic stem cell transplant, whereas acquired HLH is treated by mitigating the underlying condition. There are two therapeutic protocols for HLH: HLH-94 and HLH-2004.

Both protocols are derived from pediatric clinical trial data and involve a combination of medications, including steroids, etoposide, cyclosporin, intrathecal methotrexate, and intravenous immunoglobulin. The HLH-94 protocol (Fig. 7.1) includes gradually tapering doses of dexamethasone and etoposide, with hematopoietic stem cell transplant as a subsequent treatment option for refractory cases [3]. The HLH-2004 protocol initiates cyclosporina A earlier than HLH-94 and includes regular cerebrospinal fluid analysis and a corticosteroid with intrathecal therapy [4]. In adults, treatment is based on expert opinion and retrospective studies, with additional medications, such as rituximab and IL-1– and IL-6–receptor inhibitors, used in conjunction with the above agents. Rituximab is particularly useful for treating EBV-associated HLH. Treatment algorithm for HLH is summarized as below (Fig. 7.2).

There are few treatment options available for relapsed or refractory HLH. However, emapalumab, a monoclonal immunoglobulin G1 antibody that targets interferon gamma, was approved by the FDA in 2018 as a targeted therapy for primary HLH in patients with refractory, recurrent, or progressive disease or for those who are intolerant to conventional HLH treatment protocol.

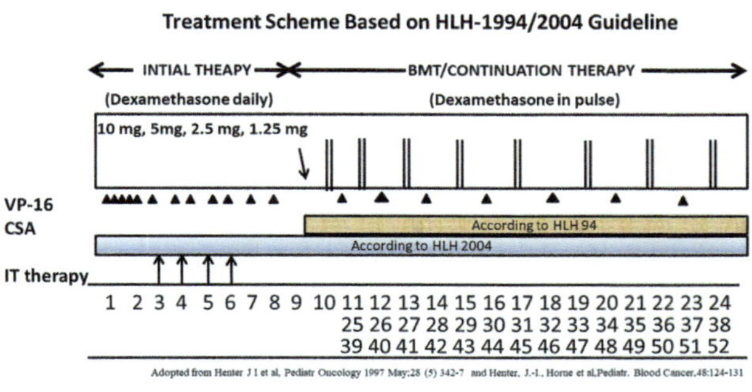

Fig. 7.1 Treatment scheme based on HLH-94 protocol. BMT bone marrow transplant, HLH hemophagocytic lymphohistiocytosis, IT MTX intrathecal methotrexate, VP-16 etoposide, CSA cyclosporin A

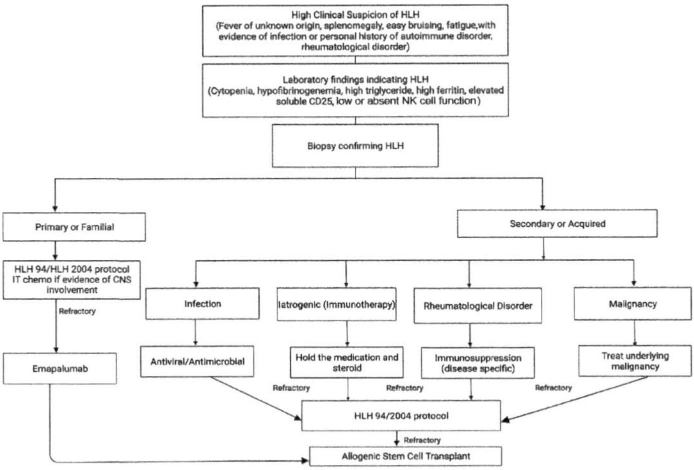

Abbreviations: CNS, central nervous system; HLH, hemophagocytic lymphohistiocytosis; IT, intrathecal; NK, natural killer.

Fig. 7.2 Treatment algorithm for HLH. CNS central nervous system, HLH hemophagocytic lymphohistiocytosis, IT intrathecal, NK natural killer

Prognosis

HLH is a life-threatening disorder with a mortality rate of 66%. Increasing age, male sex, low platelet count, organomegaly, disseminated intravascular coagulation, active EBV infection, ferritin levels >50,000 ng/mL, hypoalbuminemia, and multiorgan failure are considered poor prognostic factors.

Promising Clinical Studies

Clinical trials for HLH are limited because of the rarity of the disease. One ongoing clinical trial, NCT02385110, is investigating the addition of tocilizumab and alemtuzumab (an anti-CD52 monoclonal antibody) to standard induction chemotherapy to reduce treatment-induced cytopenia. Another ongoing phase 2 clinical trial, NCT02400463, is examining the utility of ruxolitinib, an oral JAK1/2 inhibitor. An ongoing phase 3 trial,

NCT04084626, is evaluating the efficacy of anti–PD-1 antibodies and lenalidomide for EBV-associated HLH.

Board Questions

1. Which of the following is the most specific marker to follow severity and progression of HLH?

   a. Ferritin
   b. Fibrinogen
   c. Soluble CD25
   d. Function of NK cells
   e. Cytopenia

   Answer: c. Soluble CD25 is considered the most specific marker predicting the prognosis of HLH.

2. A 55-year-old male with a history of deceased donor renal *transplantation* 2 years ago is admitted with a high-grade fever for 10 days. Posttransplant patient was on tacrolimus, mycophenolic acid, and prednisone. On admission, he has temperature of 102 °F. Laboratory evaluation revealed a white blood cell (WBC) count of 2.1×10^9/L, hemoglobin (Hb) level of 9 g/dL, platelet count of 1.97×10^{11}/L, erythrocyte sedimentation rate (ESR) of 62 mm/hour, C-reactive protein (CRP) level of 12 mg/dL, and ferritin level of 7620 ug/L. Triglycerides and soluble CD25 are pending, and cultures were sent out. What is the next best step?

   a. Serum EBV DNA titers
   b. Treat with high-dose steroid
   c. Bone marrow biopsy
   d. CT scan of the chest, abdomen, and pelvis

   Answer: a. EBV infection can trigger HLH in patients who have underlying neoplastic process or immunosuppressive state. PCR will show high EBV DNA titers and serology test may be positive for both IgM and IgG antibodies. PCR test confirms active EBV infection.

References

1. Egan C, Jaffe ES. Non-neoplastic histiocytic and dendritic cell disorders in lymph nodes. Sem Diag Pathol. 2018;35:20–33. https://doi.org/10.1053/j.semdp.2017.11.002.
2. Fardet L, Galicier L, Lambotte O, Marzac C, Aumont C, Chahwan D, Coppo P, Hejblum G. Development and validation of the HScore, a score for the diagnosis of reactive hemophagocytic syndrome. Arthritis Rheumatol. 2014;66:2613–20. https://doi.org/10.1002/art.38690.
3. Henter J-I, Samuelsson-Horne A, Aricò M, Egeler RM, Elinder GR, Filipovich AH, Gadner H, Imashuku S, Komp D, Ladisch S, et al. Treatment of hemophagocytic lymphohistiocytosis with HLH-94 immunochemotherapy and bone marrow transplantation. Blood. 2002;100:2367–73. https://doi.org/10.1182/blood-2002-01-0172.
4. Henter JI, Horne A, Aricó M, Egeler RM, Filipovich AH, Imashuku S, Ladisch S, McClain K, Webb D, Winiarski J, et al. HLH-2004: diagnostic and therapeutic guidelines for hemophagocytic lymphohistiocytosis. Pediatr Blood Cancer. 2007;48:124–31. https://doi.org/10.1002/pbc.21039.

Part II

Disorders of Red Blood Cells

Iron Deficiency Anemia

8

Nagehan Pakasticali and Jesse M. Jaso

Introduction

Iron Deficiency Anemia (IDA) is the most common cause of anemia worldwide. IDA impacts cognitive development in children, increases the risk of adverse outcomes in pregnancy, limits the physical health of adults, and worsens cognitive decline in geriatric patients. Women, children, and the elder are the most affected populations.

The body has access to both nutritional and storage iron, with the latter representing the body's main source of iron for hematopoiesis. Iron metabolism involves numerous processes working together to either promote or inhibit nutritional iron absorption and storage iron release, based on the body's current level of iron availability.

Nutritional iron is ingested in the ferric (Fe^{+++}) state and undergoes reduction to the ferrous (Fe^{++}) state in the low pH environment of the stomach. Ferrous iron is absorbed by intestinal

N. Pakasticali (✉)
Department of Pathology, University of South Florida, Tampa, FL, USA

J. M. Jaso
Department of Hematopathology, University of Texas Southwestern Medical Center, Dallas, TX, USA
e-mail: jesse.jaso@utsouthwestern.edu

L. Sokol, L. Zhang (eds.), *Non-Neoplastic Hematologic Disorders*,
https://doi.org/10.1007/978-3-031-62373-8_8

epithelial cells (enterocytes) in the duodenum, the main site of iron absorption. Cytochrome B provides ferrous iron to divalent metal transporter-1(DMT-1) on the apical surface of enterocytes. Ferroportin-1 (FPN1), on the basolateral surface, transports iron from the enterocyte into the circulation. Iron binds to transferrin-1 (TFR1) in the ferric state (Fe^{+++}), allowing it to circulate into various iron storage "pools." The main iron pool (~2/3 of total body iron) is the erythron, referring to the iron stored in erythroid precursors in the bone marrow. The second major pool for iron storage is found in histiocytes in the liver, spleen, and bone marrow. This "storage pool" is the major source of iron used for hematopoiesis.

Iron is primarily stored as Ferritin, a water-soluble compound composed of ferric salts and apoferritin. In the absence of concurrent inflammation, serum ferritin provides a sensitive measure of iron stores. Transferrin receptor-1 (TFR-1, CD71), present in erythroid cells and most cells of the body, is used to transport iron back and forth from storage pools into cells as needed. Before binding with TFR-1, iron must be converted from the ferrous (Fe++) state to the ferric (Fe^{+++}) state by various ferroxidases, such as Hephaestin and Ceruloplasmin. Of note, both are copper-containing molecules. As such, copper deficiency may negatively impact iron release and can cause secondary IDA (see Table 8.1).

The master regulator of iron metabolism, hepcidin, is produced by the liver. By binding and occluding ferroportin-1 (FPN-1) on enterocytes and macrophages, hepcidin simultaneously inhibits nutritional iron absorption and release of storage iron, leading to decreased iron availability. Accordingly, hepcidin production is decreased when iron availability is low and increased when it is adequate or increased. Iron availability is monitored by several "iron sensing" proteins in the liver (human hemochromatosis protein (HFE), hemojuvelin (HJV), and transferrin receptor-2 (TFR-2)). Hepcidin is also an acute phase reactant and is elevated in the presence of inflammation. Sustained states of chronic inflammation may result in "anemia of chronic disease" (Table 8.1).

Table 8.1 Common laboratory findings in IDA and major differential diagnosis

Lab parameters	IDA	Anemia of chronic disease	Thalassemia	Copper deficiency	Lead poisoning
Hb	Low	Low	Low	Low	Low
MCV	Low	Normal or low	Low	Low	Low
MCHC	Low	Normal or low	Low	Low	Low
Serum iron	Low	Low	Normal to high	High	Variable
Serum ferritin	Low	Normal to high	Normal to high	High	Normal
TIBC	High	Low	Normal	Normal or low	Normal
Transferrin	Low	Normal or low	Normal to high	Normal to high	Normal to high

IDA iron deficiency anemia, *Hb* hemoglobin, *MCV* mean cell volume, *MCHC* mean cell hemoglobin concentration, *TIBC* total iron-binding capacity

Pathogenesis

Development of Iron Deficiency and Iron Deficiency Anemia

If iron levels are insufficient for the body's needs, a state of "iron imbalance" exists, and the body will respond by decreasing hepcidin production. As iron is mobilized from various storage pools, serum ferritin and transferrin saturation decrease, prompting further decrease of hepcidin and release of storage iron. Continued iron imbalance results in hypoxia which stimulates production of erythropoietin (EPO) and erythropoiesis. Increased erythropoiesis in the presence of decreased iron stores ("iron-deficient erythropoiesis") results in production of small RBCs with decreased hemoglobin content (microcytic and hypochromic) (Fig. 8.1). Rarely, patients have decreased iron levels without laboratory evidence of anemia. This state, known as "Iron Deficiency without

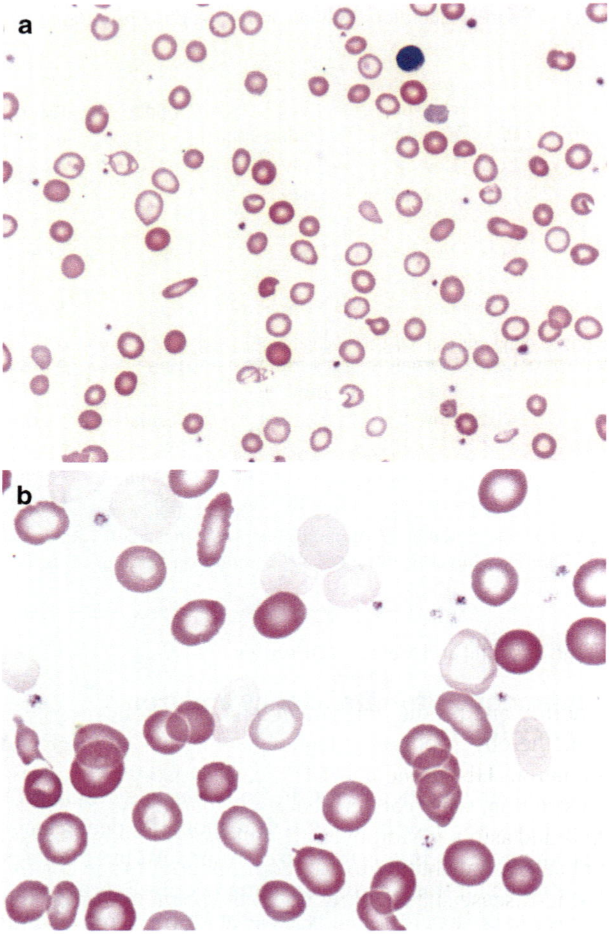

Fig. 8.1 (**a**) Peripheral blood smear from a patient with iron deficiency anemia shows numerous small, hypochromic RBCs with marked variable size and shape (anisopoikilocytosis). Note the presence of elongated, pencil-shaped cells, which are frequently encountered. (Wright-Giemsa, 50×). (**b**) High power view of severe iron deficiency, note the prominent central pallor resulting from iron-deficient hematopoiesis. (Wright-Giemsa, 100×)

Anemia," can present with subtle musculoskeletal and/or neurocognitive symptoms. Resolution of symptoms after a trial of iron therapy confirms the diagnosis.

The main causes of IDA can be broadly grouped into four broad categories:

1. **Increased iron requirements**
    (a) Typically, during periods of rapid growth such as infancy, childhood, adolescence, and pregnancy.
2. **Insufficient intake or impaired absorption**.
    (a) In developing nations, insufficient intake and parasites (Hookworm infection) may cause IDA.
    (b) In developed nations, insufficient intake is rarely seen. Impaired absorption may be due to inflammatory bowel disease, partial gastrectomy, and other causes.
3. **Chronic blood loss/hemorrhage**
    (a) Often associated with heavy menstruation and/or abnormal uterine bleeding in female patients.
    (b) Frequently associated with chronic gastrointestinal (GI) bleeding due to benign or malignant GI lesions in male patients.
4. **Iron Refractory Iron Deficiency Anemia (IRIDA)**
    (a) Caused by inherited mutation of the *TMPRSS6* gene, which encodes an enzyme promoting downregulation of hepcidin. The mutation results in abnormally high hepcidin levels and IDA that shows poor, or no, response to oral iron therapy.

Diagnosis

Clinical Presentation

The signs and symptoms of IDA are the results of insufficient tissue oxygenation and include fatigue, dyspnea on exertion, syncope, and pallor. Tachycardia, palpitations, hypotension, edema, and heart murmurs may also be encountered. IDA may also cause the compulsive eating of nonnutritive substances (pica), paresthesia, restless legs syndrome, and delayed neurologic and motor development in pediatric patients. Other findings include epithelial cell changes such as koilonychia, atrophy/fissuring of the tongue, angular stomatitis, and difficulty swallowing due to esophageal webs/strictures. Of note, the degree of symptoms may not directly correspond to the degree of anemia. The slow, gradual development of IDA may be minimally symptomatic, whereas faster development is less well-tolerated.

Laboratory Findings

Initial laboratory testing should include a complete blood count (CBC), peripheral blood smear examination, serum iron, serum total iron-binding capacity, and serum ferritin. (Table 8.1).

1. ***Complete blood count***: Hemoglobin, hematocrit, and RBC counts are decreased. MCV (mean cell volume) and MCH (mean cell hemoglobin) are variably decreased. RDW (red cell distribution width) is characteristically increased, indicating anisocytosis. Secondary reactive thrombocytosis may occur in some patients [1].
2. ***Peripheral blood smear***: Peripheral blood findings include hypochromic and microcytic RBCs. RBCs typically show variation in size and shape (anisopoikilocytosis), including the presence of elongated elliptocytes termed "pencil cells" (Fig. 8.1).
3. ***Serum iron***: Serum iron is decreased.
4. ***Total iron-binding capacity (TIBC)***: TIBC is increased, which allows for differentiation with ACD, which shows normal or elevated TIBC. In the absence of concurrent inflammation, the combination of decreased serum iron and increased TIBC is specific for iron deficiency anemia.
5. ***Transferrin saturation***: Measures functional iron supply available for erythropoiesis, defined as the ratio of serum iron to serum TIBC (Serum Iron/TIBC). In the absence of inflammatory and other diseases, percent saturation <15% is highly indicative of iron deficiency anemia.

6. ***Serum ferritin***: In the absence of concurrent inflammation, decreased serum ferritin level (<15 μg/L) is highly indicative of iron deficiency. However, ferritin is an acute phase reactant and will be elevated in geriatric patients and patients with inflammatory conditions. Serum ferritin <100 ng/mL, combined with transferrin saturation of <20%, suggests IDA in these patients.
7. ***Zinc protoporphyrin (ZPP)*:** Heme is formed from the combination of protoporphyrin IX and ferrous iron. Protoporphyrin builds up during iron-deficient erythropoiesis and binds with zinc. ZPP levels are increased in IDA, ACD, and lead poisoning but are normal in thalassemia. However, this test is not yet routinely available in most laboratories.
8. ***Serum transferrin receptor level (sTFR)*:** Iron deficiency and increased erythropoiesis may increase the production of soluble sTFRs. Levels are increased in patients with IDA. Levels are not affected by concurrent inflammation.
9. ***Hepcidin*:** Not commonly tested, but demonstration of increased hepcidin levels in patients with poor/no response to iron therapy suggests Iron Resistant Iron Deficiency Anemia (IRIDA).
10. ***Bone marrow examination*:** Not generally indicated for diagnosis of IDA.

Prognosis

With treatment, reticulocyte levels increase in 4 to 5 days, and hemoglobin levels improve by 2 weeks. Three to 6 months may be required to completely replete iron stores.

Treatment

Identification and treatment of the underlying cause of IDA is mandatory. Clinical judgment, along with the patient's symptoms, degree of anemia, underlying condition, age, sex, pregnancy status, and presence of comorbid conditions, determines the best course of treatment. General strategies are discussed below.

Nutritional Intake

Optimizing nutritional intake improves iron therapy's effectiveness and hastens iron stores' recovery. Nutritional iron is found in heme iron and inorganic/nonheme iron. Heme iron is bound to hemoglobin and is thus only found in meat. Nonheme iron is generally found in vegetables, grains, legumes, and iron supplements. Heme iron is more efficiently absorbed than nonheme iron, but intake of both types is encouraged. Citric and ascorbic acids improve iron absorption, while calcium, fiber, tea, and coffee inhibit its absorption. Of note, optimizing intake alone is insufficient for the treatment of IDA.

Oral Iron Therapy

Oral iron therapy with iron salts such as iron sulfate, fumarate, and gluconate is the mainstay for the treatment of mild to moderate IDA and shows similar efficacy (Table 8.2). Side effects are unfortunately common with oral therapy, leading to poor compliance and partially treated disease in many patients. In contrast, parental iron therapy is associated with fast and efficient recovery of iron stores without the common side effects or oral iron.

Table 8.2 List of commonly used agents for oral iron therapy

<table>
<tr><th>Name</th><th>Route</th><th>Preparation</th><th>Potential side effects</th></tr>
<tr><td>Ferrous Sulfate</td><td>Oral</td><td>Tablet (200 mg)
Drops (125 mg/mL)</td><td rowspan="3">Nausea
Vomiting
Constipation
Diarrhea</td></tr>
<tr><td>Ferrous gluconate</td><td>Oral</td><td>Tablet (300 mg)</td></tr>
<tr><td>Ferrous fumarate</td><td>Oral</td><td>Tablet (210 mg)
Capsule (305 mg)
Liquid (45 mg/mL)</td></tr>
</table>

Parental Iron Therapy

Patients who cannot tolerate oral iron or have concurrent inflammatory disease or malabsorption should be considered for parental iron therapy. There are several approved preparations for parental iron therapy [2]. Side effects are similar to those for oral preparations, but also include potential for a "hypersensitivity reaction", which is an anaphylactic-like response to iron particles in the preparation.

Dosages are dependent on numerous factors such as patient age, weight, calculation of total iron deficit, and presence of acquired conditions such as heart failure and chronic kidney disease. Total body iron deficit can be calculated using the *Ganzoni* formula (Total iron deficit [mg] = Body weight [kg] × (Target Hb – Actual Hb) [g/dL] × 2.4 + iron depot [mg]). In overweight patients, the ideal body weight should be used as body weight. If the body weight is <35 kg, iron depot is 15 mg/kg; if ≥35 kg, the iron depot is 500 mg.

Red Blood Cell Transfusion

RBC transfusion is rarely indicated and should only be considered for severely symptomatic patients and for those with severe anemia (Hb<7 g/dL or 8 g/dL if symptomatic).

Promising Clinical Studies

Recombinant human erythropoietin-related products (erythropoiesis-stimulating agents, ESAs) have been used to treat IDA in patients with chronic kidney disease in combination with iron replacement. However, many side effects have been reported regarding the use of ESAs. As a result, new therapeutic agents have been studied. One is prolyl hydroxylase domain (PHD) enzyme inhibitor, which stabilizes hypoxia-inducible factor (HIF), a crucial compound to produce erythropoietin. In clinical trials, it has been found that PHD inhibitors enhanced erythropoiesis and improved IDA compared with ESAs [3].

Board Questions

1. In the absence of concurrent inflammation, which of the following is the most sensitive test for iron deficiency anemia?

   A. Serum iron level.
   B. Total iron-binding capacity.
   C. Soluble serum transferrin receptor.
   D. Serum ferritin level.

   Answer: D. Serum ferritin level.

2. A 73-year-old male presents with complaints of progressive fatigue and shortness of breath. He is a vegetarian and describes his typical daily meal as tea and toast for breakfast, with a jelly sandwich for lunch and dinner. He also reports drinking 3–4 cups of coffee daily. Laboratory investigation shows Hb 10 g/dL, Hematocrit 24%, and MCV 72 fL. Serum ferritin and serum iron levels are decreased, and serum total iron-binding capacity (TIBC) is increased. Which of the following statements is most correct?

   A. This patient will need bone marrow biopsy to confirm iron deficiency anemia.
   B. In addition to iron replacement therapy, the patient should receive nutritional counseling to optimize iron intake.
   C. Optimizing nutritional iron intake alone will be sufficient treatment for this patient.
   D. No additional testing is required for this patient.

Answer: B. The clinical and laboratory findings are consistent with IDA. Invasive studies, such as bone marrow biopsy, are rarely indicated for diagnosis. In addition to iron replacement therapy, this patient will require nutritional counseling to optimize dietary intake of iron, as failure to do may slow recovery.

His diet is deficient in iron-rich foods. In addition, excessive intake of tea and coffee can inhibit iron absorption. Nevertheless, increased dietary intake alone is insufficient for restoring storage iron levels. Further workup (e.g., screening for underlying malignancy) is indicated, especially given the patient's gender and advanced age.

References

1. Evstatiev R, et al. Iron deficiency alters megakaryopoiesis and platelet phenotype independent of thrombopoietin. Am J Hematol. 2014;89(5):524–9. https://doi.org/10.1002/ajh.23682. Epub 2014 Feb 24. PMID: 24464533.
2. Camaschella C. Iron-deficiency anemia. N Engl J Med. 2015;372(19):1832–43. https://doi.org/10.1056/NEJMra1401038. PMID: 25946282.
3. Chou Y-H, Pan S-Y, Lin S-L. Pleotropic effects of hypoxia-inducible factor-prolyl hydroxylase domain inhibitors: are they clinically relevant? Kidney Res Clin Pract. 2023;42(1):27–38. https://doi.org/10.23876/j.krcp.22.118. Epub 2022 Nov 21. PMID: 36634968.

Anemia of Inflammation 9

Udhayvir Singh Grewal, Prerna Rastogi,
and Sabarish Ayyappan

Introduction (Definition, Epidemiology, Etiology, Novel Findings)

Anemia of inflammation (AI, formerly known as anemia of chronic disease) is a common, usually mild form of normocytic normochromic anemia (hemoglobin typically >8.0 g/dL), which is caused by an underlying inflammatory or autoimmune disease, infection, or neoplasm. AI is the second most prevalent cause of anemia worldwide (after iron-deficiency anemia [IDA]) and is also the most common cause of anemia among hospitalized or chronically ill patients. Primarily, AI was attributed to chronic illnesses with sustained inflammatory states like infections, malignancies, and

U. S. Grewal
Division of Hematology–Oncology, University of Iowa Hospitals and Clinics, Iowa City, IA, USA

P. Rastogi (✉)
Department of Pathology, University of Iowa, Carver College of Medicine, Iowa City, IA, USA
e-mail: prerna-rastogi@uiowa.edu

S. Ayyappan
Division of Hematology–Oncology, University of Iowa Hospitals and Clinics, Iowa City, IA, USA

Department of Internal Medicine, University of Iowa, Carver College of Medicine, Iowa City, IA, USA

L. Sokol, L. Zhang (eds.), *Non-Neoplastic Hematologic Disorders*,
https://doi.org/10.1007/978-3-031-62373-8_9

autoimmune diseases. Recently, other chronic conditions, including chronic obstructive pulmonary disease, obesity, chronic liver disease, congestive heart failure, and advanced atherosclerosis, including stroke and coronary artery disease, have been related to causation of AI. Patients with AI may also have concomitant true iron deficiency. Identification of superimposed iron deficiency among these patients is important as iron replacement reduces the need for frequent transfusions and helps improve overall quality of life. Management primarily focuses on treating the underlying cause of systemic inflammation, which often varies with the severity of the underlying condition and therapeutic options available. Beside additional therapies, such as iron replacement and blood transfusions, novel treatment options targeting hepcidin and iron trafficking are currently in the pipeline.

In this chapter, we discuss the pathophysiology, clinical features, diagnosis (including differential diagnosis), and treatment of patients with AI. Although several pathophysiological mechanisms are shared between anemia of chronic kidney disease and AI associated with other chronic conditions, the diagnosis and treatment may vary significantly. Therefore, the current chapter will focus only on AI associated with conditions other than chronic kidney disease.

Pathophysiology

The pathophysiology of AI is complex and poorly understood. Three major pathophysiological mechanisms for AI have been described in literature. These mechanisms may contribute to the development of anemia in chronic inflammatory states in variable proportions and patterns (Fig. 9.1).

(i) *Increase in hepcidin level*

The impact of chronic inflammation on iron trafficking is mediated by a complex interplay between various cytokines, out of which interleukin-6 (IL-6) is the most significant player. IL-6

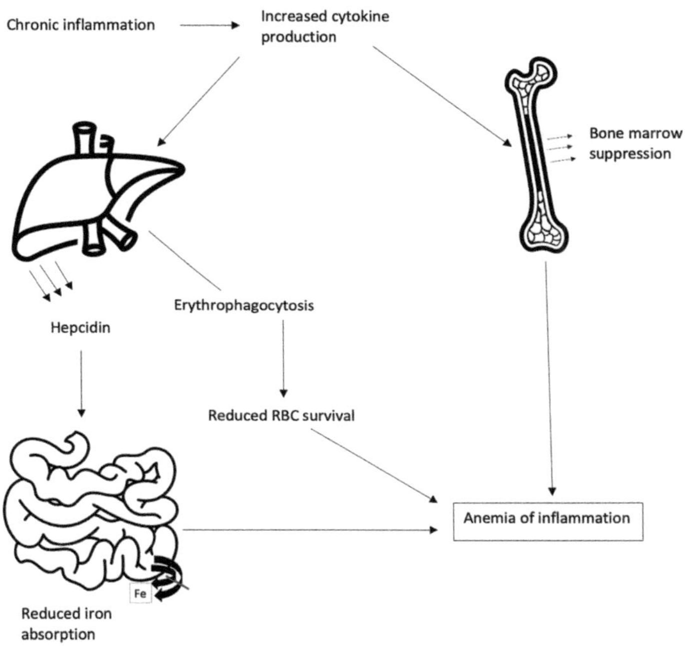

Fig. 9.1 Pathophysiology of AI. AI anemia of inflammation, Fe iron, RBC red blood cell

promotes the production of hepcidin by hepatocytes, which further binds to the intestinal transmembrane iron exporter known as ferroportin. This binding leads to internalization and degradation of ferroportin, thereby restricting the duodenal absorption of iron. Hepcidin also limits the release of iron from macrophages, resulting in an overall *iron-restricted* state, thereby limiting the mobilizable iron stores available for erythropoiesis resulting in anemia.

(ii) *Suppression of erythropoiesis*

Chronic inflammation also leads to impairment of erythropoiesis by a reduction in the production of erythropoietin. This effect is primarily mediated by interleukin-1 (IL-1) and tumor-necrosis factor. Additionally, hyporesponsiveness to erythropoietin has also been observed among patients with AI. This effect is driven by impairment in erythropoietin-mediated signaling caused by elevated levels of IL-1 and IL-6. Iron restriction and suppression of erythropoiesis (both direct suppression and via impaired erythropoietin-mediated signaling) result in impaired erythroid-cell proliferation and differentiation. Alternate pathways of erythropoiesis inhibition have been identified like high-mobility group box-1 protein, which is secreted during sepsis from dying cells and activated immune cells. Upon binding to surface receptors, this reduces the growth and causes increased destruction of erythropoietin-sensitive precursors [1]. This has been speculated to influence the chronic phase of AI and antibodies to high-mobility group box-1 in vivo have shown to partially restore the erythropoietin signaling.

(iii) *Reduced erythrocyte survival*

Erythrophagocytosis in hepatic and splenic macrophages has been extensively studied and noted among patients with AI, which contributes to reduced erythrocyte survival. However, this does not appear to play a dominant role in driving anemia in chronic inflammation. The reduced erythrocyte survival may become particularly important in acute illness such as infections, sepsis, acute flare of underlying autoimmune conditions, etc.

Diagnosis

AI tends to be very similar and sometimes indistinguishable from IDA in terms of clinical features and presentation. Patients may present with symptoms such as fatigue, generalized weakness, exercise intolerance, aprosexia (reduced ability to concentrate), memory loss, and dyspnea on exertion. Some of these symptoms may also appear to be related to underlying diseases, such as autoimmune disease and chronic infections, which may delay their clinical identification.

Any individual with anemia (hemoglobin <12 mg/dL in females and <13 mg/dL in males) along with clinical or laboratory supporting evidence may be diagnosed with AI, provided important alternate causes of anemia have been excluded. These alternate causes include, but are not limited to, the following:

1. Occult blood loss (gastrointestinal or genitourinary blood loss)
2. Micronutrient or vitamin deficiency (nutritional deficiency of iron, folate, vitamin B12, or vitamin D)
3. Renal dysfunction (chronic kidney disease or end-stage renal disease)
4. Drug-induced anemia (cytotoxic chemotherapy, nonsteroidal anti-inflammatory drugs, proton-pump inhibitors, etc.)
5. Underlying hematological malignancies (myelodysplastic syndrome, undiagnosed multiple myeloma, etc.)
6. Hemolytic anemia (associated with infections, neoplasms, or autoimmune conditions)

Differential Diagnosis

Anemia in AI tends to be mild to moderate and normocytic and normochromic; however, among about 25% patients, it may be microcytic (mean corpuscular volume is rarely below 70). This is in contrast with the characteristic microcytic and hypochromic picture with distinct anisopoikilocytosis seen among patients with IDA. Iron studies are a valuable tool for distinguishing iron anemia (IA) from IDA (also see Table 9.1). Checking serum copper level would be useful for detection of patients with copper deficiency.

Use of hepcidin levels as a surrogate marker for iron deficiency is confounded by diurnal variations, fluctuations with dietary iron content, and lack of standardized assays in the clinical setting. Patients with AI may also have concomitant true iron deficiency, which is often referred to as AI with superimposed iron deficiency or AI/IDA. Soluble transferrin receptor levels may be helpful in identifying patients with AI/IDA. Because of a

Table 9.1 Differential diagnosis between AI and IDA

	AI	IDA
Hemoglobin	Decreased	Decreased
MCV/MCH	Decreased to normal	Decreased
Serum ferritin	Normal or increased (>100 g/ml)	Decreased (<30 g/ml)
Serum hepcidin	High	Low
Serum iron concentration	Decreased	Significantly decreased
Transferrin	Decreased to normal	Increased
Serum-transferrin saturation	Decreased	Decreased
Serum transferrin receptor*	Normal	Increased
Serum transferrin receptor index	<1	>2
EPO	Decreased	Increased
TIBC	Decreased	Increased

*The assay unreliable for use in identification of superimposed IDA
AI anemia of inflammation, *EPO* erythropoietin, *IDA* iron-deficiency anemia, *MCH* mean corpuscular hemoglobin, *MCV* mean corpuscular volume, *TIBC* total iron-binding proteins

decrease in availability of iron among patients with IDA, soluble transferrin receptor levels are increased in IDA, as opposed to AI, in which serum-transferrin receptor levels are expected to be normal. However, soluble transferrin receptor levels can be confounded by several cytokines in the setting of underlying inflammation, which may render the assay unreliable for use in identification of superimposed IDA. In some studies, ferritin index (soluble transferrin level/log ferritin levels) has shown promise in allowing better differentiation between patients with AI and AI/IDA. There is a growing need to develop better and more reliable biomarkers that may allow discrimination between patients with AI and AI/IDA, allowing personalization of treatment and response monitoring.

There is a list of diseases that can manifest with anemia resembling AI. These common diseases associated with, or mimic AI, are selected in Table 9.2.

Table 9.2 Diseases associated with or mimic AI

Conditions	Samples
Infections	Viral, bacterial, fungal, parasitic Infection, e.g., HIV, parvovirus B19, malaria or leishmaniasis, as causes of anemia secondary to bone marrow suppression. Virology, serology, parasitic tests are considered
Autoimmune disorders	Systemic lupus erythematosus, Rheumatoid arthritis, Sarcoidosis, and Inflammatory bowel disease can also be mimickers. Additional laboratory study and tissue biopsy would help diagnosis
Endocrine disorders	Hypothyroidism, hyperthyroidism, panhypopituitarism, or hyperparathyroidism. Laboratory testing may be considered in the appropriate clinical setting
Chronic kidney disease	Key differences between AI and anemia associated with chronic kidney disease are low erythropoietin levels and abnormal renal function tests
Underlying hematological conditions	Myelodysplastic syndrome, aleukemic leukemia, pure red cell aplasia, etc. can manifest with anemia. A bone marrow biopsy with molecular testing is required for accurate diagnosis
Drug-induced anemia	It is important to review the list of medications to ensure potential culprit agents, such as proton-pump inhibitors, nonsteroidal anti-inflammatory drugs, etc., which may explain a component of the anemia

AI anemia of inflammation, *MDS* myelodysplastic syndromes

Prognosis

AI is a widely prevalent subtype of anemia, with an estimated 40% of all anemias worldwide, and comprises either AI or combined anemias with an AI component, afflicting a population of almost more than 1 billion cases [2]. There has been an improved understanding of the iron metabolism and interplay of numerous factors in the pathogenesis of AI, but the impact of anemia on the disease trajectory and long-term outcomes and the influence of anemia treatment on patients' prognosis in different diseases remain to be studied. A prospective population-based study of 138,670 subjects in The Netherlands demonstrated that anemia was associated with worsened overall survival and health-related quality of life among older subjects (age >60 years) [3]. In this cohort, AI, although poorly defined, was shown to have worsened overall survival and health-related quality of life. Whether AI is a marker for poorer outcomes among subjects with chronic disease, or the presence of AI contributes to adverse outcomes from chronic illness remains to be explored. Recent advances in understanding the pathophysiology and underlying interactions between complex pathways might help elucidate individualized diagnostic algorithm and therapeutic approach for each variety of AI.

Treatment

Treatment of AI is primarily aimed at treating the underlying conditions, such as infections, neoplasms, or autoimmune conditions. However, because of the chronic nature of these conditions, treatment may not always be feasible and may often be long term. Improvement in anemia among these patients may not just be of prognostic significance, but may also improve overall quality of life.

Identification of superimposed iron deficiency (AI/IDA) is paramount for treating anemia among these patients. Even in the absence of obvious signs of bleeding, a referral to a gastroenterologist for possible occult gastrointestinal bleeding is important to help identify the cause and limit further blood loss. Treatment of AI/IDA with iron replacement may lead to an improvement in clinical symptoms and a reduction in the need for transfusions. Overall, intravenous iron therapy is preferred as elevated hepcidin levels in these patients may limit intestinal absorption of iron. Of note, oral iron therapy has been shown to be equally efficacious as intravenous iron therapy for patients with AI/IDA with mild inflammation. However, the use of intravenous iron therapy is recommended despite mild inflammation among patients with chronic heart failure. For patients who do need transfusions (such as hospitalized patients with severe anemia), a goal of hemoglobin >7.0 g/dL may be appropriate, unless there is a history of coronary artery disease (in which case the target hemoglobin level would be >8.0 g/dL).

It is important to be mindful of and educate patients about the complications associated with frequent blood transfusions, such as iron overload and alloimmunization. Several studies have investigated the use of erythropoietin-stimulating agents (ESAs) in the management of anemia with underlying conditions, such as cancer and liver cirrhosis. However, because of a lack of clear benefit and potential adverse effects, such as increased risk of thromboembolic events and worsening hypertension, their use remains limited. There is theoretical benefit associated with using ESAs in iron-refractory severe IDA/IA, when ESAs may help by stimulating erythropoiesis and suppressing hepcidin. There is a high prevalence of vitamin-D deficiency among patients with AI. Interestingly, vitamin-D supplementation has been shown to be associated with a reduction in the hepcidin levels. Therefore, checking vitamin-D levels and appropriate supplementation may be helpful for these patients.

Promising Clinical Studies

Because of the limitations associated with the use of the above therapies, several novel therapeutic strategies are currently being developed for managing patients with AI. Prolyl-hydroxylase inhibitors (e.g., Roxadustat) stabilize hypoxia-inducible factors, resulting in an increase in erythropoietin production and mobilization of iron from macrophages and enterocytes. These agents have shown promise in ameliorating anemia of chronic kidney disease; however, there is a growing interest in their use as therapeutic agents for AI. There are several novel therapeutic agents that are currently being developed to target increased hepcidin levels in AI. Antihepcidin monoclonal antibodies that bind to hepcidin and prevent its binding to ferroportin are being investigated for ameliorating anemia in AI. Hepcidin-modifying therapies may have a role in combination with ESA, when the increased endogenous availability of iron may reduce the need for ESA and minimize the ESA side effects [4]. With a similar rationale, hepcidin-binding proteins, such as anticalins and spiegelmers, are also being developed and investigated for use among patients with AI. Similarly, ferroportin-stabilizing antibodies that impair the interaction between ferroportin and hepcidin are also being investigated for use in AI.

Caveats

1. AI tends to be very similar and sometimes indistinguishable from IDA in terms of clinical features and presentation.
2. Before a diagnosis of AI is made in any individual (hemoglobin <12 mg/dL in females and <13 mg/dL in males), it is important to rule out alternate causes of anemia, as described in this chapter.
3. There is a high prevalence of vitamin-D deficiency among patients with AI. Vitamin-D supplementation reduces hepcidin levels and may be useful in treating AI.

Board-Style Question

1. A 69-year-old patient with chronic lymphocytic leukemia is currently on therapy for his malignancy and has progressive anemia with a change in his hemoglobin from 12 to 9.6 over 6 months. His chronic lymphocytic leukemia is under control with no detectable disease in the blood and bone marrow. His blood tests show:

	Result	Normal range
White cell count (× 10^9/L)	4.8	4.0–11.00
Hemoglobin (g/dL)	9.6	14 to 18 (male); 12 to 16 (female)
MCV (fL)	87	80–100
Ferritin (ng/mL)	658	30–400
Serum iron (μg/dL)	32	59–158
Iron saturation (%)	14	20–50%
Transferrin (μg/dL)	192	200–360
TIBC (μg/dL)	224	235–451

MCV mean corpuscular volume, *TIBC* total iron-binding capacity

Which of the next tests would be helpful in the diagnosis?

A. Gastrointestinal workup including endoscopy and colonoscopy.
B. Bone marrow stain for iron
C. Soluble transferrin receptor
D. Serum B12 and folate levels

Answer C: This patient has AI and possibility of concomitant iron deficiency with depleted iron stores. Soluble transferrin receptor levels can help distinguish between AI and AI in combination with IDA. Bone marrow stain can assess bone marrow iron stores, but correlation with iron stores is inconsistent and may not help iron-deficiency evaluation. Gastrointestinal workup for bleeding could be considered if iron stores are not improved with supplementation or concomitant IDA is confirmed with soluble transferrin receptor testing.

2. Which laboratory parameter is elevated in anemia of inflammation (AI).

   A. Iron
   B. Erythropoietin
   C. Hepcidin
   D. TIBC
   E. Soluble transferrin receptor

Answer C: Hepcidin is elevated in anemia of inflammation secondary to increased production of IL-6 due to inflammation. Iron, erythropoietin, TIBC, and soluble transferrin receptor levels are low or normal in AI.

References

1. Dulmovits BM, et al. HMGB1-mediated restriction of EPO signaling contributes to anemia of inflammation. Blood. 2022;139(21):3181–93.
2. Kassebaum NJ, et al. A systematic analysis of global anemia burden from 1990 to 2010. Blood. 2014;123(5):615–24.
3. Wouters H, et al. Association of anemia with health-related quality of life and survival: a large population-based cohort study. Haematologica. 2019;104(3):468–76.
4. Theurl M, et al. Hepcidin as a predictive factor and therapeutic target in erythropoiesis-stimulating agent treatment for anemia of chronic disease in rats. Haematologica. 2014;99(9):1516–24.

Megaloblastic Anemia

10

Olger Nano, Meri Muminovic,
Amalia Bonano-Rios,
and Fernando Vargas Madueno

Introduction

Macrocytes are defined as RBCs with a mean corpuscular volume (MCV) >100 femtoliter (fL). Megaloblastic anemia (MA) is a form of anemia that results from a variety of reasons, which produce enlarged red blood cell (RBC) precursors in the bone marrow, namely megaloblasts, and macrocytes in peripheral blood. Megaloblasts occur because of asynchronous maturation between the nucleus (dependent on DNA synthesis) and cytoplasm (dependent on RNA and protein synthesis), during which the cytoplasm increases more rapidly than the nucleus, leading to an increase in cell size [1]. The leading causes of MA include deficiencies in cobalamin (vitamin B12) and folate [2]. These two nutrients are essential in biochemical processes that lead to ATP generation (Krebs Cycle) and DNA synthesis, both of which are critical for cell growth and tissue generation (Fig. 10.1). The other etiologies leading to MA include myelodysplastic syndrome (MDS), liver dysfunction, alcoholism, hypothyroidism, copper deficiency, and certain drugs that interfere with DNA synthesis (Table 10.1).

O. Nano (✉) · M. Muminovic · A. Bonano-Rios · F. V. Madueno
Memorial Cancer Institute at Memorial Healthcare System,
Pembroke Pines, FL, USA
e-mail: ONano@mhs.net; MMuminovic@mhs.net;
ABonanoRios@mhs.net; FVargasMadueno@mhs.net

L. Sokol, L. Zhang (eds.), *Non-Neoplastic Hematologic Disorders*,
https://doi.org/10.1007/978-3-031-62373-8_10

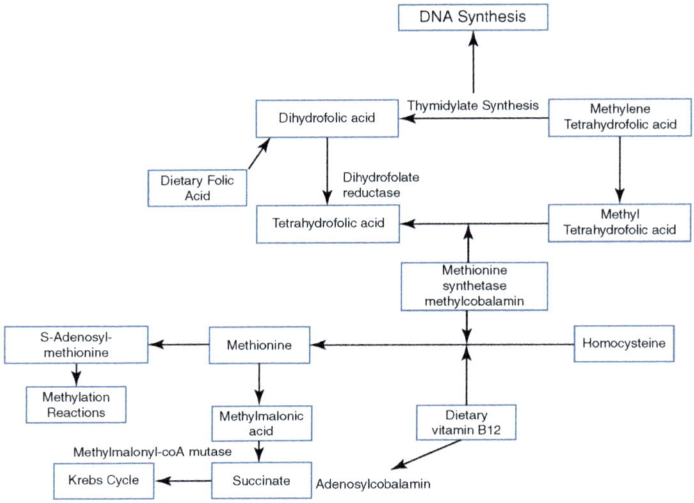

Fig. 10.1 Biochemical pathways involving folic acid and vitamin B12

Table 10.1 A list of drugs that cause megaloblastic anemia

Drug induced megaloblastic anemia	
Interfering bone marrow progenitors	*Decreased intestinal absorption*
Allopurinol	Aminosalicyclic acid
Azathioprine	Antacids
Capecitabine	Proton Pump Inhibitors
Cladribine	Pencillin
Fludarabine	Chloramphenicol
Fluorouracil	Erythromycin
Gadolinium	Oral contraceptives
Gemcitabine	Metformin
Hydroxyurea	Phenytoin
Lamivudine	Tetracyclines
Leflunomide	Valproic acid
Mercaptopurine	
Methotrexate	
Mycophenolate mofetil	
Trimethoprim	
Zidovudine	

Rarely, it is caused by a hereditary disorder called thiamine-responsive megaloblastic anemia (TRMA) [3].

Etiology

There is a variety of etiology of MA, which can be classified into nutritional (deficiencies of nutritional compounds, e.g., Vitamin B12) or non-nutritional due to endocrine, liver disease or MDS, etc.

Folic Acid (FA) Deficiency

FA is absorbed in the upper jejunum by active absorption or passive diffusion, and the body stores are about 5 to 20 μg in the liver. This can suffice for about 3 to 4 months and be used in DNA synthesis. The recommended daily requirement for folate is about 50 to 100 μg (up to 400 μg) for adults and 600 μg for pregnant females [4]. It is found in leafy green vegetables, meats, fruits, and liver. Folate deficiency is caused by decreased folate intake, e.g., nutritional deficiency including alcohol abuse, poor diet, or malabsorption (e.g., celiac disease, inflammatory bowel disease), increased demand (e.g., pregnancy, hemolysis; lactation), or exposure to medication that interferes with DNA synthesis e.g., methotrexate, trimethoprim, phenytoin [4].

Cyanocobalamin (Vitamin B12)

Vitamin B12 is absorbed in the duodenum and jejunum where it is bound to intrinsic factor (IF), a carrier protein produced by gastric parietal cells, and then it is absorbed in the terminal ileum. Daily requirements are 1 to 3 μg, and the body stores about 2 to 3 μg in the liver, which is sufficient for 2 to 4 years [3]. It is found in meats, fish, egg, and dairy products. Common causes of vitamin B12 deficiency are strict adherence to a vegetarian or vegan diet, surgical procedures (gastrectomy, ileal resection), ileitis, Zollinger-Ellison syndrome, tapeworm infestation, pancreatic insufficiency, and blind-loop syndrome. Transcobalamin II deficiency, a congenital disorder, or exposure to nitrous oxide can also result in vitamin B12 deficiency.

Worthy of mention is that 20–50% of patients with vitamin B12 deficiency suffer from pernicious anemia. Pernicious anemia is an autoimmune process that destructs gastric parietal cells and results in loss of intrinsic factor (IF), a key factor involving in Vitamin B12 absorption.

Vitamin B12 also helps to convert inactive folic acid to active form via its coenzymatic reaction (Fig. 10.1). Thus, deficiency of vitamin B12 accompanies with deficiency of active folic acid.

Drugs

A list of medications [5] that can lead to MA are listed in Table 10.1.

Copper Deficiency

Copper can be found in whole grains, nuts, seeds, meats, and fish. It is absorbed in the duodenum and small intestine. Copper deficiency can lead to any microcytic, normocytic, or macrocytic anemia and coexist with neutropenia and/or thrombocytopenia. Similar to Vitamin B12 deficiency, patients with copper deficiency could clinically manifest with neurological symptoms due to demyelinating neuropathy. Several clinical conditions such as gastric surgery and high doses of zinc supplementation can result in copper deficiency. A bone marrow biopsy from the patients with copper deficiency demonstrates unique cytoplasmic vacuoles present in all lineage cells and increased ring sideroblasts.

Pathogenesis

MA primarily involves ineffective erythropoiesis caused by apoptosis of hematopoietic precursors in the bone marrow secondary to decreased DNA synthesis and DNA replication errors. Even though DNA synthesis is significantly reduced, protein and RNA syntheses are not affected, creating an imbalance between the cytoplasm and nuclear growth, otherwise known as nuclear-cytoplasm asynchrony.

Furthermore, the increased number of immature cells could lead to a decrease in all blood counts, manifesting as cytopenia or pancytopenia. At the cell level, the initial mechanism starts with impaired DNA synthesis, leading to an arrest in the S phase of the cell cycle and cell maturation. Ineffective erythropoiesis results in intravascular and extravascular hemolysis [6]. The role of folate is to donate methyl groups that contribute to DNA methylation. Vitamin B12, by contrast, is a cofactor in the reaction that regenerates tetrahydrofolate (THF) (Fig. 10.1). To make THF, homocysteine is converted to methionine; hence, if there is no vitamin B12, folate is trapped in the 5-methyl-THF form and methionine becomes deficient. If the deficiency occurs for extended periods of time, hematopoietic precursors (myeloid and erythroid lineages) in bone marrow show megaloblastic changes. Macrocytic RBCs and hypersegmented neutrophils appear on peripheral smear (Fig. 10.2a, b). At this stage, laboratory results would be indicative of hemolysis and low reticulocyte count. By contrast, pernicious anemia involves an autoimmune process, with formation of autoantibodies against intrinsic factor or gastric parietal cell antigens, thereby leading to a functional vitamin B12 deficiency state.

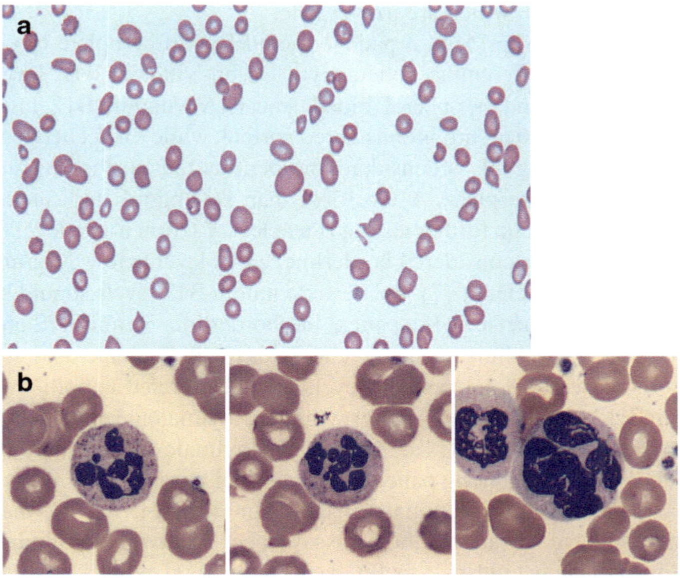

Fig. 10.2 (**a**) Megaloblastic Anemia Peripheral Smear. (Courtesy of Memorial Hospital West Pathology Department). (**b**) Megaloblastic Anemia Peripheral Smear (hypersegmented neutrophils)

Diagnosis

Patients should be evaluated for MA if there is anemia with macrocytosis (mean corpuscular volume > 100 fL) or if they present with hypersegmented neutrophils, which could also be noted on examination of peripheral smear. At times, patients may have a normal MCV with MA, but often it is greater than 115 fL, especially in folate and vitamin B12 deficiencies than other causes of macrocytosis. Clinically, patients may have symptoms of anemia (e.g., headache, palpitation, and dyspnea) or neuropsychiatric manifestations (e.g. ataxia, numbness, difficult speaking or walking, impaired concentration, insomnia, delusions, hallucinations) in cases with vitamin B12 or copper deficiencies. Among patients with B12 deficiency, lower extremity peripheral neuropathy can present with symptoms of paresthesia and imbalance. Neurologic examination findings are consistent with decreased proprioception and positive Romberg test. Optic nerve demyelination cases have also been documented. Neuropsychiatric disturbances have been described, which are irreversible.

To evaluate for MA, a patient should have a complete blood count with differential, reticulocyte count, vitamin B12 level, folate level, and peripheral blood smear. A vitamin B12 level greater than 300 pg/mL is considered normal, while a level between 200 and 300 pg/mL is considered borderline, thus further evaluation should take place. A level less than 200 pg/mL indicates a deficiency, and no further testing is needed. A serum folate level of 2 to 4 ng/mL is considered borderline, and a level below 2 ng/mL indicates a deficiency [7]. Folate and vitamin B12 levels should be obtained concurrently. If a patient has borderline vitamin B12 and folate levels, a clinician should check for methylmalonic acid and homocysteine. Homocysteine levels may be elevated in both vitamin B12 and folate deficiencies, while methylmalonic acid is only elevated in vitamin B12 deficiency. Methylmalonic acid may be falsely elevated among patients with renal disease.

Once a patient is found to be vitamin B12-deficient, they should have an autoantibody assay to evaluate for antibodies directed against intrinsic factor or gastric parietal cells. A positive result indicates pernicious anemia.

The diagnosis of concomitant microcytic and macrocytic anemia could represent a diagnostic dilemma. The microcytic component could be caused by iron deficiency anemia, thalassemia, lead poisoning, or anemia of chronic disease. In ethnic groups with a high prevalence of thalassemia, normocytic anemia should raise suspicion of concomitant B12 deficiency. Special attention should be paid to patients with a history of Helicobacter pylori (*H. pylori*), since this can cause chronic inflammation and damage the stomach lining, leading to decreased absorption of both iron and vitamin B12. Additionally, *H. pylori* produces the substance urease which neutralizes stomach acid and reduces the ability of the stomach to release vitamin B12 from food. In addition, this could be a complication from weight loss surgery. A bone marrow biopsy is only indicated for MA patients with clinically high suspicion for MDS.

Differential Diagnosis

Besides the etiologies leading to MA, other diseases could also result in decreased vitamin B12. Low levels of vitamin B12 are commonly found in multiple myeloma, pregnancy, HIV, pregnancy, and oral contraceptive usage. Many hematologic disorders such as MDS, hemolytic anemia, and thrombotic thrombocytopenic purpura can manifest with MA. Certain diseases or situations (e.g., infection, diabetes mellitus, medications, carpal tunnel syndrome alcoholism) can develop neurologic signs that could mimic vitamin B12 deficiency. Inaccurately elevated levels of B12 may be seen in renal disease, myeloproliferative neoplasms, and alcoholic liver disease [8].

Prognosis

The outcome of MA is upon its underlying disease. Nutritional deficiencies or drug-induced MA have good prognosis, while MDS-related MA should be managed appropriately, otherwise one-third of them will transfer to acute myeloid leukemia. In general, B12 supplementation can improve symptoms and/or signs of pernicious anemia. However, patients in later stage with subacute combined degeneration of the spinal cord show less optimal outcome, and only a small subset of them has complete resolution. Neurological symptoms persistent for more than 12 months after starting parenteral therapy with vitamin B12 are usually considered irreversible.

[https://www.ncbi.nlm.nih.gov/books/NBK540989/].

Treatment

FA can be supplemented with a dose of 1 mg by mouth daily until the cause of the deficiency is reversed. For patients with increased FA requirements, or if the cause is irreversible, supplementation should continue indefinitely. According to WHO guidelines and American Pediatric Association, all women of reproductive age should receive 400 micrograms (mcg) of FA each day to prevent neural tube defects. Pregnant women with malabsorption or prior history of children with neural tube birth defect are recommended to use higher FA doses such as 5 mg daily.

Pernicious anemia. Vitamin B12 can be administered intramuscularly or subcutaneously with dose of 1000 μg every other day for 1–2 weeks, then weekly for 4 weeks, and subsequently monthly indefinitely. For patients with B12 deficiency due to malabsorption but no evidence of anemia or neurological symptoms, either intramuscular or sublingual formulations can be administered. Reticulocytosis in peripheral blood usually occurs within 24–48 hours posttreatment initiation. Hemolytic parameters are expected to improve within 1 week of starting treatment in cases of intramedullary hemolysis [8].

Promising Clinical Studies

NA.

Caveats

1. There are multiple factors that can lead to MA, nutritional (vitamin B12, folate, copper) or non-nutritional (endocrine, liver disease, MDS)
2. Homocysteine levels may be elevated in both vitamin B12 and folate deficiency. However, methylmalonic acid is only elevated in vitamin B12 deficiency. Methylmalonic acid may be falsely elevated among patients with renal disease.
3. Ani-intrinsic factor or gastric parietal cells should be ordered in patients with vitamin B12 deficiency. A positive result indicates pernicious anemia.
4. Abnormal bone marrow hematopoiesis associated with pernicious anemia can be replaced within 24–48 hours after starting parenteral administration of vitamin B12. Such rapid hematopoietic cell renewal can result in consumption of the large amount of potassium and development of cardiac arrhythmias such as atrial fibrillation, warranting close cardiac monitoring.

Questions

1. The administration of which of the following agents does not lead to development for red cell macrocytosis?

   A. Methotrexate
   B. Zidovudine
   C. Alcohol
   D. Lead
   E. Hydroxyurea

Correct answer D: Lead poisoning results in iron deficiency and microcytic anemia. Administration or intake of methotrexate, zidovudine, alcohol, and hydroxyurea can result in macrocytosis.

2. Which of the following conditions does not lead to Vitamin B12 deficiency?

   A. Gastric bypass surgery
   B. Vegetarian diet
   C. Imerslund-Gräsbeck Syndrome
   D. Mutation in *SLC19A2* gene
   E. Infection with Diphyllobothrium latum

Correct answer: D. Inherited mutation in *SLC19A2* gene, encoding a high-affinity *thiamine* transporter 1, results in thiamine-responsive megaloblastic anemia syndrome. Gastric bypass surgery can lead to development of B12 deficiency. Mutations in cubilin gene, which encodes the intrinsic factor-vitamin B12 receptor, result in hereditary megaloblastic anemia 1. Infection with *Diphyllobothrium latum* results in development of B12 deficiency.

References

1. Green R, Datta MA. Megaloblastic anemias: nutritional and other causes. Med Clin North Am. 2017;101(2):297–317.
2. Stouten K, Riedl JA, Droogendijk J, et al. Prevalence of potential underlying aetiology of macrocytic anaemia in Dutch general practice. BMC Fam Pract. 2016;17(1):113.
3. Borgna-Pignatti C, Azzalli M, Pedretti S. Thiamine-responsive megaloblastic anemia syndrome: long term follow-up. J Pediatr. 2009; 155(2):295–7.
4. Stamm RA, Houghton LA. Nutrient intake values for folate during pregnancy and lactation vary widely around the world. Nutrients. 2013; 5(10):3920–47.
5. Hesdorffer CS, Longo DL. Drug-induced megaloblastic anemia. N Engl J Med. 2015;373:17 nejm.org October 22.
6. Green R. Vitamin B12 deficiency from the perspective of a practicing hematologist. Blood. 2017;129(19):2603–11.
7. Gudgeon P, Cavalcanti R. Folate testing in hospital inpatients. Am J Med. 2015;128(1):56–9.
8. Green R, Mitra A. Folate, cobalamin, and megaloblastic anemias. In: Kaushansky K, Prchal JT, Burns LJ, Lichtman MA, Levi M, Linch DC, editors. Williams hematology. 10th ed. McGraw Hill; 2021.

Sideroblastic Anemia

11

Yulan Jin and Natasha M. Savage

Introduction

Sideroblastic anemia (SA) is a familial or congenital or acquired anemia, which represents a diverse group of disorders characterized by increased ring sideroblasts in bone marrow. Ring sideroblasts are erythroblasts with pathogenic iron-laden mitochondria encircling their nucleus. Morphologically, ring sideroblasts are defined by having a minimum of 5 siderotic granules covering at least one-third of the circumference of the nucleus of erythroblasts [1] (Fig. 11.1a). Ring sideroblasts should be distinguished from sideroblasts. The latter is iron deposition inside cytoplasm of erythroblasts, usually not riming nuclei and does not meet the above criteria to be called ring sideroblasts (Fig. 11.1b).

Y. Jin
Department of Pathology, H.Lee Moffitt Cancer Center and Research Institute, University of South Florida, Tampa, FL, USA

N. M. Savage (✉)
Department of Pathology, Medical College of Georgia, Augusta University, Augusta, GA, USA
e-mail: NSAVAGE@augusta.edu

L. Sokol, L. Zhang (eds.), *Non-Neoplastic Hematologic Disorders*,
https://doi.org/10.1007/978-3-031-62373-8_11

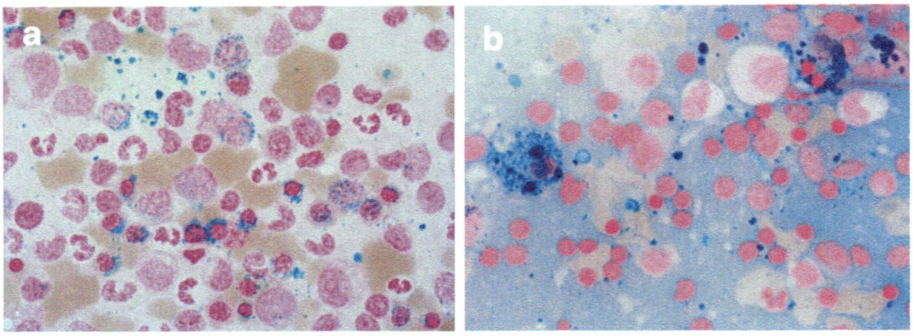

Fig. 11.1 (**a**, **b**) Bone marrow histomorphology in sideroblastic anemia [including ring sideroblasts. Left (**a**) and sideroblasts, right (**b**)]

Iron is the key element for heme synthesis. The structure of heme is ring-shaped molecular, which is made by 4 pyrroles connected by 4 methine bridges holding with an iron atom at the center of the ring. Heme is commonly (85%) synthesized in the cytoplasm and mitochondria of the erythroblast cells with multiple critical enzymes involved in its biosynthesis pathway (Fig. 11.2a). Multiple genetic and environmental factors, directly or indirectly contributing to defective heme biosynthesis and/or iron metabolism within mitochondria, can lead to ring sideroblasts and result in ineffective erythropoiesis.

There are several key enzymes involving heme synthesis: aminolevulinic acid synthase, porphobilinogen synthase, porphobilinogen deaminase, uroporphyrinogen III synthase, uroporphyrinogen decarboxylase, coproporphyrinogen oxidase, protoporphyrinogen oxidase, and ferrochelatase (Fig. 11.2a) [2].

The prevalence of SA (including both congenital and acquired) is rare, affecting fewer than 200,000 people in the United States [3]. Congenital SA (cSA) affects not only infants and children, but also adults with a variable degree of anemia, while acquired SA (aSA) occurs often among adults who have a diagnosis of myelodysplastic syndromes/neoplasms (MDS) or exposure to certain medications, metals, or minerals. There is a wide spectrum of natural history, clinical presentation, anemia severity, and prognosis among SA patients because of various pathogenesis. The treatment of SA largely depends on the underlying etiologies, but mainly relies on supportive care.

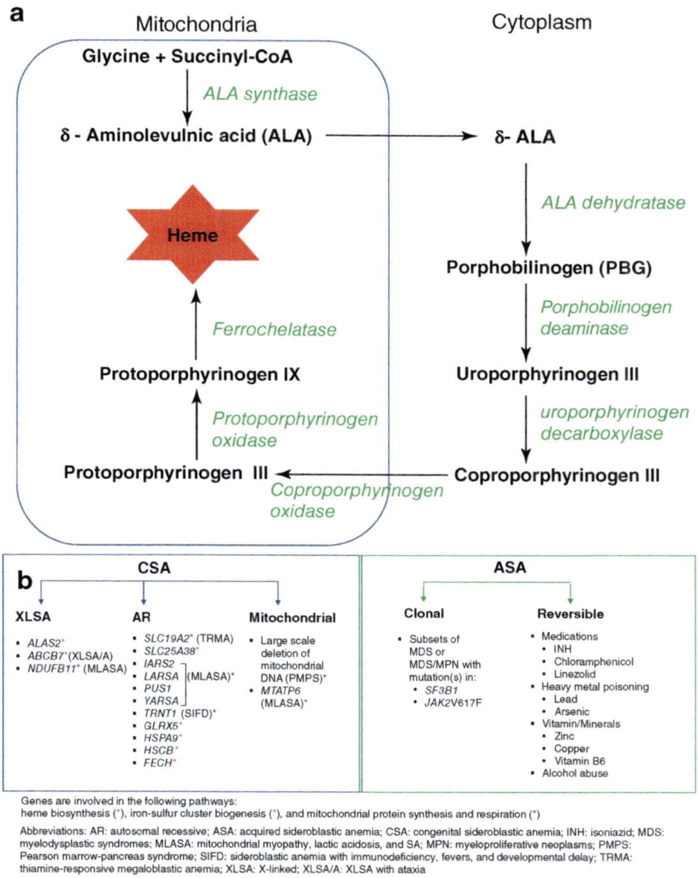

Fig. 11.2 (**a**) Heme synthase pathway. (**b**) Summary of pathogenesis of different subtypes of sideroblastic anemia. Genes are involved in the following pathways: heme biosynthesis (*), iron-sulfur cluster biogenesis (*), and mitochondrial protein synthesis and respiration (*). AR autosomal recessive, ASA acquired sideroblastic anemia, CSA congenital sideroblastic anemia, INH isoniazid, MDS myelodysplastic syndromes, MLASA mitochondrial myopathy, lactic acidosis, and SA, MPN myeloproliferative neoplasms, PMPS Pearson marrow-pancreas syndrome, SIFD sideroblastic anemia with immunodeficiency, fevers, and developmental delay, TRMA thiamine-responsive megaloblastic anemia, XLSA X-linked, XLSA/A XLSA with ataxia

Pathogenesis

The causes of SA can be congenital (cSA) or acquired (aSA), with the latter being vastly more common. Most of the causative factors are involved in the following three mitochondrial interrelated pathways: heme biosynthesis, iron-sulfur cluster biogenesis, and mitochondrial protein synthesis and respiration (Fig. 11.2b).

cSA

There are three ways of inheritance of cSA: X-linked (XLSA), autosomal recessive (ARCSA), and mitochondrial/maternal. cSA presents as either non-syndromic (with isolated anemia) or as syndromic disorders (involving other organ systems), with the former as more common.

XLSA is the most common inheritance mode, first described in the 1940s. Although XLSA typically affects males, nearly one-third of cases present among females mainly because of skewed X-chromosome inactivation.

- Mutations in *ALAS2* gene located on Xp11.21 chromosome are most commonly found in patients with cSA, representing 40% of all cSA cases. This type of cSA is non-syndromic. *ALAS2* encodes 5-aminolevulinate synthase, the first and rate-limiting enzyme in the heme biosynthesis pathway. More than 100 distinct mutations in *ALAS2* gene have been identified mainly at the catalytic domain, but also at the pyridoxal phosphate (active vitamin B6 cofactor) binding domain, promoter, and enhancer gene regions.
- Mutations in *SLC19A2* gene (1q23.3) lead to downregulation of cell membrane thiamine transporter, resulting in thiamine-responsive megaloblastic anemia. TRMA, also known as Rogers syndrome, is inherited in autosomal recessive fashion and comprises about 26% of all cSA. Thiamine is well-known as an important cofactor for enzymes involving cellular metabolism and DNA, RNA, and heme biosynthesis. Clinically, TRMA manifests with megaloblastic anemia, ringed

sideroblasts, progressive sensorineural hearing loss, and diabetes mellitus.

- *ABCB7* and *NDUFB11* are two less frequently mutated genes associated with syndromic forms of XLSA. *ABCB7* encodes an essential mitochondrial membrane transporter, through which iron-sulfur (Fe-S) clusters are transferred into the cytoplasm for assembling Fe-S cluster-containing proteins such as hemoglobin. *ABCB7* mutations are associated with "XLSA with ataxia" syndrome (XLSA/A) (PMID: 17192398). *NDUFB11* encodes NADH: ubiquinone oxidoreductase subunit B1 and is associated with syndrome of "mitochondrial myopathy, lactic acidosis, and SA" (MLASA) (PMID: 30588737).

ARCSA is the second most common subtype, representing 35% to 40% of all cSA cases.

- *ARCSA* gene, *SLC25A38* (3p22.1), encodes the transporter of glycine, an essential amino acid for producing heme synthesis enzymes. *SLC25A38* mutations occur among about 10% of cSA patients and is non-syndromic.
- Other rare ARCSA genes include syndromic types: *IARS2*, *LARS2*, *PUS1*, *YARS2* (all associated with MLASA), and *TRNT1* (*SA with immunodeficiency, fevers, and developmental delay*); and non-syndromic types: *GLRX5*, *HSPA9*, *HSCB*, and *FECH*.

Mitochondrially inherited forms constitute about 20% of all cSA cases.

- Large scale deletion of mitochondrial DNA is associated with Pearson syndrome, also named Pearson marrow-pancreas syndrome, characterized by severe SA, milder neutropenia and thrombocytopenia, pancreatic insufficiency, lactic acidosis, and failure to thrive from infancy or early childhood.
- In addition to the above-mentioned X-linked and ARCSA forms, a mitochondrial gene mutation, *MTATP6*, is also associated with the MLASA phenotype. *MTATP6* encodes ATPase6,

a component of mitochondrial respiratory chain complex. Anemia is typically severe and usually transfusion-dependent.

Acquired Sideroblastic Anemia (aSA)

Acquired SA is a diverse group that includes clonal and reversible forms.

- Ring sideroblasts are seen in some clonal hematopoietic disorders, specifically MDS and myelodysplastic/myeloproliferative neoplasms (MDS/MPN). A subtype of MDS with low blast count, MDS with ring sideroblasts, and single or multilineage dysplasia with RS phenotype and low blasts (<5%) are often associated with mutation in the *SF3B1* gene (>90% cases), which forms a new sub-entity under the 5th edition of WHO classification, namely MDS with *SF3B1* mutation with better clinical outcome when compared with other MDS subtype [4]. Cases with high blasts (>5%), presence of del(5q), monosomy 7/del(7q), complex karyotype, or *biallele-TP53* mutations should be excluded from the entity (MDS-*SF3B1* mutated). *SF3B1* with *JAK2*V617F or *CALR* or *MPL* co-mutations are more commonly associated with MDS/MPN with *SF3B1* mutation and thrombocytosis according to the new WHO classification [4]. *SF3B1* encodes an mRNA splicing component, where defects may affect erythroid-iron handling pathway and induce RS in human cells.
- Reversible aSA is caused by various environmental factors, including medications (such as isoniazid [INH], linezolid, and chloramphenicol), heavy metal poisoning (lead, arsenic), overdose or deficiency of vitamins and/or minerals (zinc, copper, vitamin B6), and alcohol abuse. These factors are directly or indirectly involved in the mechanisms of disturbed heme biosynthesis and ring sideroblast formation. For instance, both INH and alcohol consumption can impair heme synthesis through altering metabolism of pyridoxine and thus impairing the function of the ALAS2 enzyme. Chloramphenicol and linezolid can

impair heme biosynthesis with their dose-dependent mitochondrial toxicity and their suppressive role on mitochondrial protein synthesis. As an essential cofactor for superoxide dismutase, copper deficiency can suppress activity of this mitochondrial enzyme and then lead to mitochondrial iron accumulation. Zinc acts as a catalytic cofactor for the enzyme ALSL in heme synthesis and plays a competitive role in incorporation of iron to protoporphyrin and reduces absorption of copper. Lead poisoning has been associated with inhibition of various enzymes within heme synthesis pathway including FECH and ALAD, leading to increased ring sideroblasts.

- In addition to the above-mentioned well-established ASA-related medications, some others are also reported in small sets of studies, including busulfan, cycloserine, fusidic acid, melphalan, penicillamine, pyrazinamide, and trientine.

Diagnosis

SA should be considered as a differential diagnosis of unexplained anemias when other more common forms, for example, iron deficiency and thalassemia, are excluded. Identification of RS in bone marrow–aspirate smear by Prussian blue–iron staining provides a definite diagnosis of SA (Fig. 11.1). A recent molecular study shows that the presence of an *SF3B1* gene mutation is strongly associated with RS in MDS bone marrow [5].

Given the large diversity and distinction among the SA subtypes which determine specific managements, subclassification of SA will be based on all of the following factors: clinical features (age, gender, family history, and syndromic features); laboratory/pathology data (complete blood count, red blood cell film, and bone marrow morphology); and genetic testing (for diagnostic algorithm, see Fig. 11.3).

For the majority of reversible aSA, a bone marrow biopsy to identify the presence of ring sideroblasts is usually not required because of the reversibility of anemia following correction of underlying causes. However, when cSA and clonal SA (e.g., MDS

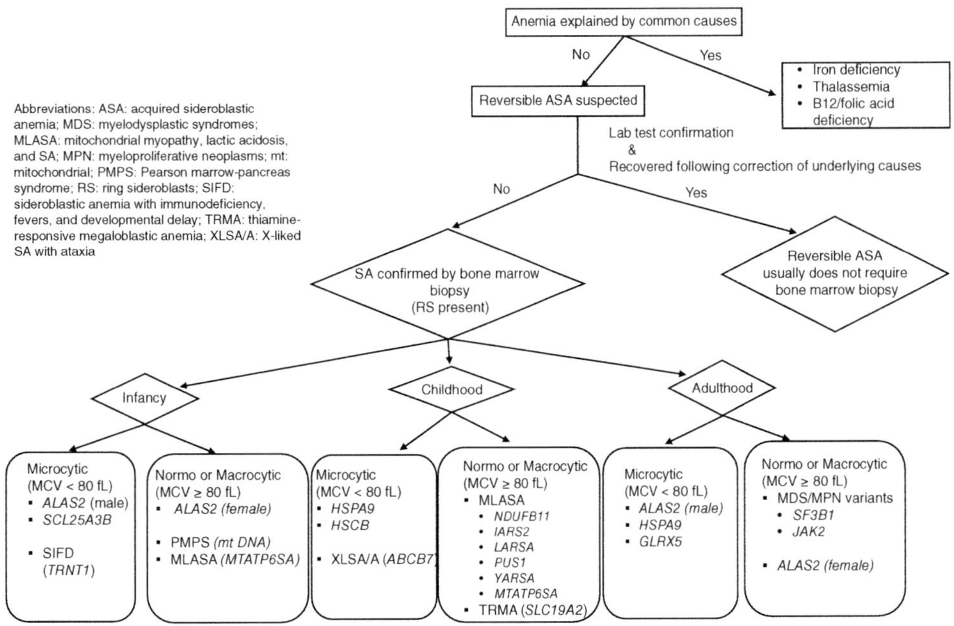

Fig. 11.3 Diagnostic algorithm for sideroblastic anemia. ASA acquired sideroblastic anemia, MDS myelodysplastic syndromes, MLASA mitochondrial myopathy, lactic acidosis, and SA, MPN myeloproliferative neoplasms, mt mitochondrial, PMPS Pearson marrow-pancreas syndrome, RS ring sideroblasts, SIFD sideroblastic anemia with immunodeficiency, fevers, and developmental delay, TRMA thiamine-responsive megaloblastic anemia, XLSA/A X-liked SA with ataxia

or MDS/MPN) are suspected in clinic, a bone marrow biopsy, in conjunction with cytogenetics and a next-generation sequencing study, is necessary to establish diagnosis and subclassification.

Differential Diagnosis

Iron deficiency anemia: SA often (but not exclusively) presents as microcytic anemia. Obtaining a clinical history and laboratory iron profile would be helpful in differentiation between the two entities. The presence of Pappenheimer bodies on peripheral blood smear may favor SA over iron deficiency anemia. Routine Prussian blue–iron staining on bone marrow aspirate smear would provide a definite clue.

Megaloblastic anemia: A small subset of SA (mutations in mitochondria, *SLC19A2*, *PUS1*, *YARS2*, and *TRNT1*) presents as macrocytic anemia. In addition to laboratory evaluations, hypersegmented neutrophils in peripheral blood and megaloblastic changes rather than ring sideroblasts in the bone marrow are typical features of megaloblastic anemia, such as giant bands caused by deficiency of vitamin B12 or folic acid. Careful clinical inquiry and ancillary tests, including a next-generation sequencing study, would be useful for distinguishing cSA and aSA from a vast variety of etiologies, leading to megaloblastic anemia, for example, drug-induced megaloblastic anemia.

Erythropoietic protoporphyria (EPP): This disorder is characterized by deficiency of ferrochelatase, the enzyme-catalyzing final step of heme synthesis (iron incorporation) in mitochondria. Although mild microcytic anemia and ring sideroblasts can be detected in EPP, extreme sun sensitivity is the significant and unique symptom of EPP.

Prognosis

The prognosis of SA varies based on the underlying causes. In secondary aSA, the prognosis will usually be good when the overdose or deficiency is corrected. However, in patients with aSA due to myeloid malignancies, these disorders usually dictate long-term prognosis. In a subset of patients with X-linked SA, the prognosis can be improved by proper pyridoxine replacement therapy and iron-overload management with iron chelation. However, in some patients with severe transfusion-dependent SA, iron overload may not be easily controlled resulting in poor prognosis.

Treatment

Treating anemia depends on the underlying etiologies, severity, and associated symptoms, and thus, it mainly includes supportive care [6]. The goal of therapy is to achieve a safe hemoglobin level and reduce symptoms associated with anemia.

- For secondary aSA, withdrawal of a drug (e.g., INH) or supplementation in deficiencies (e.g., vitamin B6 or copper) can fully reverse anemia.
- Vitamin B6 (pyridoxine) therapy is effective in subset of XLSA patients; thiamin is used to treat TRMA.
- MDS/MPN variants: erythroid maturation agent (luspatercept) may be used in low-risk MDS to improve anemia.
- Blood transfusions are indicated in all symptomatic patients with cSA or aSA along with chronic iron chelation therapy to control iron overload.
- Genetic counseling and testing should be recommended for first relatives of cSA patients.

Promising Clinical Studies

- H3B-8800, a novel-identified splicing modulator, has demonstrated therapeutic potential in myeloid disorders harboring *SF3B1* mutations. It is currently under a phase I clinical trial (NCT02841540).
- Antitumor necrosis factor therapy, along with infliximab and etanercept, has showed promising effects among four patients with SA *with immunodeficiency, fevers, and developmental*

delay by suppressing fevers and inflammation and reducing the need for transfusion.

- Allogeneic hematopoietic stem cell transplantation has showed curative effect in a very small number of congenital SA patients ($n = 2$), but this procedure needs to be performed before significant iron overload of organs such as liver, heart, and pancreas occurs.

Caveats

1. Sideroblastic anemia can be inherited or acquired. The X-linked SA is predominant hereditary mode, followed by autosomal recessive and mitochondrial/ maternal pattern.
2. The most often X-linked mutations occur in the ALAS2 gene on Xp11.21, which is responsive to B6 therapy in 40% of all cSA cases
3. Mutations of *SLC19A2* gene are associated with thiamine-responsive megaloblastic anemia (TRMA), also known as Rogers syndrome. However, bone marrow demonstrates the presence of ring sideroblasts.
4. aSA can be associated with drugs such as lead/arsenic poisoning, copper deficiency, and alcohol abuse, which is usually reversible after cessation of exposure as well as MDS or MDS/ MPN, often associated with *SF3B1* mutation.

Board Questions

1. Ring sideroblasts are erythroblasts with pathogenic iron-laden mitochondria and morphologically are formed when:

   A. More than 5 siderotic granules are in the cytoplasm.
   B. Fewer than 5 siderotic granules but no perinuclear distribution.
   C. More than 5 siderotic granules in a perinuclear position, covering at least one-third of the nuclear circumference.
   D. More than 5 siderotic granules in a perinuclear position, covering at least one-half of the nuclear circumference.

Answer: C. Confirming ring sideroblasts requires more than 5 siderotic granules in a perinuclear position, covering at least one-third of the nuclear circumference. Other answers are inaccurate or incorrect.

2. The presence of which gene mutation is strongly associated with ring sideroblasts in MDS bone marrows:

   A. *JAK2*
   B. *CALR*
   C. *NPM1*
   D. *SF3B1*

Answer D. *SF3B1* mutation is strongly associated with the presence of ring sideroblasts in patients with MDS.

References

1. Cazzola M, Invernizzi R. Ring sideroblasts and sideroblastic anemias. Haematologica. 2011;96(6):789–92. PMID: 21632840.
2. Fujiwara T, Harigae H. Molecular pathophysiology and genetic mutations in congenital sideroblastic anemia. Free Radic Biol Med. 2019;133:179–85. PMID: 30098397.
3. Abu-Zeinah G, DeSancho MT. Understanding sideroblastic anemia: an overview of genetics, epidemiology, pathophysiology, and current therapeutic options. J Blood Med. 2020;11:305–18.
4. Khoury JD, Solary E, Abla O, et al. The 5th edition of the World Health Organization classification of haematolymphoid tumours: myeloid and histiocytic/dendritic neoplasms. Leukemia. 2022;36(7):1703–19.
5. Rodriguez-Sevilla JJ, Calvo X, Arenillas L. Causes and pathophysiology of acquired sideroblastic anemia. Genes (Basel). 2022;13(9):1562.
6. Bottomley SS. Sideroblastic anemias: diagnosis and management. In: Post TW, editor. UpToDate. Wolters Kluwer. Accessed 28 Nov 2023.

Hemoglobin Disorders 12

Ziad Abuhelwa, Jinjun Cheng,
and Julie Li

Hemoglobin disorders are a group of genetic disorders that affect the structure and production of hemoglobin. They can be either quantitative, with decreased production of globin chains, as in thalassemia, or qualitative, with structural abnormalities in the affected globin chains, as in sickle cell syndromes and hemoglobin C, E, and M disorders.

Hemoglobin (Hb) is a tetramer of two pairs of globin polypeptide chains connected to iron-containing tetrapyrroles. A series of normal hemoglobins is created during the embryonic, fetal, and postnatal periods. Embryonic hemoglobins (Gower I $\zeta_2\varepsilon_2$, Gower II $\alpha_2\varepsilon_2$, and Portland $\zeta_2\gamma_2$) are detectable during the earliest stages of embryogenesis. By approximately the 14th week of gestation, embryonic hemoglobins are completely replaced by fetal Hb (Hb F $\alpha_2\gamma_2$). At the age of 6 months, production of β-globin chain starts, and by the first year of life, normal adult hemoglobins will

Z. Abuhelwa
Department of Hematology/Oncology, Moffitt Cancer Center/University of South Florida, Tampa, FL, USA

J. Cheng
Department of Pathology and Laboratory Medicine, Children's National Hospital, Washington, DC, USA

J. Li (✉)
Department of Pathology, Moffitt Cancer Center, Tampa, FL, USA
e-mail: julie.li@moffitt.org

L. Sokol, L. Zhang (eds.), *Non-Neoplastic Hematologic Disorders*,
https://doi.org/10.1007/978-3-031-62373-8_12

be Hb A ($\alpha_2\beta_2$), making up about 95% to 98%; Hb A2 ($\alpha_2\delta_2$) makes up 2% to 3%; and Hb F ($\alpha_2\gamma_2$) makes less than 2%.

Diagnosis of hemoglobin disorders typically involves clinical history with a combination of tests: [1] complete blood count and peripheral blood smears. A complete blood count can suggest anemia and other abnormalities that may be indicative of red blood cell (RBC) disorder. Peripheral blood smear is a powerful tool to assess blood cell morphology; [2] Hb electrophoresis and high-performance liquid chromatography (HPLC); [3] molecular studies to detect specific mutations associated with certain Hb disorders; and [4] newborn screening for certain Hb disorders shortly after birth.

Thalassemia

Introduction

There are approximately 80 million to 90 million thalassemia carriers worldwide, with around 60,000 affected individuals born each year. While the exact prevalence of thalassemia in the United States is unknown, it is estimated to affect 2000 individuals annually [1]. Thalassemia is more common in African and Mediterranean countries, India, Southeast Asia, and China, although its epidemiology has changed because of immigration and shifting demographics.

Pathogenesis

Thalassemia is an inherited disorder caused by the deletion of a large part or all of a gene, or by a small deletion or other mutation of a gene. The production of α-globin chains occurs from genes located on chromosome 16, and production of β-globin chains occurs from genes located on chromosome 11. If there is a decreased synthesis in β-globin chains, excess α-globin chains will be formed, and vice versa. Intramedullary, the excess globin chains precipitate in the RBC precursors forming inclusion bodies, leading to apoptosis of these cells and resulting in ineffective erythropoiesis. Additionally, the excess globin chains alter the mechanical prosperities and the stability of RBCs membrane, causing extramedullary hemolysis. The greater the imbalance between α and β chains, the more severe the disease.

α-thalassemia

α-thalassemia occurs if there is a decrease in α-globin chain synthesis. Deletional mutations (90%) in all or part of the α-globin gene or nondeletional abnormalities (10%) can lead to α-thalassemia. Normally, there are four α-globin gene loci on chromosome 16. The clinical presentation and severity depend on the number of affected α-globin genes (Table 12.1).

Table 12.1 α-Thalassemia

Phenotype	Genotype	Features	Diagno	Treatment
Silent	−α/αα	Asymptomatic	Normal Hb Normal to slightly low MCV Normal Hb electrophoresis and HPLC Molecular studies	None
Trait	trans −α/−α cis αα/–	Mild microcytic hypochromic anemia Can be mistaken for IDA	Low Hb Low MCV <75 fL, low MCH Normal Hb electrophoresis and HPLC Molecular studies	None
Hb H disease (minor)	−α/–	Moderate-to-severe hemolytic anemia Ineffective erythropoiesis Splenomegaly Iron loading Anemia can be aggravated by infection, pregnancy, and oxidative stress Risk for aplastic crisis with parvovirus B19	Hb 7–11 g/dL MCV 50–65 fL Hemolytic anemia Hb electrophoresis and HPLC: high Hb H 5–40% Molecular studies	Transfusion if needed

(continued)

Table 12.1 (continued)

Phenotype	Genotype	Features	Diagno	Treatment
Hb Barts disease (major)	–/–	Hydrops fetalis Fetal death	Severely low Hb Low MCV Hydrops fetalis Hb electrophoresis and HPLC: high Hb Barts and H; absent Hb F, A, and A2 Molecular studies	In utero transfusion

Hb hemoglobin, *HPLC* high-performance liquid chromatography, *IDA* iron deficiency anemia, *MCV* mean corpuscular volume, *MCH* mean corpuscular hemoglobin, *PBS* peripheral blood smear, *RBCs* red blood cells

Treatment for α-thalassemia depends on the clinical severity of the disease. In silent carriers and those with the α-thalassemia trait, usually no treatment is required. In Hb H disease, most individuals are symptomatic at birth but typically do not require regular transfusions. Intermittent transfusions may be needed for symptomatic management or under stressful conditions; hence it is called *nontransfusion-dependent thalassemia (NTDT)*. Among some patients, the disease can deteriorate, requiring regular transfusions, and now will be called *transfusion-dependent thalassemia (TDT)*. Hb Barts disease is a *transfusion-dependent thalassemia*; intrauterine and regular transfusions can help reverse the anemia, preventing growth restriction and hydrops fetalis. The improvement in survival is due to the advancement of intrauterine interventions and curative stem cell transplantation.

β-Thalassemia

β-Thalassemia occurs if there is a decrease in the synthesis of β-globin chains, often resulting from mutations in the β-globin gene. There are 2 β-globin loci on chromosome 11. The clinical presentation depends on whether the mutations reduce β-globin production (β^+) or abolish it (β^0) (Table 12.2).

Treatment of β-thalassemia depends on the clinical severity. In β-thalassemia minor, usually no interventions are needed other

Table 12.2 β-Thalassemia

Phenotype	Genotype	Features	Diagnosis	Treatment
Minor (trait)	β^0/β β^+/β	Mild anemia	Normal or low Hb Low MCV PBS: target cells Hb electrophoresis and HPLC: **High Hb A2 (>3.5%)**, normal Hb A and Hb F Molecular studies	None
Intermediate	Variable: mild forms of β^+/β^+ or $\beta0/\beta^+$	Moderate anemia: severity may worsen with age	Low Hb Low MCV Hb electrophoresis and HPLC: **Hb A2 variable Hb F up to 100%** Molecular studies	Transfusion if needed
Major	β^+/β^+ β^0/β^+ β^0/β^0	Severe hemolytic anemia during first year of life Ineffective erythropoiesis Extramedullary hematopoiesis Splenomegaly Bone deformities Iron overload	Hb <6 g/dL Low MCV PBS: anisopoikilocytosis, microcytosis, target cells, nucleated red cells Hb electrophoresis and HPLC**: absent Hb A, Hb A2 variable, Hb F > 95%** Molecular studies	Transfusion

Hb hemoglobin, *HPLC* high-performance liquid chromatography, *MCV* mean corpuscular volume, *PBS* peripheral blood smear

than partner testing and genetic counseling. In more severe cases, as in β-thalassemia major, usually regular blood transfusions, at 2- to 4-week intervals, are needed to maintain a Hb of 9–10.5 g/dL (*transfusion-dependent thalassemia, TDT*). β-thalassemia intermedia may require intermittent blood transfusions if Hb drops with acute infections, surgery, or pregnancy (*non-transfusion-dependent thalassemia, NTDT*). Hydroxyurea has shown promise in improving Hb levels and disease-related complications among patients with *non-transfusion-dependent thalas-*

semia [4]. Stem cell transplantation is still the only curative option. Gene therapy with gene addition or gene editing may be a curative option in selected patients, but cost may be prohibitive for patients living in countries with lower socioeconomic status; clinical trials with novel agents are undergoing [5].

Sickle Cell Hemoglobinopathy

Introduction

Sickle cell hemoglobinopathy is characterized by the presence of Hb S (β^S) that results from a genetic mutation at codon 6 in the β-globin allele, which substitutes valine for glutamic acid. It can manifest as either sickle cell trait (Hb AS) or sickle cell anemia (Hb SS). The β^S gene could be inherited with another β-chain variant, leading to a range of mixed heterozygous hemoglobinopathies. The term *sickle cell disease* includes sickle cell trait (Hb AS) and sickle cell anemia (Hb SS) and a range of mixed heterozygous hemoglobinopathies, such as Hb S combined with β-thalassemia (Hb $S\beta^0$ or Hb $S\beta^+$), hemoglobin sickle C (SC) disease (Hb SC), and other variants (Table 12.3).

Table 12.3 Sickle cell disease

	Sickle trait	Sickle cell anemia	HbS combined with other variant Hb		
	Hb AS	Hb SS	Hb $S\beta^0$	Hb $S\beta^+$	Hb SC
Severity	Asymptomatic	Severe	Moderate to severe	Mild to moderate	Mild to moderate
Hb (g/dL)	Normal	6–9	6–9	9–12	10–15
MCV (fL)	Normal	Normal	<70	<75	75-normal
Reticulocyte	Normal	5%-20%	5%-20%	3%-10%	5–10%
Hb S	40%	>90%	>80%	>60%	50%
Hb A	60%	0	0	10%-30%	0
Hb A2	<3.5%	<3.5%	>3.5%	>3.5%	0
Hb C	0	0	0	0	50%

Hb hemoglobin, *MCV* mean corpuscular volume

Pathogenesis

Among patients with sickle cell trait (Hb AS), β^S has less affinity than normal β for α chains. Instead of equal amounts of Hb A and Hb S, typical cases show 60% Hb A and 35% to 40% of Hb S. Abnormal Hb S causes rigid RBCs with a shorter lifespan, increased susceptibility to hemolysis, and accelerated turnover, leading to the characteristic anemia. α-globin exhibits stronger affinity for normal β-globin than mutant β^S-globin. In alpha thalassemia, relative alpha globin deficiency intensifies this effect, lowering Hb S levels (<30–35%) in coexisting HBAS with α-thalassemia. Conversely, β-thalassemia reduces normal β-globin quantitatively, leading to normal α-globin excess. Additional α-globin binds to β^S-globin, increasing Hb S level (>50%), and maybe slightly elevated HbA2 when HbAS coexists with β-thalassemia.

Patients with sickle cell anemia (Hb SS) have predominant Hb S, a small proportion of Hb A2, variable Hb F, and absent Hb A. The Hb S percentage correlates inversely with Hb F percentage. Newborns are asymptomatic with major Hb F, and begin to have symptoms after 6 months. Hb S has decreased oxygen affinity, and under stressful situations, such as hypoxia, acidosis, dehydration, or cold, it polymerizes to form elongated fibers, leading to distortion of the affected RBCs and their membranes, ultimately causing hemolysis.

Coexistence of α-thalassemia trait with Hb SS reduces mean corpuscular volume (MCV) and Hb S percentage, prolonging RBC survival. Hb H with Hb SS reduces Hb S (10% to 25%). The clinical impact can be complicated due to improved RBC survival and hemolysis.

Sickle cell/β-thalassemia is a compound heterozygous state for β^S with either β^+ or β^0 thalassemia. There is variable Hb A in Hb $S\beta^+$ and complete loss of Hb A in Hb $S\beta^0$. Individuals present milder anemia with decreased mean corpuscular volume (MCV), mean corpuscular hemoglobin (MCH), and mean corpuscular hemoglobin concentration (MCHC). The clinical presentations depend on the HbA level. Hb $S\beta^0$ presents similar symptoms to HbSS, while Hb $S\beta^+$ typical results in moderate anemia and less frequent pain crisis than Hb SS.

Sickle cell/Hb C disease (Hb SC) is the consequence of coinheritance of β^S and β^c genes. There is 50% of Hb S and 50% of Hb C, without Hb A (no normal β-chain). Patients with Hb SC have mild chronic hemolytic anemia and intermittent sickle cell crisis, less frequent than Hb SS. Hb SC is a hypercoagulable state with increased venous thromboembolism and arterial thrombosis.

Diagnosis

Diagnosis of sickle cell disease is based on hemoglobin electrophoresis, HPLC, or molecular study. Peripheral blood smear is useful for detection of Hb SS (Fig. 12.1), especially at crisis. The clinical severity of SCD depends on the amount of Hb S. People with sickle cell trait are usually asymptomatic. However, spontaneous sickle cell formation can occur in renal papillae, leading to renal papillary necrosis and episodes of hematuria. Renal medullary carcinoma is highly associated with Hb AS. Definitive diagnosis of the most common hemoglobinopathies is usually determined using Hb electrophoresis or HPLC (Fig. 12.2).

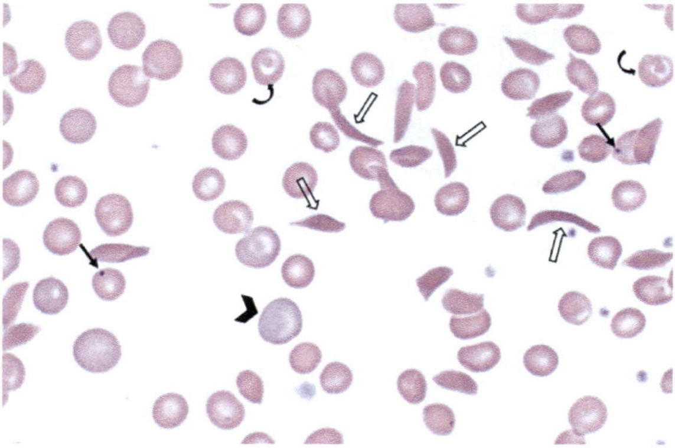

Fig. 12.1 Peripheral blood smear (1000×) of a patient with sickle cell anemia (Hb SS) shows sickle cells (hollow arrows), Howell-Jolly body (arrows), target cells (curved arrows), and polychromasia (arrowhead)

a

b

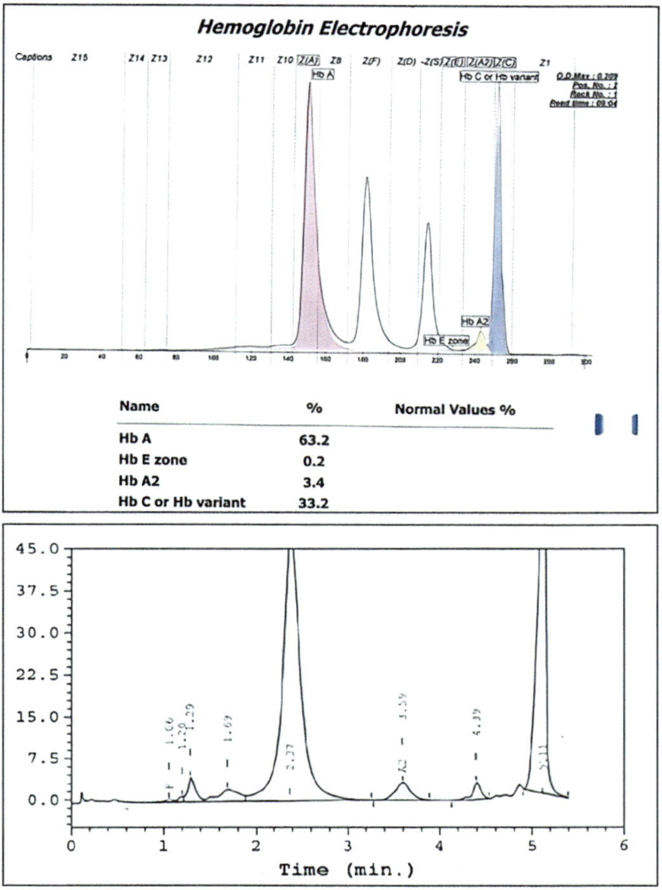

Fig. 12.2 (**a**) Capillary electrophoresis electropherogram (Sebia Capillary 3) from an adult, a patient with Hb AC, showing hemoglobin A, A2, and Hb C. The small peak Hb E represents a small amount of degraded hemoglobin C. (**b**) High-performance liquid chromatograph chromatogram (Bio-Rad Variant II). Confirmation of Hb AC in an adult with Hb A and Hb C suggests Hb C trait

The clinical hallmarks of Hb SS are hemolytic anemia and vaso-occulsion. HbS polymerization increases RBCs' adherence to the vascular endothelium and decreases nitric oxide availability, causing vaso-occlusion and vasoconstriction, which can lead to splenic, pulmonary, pituitary, cerebral, retinal, renal, and bone infarcts and to priapism.

Treatment

1. **Disease-modifying therapies**

   (a) **Hydroxyurea:** can increase Hb F and reticulocyte count and decrease white blood cells (WBC), neutrophils, and platelet count as a consequence of the cytotoxic effect, resulting in decreased vaso-occlusive events [6].
   (b) **L-glutamine:** an antioxidant that can reduce RBCs susceptibility to oxidative stress [7].
   (c) **Crizanlizumab:** monoclonal antibody against P-selection (adhesion molecule); interferes with sickled RBCs adhesion on the endothelium [8].
   (d) **Voxelotor:** Hb S polymerization inhibitor by increasing Hb S oxygen affinity. In the phase III clinical trial, 1500 mg of oral voxelotor administered daily showed a significant increase in Hb level and acute coronary syndrome reduction in hemolysis markers compared to placebo [9].

2. **RBC Transfusion**
Acute Transfusion

   (a) **Simple transfusion** (to correct acute anemia if Hb drops >2 g/dL from baseline) such as in red cell aplasia, splenic or hepatic sequestration, mild acute coronary syndrome, complicated painful crisis, or acute blood loss anemia.
   (b) **Red cell exchange** (to decrease Hb S < 30% and to keep target Hb at 9–10 g/dL) such as in acute stroke, acute mul-

tiorgan failure, acute intrahepatic cholestasis, and acute ocular vaso-occlusive events.

Chronic transfusion: to keep Hb S < 30% and Hb from 9 to 10 g/dL.

3. **Supportive and Preventive Measures**

   (a) Management of acute and chronic pain.
   (b) Vaccinations: influenza annually, pneumococcal every 5 years, meningococcal, and hepatitis A and B vaccines.
   (c) Screening and managing acute and chronic complications.

4. **Curative therapies: hematopoietic** stem cell transplantation has been the only approved curative therapy for patients with sickle cell disease until now. Recently, FDA approved two different gene-based cells therapies for patients with hemoglobinopathies. Exagamglogene autotemcel (Casgevy) therapy is based on autologous stem cell transplantation using ex vivo genetically modified CD34+ cell population of hematopoietic stem cells and progenitor cells edited by CRISPR/Cas9 at the erythroid-specific enhancer region of the transcription factor BCL11A, which is a critical HbF silencer [10]. Gene editing of the enhancer results in downregulation of BCL11A, leading to increased production of HbF in mature erythrocytes. Exagamglogene autotemcel is FDA-approved for patients 12 years of age and older with transfusion-dependent beta-thalassemia and sickle cell disease.

Lovotibeglogene autotemcel (Lyfgenia) is an autologous stem cell transplantation-based gene therapy using lentiviral vector with insertion of a genetically modified normal beta-globin gene (substitution of threonine to glutamine at amino acid position 87), which becomes a part of HbA^{T87Q} [11]. Erythrocytes containing this modified HbA have a lower propensity for sickling and vaso-occlusion. This therapy is FDA-approved for the treatment of patients 12 years of age and older with sickle cell disease and a history of vaso-occlusive events.

Other Hemoglobin Disorders

1. **Hereditary persistence of fetal hemoglobin (HPFH):** Patients with HPFH present a significantly increased amount of Hb F in adulthood with normal Hb A2. HPFH can be categorized into two groups: (1) deletional HPFH: caused the variable length of deletion in δ and β genes leading to decreased/absent β globin and increased γ-globin synthesis with a pancellular homogenous Hb F distribution. (2) Nondeletional HPFHs are a heterogeneous group of disorders, with increased Hb F heterocellular distribution. Heterocellular distribution can also be seen in β thalassemia and βδ thalassemia. Individuals with homozygous HPFH may show 100% Hb F, and with heterozygous HPFH typically show 15% to 25% Hb F [12]. Patients are asymptomatic in either heterozygous or homozygous HPFH state. Patients with coinheritance of Hb S and HPFH experience fewer sickle cell disease-related complications.
2. **Hemoglobin C (〈$_2$®$_2$ $^{(6Glu\text{-}lys)}$):** ®-globin chain variant characterized by lysine amino acid substitution for glutamic acid at position 6 of the ®-globin chain. The clinical severity is variable (Table 12.4).
3. **Hemoglobin E (〈$_2$®$_2$ $^{(26Glu\text{-}lys)}$):** ®-globin chain variant similar to Hb C characterized by lysine amino acid substitution, at position 26, for glutamic acid (Table 12.4).
4. **Hemoglobin M disorder:** autosomal dominant hereditary disorder of hemoglobin resulting in methemoglobinemia. Variety of mutations usually due to tyrosine amino acid substitutions in 〈, β, or ©-globin chains, lead to iron oxidation from ferrous (Fe^{+2}) to ferric (Fe^{+3}) heme and make the oxidized variant chain nonfunctional for oxygen transport. Affected patients usually present with asymptomatic cyanosis and slate-gray or brownish skin. Serum Hb will be normal or high, but methemoglobin level will be elevated (usually <30%). Hereditary methemoglobinemia should be distinguished from other congenital and acquired methemoglobinemias as no treatment is needed. The cyanosis is not reversible with vitamin C or methylene blue, and patients will have normal life expectancy.

Table 12.4 Common Hb C and Hb E disorders

Phenotype	Genotype	Features
Hb C disorders		
Hb C trait	A/C	Asymptomatic Normal Hb Normal or low MCV Hb C 45–50%
Hb C homozygosity	C/C	Mild hemolytic anemia, gallstones, splenomegaly Normal-to-mild low Hb Low MCV Hb C almost 100%
Hb C/β--thalassemia	C/β^+ C/β^0	Thalassemia intermedia: moderate-to-severe hemolytic, gallstones, splenomegaly Hb 7–10 g/dL Low MCV Hb C > Hb A
Hb SC disease	S/C	HbSC Hb C 50%, Hb S 50%
Hb E disorders		
Hb E trait	A/E	Asymptomatic Normal-to-low MCV Hb E 30–35%
Hb E homozygosity	E/E	Asymptomatic Low MCV Hb E 90%
Hb E/ β-thalassemia	E/β^+ E/β^0	Variable presentation: thalassemia intermedia or major (TDT or NTDT) Low Hb Low MCV Hb E 40–85%, Hb F 10–60%

Hb hemoglobin, *MCV* mean corpuscular volume, *NTDT* non-transfusion-dependent Thalassemia, *SCD* sickle cell disease, *TDT* transfusion-dependent thalassemia

5. **Hemoglobin variants with altered oxygen affinity:** alteration in ⟨- or β-globin chains can result in Hb variants with either high or low oxygen affinity. High oxygen affinity Hb variants cause left shift in the oxygen-dissociation curve and relative tissue hypoxia, leading to increased erythropoietin and secondary polycythemia. By contrast, low oxygen affinity Hb

variants cause right shift in oxygen-dissociation curve and affected individuals have asymptomatic anemia and cyanosis. Molecular studies are helpful in establishing the diagnosis. No treatment is required in either situation.

Promising Clinical Studies

NA.

Caveats

1. α-thalassemia occurs because of gene mutation or alteration in the α-globin gene, leading to decrease in α-globin chain synthesis. The entity manifests with various phenotypes (silent, trait, Hb-H, Hb-Barts disease).
2. β-Thalassemia often results from mutations in the β-globin gene, leading to a decrease in the synthesis of β-globin chains. The entity includes three phenotypes: minor, intermediate, and major.
3. Mildly elevated Hb A2 (>3.5%) is observed in β thalassemia trait by Hb electrophoresis and HPLC along with normal Hb A and Hb F and microcytic anemia.
4. Hb SC is a hypercoagulable state with increased venous thromboembolism and arterial thrombosis.

Board Questions

1. Which therapy has not been approved for patients with sickle cell disease:

   A. Voxelotor
   B. Hydroxyurea
   C. Crizanlizumab
   D. L-glycin
   E. Lovotibeglogene autotemcel

Answer: L-glutamine, not L-glycin, has been FDA-approved for adult and pediatric patients, age 5 and older, to decrease severe complications associated with sickle cell disease. L glutamine reduces red cell oxidative injury by improving the redox potential of nicotinamide adenine dinucleotide (NAD). Voxelotor, hydroxyurea, crizanlizumab, and lovotibeglogene autotemcel have been FDA-approved for management of sickle cell disease.

2. Which complication of HbSS disease requires therapy with exchange transfusions?

   A. Chronic renal insufficiency
   B. Sickle cell pain crisis
   C. Acute CVA
   D. Avascular hip necrosis
   E. Chronic osteomyelitis

Answer: Acute CVA is an indication for exchange transfusions. Randomized controlled studies have shown that a transfusion target of HbS $\leq$30% (compared with no transfusion) is effective in reducing incidence rates of CVA. Other complications of sickle cell disease such as chronic renal insufficiency, sickle cell pain crisis, avascular hip necrosis, and chronic osteomyelitis can be managed with a simple blood transfusion and supportive care including pain medications, antibiotics, IV fluids, antihypertensive therapy, elective surgical procedures, etc.

References

1. Weatherall DJ. The thalassaemias. BMJ. 1997;314(7095):1675–8.
2. Cohen AR, Galanello R, Pennell DJ, Cunningham MJ, Vichinsky E. Thalassemia. Hematology. 2004;2004(1):14–34.
3. Schrier SL, Bunyaratvej A, Khuhapinant A, Fucharoen S, Aljurf M, Snyder LM, et al. The unusual pathobiology of hemoglobin constant spring red blood cells. Blood. 1997;89(5):1762–9.
4. Cappellini MD, Viprakasit V, Taher AT, Georgiev P, Kuo KHM, Coates T, et al. A phase 3 trial of luspatercept in patients with transfusion-dependent β-thalassemia. New Engl J Med. 382(13):1219–31.

5. Thompson AA, et al. Gene therapy in patients with transfusion-dependent β-thalassemia. N Engl J Med. 2018;378(16):1479–93.
6. Charache S, Terrin ML, Moore RD, Dover GJ, Barton FB, Eckert SV, et al. Effect of hydroxyurea on the frequency of painful crises in sickle cell anemia. Investigators of the Multicenter Study of Hydroxyurea in Sickle Cell Anemia. N Engl J Med. 1995;332(20):1317–22.
7. Niihara Y, Miller ST, Kanter J, Lanzkron S, Smith WR, Hsu LL, et al. A phase 3 trial of l-glutamine in sickle cell disease. New Engl J Med. 2018;379(3):226–35.
8. Ataga KI, Kutlar A, Kanter J, Liles D, Cancado R, Friedrisch J, et al. Crizanlizumab for the prevention of pain crises in sickle cell disease. N Engl J Med. 2017;376(5):429–39.
9. Vichinsky E, Hoppe CC, Ataga KI, Ware RE, Nduba V, El-Beshlawy A, et al. A phase 3 randomized trial of voxelotor in sickle cell disease. New Engl J Med. 381(6):509–19.
10. Sharma A, Boelens J-J, Cancio M, et al. CRISPR-CAS9 editing of the HBG1 and HBG2 promoters to treat sickle cell disease. N Engl J Med. 2023;389:820–32.
11. Kanter J, Walters MC, Krishnamurti L, et al. Bilologic and clinical efficacy of LentiGlobin for sickle cell disease. N Engl J Med. 2022;386:617–28.
12. Bain BJ. Haemoglobinopathy diagnosis. 3rd ed. Hoboken: Wiley-Blackwell; 2020.

Red Blood Cell Enzymopathies

13

Clark R. Robinson, Aaron B. Boothby, and Kleber Y. Fertrin

Introduction

Red blood cell (RBC) enzymopathies are a class of genetic disorders that affect the enzymes responsible for RBC metabolism. They present with non-spherocytic hemolytic anemia (NSHA) because of RBC's decreased ability to manage oxidative stress and/or keep up with metabolic demands. The diagnosis of an RBC enzymopathy usually requires laboratory evidence of a nonimmune (i.e., negative direct antiglobulin test [DAT] or "Coombs test") hemolytic anemia in association with a screening tool such as a quantitative spectrophotometric assay of the suspected enzyme deficiency that may then be confirmed by molecular testing finding a known pathogenic mutation. Severity is highly variable; however, the prognosis of RBC enzymopathies is typically favorable as the treatment is most often supportive care with packed red blood cell transfusions and management of the complications from chronic hemolysis.

C. R. Robinson (✉)
University of Texas Southwestern Medical Center, Dallas, TX, USA

A. B. Boothby
University of Washington, Seattle, WA, USA

K. Y. Fertrin
Fred Hutchinson Cancer Center, Seattle, WA, USA

L. Sokol, L. Zhang (eds.), *Non-Neoplastic Hematologic Disorders*,
https://doi.org/10.1007/978-3-031-62373-8_13

Table 13.1 Red blood cell enzymopathies

Enzyme	Pathway	Inheritance	Frequency
Glucose-6-Phosphate Dehydrogenase	Pentose Phosphate	X-linked Recessive	2.9–7.5% of world population [6]
Pyruvate Kinase Deficiency	Glycolytic	Autosomal Recessive	3.2 to 8.5 per million [2]
Pyrimidine-5′-Nucleotidase	Nucleotide Salvage	Autosomal Recessive	20 cases described [4]
Glucose Phosphate Isomerase	Glycolytic	Autosomal Recessive	30 cases described [4]
Triosephosphate Isomerase	Glycolytic	Autosomal Recessive	20 cases described [4]
Phosphoglycerate Kinase	Glycolytic	X-linked Recessive	12 cases described [4]
Adenosine Deaminase Hyperactivity	Nucleotide Salvage	Autosomal Dominant	3 known families described [4]
Adenylate Kinase Deficiency	Nucleotide Salvage	Autosomal Recessive	Ultra rare [1]

Glucose-6-phosphate dehydrogenase (G6PD) deficiency is by far the most common RBC enzymopathy with a global prevalence estimated at over 500 million and annually more than 200,000 cases in the USA [1]. It is most commonly found in people of African, Mediterranean, or Asian descent. Pyruvate kinase (PK) deficiency is the second most common RBC enzymopathy with a global incidence at birth of between 3.2 and 51 per million [2]. Other very rare types of RBC enzymopathies can be found in Table 13.1 [3, 4]. All RBC enzymopathies are autosomal recessive, except for G6PD deficiency and phosphoglycerate kinase deficiency, which are both X-linked recessive, and ADA hyperactivity, which is autosomal dominant [3, 5, 6].

Pathogenesis

Because RBCs lack nuclei and are obligate anaerobes without mitochondria or ribosomes, they are unable to synthesize new proteins, and therefore, depend on prepackaged enzymes left over after completing their maturation for their metabolism [5]. Most RBC enzymopathies affect one of three well-defined metabolic pathways (Fig. 13.1):

1. The pentose phosphate pathway
2. The glycolytic pathway
3. The nucleotide salvage pathway

Enzymatic deficiencies in those pathways lead to a shortened lifespan of RBCs via inability to deal with oxidative stress or

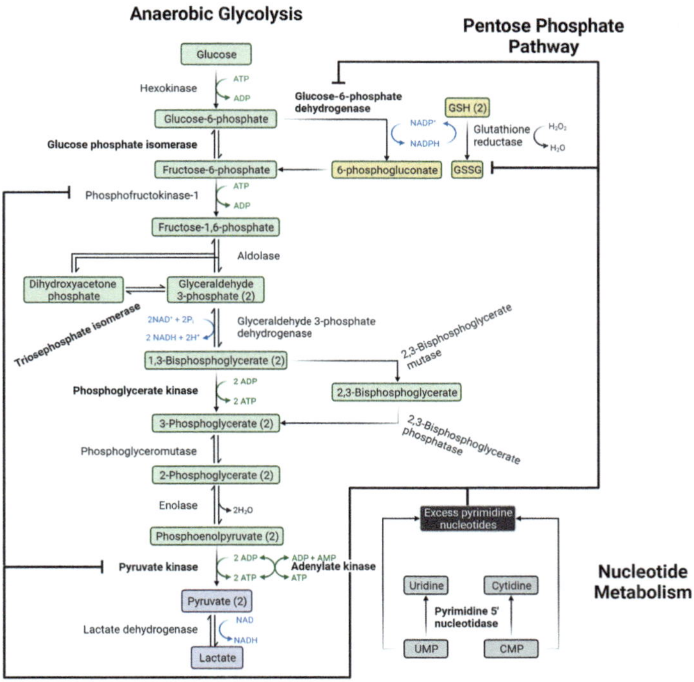

Fig. 13.1 Red blood cell metabolic pathways. ADP adenosine diphosphate, AMP adenosine monophosphate, ATP adenosine triphosphate, CMP cytidine monophosphate, GSH glutathione, GSSG glutathione disulfide, NAD+ nicotinamide adenine dinucleotide (oxidized), NADP+ nicotinamide adenine dinucleotide phosphate (oxidized), NADPH nicotinamide adenine dinucleotide phosphate, UMP uridine monophosphate. (Created with BioRender.com)

insufficient generation of adenosine triphosphate (ATP), which clinically manifests as a hemolytic anemia without apparent morphologic abnormalities on peripheral smear. Very rarely, RBC enzymopathies may present as methemoglobinemias, immunodeficiencies, neuropathies, and myopathies, which will not be covered in this chapter [4]. In this section, we will detail the pathogenesis behind the three most common RBC enzymopathies.

G6PD deficiency arises from a defect in the pentose phosphate pathway. The pentose phosphate pathway is the only source of nicotinamide adenine dinucleotide phosphate (NADPH) in the RBC. NADPH regenerates glutathione, a reducing agent that protects the hemoglobin protein from oxidative stress. Without glutathione, oxidation of the sulfhydryl and beta sheets leads to denaturation of globin chains [6]. Aggregates of denatured globins adhere to the red cell membrane and are known as Heinz bodies. When Heinz bodies are phagocytosed by macrophages, the resulting deformed RBC is called a "bite cell" or "blister cell." [6] These forms may be seen in the peripheral blood smear and provide an important clue to oxidative stress as a cause for hemolysis.

G6PD has over 300 allelic variants that have been categorized by the World Health Organization into different classes (Table 13.2). Because of that variability, G6PD deficiency may present as episodes of acute NSHA, as neonatal jaundice, and/or chronic NSHA. The various subtypes can range in their clinical severity from episodes of acute hemolytic anemia in asymptomatic adults who are self-limiting (e.g., G6PD A- or G6PD Canton) to severe episodes of acute hemolytic anemia with an acute kidney injury that may require hospitalization for supportive care (e.g., G6PD Mediterranean). Examples of oxidative agents that can trigger these episodes of acute hemolytic anemia in patients with G6PD deficiency include medications, herbal remedies, infections, exposure to certain substances such as naphthalene mothballs, or consumption of fava beans (Table 13.3) [1, 4, 6]. The enzymatically normal form of G6PD ("wild type") is variant B (Class IV) [1]. Variant G6PD A is

Table 13.2 G6PD enzyme variants and classes

Variant	Class*	Enzymatic activity	Geographic distribution	Clinical features
G6PD B	IV	100%	Worldwide	None
G6PD A	IV	85%	Africa	None
G6PD A-	III	10–23%	Africa, Latin America	Mild acute hemolytic anemia
Canton	II	4%	China	Severe acute hemolytic anemia
Mediterranean	II	<5%	Mediterranean	Severe acute hemolytic anemia
Santiago	I	<1%	Sporadic	Neonatal Jaundice, NSHA

G6PD classification is based on residual enzymatic activity of the G6PD enzyme as follows:
Class I associated with chronic NSHA
Class II: <10% residual activity
Class III: 10–60% residual activity
Class IV: Normal activity

Table 13.3 G6PD deficiency: hemolytic risk of exposure

High risk		Possible risk	Less likely
Dapsone	Phenazopyridine	Aspirin (>100 mg)	Aspirin (<100 mg)
Fluoroquinolones	Rasburicase	Chloroquine	Chloramphenicol
Glyburide	Sulfamethoxazole	Quinidine	Dimercaptosuccinic acid (DMSA)
Methylene blue	Tafenoquine	Quinine	
Niridazole	Fava beans	Sulfadiazine	Mepacrine
Nitrofurantoin	Henna compounds	Sulfasalazine	Vitamin K
Pegloticase	Naphthalene	Sulfonylureas	
Primaquine	Phenylhydrazine	Tolonium chloride	

Adapted from Luzzatto et al. [1]

phenotypically normal, but electrophoretically different from G6PD B with 85% enzymatic activity and is found in about 40% of the African population [1, 6]. G6PD variants tend to be most prevalent in malaria endemic areas and confer protection to the RBC against *Plasmodium falciparum*.

PK deficiency is the most common RBC enzymopathy involving the glycolytic pathway. PK is the final enzyme in glycolysis that hydrolyzes phosphoenol pyruvate (PEP) to make ATP and is encoded by the *PKLR* gene [5]. Decreased PK activity results in lower intracellular ATP and an increase in 2,3 diphosphoglycerate (2,3-DPG). ATP powers sodium/potassium membrane pumps that maintain the RBC membrane's flexibility and integrity. Without ATP, RBCs are more susceptible to hemolysis. Increased 2,3-DPG also lowers hemoglobin's affinity for oxygen.

PK deficiency is an autosomal recessive condition and can arise from either a homozygous pathogenic mutation or compound heterozygosity (two different pathogenic variants in trans orientation). Over 200 mutations have been described and may affect the protein's affinity for enzyme substrates (i.e., PEP), protein stability, or protein production. Because of that underlying genetic variability, the anemia in PK deficiency can vary from mild and asymptomatic to severe with transfusion dependence.

The hemolysis in PK deficiency is primarily extravascular; however, red cell destruction is not entirely explained by shortened lifespan of RBC due to lack of ATP. PK deficiency may also affect the maturation of erythroid progenitors leading to ineffective erythropoiesis, which is believed to be the cause of increased absorption of iron, extramedullary hematopoiesis, and a propensity to bone fractures [7]. Iron overload is a significant feature in PK deficiency and occurs regardless of transfusions. The higher incidence of bone fractures cannot be directly explained by the enzymatic defect itself, but may be caused by a higher cell turnover with bone marrow expansion.

Pyrimidine-5′-Nucleotidase (P5′N) deficiency is the third most common RBC enzymopathy associated with a chronic NHSA and involves the nucleotide salvage pathway. P5′N hydrolyzes the pyrimidines into nucleosides and free phosphates for future nucleotide metabolism. Without P5′N, RBCs accumulate pyrimidine aggregates that decrease the RBC cell membrane stability and lead to a chronic hemolysis. Those pyrimidine aggregates are seen as coarse basophilic stippling in the RBCs on a routine peripheral blood smear (Of note, basophilic stippling is also seen in RBCs with lead poisoning, likely related to the fact that lead inhibits P5′N) [4, 5].

Diagnosis

A general diagnostic approach to hemolytic anemias is depicted in Fig. 13.2 and highlights where RBC enzymopathies are considered. Clinical symptoms of RBC enzymopathies include fatigue, jaundice (including neonatal), and splenomegaly. An RBC

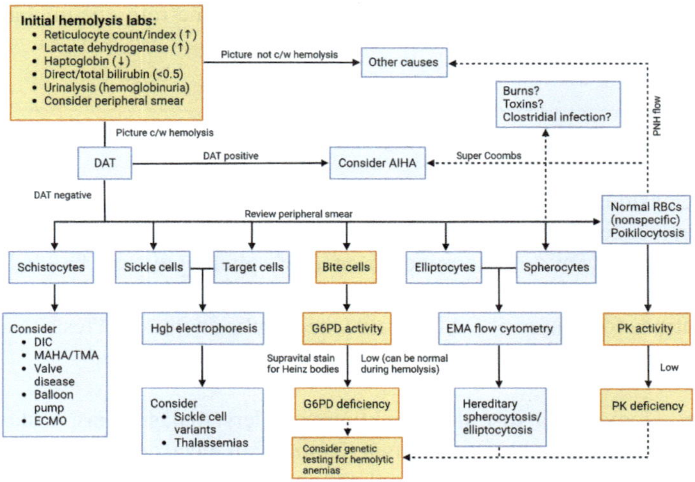

Fig. 13.2 Diagnostic algorithm for hemolytic anemia. AIHA autoimmune hemolytic anemia, DAT direct antiglobulin test, DIC disseminated intravascular coagulation, ECMO extracorporeal membrane oxygenation, EMA Eosin-5′-maleimide, G6PD glucose-6-phosphate dehydrogenase, MAHA microangiopathic hemolytic anemia, PNH paroxysmal nocturnal hemoglobinuria, PK pyruvate kinase' RBCs red blood cells, TMA thrombotic microangiopathy (Created with BioRender.com)

enzymopathy should always be considered in the differential diagnosis of a hemolytic anemia without evidence of an autoimmune cause, i.e., labs confirming evidence of hemolysis – elevated bilirubin (indirect predominant), elevated lactate dehydrogenase (LDH) level, low haptoglobin, and elevated reticulocyte count – with a negative DAT [4]. Quantitative spectrophotometric assays measuring the specific enzyme activity in question are useful screening steps in the diagnosis of RBC enzymopathies, but are only more widely available for G6PD and PK deficiencies. For P5′N deficiency, the biochemical evidence is the demonstration of a shift in the ultraviolet spectral absorption curve of the RBC lysate due to accumulation of pyrimidine nucleotides. Molecular testing can confirm the diagnosis of an RBC enzymopathy by demonstrating a known pathogenic variant in a gene encoding a specific RBC enzyme. Molecular testing may be employed as diagnostic follow-up to an abnormal biochemical assay, or as the only diagnostic option in some rare enzymopathies [8].

Major Differential Diagnosis

Consideration of an RBC enzymopathy should arise when there is evidence of nonimmune hemolytic anemia. Given that peripheral smear review to determine absence of spherocytes can be challenging in certain settings, the following are the major considerations for causes of DAT-negative hemolytic anemia and tests that may help exclude them from your differential diagnosis.

- Hemoglobin disorders (sickling disorders, thalassemias, unstable hemoglobins): abnormal hemoglobin electrophoresis
- Infection (bacterial: e.g., clostridium; viral: hepatitis A, cytomegalovirus, influenza; parasitic: malaria): positive blood cultures, positive serum polymerase chain reaction testing for infectious organisms
- Disseminated intravascular coagulation (DIC): low fibrinogen, low platelets, elevated d-dimer, and extended prothrombin (PT)/international normalized ratio (INR)

- Mechanical valve causing hemolysis: echocardiogram
- Thrombotic microangiopathy/Microangiopathic hemolytic anemia (TMA/MAHA): elevated creatinine, elevated LDH, thrombocytopenia, and schistocytes on peripheral smear (aka PLASMIC score)
- Membranopathies (hereditary spherocytosis, Southeast Asian ovalocytosis, and some types of elliptocytosis): low expression on flow cytometry with EMA (eosin-5-maleimide) and red cell membrane electrophoresis (specialized labs only)
- Paroxysmal nocturnal hemoglobinuria: positive for PNH clone on flow cytometry for CD55 and CD59
- DAT-negative autoimmune hemolytic anemia: positive "Super Coombs" despite initial negative DAT

Prognosis

The prognosis of RBC enzymopathies varies depending on the degree of anemia, with phenotypes ranging from clinically silent to life threatening, and on comorbidities in syndromic cases. Most patients have a good prognosis as long as the sequelae of chronic hemolysis, such as nutritional need, iron overload, and propensity for gallstones, are well-managed [6]. The main exception is triosephosphate isomerase (TPI) deficiency, which is almost universally fatal within 20 years of age due to the associated neurological complications. G6PD deficiency usually has rapid recovery after removing the triggering agent and is not expected to shorten lifespan [1].

Treatment

The staple of management for RBC enzymopathies that cause hemolytic anemia is supportive care with folate supplementation, transfusions, and ultrasound screening for gallstones [5]. Since hemolysis in RBC enzymopathies is largely extravascular, splenectomy may be considered in severe cases, but often, only partially normalizes hemoglobin levels [5]. Management of neonatal jaundice from RBC enzymopathies includes phototherapy and exchange transfusion in severe cases [1]. All patients should be referred to genetic counseling if a diagnosis of hereditary hemolytic anemia is made. Oxidant triggers should be avoided specifically in G6PD deficiency (Table 13.3) [1]. Iron chelation plays an important role in patients who are dependent on transfusions, or any patient with PK deficiency, in whom iron overload may develop spontaneously. In 2022, mitapivat (a first-in-class, oral, allosteric activator of PK) was approved by the Federal Drug Administration for treatment of PK deficiency. Use of mitapivat significantly improves hemoglobin levels in 40% of patients who are not transfusion-dependent and significantly reduces transfusion burden in 33% of patients treated [9, 10]. Allogeneic stem cell transplantation remains as a possible treatment option for hematologists in patients with severe disease and has been done in a limited number of PK deficiency patients with its best results in patients under the age of 16. (Table 13.4)

Table 13.4 Management of clinical manifestations of RBC enzymopathies

Clinical manifestation	Enzyme deficiency	Management
Neonatal jaundice	All	Phototherapy Exchange transfusion if severe
Acute hemolysis	G6PD	Folate supplementation Transfusion support as needed Intravenous hydration (if acute kidney injury) Avoid exposure to triggers
Chronic hemolysis	All (only class I variants in G6PD)	Folate supplementation Monitor for gallstones Transfusion (as needed or chronic transfusion for hemoglobin <7 g/dL) Consider splenectomy for severe cases Consider hematopoietic cell transplant for severe cases age < 16 (PK deficiency) Monitor for iron overload and chelate as needed (all, includes transfusion-naive PK deficiency) PK activator: mitapivat (FDA-approved for PK deficiency) Monitor bone mineral density (PK deficiency)

Promising Clinical Studies

More pharmaceuticals are being developed for PK deficiency and may expand to other RBC enzymopathies. Gene therapy is under investigation for PK deficiency (NCT04105166) and may pave the way for its use in other RBC enzymopathies.

Clinical studies of G6PD deficiency tend to focus on studying incidence of hemolytic events in response to suspected triggers as well as improving diagnostics. However, there has been some consideration using histone deacetylase inhibitors, butyrate, and valproate to induce G6PD synthesis [1].

Caveats and Medical Pearls

- G6PD deficiency is inherited in an X-linked recessive pattern, and therefore, more common in males
- G6PD levels may appear normal during hemolytic episodes due to the increased proportion of reticulocytes (which are relatively rich in G6PD) or donor RBCs if the patient has received transfusions
- Supravital staining with new methylene blue, crystal violet, or brilliant cresyl blue is required to detect Heinz bodies, which are classically seen in G6PD deficiency [1]
- G6PD deficiency may exhibit chronic non-spherocytic hemolytic anemia in rare cases caused by class I variants [1]
- Patients with PK deficiency display a paradoxical increase in reticulocyte count (sometimes above 50%) after splenectomy
- Spontaneous iron overload, extramedullary hematopoiesis, and increased incidence of bone fractures have been observed in PK deficiency patients.

Board Questions

1. A 34-year-old, Ethiopian man presents to his primary care physician complaining of fatigue and dark urine without fevers. He reports he has just returned from a trip to his home country, where he took antimalarial prophylaxis while abroad. Labs are shown below.

White blood cells 11,000 cells/μL,
Hemoglobin 7.8 g/dL (Mean Corpuscular Volume 104 fl)
Platelet count 204,000 cells/μL
Total bilirubin 6.2 mg/dL (direct bilirubin 1.3 mg/dL)
LDH 450 units/L and haptoglobin undetectable

You suspect G6PD deficiency underlying the hemolytic anemia. Which of the following medications is most likely implicated and what do you expect a G6PD activity to be?

A. Primaquine, normal G6PD activity
B. Doxycycline, low G6PD activity
C. Atovaquone, elevated G6PD activity
D. Levofloxacin, low G6PD activity

Answer: A. Primaquine is a commonly used antimalarial which can cause a hemolytic crisis in people with G6PD deficiency. During hemolysis, levels of G6PD activity may normalize due to the increased numbers of reticulocytes, which have higher levels of G6PD activity. Doxycycline, atovaquone, and levofloxacin are not associated with acute hemolytic episodes in patients with G6PD deficiency.

2. A young man with newly diagnosed Human Immunodeficiency Virus, and a CD4 cell count of 112 cells/μL, has intolerance to trimethoprim/sulfamethoxazole and was recently started on dapsone for *Pneumocystis* prophylaxis in the hospital. Testing for G6PD deficiency was pending at the time of discharge. What finding on a follow-up on a routine Wright-stained peripheral blood smear is most suggestive of a diagnosis of G6PD deficiency?

   A. Coarse basophilic stippling
   B. Howell-Jolly bodies
   C. Bite cells
   D. Heinz bodies

Answer C – Certain medications, including dapsone, can cause increased oxidative stress, causing hemolysis in G6PD deficiency. Bite cells are caused by phagocytosis of the precipitates of denatured hemoglobin attached to parts of the red cell membrane and may be the first clue to a hemolytic anemia due to oxidant sensitivity. Coarse basophilic stippling can be caused by acute oxidative stress in G6PD deficiency, but is also generated by nucleotide aggregates seen in P5′N deficiency and lead toxicity (lead acutely inhibits P5′N). Howell-Jolly bodies are DNA remnants from the nuclei seen in asplenic patients, not expected in G6PD deficiency alone. Heinz bodies are the red cell inclusions of denatured hemoglobin in G6PD deficiency, but can only be seen on supravital staining (new methylene blue, brilliant cresyl blue, or crystal violet).

References

1. Luzzatto L, Ally M, Notaro R. Glucose-6-phosphate dehydrogenase deficiency. Blood. 2020;136(11):1225–40.
2. Secrest MH, Storm M, Carrington C, et al. Prevalence of pyruvate kinase deficiency: a systematic literature review. Eur J Haematol. 2020; 105(2):173–84.
3. Luzzatto L, Notaro R. Red cell enzymopathies. In: Jameson JL, editor. Principles of molecular medicine. Totowa: Humana Press; 1998.
4. Dreyfus JC, Kahn A. Red cell enzymopathies: molecular mechanisms. Clin Biochem. 1984;17(6):331–40.
5. Koralkova P, van Solinge WW, van Wijk R. Rare hereditary red blood cell enzymopathies associated with hemolytic anemia – pathophysiology, clinical aspects, and laboratory diagnosis. Int J Lab Hematol. 2014;36(3):388–97.
6. WHO Working Group. Glucose-6-phosphate dehydrogenase deficiency. Bull World Health Organ. 1989;67(6):601–11.
7. Grace RF, Bianchi P, van Beers EJ, et al. Clinical spectrum of pyruvate kinase deficiency: data from the Pyruvate Kinase Deficiency Natural History Study. Blood. 2018;131(20):2183–92.
8. Kim Y, Park J, Kim M. Diagnostic approaches for inherited hemolytic anemia in the genetic era. Blood Res. 2017;52(2):84–94.
9. Al-Samkari H, Galactéros F, Glenthøj A, et al. Mitapivat versus Placebo for Pyruvate Kinase Deficiency. N Engl J Med. 2022;386(15):1432–42.
10. Glenthøj A, van Beers EJ, Al-Samkari H, et al. Mitapivat in adult patients with pyruvate kinase deficiency receiving regular transfusions (ACTIVATE-T): a multicentre, open-label, single-arm, phase 3 trial. Lancet Haematol. 2022;9(10):e724–32.

Red Blood Cell Membrane Disorders

14

Shivani M. Dalal, Olger Nano, and Michel Vulfovich

Introduction

The process of erythropoiesis, which produces around 2 million red blood cells (RBCs) per second, is intricate. These RBCs deform their normal shape to pass through the 3-μm diameter capillaries and the 1-μm to 2-μm-wide endothelial slits in the spleen. Normal RBCs are 7–8 μM in size with a complexly regulated ratio of their membrane surface area to cytoplasmic volume, which gives them the classic biconcave disc shape. The RBC membrane consists of an array of lipids and proteins. The membrane proteins can be classified into two general groups: (1) integral proteins: band 3, aquaporin 1, GLUT1, PIEZO1, glycophorins; and (2) peripheral proteins: ankyrin, spectrin, band 4.2, actin, tropomyosin, and tropomodulin, protein 4.1, adductin, sematin [1]. Conditions that can interfere with normal membrane deformability and stability of RBCs can decrease the normal surface membrane area-to-volume ratio, thereby altering RBC shape, inducing hemolysis, and shortening the lifespan of the RBC. Hemolytic anemias resulting from defects in the RBC membrane are an important group of hereditary anemias.

S. M. Dalal (✉) · O. Nano · M. Vulfovich
Memorial Cancer Institute at Memorial Healthcare System, Pembroke Pines, FL, USA
e-mail: SDalal@mhs.net

L. Sokol, L. Zhang (eds.), *Non-Neoplastic Hematologic Disorders*, https://doi.org/10.1007/978-3-031-62373-8_14

Hereditary Spherocytosis

Introduction and Epidemiology

Hereditary spherocytosis (HS) is the most comment hereditary RBC-membrane disorder leading to hemolytic anemia. It is prevalent among people of northern European descent, where HS can affect as many as 1 in 2000 to 1 in 5000 individuals. Approximately 75% of HS follow an autosomal-dominant inheritance pattern.

Pathophysiology

Patients with HS harbor mutations of genes encoding the RBC-membrane proteins that participate in vertical associations which are critical in linking the membrane cytoskeleton to the lipid bilayer: for example, spectrin encoded by the genes *SPTA1* and *SPTB (20%)*; ankyrin encoded by the ANK1 gene (50%); and band 3 encoded by the *SLC4A1* gene (25%). These proteins play different roles. Ankyrin allows mechanical coupling between the plasma membrane of RBCs and underlying cytoskeleton. Spectrin is a flexible, rod-like protein that binds ankyrin [1]. Spectrin helps maintain the composition of proteins and lipids in the RBC membrane, confers the biconcave disc shape of the RBCs, and allows them to undergo deformations as they traverse the microvasculature throughout the human body. Band 3 allows cohesion between the RBC plasma membrane and cytoskeletal proteins. It prevents membrane-surface loss, maintains RBC water content, and prevents dehydration by exchanging bicarbonate for chloride ions. Band 4.2 forms a strong link between band 3 and ankyrin. Deficiencies and qualitative defects in these proteins affect the RBC-membrane structure by reducing the vertical association between the cytoskeleton and membrane, causing reduced deformability, and thereby impair passage through vasculature in the microcirculation. This leads to splenic trapping and phagocytosis by splenic macrophages. Loss of spectrin is correlated with the severity of hemolysis.

Clinical Presentation

HS can present signs and symptoms of hemolysis at any age with any severity. Commonly noted signs and symptoms may include splenomegaly; deficiencies of iron, vitamin B12, and folate; jaundice from hyperbilirubinemia secondary to hemolysis; and formation of pigment gallstones.

Evaluation

All individuals with high suspicion of HS based on family history or signs and symptoms should be tested. As per the guidelines of the International Council for Standardization in Haematology, complete blood count with differential is commonly tested for diagnosis of nonimmune hereditary RBC-membrane disorders. Mean corpuscular hemoglobin concentration (MCHC) >36 g/dL is consistent with spherocytosis [2]. Peripheral smear review will demonstrate increased spherocytes with loss of normal central pallor. Laboratory tests for hemolysis panel should be performed which show elevated lactate dehydrogenase (LDH), decreased haptoglobin, increased reticulocyte count, and elevated indirect bilirubin. Coombs testing is usually negative in HS, while it is positive for autoimmune etiology of hemolytic anemia. Specialized confirmatory testing includes the eosin-5′-maleimide (EMA) binding test, which is highly sensitive and specific. EMA is an eosin-based fluorescent dye that binds to band 3 and Rh-related RBC-membrane proteins. When HS is caused by deficiencies of band 3, ankyrin, or spectrin, reduction in EMA binding is noted in RBCs [3]. The osmotic fragility test is another special test; however, its use is limited because of being less sensitive and specific. In this osmotic fragility test, fresh RBCs are incubated in hypotonic-buffered salt solutions of various osmolarities. The fraction of hemoglobin released because of hemolysis is measured. However, it may fail to identify a substantial number of individuals with HS, particularly the newborns; it may also be positive in other conditions, including immune hemolytic anemia and other RBC-enzyme defects, such as glucose-6-phosphate dehydrogenase deficiency, hemolytic-transfusion reactions, and unstable hemoglobin variants. Other infrequently used tests are glycerol-lysis and acidified glycerol-lysis test.

Because of the cost reduction, the targeted next-generation sequencing-based panels of the known genes have decreased the number of undiagnosed cases and contributed to the accurate diagnosis of the patients. Targeted next-generation sequencing will continue to evolve into an important test for diagnosing RBC membranopathy.

Management

HS treatment is mainly supportive and aims to minimize the chronic hemolysis and anemia complications. This may include treatment of hyperbilirubinemia and transfusions for neonates with HS. Folic acid supplementation can be used as a supportive measure. Erythropoietin can be helpful in certain situations to avoid the need of transfusions. For individuals with severe hemolysis and chronic transfusion dependence, splenectomy is a feasible option. It is prudent to ensure that appropriate vaccinations for encapsulated organisms have been administered well in advance to allow time for formation of the antibodies before splenectomy is performed.

Hereditary Stomatocytosis

Introduction

Hereditary stomatocytosis (HSt) (also namely hereditary hydrocytosis or overhydrated stomatocytosis) is characterized by red cell overhydration and macrocytosis due to passive sodium leak from the RBC membranes. This rare disorder is associated with defects in RBC hydration and presents with a variable degree of hemolysis. It is an autosomal-dominant inherited disorder. It is classified into four disorders: overhydrated HSt, dehydrated HSt, cryohydrocytosis, and familial pseudohyperkalemia [4].

Pathogenesis

Some cases are attributed to pathogenic variants in the *PEIZO* gene, *RHAG* gene, and *SLC4A1* gene. The membrane of stomatocytes has enhanced permeability toward monovalent cations such as sodium ions (Na^+). Overhydration occurs when cellular permeability to Na^+ increases, leading to a marked increase in intracellular Na^+ that cannot be compensated for by the Na±K±ATPase pump. This is followed by an increase in cell water caused by osmosis. Multiple theories propose that a relative expansion of the inner leaflet to the outer leaflet of the bilayer may be responsible.

Clinical Features

The patients can be completely asymptomatic or have varying degrees of chronic hemolysis and thereby have side effects from chronic hemolysis, such as splenomegaly, pigmenturia, pigmented gallstones, and anemia. Iron overload is frequently observed. Rare cases of patients with HSt with vaso-occlusive symptoms have been reported with symptoms such as short of breath, chest pain, and abdominal pain. Some patients may develop thrombosis, which may lead to pulmonary hypertension [5].

Diagnosis

Diagnosis of HSt requires a high index of clinical suspicion—positive family history, especially among first-degree relatives, elevated MCHC and MCH, nonimmune hemolysis of unknown etiology, history of unexplained neonatal anemia, and hyperbilirubinemia should prompt evaluation for HSt. Testing for HSt should include CBC, peripheral smear, LDH, haptoglobin, reticulocyte count, bilirubin levels, reticulocyte count, Coombs test, and osmotic fragility. Genetic testing needs to be individualized based on clinical severity, family history, and prenatal testing of family members.

Treatment

Limited data are available on management of HSt. Patients with chronic hemolysis are recommended to be on folate supplementations. One should be mindful of the possibility of iron overload with the frequency of blood transfusions. Patients should be aware of the possibility of pigment gallstones. Splenectomy is usually reserved as the last resort because there is limited evidence of treatment benefit. There is an increased risk of developing catastrophic thrombosis in patients postsplenectomy because of hypercoagulable state after the procedure [6].

Hereditary Xerocytosis

Introduction

Hereditary xerocytosis, also called dehydrated HSt, is the most common disorder with cation-permeability defects and inhered in an autosomal-dominant model. Xerocytes are dense hyperchromic RBCs. Loss of cell solute followed by osmotic water loss leads to formation of xerocytes. Clinically, it manifests with hemolytic anemia secondary to an efflux of potassium (K^+) from RBCs and RBC dehydration.

Pathophysiology

Some cases are attributed to pathogenic variants in the *PIEZO1* gene. This gene encodes subunits of the PIEZO1 channel. The underlying membrane-permeability defect is complex. There is a net loss of K^+ from the RBCs that is not accompanied by a proportional gain of Na^+, subsequently causing a decrease in the net intracellular cation and cell water content.

Clinical Features

Patients may present with classic symptoms of hemolytic anemia, such as jaundice, splenomegaly, and gallstones. A subset of patients may also demonstrate pseudohyperkalemia, perinatal edema, and even hydrops fetalis in rare cases.

Diagnosis

Diagnosis is typically made by the presence of pathognomonic RBC morphology in conjunction with features of hemolytic anemia, such as elevated LDH, bilirubin, and reticulocyte count and low haptoglobin. Though blood smear examination is helpful in some cases, RBC morphology can interfere with coinheritance of more than one RBC defect, overlapping clinical variability, reticulocytosis, and frequent blood transfusions. Specialized gene panels, including the PIEZO1, KCNN4, and RHAG genes, should be performed along with osmotic fragility testing.

Treatment

Treatment is not required for patients who experience only mild anemia. Folate supplementation is recommended and patients are monitored for complications of hemolysis. Given a high risk of hypercoagulability and life-threatening thrombotic episodes after the procedure, splenectomy is contraindicated for these patients [6].

Hereditary Elliptocytosis (HE)

Hereditary elliptocytosis (HE) is an RBC-membrane disorder inherited in an autosomal-dominant fashion. It is characterized by oval- and elliptical-shaped cells that are elongated. HE occurs when genetic alterations lead to structure and function changes of several interconnected structural proteins of the RBC cytoskeleton, such alpha and beta spectrin, protein 4.1, band 3, and, on rare occasions, glycophorin C. The most common mutations are those in the gene encoding for alpha-spectrin SPTA1 (65%), the gene encoding for beta-spectrin SPTB (30%), and the gene encoding for protein 4.1 EPB41 (5%). HE is also known as hereditary ovalocytosis because of its typical egg-shaped form, which results from the elastic recoil properties of the RBCs being lost or diminished in the peripheral circulation. Because of their faulty shape, these distorted cells are sequestered to the spleen and eliminated, subsequently leading to hemolytic anemia. Other subtypes of HE included hereditary pyropoikilocytosis and Southeast Asian ovalocytosis (SAO).

Epidemiology

It is unknown what the true prevalence of HE is around the world. It is most prevalent among the population of Africa, Southeast Asia, and the Mediterranean, which not surprisingly correlates with areas where malaria is endemic. An estimated prevalence is 1 in 2000 to 1 in 4000 individuals in the world. The subtype of HE, SAO, is common among people in Malaysia, Philippines, Indonesia, and Papua New Guinea.

Pathophysiology

The proteinaceous cytoskeleton underneath the lipid bilayer of the RBC helps maintain the typical biconcave shape of the cell by providing membrane structural integrity and surface area. The genetic alterations cause defects in the RBC, leading to instability and rendering the membrane to be deformed as it passes through microvasculature. The cells do not resume their biconcave shape since the altered proteins do not allow for elastic recoil and the elliptical morphology remains. These elliptocytes are subsequently sequestered to the spleen and destroyed there prematurely, and hence, have a shortened lifespan fewer than 120 days. The result is intravascular hemolysis, which is characteristic in HE. This hemolysis can range from being asymptomatic in those who may be heterozygous for other variants of elliptocytes to severe in those who are homozygous.

Evaluation

HE and its variants are mostly asymptomatic and usually incidentally found during laboratory workup for anemia. Symptoms are typical of the other anemias, including reduced exercise tolerance and fatigue. When elliptocytes are noted on the peripheral smear, it is important to focus on family history. Often, family members are misdiagnosed with other conditions like iron-deficiency anemia. A physical exam should be performed to evaluate for splenomegaly and right-upper-quadrant pain for gall stones. Laboratory evaluation with CBC with differential, a peripheral smear, hemolysis labs including lactate dehydrogenase, and direct and indirect bilirubin should be performed. Hemolysis profile like reticulocyte count, lactate dehydrogenase, and haptoglobin should also be conducted. If there is high suspicion, check for protein 4.1 and spectrin analysis.

1. **HE:** It is asymptomatic. If severe, it presents in very early childhood and neonates with hemolysis in the first year of life which does resolve on its own. Mean corpuscular volume is low, in the 50–70 range. The patients may require transfusions and/or phototherapy if found to have severe hemolytic anemia or jaundice. Elliptocytes on peripheral smear are pathognomonic and typically range from 15% to 100%, depending on severity.
2. **Hereditary pyropoikilocytosis:** This entity is often grouped with HE because of the same genetic anomalies as HE. It is the most severe form and commonly affects neonates with jaundice and hemolytic anemia, persisting past the first year of life. These patients have the most complications of persistent hemolysis, including splenomegaly, pigmented gallstones, frequent transfusions, and early splenectomy. The peripheral smear shows a mix of poikilocytes, occasional elliptocytes, and spherocytes.
3. **Southeast Asian ovalocytosis (SAO):** As the name suggests, this is more common among patients of Southeast Asian

descent and seen in areas where malaria is endemic. Symptoms are often mild. The peripheral blood smear shows stomatocytes and ovalocytes.

Differential Diagnosis

Iron-deficiency anemia, hereditary spherocytosis, thalassemia, glucose-6-phosphate dehydrogenase deficiency, sickle-cell disease, myelofibrosis, or myelodysplastic syndrome. In addition, the other RBC-membrane deficiencies are mentioned earlier.

Treatment

- Asymptomatic patients with no stigmata or hemolysis: no treatment or follow-up. Provide education and documentation to prevent future unnecessary testing.
- Intermittent hemolysis of anemia: If the patient is symptomatic or if the hemoglobin drops below the required threshold, provide transfusions. Continue to monitor splenomegaly and gallstones.
- Severe hemolysis and anemia: splenectomy. Provide necessary vaccinations before the procedure.

RBC-membrane protein	Inherited disorder
Band 3	HAc, SAO, HS
Ankyrin	HS
β spectrin	HE, HPP, HS
α spectrin	HE, HS, HPP
GPC	HE
Protein 4.1	HE
Protein 4.2	HS

GPC glycophorin C, *HAc* Hereditary Acanthocytosis, *HE* hereditary elliptocytosis, *HPP* hereditary pyropoikilocytosis, *HS* hereditary spherocytosis, *SAO* Southeast Asian ovalocytosis

Promising Clinical Trials

Not applicable

Caveats

1. There are varieties of RBC-membrane disorders that manifest with hemolysis due to structural alteration or transport dysfunction derived from intrinsic gene mutations.
2. Application of next-generation sequencing study will facilitate accurate diagnosis. Approximately 65–70% of autosomal HS patients harbor heterozygous mutations of *ANK1, SLC4A1,* and *SPTB* genes. Additionally, PIEZO1 mutation results in HX, *SPTA1* mutation causes HE, and hereditary pyropoikilocytosis (HPP) shares the same genetic anomalies with HE.

Questions

1. A 40-year-old female with a medical history of hypertension, diabetes, and chronic anemia seeks evaluation for right-upper-quadrant abdominal pain. She reports being chronically anemic and having occasional bouts of jaundice. She states that anemia "runs in her family." Her blood tests are remarkable for hemoglobin of 8.6 (12–15 g/dl), MCV of 105 (80–95 fL), MCHC of 38 (32–35 g/dl), platelets 180 (150–450 × 10^9/L), and white blood cells of 5.4 (4.5–10 × 10^9/L). Her indirect bilirubin is 3.2 (0.2–0.8 mg/dL); LDH is 400 (140–280 U/L); and reticulocyte count is 4%. She is afebrile and vitally stable. What is the most likely etiology of her right-upper-quadrant abdominal pain?

   A. Liver abscess
   B. Portal vein thrombosis
   C. Symptomatic pigment gallstones
   D. Acute hepatitis
   E. Pyelonephritis

Answer: C. Symptomatic pigment gallstones. The patient most likely has inherited RBC-membrane disorder, leading to chronic hemolysis given her family history of chronic anemia, occasional bouts of jaundice, evidence of hemolysis based on laboratory tests, elevated LDH, reticulocyte count, and indirect bilirubin. Elevated MCHC is classically seen among patients with HS. Patients with HS are prone to develop pigment gall stones in the setting of chronic hemolysis.

2. A 55-year-old male with hereditary stomatocytosis is admitted to the hospital for his fifth episode of hemolysis in the last year. He is ill-appearing and jaundiced. Given his recurrent episodes of hemolysis requiring frequent blood transfusions, he was offered outpatient splenectomy as the last resort. He tolerated this surgical procedure without any major side effects and was discharged home safely. He returned to the emergency department with shortness of breath at rest that became worse with exertion. What is the most likely cause of his symptoms?

   A. Postoperative pneumonia
   B. Postsurgical atelectasis of lung
   C. Pulmonary embolism
   D. Heart failure
   E. Acute chest syndrome

Answer: C. Pulmonary embolism. Patients with HSt should be offered splenectomy as the last resort. These patients are prone to develop catastrophic venous thromboembolism events postoperatively as they become more hypercoagulable after the splenectomy.

References

1. Narla J, Mohandas N. Red cell membrane disorders. Int J Lab Hematol. 2017;39(Suppl 1):47.
2. King MJ, Garçon L, Hoyer JD, et al. ICSH guidelines for the laboratory diagnosis of nonimmune hereditary red cell membrane disorders. Int J Lab Hematol. 2015;37:304.

3. Ciepiela O, Kotuła I, Górska E, et al. Delay in the measurement of eosin-5′-maleimide (EMA) binding does not affect the test result for the diagnosis of hereditary spherocytosis. Clin Chem Lab Med. 2013;51:817.
4. Andolfo I, Russo R, Gambale A, Iolascon A. Hereditary stomatocytosis: an underdiagnosed condition. Am J Hematol. 2018;93:107.
5. Yoshimoto A, Fujimura M, Nakao S. Pulmonary hypertension after splenectomy in hereditary stomatocytosis. Am J Med Sci. 2005;330:195.
6. Stewart GW, Amess JA, Eber SW, et al. Thrombo-embolic disease after splenectomy for hereditary stomatocytosis. Br J Haematol. 1996;93:303.

Congenital Dyserythropoietic Anemias

15

Alexandra Dreyzin, Julie Li,
and Jinjun Cheng

Introduction

Congenital dyserythropoietic anemias (CDAs) are a heterogenous group of disorders which are caused by a disruption of normal erythropoiesis [1]. Their clinical presentation, which typically involves anemia with some degree of hemolysis, ranges in severity and has overlapped with other hereditary hemolytic anemias. Management and prognosis of CDAs, however, do have some differences from other hemolytic anemias; therefore, it is important to consider this diagnosis and pursue further diagnostic testing when appropriate [1]. Furthermore, gathering accurate diagnostic information and studying the natural history of patients with CDAs will help characterize these rare disorders and optimize treatment.

A. Dreyzin
Center for Cancer and Blood Disorders, Children's National Hospital, Washington, DC, USA

J. Li
Department of Pathology, Moffitt Cancer Center, Tampa, FL, USA

J. Cheng (✉)
Department of Pathology and Laboratory Medicine, Children's National Hospital, Washington, DC, USA
e-mail: jcheng2@childrensnational.org

L. Sokol, L. Zhang (eds.), *Non-Neoplastic Hematologic Disorders*,
https://doi.org/10.1007/978-3-031-62373-8_15

Pathogenesis

CDAs have historically been separated into categories based on morphologic findings of the erythroblasts. With the advent of genetic testing, these phenotypical categories have been found to correlate with genotypes as well.

CDA Type I

CDA type I (CDA I) typically presents in the newborn period with moderate-to-severe macrocytic anemia and decreased reticulocyte count. Some patients also have associated skeletal and distal limb anomalies. On morphologic examination of bone marrow biopsies, 2% to 10% of erythroblasts are binucleate, classically with a chromatin bridge connecting the nuclei of two erythroid precursors [2]. Electron microscopy, if performed, shows a characteristic spongy appearance of nuclei with dense heterochromatin and vacuoles. Inheritance is in an autosomal recessive pattern. The genetic mutations most commonly associated with CDA I are *CDAN1* at 15q15.2 and *C15orf41* at 15q15, which encode proteins responsible for DNA repair and chromatin assembly [2]. Interestingly, loss of these proteins is incompatible with life, but alterations predominantly affect erythroid lineage cells, possibly because of their faster cell cycle or need for nuclear extrusion.

CDA Type II

The most common of the CDAs is CDA type II (CDA II), which has a milder phenotype with normocytic anemia, normal-to-elevated reticulocyte count, occasional microspherocytes, and signs of hemolysis, such as jaundice and splenomegaly [1]. Approximately 10% of patients are asymptomatic, while about 20% eventually require chronic transfusions. Bone marrow examination reveals erythroid hyperplasia with >10% binucleate cells, karyorrhexis, and erythroblasts whose nuclei have a discontinuous double membrane. A hypoglycosylated band 3 is pathognomonic for CDA II. Inheritance is autosomal recessive, and the most common mutation is in *SEC23B* gene at 20q11.2, which is responsible for vesicle trafficking. As with the genetic mutations responsible for CDA I, it is unclear why *SEC23B* mutations affect the erythroid lineage more than other cell types.

Patients with CDA II are also particularly susceptible to iron overload, which may occur out of proportion to their transfusion needs. The accumulation of erythroblasts in the bone marrow leads to production of the hormone, erythroferrone (ERFE), which then suppresses hepcidin production in the liver, leading to hepatic iron overload.

CDA Type III

CDA III is exceedingly rare and has only been reported in a few sporadic cases and four families at the time of this writing. It presents with mild macrocytic anemias and intravascular hemolysis. Some associated disorders have also been reported, including angioid streaks, macular degeneration, monoclonal gammopathy, and multiple myeloma. Erythroid hyperplasia with giant, multinucleated erythroblasts is seen on bone marrow examination [1]. Inheritance is autosomal-dominant, with mutation of the *KIF23/MKLp1* gene at 5q23. This gene encodes for a protein necessary to the formation of the mitotic spindle, thus the interruption of normal mitosis leads to large, multinucleated cells. Mutations in the *RACGAP1* gene at 12q13.12 have recently been reported in autosomal recessive congenital dyserythropoietic anemia type III [3].

CDA IV

CDA IV is also known as transcription factor-related CDA. Only a few patients with this variant have been reported, and they have had presentations ranging from fetal hydrops to transfusion-dependent hemolytic anemia. All of these patients also have elevation of hemoglobin F [1]. Bone marrow morphology, similar to other CDA variants, shows a hypercellular marrow with binucleated or multinucleated erythroblasts. It has an autosomal-dominant inheritance, with mutations in the *KLF1* gene which affect erythroid differentiation and the switch from fetal to adult hemoglobin.

Another CDA Variant

Another CDA variant, also known as X-linked thrombocytopenia with or without dyserythropoietic anemia (XLTDA), presents with a variable degree of anemia as well as thrombocytopenia and bleeding symptoms. It is caused by *GATA1* mutations which lead to impaired megakaryopoiesis with or without dyserythropoiesis [1].

Diagnosis

Clinical suspicion for CDA is initially based on presentation with hemolytic anemia and erythroblast morphology on bone marrow evaluation. Family history of anemia or associated findings, such as skeletal anomalies found in CDA I, can also guide diagnostic evaluation [1].

Some additional laboratory tests may also be useful. The mean corpuscular volume, reticulocyte count, platelet count, and hemoglobin F percentage can all help distinguish CDA variants. Increased osmotic fragility can also be found among many patients with CDA, and ektacytometry can help distinguish CDA from hereditary spherocytosis. As mentioned above, testing for hypoglycosylated band 3 can also be used to diagnose CDA II.

Genetic testing is increasingly important in diagnosing CDA. While some variants in CDA-related genes are known to be pathogenic, about 50% of patients who are diagnosed with CDA are found to have novel mutations. This means that single-gene testing or hereditary anemia gene panels are frequently negative among patients who have clinical presentations consistent with CDA, and whole exome or genome sequencing is needed for further characterization (see the summary Table 15.1).

Table 15.1 Clinical summary of multiple types of congenital dyserythropoietic anemias

Parameter	CDA-I	CDA-II	CDA-III	CDA-IV	Other CDA
Peripheral blood count					
Anemia	Moderate-severe	Severe	Moderate	Severe	Mild
MCV	↑	nL – ↑	↑	nL – ↑	nL
Reticulocyte count	↑	nL – ↑	nL – ↑	nL – ↑	
Platelet count	nL	nL	nL	nL	Decreased
Smear findings	All: Anisopoikilocytosis, elevated RDW, basophilic stippling				
Other laboratory values					
Hemolysis markers	All: Elevated LDH and bilirubin				
Hgb F	↑	↑	↑	↑↑	Variable
Ham's test	Negative	Positive	Negative	Negative	Negative
Known Genetics	CDAN1; C15orf41	SEC23B	KIF23	KLF1	GATA1

(continued)

Table 15.1 (continued)

Parameter	CDA-I	CDA-II	CDA-III	CDA-IV	Other CDA
Bone marrow morphology	Erythroid hyperplasia, multinucleated erythroblasts; Chromatin bridges with binucleation	Erythroid hyperplasia, multinucleated erythroblasts; Rare pseudo Gaucher macrophages	Erythroid hyperplasia, multinucleated erythroblasts	Erythroid hyperplasia, multinucleated or bi-nucleated erythroblasts	Megakaryocytic hypoplasia and dysplasia; erythroid hyperplasia with variable nuclear aberrancy
Inheritance pattern	Autosomal recessive	Autosomal recessive	Autosomal dominant or sporadic	Autosomal dominant	Autosomal recessive, X-linked, other
Clinical Symptoms	Usually present in neonatal period; skeletal dysmorphism; HSM; jaundice	Often young children; HSM; jaundice; iron overload	Variable age presentation; mild iron overload; angioid streak, occasional lymphoproliferative disorder	Variable age presentation; HSM; jaundice; iron overload	Variable age presentation; thrombocytopenia; iron overload
Therapy	All: Transfusions as needed (many are not transfusion dependent); monitor for iron overload; consider HSCT in refractory cases; consider splenectomy in refractory cases of CDA-II				

MCV mean corpuscular volume, *nL* normal, *HSM* hepatosplenomegaly

Differential Diagnosis

The variability of presentation makes CDA difficult to distinguish from other inherited hemolytic anemias, such as hereditary spherocytosis, hereditary stomatocytosis, RBC enzyme defects such as G6PD (glucose-6-phosphate dehydrogenase), or pyruvate kinase deficiency. The absence of neutropenia, thrombocytopenia, or dysplasia in nonerythroid lineages will differentiate CDA from myelodysplastic syndrome [1, 4, 5]. As above, morphology and, increasingly, genetic testing will help distinguish CDAs from other diseases.

Prognosis

The majority of patients with CDA do well with supportive care and appropriate management of transfusions and iron overload. The most severe presentations are those that present in the newborn period or even in utero, with hydrops, and these patients may require intrauterine transfusions [1]. Some morbidity among patients with CDA can also be attributed to misdiagnoses. For example, while splenectomy is often a part of management in hereditary spherocytosis, it does not benefit patients with CDA whose hemolysis is primarily intravascular and can lead to adverse effects such as thrombosis or infectious complications. CDAs usually do not progress to myelodysplastic disease or acute myeloid leukemia.

Treatment

Treating CDA requires a balance between managing anemia and preventing iron overload. Patients with milder symptoms who do not require transfusions should be monitored with complete blood counts and iron studies on a regular basis. Transfusions are standard of care for those with severe anemia, and those who have regular transfusions will require subsequent chelation for iron overload. Patients with CDA are likely to develop iron overload out of proportion to their transfusion requirements.

Patients with severe CDA have been treated with hematopoietic stem cell transplantation [4]. Transplant can be curative for patients who would otherwise have high transfusion needs, but it can lead to considerable morbidities, including graft-vs-host disease, viral reactivation, veno-occlusive disease, and graft failure requiring second transplant. As with most transplants, matched sibling donors are preferred to unrelated donors.

While splenectomy may reduce transfusion needs among patients with CDA II, it is not helpful and may be harmful for patients with CDA I. Patients with CDA may also require cholecystectomy because they develop gallstones secondary to chronic hemolysis.

Promising Clinical Studies

Given the rarity of CDA, there have been few organized clinical studies aimed at new treatments. There are currently two registries that are working to collect data on patients with CDA to further characterize the disease course and associated genetic mutations. The CDA Registry (CDAR) was started in 2016 and includes patients from the United States, Canada, and Mexico. There is also a similar European Registry of CDA Types [5].

A few targeted therapies have been evaluated for patients with specific subtypes of CDA. For example, interferon-alpha has been shown to improve the efficiency of erythropoiesis among patients with CDA I, although the underlying mechanism is not clear [5].

CDA clinical research is limited by a notable lack of preclinical models. Because of different gene expression patterns between mice and humans, many of the mutations that preferentially affect erythroid cells in humans lead to prenatal death in mouse models. In combination with data collection from registries, further preclinical models are needed to test novel therapies for CDA.

Board Questions (Single Best Choice)

1. A 2-year-old male patient was clinically diagnosed with hemolytic anemia since birth. At birth, he showed a severe anemia (Hemoglobin 4 g/dl), hyperbilirubinemia (total bilirubin 5.5 g/dl), and elevated lactate dehydrogenase (LDH 5,908 U/L). Abdominal ultrasound showed hepatomegaly. Blood exchange transfusion was performed for severe anemia and hyperbilirubinemia. Further examination showed small left fourth toe and malposition of right fourth toe. At that time, chromosomal study revealed normal karyotype (46 XY). After intensive care, his anemia was improved (Hb of 10.9 g/dl) and patient was discharged. However, he received regular transfusion during next two years, because of low Hb levels (around 5–6 g/dl) and poor body weight gain. This patient was brought to our hospital and a bone marrow aspiration was performed, which revealed an erythroid hyperplasia and occasional dyserythropoiesis (including nuclear bridging and multinucleation). A genetic consult was recommended, and a germline next-generation sequencing (NGS) panel identified a homozygous mutation in CDAN1 gene. Based on the above information, the most appropriate diagnosis of this patient is:

   A. Congenital Dyserythroid Anemia, type I
   B. Congenital Dyserythroid Anemia, type II
   C. Congenital Dyserythroid Anemia, type III
   D. Congenital Dyserythroid Anemia, type IV
   E. Congenital Dyserythroid Anemia, other types

Answer and rational: A. The bone marrow findings and genetic mutations are diagnostic for CDA-type I.

2. A 2-month-old female baby was admitted to our hospital with anemia. The hemoglobin level was 2.6 g/dl and hematocrit was 8.3%. Both red blood cells and reticulocyte counts were reduced. The white blood cell and platelet counts were normal. Total serum bilirubin level was 0.6 g/dl. The patient received two blood transfusions immediately. Further examination

showed no jaundice. The developmental milestones were appropriate for age. Examination of other systems did not reveal any abnormalities. A bone marrow aspiration showed normocellular marrow with M: E (myeloid-to-erythroid ratio) of 58:1. Red cell precursors were markedly reduced. The other cell lines were normal. Ultrasound abdomen, Ultrasound cranium, Echocardiogram, and Magnetic Resonance Imaging (MRI) of the brain did not reveal any abnormality. Based on the above case information, which of the following is true?

A. This patient is likely to have congenital dyserythropoietic anemia (CDA)
B. This patient is likely to have a germline mutation of ribosomal protein (RPS) genes.
C. This patient is likely to have reduced red cell adenosine deaminase.
D. This patient is likely to have a recent virus infection.
E. This patient is likely to have an iron deficiency.

Answer and rational: B. The bone marrow finding of marked reduced erythroid lineage in bone marrow suggests a Diamond Blackfan Anemia (DBA), which often has elevated red cell adenosine deaminase and mutations in *RPS* genes.

References

1. Iolascon A, Andolfo I, Russo R. Congenital dyserythropoietic anemias. Blood. 2020;136(11):1274–83. https://doi.org/10.1182/blood.2019000948.
2. Niss O, Lorsbach RB, Berger M, et al. Congenital dyserythropoietic anemia type I: first report from the Congenital Dyserythropoietic Anemia Registry of North America (CDAR). Blood Cells Mol Dis. 2021;87:102534. https://doi.org/10.1016/j.bcmd.2020.102534.
3. Hernández G, Romero-Cortadellas L, Ferrer-Cortès X, et al. Mutations in the RACGAP1 gene cause autosomal recessive congenital dyserythropoietic anemia type III. Haematologica. 2022;6. https://doi.org/10.3324/haematol.2022.281277.
4. Rangarajan HG, Stanek JR, Abdel-Azim H, et al. Hematopoietic cell transplantation for congenital dyserythropoietic anemia: a report from the

Pediatric Transplant and Cellular Therapy Consortium. Transplant Cell Ther. 2022;28(6):329.e1–9. https://doi.org/10.1016/j.jtct.2022.03.007.
5. Risinger M, Emberesh M, Kalfa TA. Rare hereditary hemolytic anemias: diagnostic approach and considerations in management. Hematol Oncol Clin North Am. 2019;33(3):373–92. https://doi.org/10.1016/j.hoc.2019.01.002.

Autoimmune Hemolytic Anemia

16

Sudeepthi Bandikatla, Yumeng Zhang, and Michael Jaglal

Introduction

Autoimmune hemolytic anemia (AIHA) is a group of immune-mediated disorders caused by autoantibodies against self-RBC antigens. In the United States, the estimated incidence of AIHA in adults ranges from 0.8 to 3 per 100,000 population per year, and a prevalence of 17 cases per 100,000 people yearly. AIHA includes the following types (Table 16.1):

(a) Warm autoimmune hemolytic anemia (wAIHA) accounts for 60–70% of cases.
(b) Cold agglutinin disease (CAD) accounts for 20–25% of cases.
(c) Mixed-type AIHA accounts for 1–8% of cases.
(d) Paroxysmal cold hemoglobinuria (PCH) accounts for 1–5% of cases.

S. Bandikatla (✉)
Moffitt Cancer Center, Tampa, FL, USA
e-mail: sudeepthi.bandikatla@moffitt.org

Y. Zhang
Department of Malignant Hematology, Moffitt Cancer Center, Tampa, FL, USA

M. Jaglal
Department of Hematology and Oncology, Moffitt Cancer Center, Tampa, FL, USA

L. Sokol, L. Zhang (eds.), *Non-Neoplastic Hematologic Disorders*,
https://doi.org/10.1007/978-3-031-62373-8_16

Table 16.1 Types of autoimmune hemolytic anemia

Types of autoimmune hemolytic anemia
Warm antibody
Primary
Secondary
Lymphoproliferative disorders: CLL, lymphoma
Autoimmune: e.g., SLE
Infectious disease: HIV, CMV, HSV, Hep E, babesiosis
Immunodeficiencies: CVID
Solid tumors: Ovarian cancer
Transplant
Inflammatory disease: IBD
Drugs: Penicillins, cephalosporins, methyldopa
Cold antibody
Primary
Secondary
Infectious: mycoplasma, EBV, CMV
Autoimmune
Lymphoma: Overt B cell lymphoproliferative disorder
Mixed
Paroxysmal cold hemoglobinuria

CLL chronic lymphocytic leukemia, *SLE* systemic lupus erythematosus, *HIV* human immunodeficiency virus, *CMV* cytomegalovirus, *HSV* herpes simplex virus, *Hep E* hepatitis E, *CVID* common variable immunodeficiency, *IBD* inflammatory bowel disease, *EBV* Epstein–Barr virus

These classifications can be further divided based on the pathogenesis. Primary AIHA has no apparent inciting or associated disease. In contrast, secondary AIHA occurs when the AIHA is associated with an underlying condition, such as lymphoproliferative diseases, autoimmune diseases, immunodeficiencies, infections, and solid tumors. However, these disorders may not be evident during the presentation [1, 2].

Pathogenesis (Table 16.2)

However, wAIHA occurs when autoantibodies, predominantly IgG, bind to red blood cells at a physiologic temperature (37 °C). These antibodies can induce erythrocyte destruction through a variety of mechanisms. One mechanism is opsonization, in which the autoantibodies coat the RBCs and make them more susceptible to phagocytosis by mononuclear leukocytes, particularly in the spleen. RBC destruction mostly occurs extravascularly, in reticuloendothelial macrophages. However, in severe cases or

Table 16.2 Pathogenesis of wAIHA, CAD, PCH , and mixed types

Pathogenesis				
	Autoantibody	Immunoglobulin class	Complement activation	Predominant type of hemolysis
wAIHA	Warm-reactive, panreactive, polyclonal	IgG (in rare cases, IgM or IgA)	Frequently none; classical pathway (++), terminal pathway (+)	Extravascular (mainly in the spleen)
CAD	Cold agglutinin, anti-I (in rare cases, anti-Pr or anti-IH), monoclonal	IgM (in rare cases, IgG)	Classical pathway (+++), terminal pathway (+)	Extravascular (mainly in the liver); intravascular (in acute exacerbations)
PCH	Nonagglutinating, biphasic anti-P, polyclonal	IgG (in rare cases, IgM)	Classical pathway (+++), terminal pathway (+++)	Intravascular
Mixed	Both warm- and cold-reactive antibodies	IgG plus IgM	Present, details not established	Not established

wAIHA warm autoimmune hemolytic anemia, *CAD* cold agglutinin disease, *PCH* paroxysmal cold hemoglobinuria

The designation (+) denotes weak or absent, (++) moderate, and (+++) strong

when the complement membrane attack complex is deposited on the RBC surface, intravascular hemolysis may occur. Splenic macrophages recognize and phagocytose a portion of RBC membrane with attached IgG heavy chain antibodies through the expression of the Fcγ receptor (CD16), resulting in the development of spherocytes. In addition, cytotoxic CD8+ T lymphocytes and NK cells residing in the spleen also express CD16 and can cause destruction of RBCs by means of antibody-dependent cell-mediated cytotoxicity (ADCC). Hepatic macrophages have receptors for complement C3b fragments and can phagocytose RBCs with complement on their surface.

Cold AIHA is typically mediated by IgM autoantibodies. These autoantibodies can bind to the surface of RBCs at lower temperatures, typically below 30 °C. This binding can result in the agglutination of the RBCs (cold agglutination), leading to their destruction through several mechanisms. The hemolytic process in CAD is mainly extravascular and mediated by complement. The pentameric structure of IgM allows it to agglutinate erythrocytes directly. IgM can activate complement, and this can lead to the coating of red cells with the C3b split products. Cells opsonized with C3b are susceptible to phagocytosis by the monocytes and cause RBC lysis due to the activation of terminal complement cascade.

PCH is a cold-temperature triggered autoimmune hemolytic anemia due to the production of an IgG antibody, with anti-P specificity, and detected with a positive Donath–Landsteiner test. Although the Coombs test can demonstrate positivity for complement, the titer of cold agglutinins is frequently only moderately increased. In PCH, the IgG binds to RBC in the cooler peripheral circulation, but when the RBC warms, complement-mediated destruction takes place [3, 4].

Interestingly, IgG and IgM immunoglobulins can occur simultaneously in some subjects, resulting in a disorder known as mixed AIHA.

Diagnosis

Clinical Features

- Distinct severity of symptoms such as anemia, jaundice, abdominal pain, and fever are reported. Mild splenomegaly is common. Depending on the etiology, hepatomegaly, and lymphadenopathy may be evident at presentation. The presenting complaint in secondary cases may be related to the underlying disease, such as joint pain in lupus.

Primary Evaluation

Hemolysis Screen

In the hemolysis screen test, coming in the following section are laboratory parameters serving as indicators of hemolysis: an elevated reticulocyte count, low or undetectable levels of haptoglobin in the presence of microspherocytes in the peripheral blood smear, and the possible presence of nucleated RBCs; additionally, there is an elevation in plasma-free hemoglobin, indirect bilirubin, urobilinogen, and lactate dehydrogenase (LDH) levels.

Specific Tests (Fig. 16.1)

Coombs/direct antiglobulin test (DAT): to detect surface-bound anti-RBC IgG antibodies and the complement degradation product C3d.

It is very important to mention that DAT could produce false-negative results because of the presence of IgA autoantibodies (not detectable by routine reagents), low-affinity IgG, or RBC-bound IgG with concentrations below the test threshold.

If DAT is negative, but suspicion for AIHA remains high, the following investigations might be necessary:

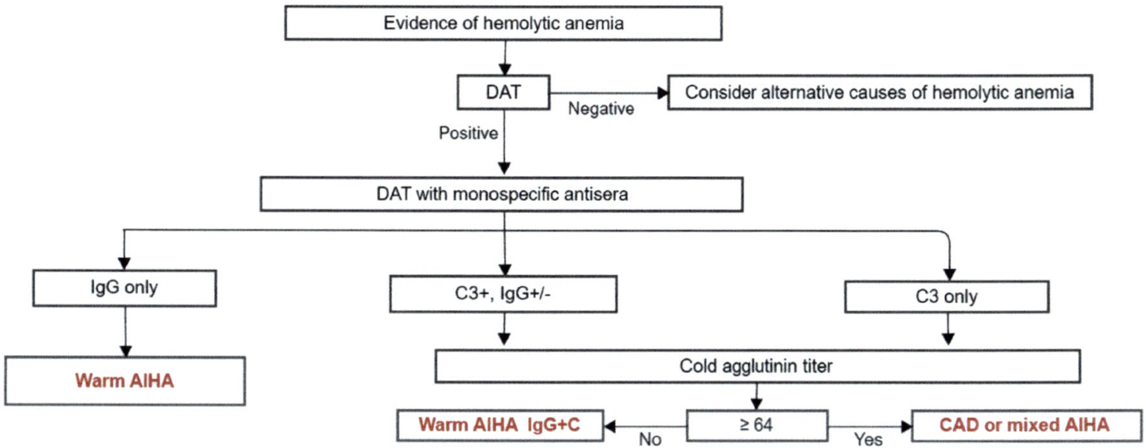

Fig. 16.1 Coombs/direct antibody test pathway. DAT direct antiglobulin test, Warm AIHA warm autoimmune hemolytic anemia, CAD cold agglutinin disease

  - To employ more sensitive DAT tests in reference labs, including microcolumn, solid phase, ELISA, flow cytometry, dual DAT, mitogen-stimulated DAT, and tests for drug-dependent and drug-independent antibodies.
- To utilize washes with cold saline, LISS (low-ionic-strength saline solution), or PEG (polyethylene glycol)
  - To perform Donath–Landsteiner biphasic hemolysin.

Approximately, 5–10% of AIHA patients have negative DAT, and the diagnosis is made after all other potential causes of hemolysis have been excluded and based on clinical response to therapy [8].

Detection of Underlying Disorders

HIV, HBV, HCV (to assess for viral infection), anti-dsDNA, ANA (to assess for rheumatologic condition), CT chest, abdomen, and pelvis (to assess for lymphoproliferative disease, splenomegaly), immunophenotyping of B-lymphocytes from peripheral blood, serum immunoglobulins, and electrophoresis with immunofixation (if a cold autoantibody is suspected, keep the sample at 37 °C until the serum has been separated).

1. Additional tests in CAD include antibody titer and thermal amplitude. Patients with CAD typically have a titer of 1:64 or greater.
2. Bone marrow examination can be useful in selected patients such as those with CAD and clinical suspicion for bone marrow disease, abnormal peripheral blood film suggesting possible marrow pathological process, presence of monoclonal gammopathy or hypogammaglobulinemia, and lymph node enlargement or splenomegaly [5–7].

Major Differential Diagnosis

DAT Positive

- Transfusion related: Acute hemolytic transfusion reaction, delayed hemolytic transfusion reaction, and delayed serologic response
- Passive transfer of antibodies in immunoglobulin preparation
- Drugs induced

DAT Negative

- Hemoglobinopathies, enzymopathies, and membrane defects
- Microangiopathic hemolytic anemias
- Drugs induced
- Toxins/Wilson's disease
- IgA- or IgM-dependent hemolysis
- Low-affinity antibody

Prognosis

The prognosis depends on the underlying condition and other factors. High mortality rates can be seen in patients admitted with rapidly progressing organ failure requiring overlapping treatments.

According to a study of patients with AIHA in Denmark, 1-year survival and median survival for patients with primary AIHA were 82.7% and 9.8 years, for secondary AIHA, they were 69.1% and 3.3 years, and for CAD, they were 85.5% and 8.8 years [8].

Treatment

General Management

- Severe acute anemia from AIHA is lethal, and immediate transfusion of packed RBCs can be lifesaving. The involvement of transfusion medicine or a blood bank may be needed to minimize delays caused by serologic incompatibility expected with AIHA. If anemia is severe and symptomatic, transfusion of ABO Rh and K-matched RBCs may be favored over waiting for blood unit with full-compatibility testing.

- Secondary AIHA usually requires therapy of the underlying disorder. If the AIHA-associated condition does not need any therapy, AIHA can usually be managed similarly to primary AIHA.

wAIHA (Fig. 16.2)

Therapies are primarily indicated for symptomatic anemia in wAIHA, in particular for acute and severe state, complete remission is often not achieved or sustained. For patients with milder anemia, a "watch and wait" strategy can be considered, after evaluating the potential benefits and burdens. Participation in clinical trials should be discussed with each patient since published data on management are very limited. Spontaneous remission seems rare.

Corticosteroids (e.g., prednisone 1 mg/kg orally once daily for 3–4 weeks and then taper in 3–6 months) are the treatment of choice in wAIHA.

AIHA relapse is common, and prolonged steroid use has significant side effects; long-term control frequently necessitates using other agents. When there is no improvement after about 3 weeks of steroids, rituximab, a human monoclonal antibody against CD20, is added. In selected patients, rituximab can be administered in the first-line setting in addition to steroids. Rituximab is given as 1000 mg IV on days 1 and 15 or 375 mg/m^2 weekly for 4 weeks or fixed-dose Rituxan 100 mg weekly ×4 doses.

Once disease remission is attained, steroids can be tapered.

About 70% of patients with primary wAIHA respond to splenectomy, and it remains a viable second-line option when economic constraints limit access to rituximab.

Mycophenolate mofetil (500 mg twice daily, titrated up to 1 g twice daily), cyclosporine (2.5 mg/kg oral twice per day), azathioprine (2–2.5 mg/kg daily), cyclophosphamide (50–100 mg or

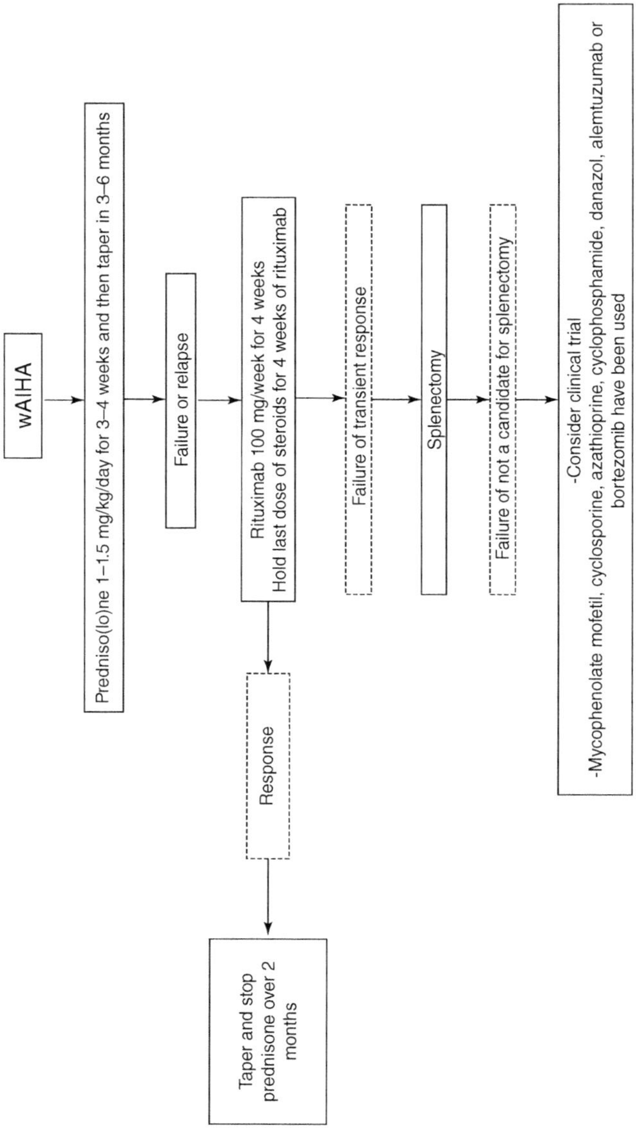

Fig. 16.2 Treatment of wAIHA. wAIHA warm autoimmune hemolytic anemia

1–2 mg/kg daily), danazol (e.g., 200 mg three times/day), alemtuzumab (IV, subcutaneous: gradually escalate to a maintenance of 10–30 mg per dose three times weekly for 4–12 weeks), bortezomib (1.3 mg/m^2 weekly for 1–4 weeks IV), and hematopoietic stem cell transplantation have all been used to treat refractory AIHA. It is challenging to determine response rates to these agents since published data are limited to small series only. However, it is estimated that they are lower than responses to rituximab or splenectomy.

Salvage Therapy for Severe Hemolysis Associated with wAIHA

Patients with severe hemolysis may not be able to maintain adequate hemoglobin levels despite transfusions.

In a few acute cases, IVIG and plasma exchange along with immunosuppressive therapy are considered as acute therapeutic approaches. Plasma exchange with human albumin replacement is used as an emergency measure to remove pathogenic immune complexes, autoantibodies, and activated complement, but its role is still being established through limited case reports, often in combination with immunosuppressive therapy.

Intravenous methylprednisolone can be considered in severe fulminant cases. Erythropoiesis-stimulating agents (ESAs) can be beneficial for patients with severe wAIHA requiring transfusions and with a low reticulocyte count. Splenectomy or partial splenic embolization may be considered for highly transfusion-dependent patients unresponsive to other therapies.

Additionally, to decrease venous thrombosis risk, thromboprophylaxis is indicated. In summary, transfusion-dependent or life-threatening wAIHA usually requires combined therapeutic approaches such as ESA ± plasma exchange and/or IVIg, active immunosuppressive therapy, and emergency splenectomy/embolization [9].

Promising Clinical Studies

Several trials include a phase II study to assess the safety, tolerability, preliminary efficacy, and pharmacokinetics of APL-2, a complement (C3) Inhibitor, in wAIHA or CAD subjects; a phase II trial with Parsaclisib, an oral PI3Kδ inhibitor, in patients with primary wAIHA.

Caveats

- DATs cannot detect less than 100 molecules in an RBC; fewer molecules can lead to clinically significant hemolysis. It will also miss IgA or IgG4. The next step will be the super Coombs test.
– Hemolysis tends to be more severe in wAIHA and can be fatal if reticulocytopenia is also present and, therefore, immediate blood transfusion should be done in such scenarios.

Board Questions

A 74-year-old female presents with fatigue for 4 weeks. Conjunctival pallor, scleral icterus, and splenomegaly are present on exam. Her recent laboratory data showed hemoglobin 6 g/dL, MCV 101 fL, platelets 300 × 10^9/L, WBC 30 × 10^9/L; reticulocyte count: 7% (0.84–2.21%), absolute reticulocyte count (absolute): 328.50 × 10^9/L (38.30–110.50). In iron studies, the serum levels of vitamin B12 and folic acid were within normal limits. Indirect bilirubin 100 μmol/L (5–25), LDH 1440 U/L (250–580), Haptoglobin <10 mg/dL (30–200). The direct antiglobulin test is strongly positive for IgG. Peripheral blood film shows spherocytes and nucleated RBCs smudge cells.

1. What is the diagnosis?

   A. Hereditary spherocytosis
   B. Autoimmune hemolytic anemia
   C. Cold agglutin disease
   D. Bone marrow failure syndrome

   Correct Answer (B). Autoimmune hemolytic anemia

A diagnosis of CLL is confirmed via immunophenotyping of the peripheral blood. Secondary warm autoimmune hemolytic anemia is diagnosed. The patient is otherwise asymptomatic and has small cervical and axillary lymphadenopathy.

2. How will you manage her wAIHA?

   A. Splenectomy
   B. Rituximab
   C. Start prednisolone 1 mg/kg
   D. Intravenous immune globulin (IVIG)
   E. Treat the underlying CLL

   Correct Answer C. Treatment with prednisolone is the most appropriate intervention

References

1. Lechner K, Jäger U. How I treat autoimmune hemolytic anemias in adults. Blood. 2010;116(11):1831–8.
2. Barcellini W, Fattizzo B. The changing landscape of autoimmune hemolytic anemia. Front Immunol. 2020;11:946. https://doi.org/10.3389/fimmu.2020.00946. Berentsen S, Barcellini W. Autoimmune hemolytic anemias. N Engl J Med 2021;385(15):1407–19.
3. Michalak SS, Olewicz-Gawlik A, Rupa-Matysek J, Wolny-Rokicka E, Nowakowska E, Gil L. Autoimmune hemolytic anemia: current knowledge and perspectives. Immun Ageing. 2020;17(1):38.
4. Hill A, Hill QA. Autoimmune hemolytic anemia. Hematology Am Soc Hematol Educ Program. 2018;2018(1):382–9.
5. Altman JK, Mandernach MW, Naik RP, Ulrickson M. American Society of Hematology self-assessment program. Washington, DC: American Society of Hematology; 2022. https://doi.org/10.1182/ashsap8. ISBN (electronic): 9780978921279.
6. Zanella A, Barcellini W. Treatment of autoimmune hemolytic anemias. Haematologica. 2014;99(10):1547–54.
7. Berentsen S, Barcellini W. Autoimmune hemolytic anemias. N Engl J Med. 2021;385(15):1407–19.
8. Hansen DL, Möller S, Frederiksen H. Survival in autoimmune hemolytic anemia remains poor, results from a nationwide cohort with 37 years of follow-up. Eur J Haematol. 2022;109(1):10–20.
9. Jäger U, Barcellini W, Broome CM, et al. Diagnosis and treatment of autoimmune hemolytic anemia in adults: recommendations from the First International Consensus Meeting. Blood Rev. 2020;41:100648.

Cryopathic Hemolytic Anemias

17

Stanislav Ivanov and Atif Hussein

Introduction

Autoimmune hemolytic anemia (AHA) is characterized by the presence of autoantibodies directed against autologous red blood cells (RBCs), leading to a shortened RBC survival. The presence of an autoantibody and/or complement on RBC membranes detected by positive direct antiglobulin test (DAT) is essential for the diagnosis. Most patients with AHA exhibit warm-reactive antibodies usually of the IgG immunoglobulin isotype, whereas the majority of the remaining AHAs demonstrate cold-reactive antibodies. These autoantibodies bind to RBCs at temperatures below 37 °C, usually below 31 °C, thus triggering a cascade of immune responses resulting in the destruction of RBCs. These types of AHA, termed cryopathic hemolytic anemias, are uncommon, at least in the classic form. Approximately, 7–25% of AHAs are cold agglutinin mediated. The incidence of cold agglutinin disease is approximately 1 in 300,000 patients. Reports demonstrate a slight predilection for female patients who are 60 years of age and older, peaking in the seventh and eighth decades of life. In this chapter,

S. Ivanov (✉) · A. Hussein
Department Hematology and Oncology, Memorial Cancer Institute, Miami, FL, USA
e-mail: SIvanov@mhs.net

L. Sokol, L. Zhang (eds.), *Non-Neoplastic Hematologic Disorders*,
https://doi.org/10.1007/978-3-031-62373-8_17

we will discuss the pathogenesis, diagnosis, prognosis, and management of these cryopathic hemolytic anemias [1, 2].

Pathogenesis

Two major cold-sensitive antibodies exist that can cause clinical manifestations of hemolytic anemia: cold agglutinins and cold hemolysins. The mechanism of how each contributes to the manifestation of symptoms is unique, but they do share a common characteristic, which is increased activity at below core body temperatures, usually below 31 °C. To understand the mechanism of these autoantibodies, we must first understand the structure of the RBC membrane as well as the role temperature plays in facilitating the interaction between the autoantibodies and RBCs.

Cryopathic autoantibodies such as cold agglutinins, cold hemolysins, or cryoglobulins tend to bind weakly to RBCs at temperatures approaching body temperature and more strongly at lower temperatures. This is because the binding of cold autoantibodies to carbohydrate antigens occurs predominantly through weak bonds such as hydrogen bonds and van der Waals forces rather than through ionic bonds. This weak interaction may be due to the nature of the antigen and the antigen-binding site on the antibody, both of which are very restricted in their chemistry. These weak forces get stronger with reduction in ambient temperature, which has the effect of reducing spontaneous Brownian movement, thus accounting for the cold-reactivity of cold autoantibodies [1, 2].

There are a multitude of antigenic epitopes on the surface of RBCs (See Fig. 17.1). Many are serologically defined as blood group antigens. These antigens contain polysaccharide epitopes on glycoprotein or glycolipids such as ceramides which are thought to contribute to the structural integrity of the cell, promote erythropoiesis, intracellular transport and immune surveillance. Two blood group antigens are implicated in the manifestation of cryopathic hemolytic anemias: "I"/ "i" and "P."

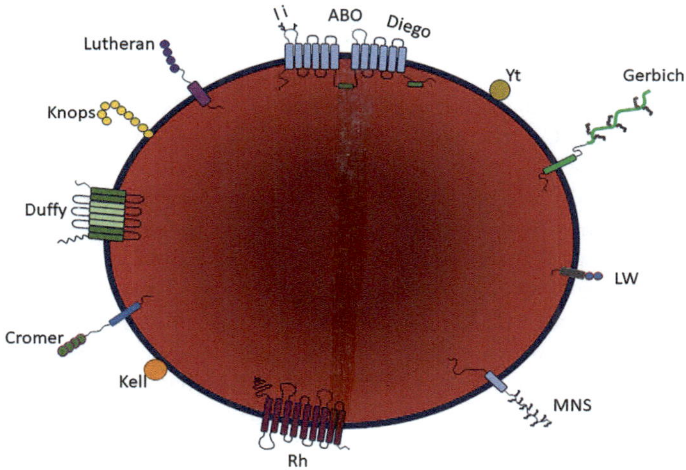

Fig. 17.1 RBC antigen epitopes

Cold Agglutinins and "I" antigen

The vast majority of cold agglutinins are directed against "I" or "i" antigens on RBCs. The "i" antigen is the predominant structure seen in fetal RBCs, however, following birth, enzymatic activity leads to the expansion and branching of the polysaccharide leading to formation of the "I" antigen which comprises ~99% of the I-blood group expression. While ubiquitous, the "I" antigens are not clearly understood but are thought to serve as precursors to the assembly of ABO and Lewis blood groups [3–5].

Cold agglutinins are autoantibodies directed against the RBC antigen. The majority of these cold agglutinins are IgM, which contribute to the antibody's ability to exert its pathologic effect. Although other isotypes have been reported, such as IgA and IgG, they are not believed to contribute markedly to the pathophysiology of cold agglutinin disease (CAD). The IgM antibodies are pentameric, which allows for the effective binding of multiple RBCs and agglutination leading to extravascular hemolysis. These antibodies can be monoclonal, derived from a single clone lymphocyte, or polyclonal, derived from multiple independent lymphocytes. This distinction can help organize cold agglutinins into (1) idiopathic or primary chronic agglutinin disease and (2) secondary cold agglutinin syndrome.

Primary CAD, characterized by RBC agglutination and extravascular hemolysis, is usually seen in patients who do not have an underlying disorder but are thought to have a low-grade clonal bone marrow disorder and thus tend to have monoclonal antibody expression. These conditions tend to be associated with a mutation in the KMT2D and CARD11 genes. Secondary cold agglutinin syndromes (CAS) can be seen in the setting of lymphoid malignancy, which is monoclonal in nature or as a sequelae of autoimmune disorders or infections (viral or bacterial) in which case polyclonal expression can be seen. The mechanism of hemolysis in both primary CAD and secondary CAS is believed to be secondary to antibody-antigen association and complement fixation. The IgM binds to antigen "I"/"i" which then serves to recruit components of the classical complement pathway (C1, C2, C4) which produce C3b-coated RBCs. These RBCs are then further phagocytosed leading to extravascular hemolysis in the reticuloendothelial system (spleen and liver). A small fraction of the remaining C3b-coated RBCs may experience dissociation of the IgM due to re-warming, causing completion of the complement cascade and formation of the membrane attack complex (MAC) leading to intravascular hemolysis.

Cold Hemolysin and "P" antigen

Cold hemolysins, like cold agglutinins, are autoantibodies that are directed toward antigen on the surface of the RBCs. Unlike cold agglutinins, cold hemolysins are primarily IgG antibodies which are polyclonal in nature. These autoantibodies, also known as Donath-Landsteiner antibodies, have increased proclivity to bind selectively to the "P" antigen, particularly when exposed to lower than core body temperatures. This antigen belongs to the GLOB blood system and has diverse expression on tissues including RBCs as well as urothelial cells. This antigen can contribute to transfusion reactions and serves as a binding site for parvovirus.

Unlike what is seen with cold agglutinins, the complement fixation in cold hemolysin-mediated disease leads to completion of the complement cascade and formation of the MAC leading to intravascular hemolysis. The primary reason for this phenomenon is that the association between the IgG and "P" antigen and subsequent complement fixation occurs in parts of the body that are experiencing low temperatures (i.e., extremities). As the blood circulates away from the cooler temperatures and closer to the core body temperature, the IgG disassociates, however, the complement fixation persists with the formation of C3b complexes that bind to cells. The C3b-coated RBCs complete the complement cascade and form the MAC (See Fig. 17.2). This manifests as intravascular hemolysis which is classic for cold hemolysin-associated hemolytic anemia. CAS caused by cold hemolysins is commonly seen in the context of recent viral or bacterial infections (particularly *Mycoplasma pneumoniae*) as well as in states of autoimmune disorders and rarely, in the context of lymphomas and lymphoid malignancies [6, 7].

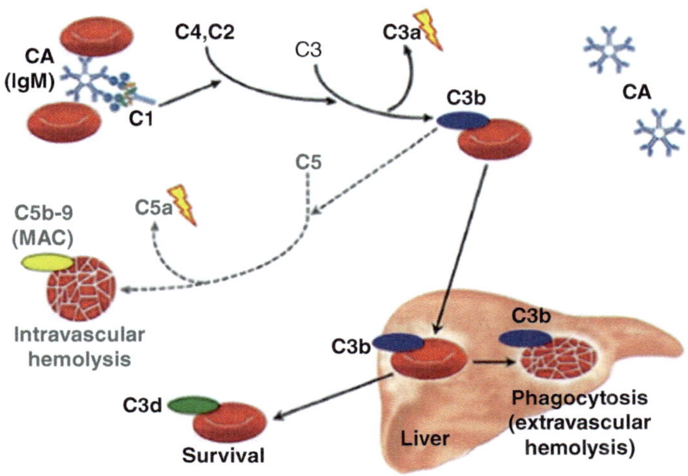

Fig. 17.2 Cold agglutinin mediated complement activation cascade

Diagnosis

Cryopathic hemolytic anemias are more commonly observed in women than men. Presentation of CAD usually occurs in the mid to late 60s, however, can broadly present between 30 and 90 years of age. In contrast, CAS, such as paroxysmal cold hemoglobinuria (PCH), is more common in the pediatric population. Generally, patients with cold autoantibodies are unaware of their condition until exposed to cold temperatures. Typical symptoms include cold-associated symptoms such as acrocyanosis, livedo reticularis, Reynaud's phenomenon, as well as skin ulcerations and pain or discomfort when consuming cold foods. These manifestations can vary in severity. Commonly patients with CAD may experience complaints of chronic fatigue likely associated with anemia. Hemolysis tends to be chronic but acute exacerbations may occur during episodes of exposure to cold. Physical examination may demonstrate evidence of splenomegaly. Laboratory evaluation usually reveals mild to moderate anemia. Peripheral smear shows evidence of agglutination as well as polychromasia and spherocytosis. Increased cellular turnover usually results in abnormal markers of hemolysis (elevated lactate dehydrogenase, reticulocytes, low haptoglobin, and elevated indirect bilirubin). Direct antiglobulin testing (Coomb's test) is usually positive for C3 alone in cryopathic hemolytic anemia. Patients with CAD will commonly have high titers of IgM antibody specific against "I/i" antigen, whereas patients with paroxysmal cold hemoglobinuria have elevated titers of IgG autoantibodies against "P antigen." The presence of these autoantibodies can be detected by biphasic Donath-Landsteiner test.

Major Differential Diagnosis

Identification of cryopathic hemolytic anemia requires that it be distinguished from other hemolytic anemias. Differential diagnoses include mixed hemolytic anemia, paroxysmal nocturnal hemoglobinuria, and drug-induced hemolytic anemia. When patients present with peripheral vaso-occlusive symptoms particularly in the context of low temperatures, consideration must be given to conditions such as Reynaud phenomena and cryoglobulinemia.

Special consideration must be given to patients with recent bouts of bacterial or viral infections. Patients with *Mycoplasma pneumoniae* and mononucleosis infections can present in a similar fashion to CAD and can often self-resolve in 3–4 weeks.

Prognosis

Generally patients with chronic presentation of CAD have stable disease and normal long-term survival. Patient with paroxysmal cold hematuria, particularly children, however, have high rates mortality due to severe acute episodes of hemolysis but can be supported through an episode if identified early. Most bouts of post-infectious PCH are self-limited and resolve on their own, although positive IgG titers may be noted for years following the acute exacerbation.

Treatment

Cryopathic hemolytic anemias are a set of autoimmune conditions that are exacerbated by low temperatures. Management of such conditions is contingent on keeping the patient warm. Such a treatment strategy may be sufficient in the management of mild cases of hemolysis. More severe cases of hemolysis require immune suppression in order to control the symptoms the patients may exhibit. Approved regimens include glucocorticoids, although may not be helpful in low titer disease. The anti-CD20 monoclonal antibodies such as rituximab are standard treatment option for CAD. Rituximab can be administered at a dose of 375 mg/m^2 weekly for a 4 weeks. Response rates usually in the range of 54% with a median time of 11 months. Alternatively, rituximab can be used in combination with chemotherapeutic agents such as bendamustine an fludarabine particularly in cases of patients with refractory disease. When given in combination with bendamustine, rituximab is given at a dose of 375 mg/m^2 on day 1, with bendamustine given at a dose of 90 mg/m^2 on days 1 and 2 for four cycles at a 28-day interval. In a prospective study involving 45 patients treated with this regimen, responses were seen in 32 individuals (71%), with complete responses in 18 (40%). Of those who had a response, only three (<10%) relapsed after 32 months. In other regimens, rituximab was given with fludarabine at a dose of 375 mg/m^2 on days 1, 29, 57, and 85, with oral fludarabine 40 mg/m^2 on days 1 through 5, 29 through 34, 57 through 61, and 85 through 89. The use of cyclophosphamide and interferon-α may be useful in the management of chronic severe cases. Surgical interventions, such as splenectomy, are usually not indicated and of little value.

Patients with PCH usually do not require treatment as most instances are limited in their course. Most cases of post-infectious PCH are treated with supportive care and do not require immune suppression. In instances where cold-induced urticarial rash manifests, the use of antihistamines can be considered [8].

Promising Clinical Studies

The pathophysiology of cryopathic hemolytic anemia includes manifestations of intravascular hemolysis which is propagated by the activation of the complement cascade. Successful interruption of this cascade has been hypothesized as an effective means of controlling the symptoms of CAD. The CARDINAL trial tested this hypothesis by enrolling 24 patients in a 26-week multicenter open label, single arm study. The patients who were enrolled in the study should have had a recent history of blood transfusion, were enrolled to receive at least a single dose of a humanized monoclonal antibody, sutimlimab, selectively targeting the C1s protein, which is responsible for activating the complement pathway. In a composite endpoint, the least-squares mean increase in hemoglobin level was 2.6 g per deciliter at the time of treatment assessment at weeks 23, 25, and 26. A mean hemoglobin level of more than 11 g per deciliter was maintained in patients from week 3 through the end of the study period of 26 weeks. The mean bilirubin levels normalized by week 3. A total of 17 patients

(71%) did not receive a transfusion from week 5 through week 26. Clinically meaningful reductions in fatigue were observed by week 1 and were maintained throughout the study. Based on this study, patients with cold agglutinin disease who received sutimlimab as a selective upstream inhibition of the classical complement pathway rapidly halted hemolysis, increased hemoglobin levels, and reduced fatigue. At least one adverse event occurred during the treatment period in 22 patients (92%), most frequent were infections and infestations, gastrointestinal disorders, and general disorders or administration-site conditions. Seven patient (29%) had at least one serious event, none of which were determined by the investigators to be related to sutimlimab. No meningococcal infections or autoimmune diseases were reported. With this data, the FDA granted approval for the use of sutimlimab in June of 2022 [9–11].

Key Teaching Points

- Cryopathic hemolytic anemias are autoimmune states that result in RBC destruction as a result of immunoglobulin induced complement activation in the setting of low temperatures.
- Two main types of cryopathic autoantibodies exist: cold agglutinins and cold hemolysins.
- Transient elevation in cold agglutinin and/or cold hemolysins can be seen in patients with acute infections with *Mycoplasma pneumoniae.*
- Primary treatment of patients with a primary cryopathic hemolytic anemia is immune suppression with an anti-CD20 agent like rituximab.
- Sutimlimab is a novel option available for the management of cryopathic hemolytic anemias.

Board Question

72 year old previously healthy woman presents to the primary care provider with fatigue, dyspnea on exertion, and intermittent dizziness. She has worsening lack of energy for 3 months and has

noticed her finger tips turn a bluish color in the winter. She denies any fevers, chills, night sweats, unintentional weight loss or lymphadenopathy. Family history is significant for coronary artery disease. A routine CBC drawn 1 year ago was normal. She is taking no medications and does not recall any recent illness. Lab results are as follows:

Hemoglobin	8.6 g/dL
Hematocrit	25.8%
White Blood Cell Count	9×10^9/L with normal differential
Platelet Count	390×10^9
MCV	112 μm^3
Vitamin B12	450 pg/mL
Folate	6.2 ng/ml
Lactate Dehydrogenase	375 U/L
Haptoglobin	<10 mg/dL
Creatinine	0.9 mg/dL
Aspartate transaminase (AST)	25 U/L
Alanine transaminase (ALT)	32 U/L
Total Bilirubin	1.8 mg/dL
Direct Bilirubin	0.3 mg/ dL
Alkaline Phosphatase	110 U/L
Direct antiglobulin test	C3 positive, IgG negative

As part of the diagnostic work up for this disorder, the next best test to order is

A. Serum protein electrophoresis (SPEP)
B. Cryoglobulin testing
C. Osmotic fragility testing
D. Antinuclear antibody testing (ANA)

Correct Answer: B

A 75 year old previously healthy woman complains of worsening fatigue and shortness of breath for the last month. She had previously been healthy and denied any recent illness or new medications. On physical examination she appears pale and is mildly dyspneic. No hepatosplenomegaly is appreciated.

Laboratory data a provided below:

WBC	5000/μL
Hemoglobin	8.0 g/dL
MCV	135 fL
Reticulocyte count	4%
Direct Coombs Test	C3+, IgG -
SPEP	M-spike 0.2 g/dL

What is the next most appropriate step in management?

A. Prednisone
B. Splenectomy
C. Rituximab
D. Erythropoietin
E. Fludarabine

Correct Answer: C

References

1. Cryopathic hemolytic anemia. In: Lichtman MA, Kaushansky K, Prchal JT, Levi MM, Burns LJ, Armitage JO, editors. Williams manual of hematology, 9e. McGraw Hill; 2017. https://hemonc.mhmedical.com/content.aspx?bookid=1889&sectionid=137388243. Accessed 04 Jan 2023.
2. Berentsen S. How I manage patients with cold agglutinin disease. Br J Haematol. 2018;181(3):320–30. https://doi.org/10.1111/bjh.15109. Epub 2018 Jan 24. PMID: 29363757.
3. Berentsen S, Barcellini W, D'Sa S, et al. Cold agglutinin disease revisited: a multinational, observational study of 232 patients. Blood. 2020;136(4):480–8.
4. Tormey CA, Hendrickson JE. Transfusion-related red blood cell alloantibodies: induction and consequences. Blood. 2019;133(17):1821–30. https://doi.org/10.1182/blood-2018-08-833962.
5. Silberstein LE, Berkman EM, Schreiber AD. Cold hemagglutinin disease associated with IgG cold-reactive antibody. Ann Intern Med.

1987;106(2):238–42. https://doi.org/10.7326/0003-4819-106-2-238. PMID: 3800184.
6. Feizi T. The blood group Ii system: a carbohydrate antigen system defined by naturally monoclonal or oligoclonal autoantibodies of man. Immunol Commun. 1981;10(2):127–56. https://doi.org/10.3109/08820138109050693. PMID: 6169630.
7. Berentsen S, Randen U, Tjønnfjord GE. Cold agglutinin-mediated autoimmune hemolytic anemia. Hematol Oncol Clin North Am. 2015;29(3):455–71. https://doi.org/10.1016/j.hoc.2015.01.002. Epub 2015 Mar 12.
8. Rosse WF, Adams JP. The variability of hemolysis in the cold agglutinin syndrome. Blood. 1980;56(3):409–16. PMID: 7407408.
9. Berentsen S, Ulvestad E, Gjertsen BT, Hjorth-Hansen H, Langholm R, Knutsen H, Ghanima W, Shammas FV, Tjønnfjord GE. Rituximab for primary chronic cold agglutinin disease: a prospective study of 37 courses of therapy in 27 patients. Blood. 2004;103(8):2925–8. https://doi.org/10.1182/blood-2003-10-3597. Epub 2003 Dec 30. PMID: 15070665.
10. Röth A, Barcellini W, D'Sa S, Miyakawa Y, Broome CM, Michel M, Kuter DJ, Jilma B, Tvedt THA, Fruebis J, Jiang X, Lin S, Reuter C, Morales-Arias J, Hobbs W, Berentsen S. Sutimlimab in Cold Agglutinin Disease. N Engl J Med. 2021;384(14):1323–34. https://doi.org/10.1056/NEJMoa2027760. PMID: 33826820.
11. Berentsen S. New insights in the pathogenesis and therapy of cold agglutinin-mediated autoimmune hemolytic anemia. Front Immunol. 2020;11:590.

Methemoglobinemia 18

Brian D. Schlick

Introduction

Methemoglobinemia is a condition of altered hemoglobin affinity for oxygen caused by oxidation of heme iron from the ferrous (Fe^{2+}) state to the ferric (Fe^{3+}) state. Although an infrequent cause of hypoxia, if left untreated, it can be deadly.

Heme ferric iron is unable to bind oxygen, thereby reducing the oxygen-carrying capacity of hemoglobin. Additionally, ferric iron stabilizes hemoglobin when the other iron molecules are bound to oxygen. This leftward shift of the oxygen-dissociation curve decreases the release of oxygen in the capillaries, furthering contributing to hypoxia.

Most cases of methemoglobinemia are secondary to exogenous substances acting as oxidizing agents. Causative agents classically include topical anesthetics, dapsone, antimalarials, rasburicase, and nitrate-containing medicines. In one retrospective study of 133 cases of methemoglobinemia, 42% of cases were attributed to dapsone, and 24% of cases were detected post-surgically. This level of methemoglobin is of minimal clinical significance and was detected incidentally on cooximetry ordered to evaluate undifferentiated postoperative dyspnea. Severe cases

B. D. Schlick (✉)
Tennessee Oncology, Nashville, TN, USA
e-mail: brian.schlick@moffitt.org

L. Sokol, L. Zhang (eds.), *Non-Neoplastic Hematologic Disorders*,
https://doi.org/10.1007/978-3-031-62373-8_18

were seen among pediatric patients with gastrointestinal induced dehydration (n = 6) and exposure to 20% benzocaine (n = 5) [1] which is commonly used in procedures such as transesophageal echocardiograms and hemorrhoidectomy. In addition to medications, other frequent causes include nitrates used as preservatives or as found in well water. Children are particularly susceptible to this last source as they are not able to reduce methemoglobin back to hemoglobin as efficiently as adults.

Pathogenesis

Although methemoglobinemia can either be congenital or acquired, both conditions share the same underlying imbalance between ferrous and ferric iron in heme.

Under normal physiologic conditions, approximately 2% of our hemoglobin exists in the methemoglobin form because of constant oxygen-induced oxidation. To prevent clinically significant levels of methemoglobinemia, red blood cells (RBCs) rely on two strategies (Fig. 18.1).

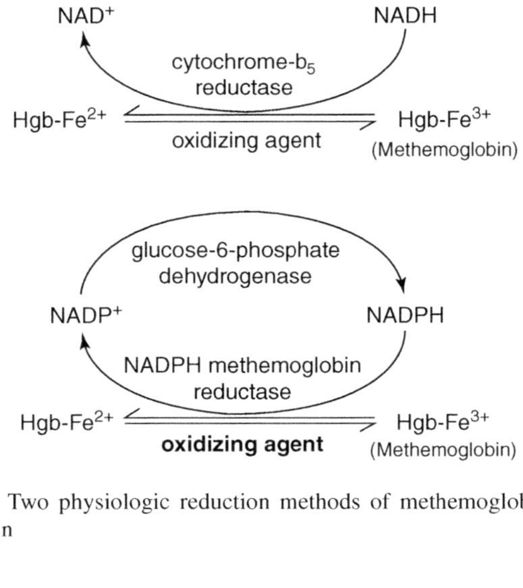

Fig. 18.1 Two physiologic reduction methods of methemoglobin back to hemoglobin

Under standard physiologic conditions, cytochrome-b5 reductase uses nicotinamide adenine dinucleotide hydrogen (NADH) formed in glycolysis to reduce iron from the ferric state back to the ferrous state. However, since RBCs do not have mitochondria to produce NADH in the Kreb's cycle, NADH is not quickly replenished when consumed under periods of oxidative stress. In these circumstances, nicotinamide adenine dinucleotide phosphate– (NADPH-) methemoglobin reductase will reduce methemoglobin back to regular hemoglobin using NADPH as a cofactor. NADPH is formed in the pentose phosphate pathway via the conversion of glucose-6-phosphate to 6-phosphogluconolactone by glucose-6-phosphate dehydrogenase.

In cases of acquired methemoglobinemia, hemoglobin oxidation overwhelms both the cytochrome-b_5 reductase and NADPH-methemoglobin reductase pathways as they are unable to replenish their respective cofactors fast enough. This prevents oxygen delivery to tissues and causes oxidative damage to the erythrocyte, leading to possible subsequent hemolysis.

Congenital methemoglobinemia is caused by either recessive mutations in enzyme cytochrome-b_5 reductase or dominant mutations in hemoglobin, which stabilize iron in the ferric state, termed as *hemoglobin M*. Mutations in cytochrome-b_5 reductase to prevent reduction of ferric iron to ferrous iron, and the erythrocyte must further rely on NADPH-methemoglobin reductase. When the cytochrome-b_5 reductase mutation is only found in erythrocytes, this is termed as *congenital methemoglobinemia type 1*, and when the mutation is found in all cells, this is termed as *congenital methemoglobinemia type 2*. Patients with congenital methemoglobinemia type 2 will have severe neurologic impairment in addition to the methemoglobin phenotype.

A diverse array of mutations leads to hemoglobin M, but all mutations stabilize heme iron in its ferric state. A mutation of histidine to tyrosine, which favors ferric over ferrous iron, in the heme binding pocket of either the α or β chains of hemoglobin is the most frequent cause of hemoglobin M [2].

Although patients with congenital methemoglobinemia will typically have methemoglobin levels from 15% to 30%, most are asymptomatic as their bodies have compensated by increasing cardiac output and RBC mass. The effect of this condition is largely cosmetic, as these patients can be visibly cyanotic. However, they are at notable risk of developing clinically significant methemoglobinemia when exposed to oxidative stress.

Diagnosis

The classic patient with methemoglobinemia has hypoxia-related symptoms, commonly headache, anxiety, and dyspnea, that are usually refractory to supplemental oxygen. When methemoglobin rise up to 15% or above, patients can demonstrate severe hypoxia related neurologic and cardiac symptoms (e.g., tachycardia, arrythmia, and confusion). Because of the rarity of this condition, a correct diagnosis may be delayed.

Methemoglobin interferes with the measurement of SpO_2 on a standard pulse oximeter, so the reported SpO_2 may not correlate with a patient's reported symptoms. A pulse oximeter emits light at two separate wavelengths—660 nm (maximally absorbed by deoxygenated hemoglobin) and 940 nm (maximally absorbed by oxyhemoglobin). The pulse oximeter uses this ratio while considering temporal differences associated with arterial pulsation to differentiate arterial from venous absorption to calculate SpO_2. Methemoglobin absorbs light at both wavelengths and thus obscures the calculated ratio between oxyhemoglobin and deoxyhemoglobin, typically giving a falsely elevated reading. Because methemoglobin cannot bind O_2, increasing levels of supplemental oxygen will not affect the measured SpO_2. As methemoglobin levels increase, the effect methemoglobin concentration has on the SpO_2 reading increases, and the SpO_2 will approach 85% because of the properties of the efficacy of methemoglobin absorbing these two wavelengths [3].

Arterial blood gas is typically obtained when evaluating a patient with undifferentiated dyspnea and cyanosis. The SaO_2 will be falsely normal but typically greater than 5% higher than the falsely elevated SpO_2. This so-called *saturation gap* is a clue to the presence of methemoglobinemia but may also be seen in carbon monoxide poisoning and sulfhemoglobinemia. To further differentiate, cooximetry is measured on the blood. Like standard pulse oximetry, cooximetry uses ratios of different absorbed wavelengths of light to calculate changes in hemoglobin oxygenation. Unlike a standard pulse oximeter, it uses multiple additional wavelengths of light to differentiate hemoglobin's varying physiologic and pathophysiologic states. Classically, the blood will also be dark brown.

Symptoms of methemoglobinemia depend on the methemoglobin level, chronicity of development of methemoglobinemia, and underlying comorbidities. Methemoglobin levels less than 15% are typically asymptomatic, while levels greater than 70% are deadly. Between these values, patients gradually developed increased symptoms of hypoxia and end-organ dysfunction. As previously discussed, patients with chronic methemoglobinemia physiologically compensate for the reduced oxygen-carrying capacity of hemoglobin. Finally, the patient's comorbidities contribute to the severity of methemoglobinemia. For instance, a patient with a baseline hemoglobin of 14 g/L and 20% methemoglobin level with have a decrease of 2.8 g/L of effective hemoglobin (notwithstanding the left shift of the oxygen-dissociation curve for simplicity), leading to an effective hemoglobin level of 11.2 g/L. On the other end of the spectrum, a patient with end-stage renal disease and a hemoglobin of 8.0 g/L and 20% methemoglobin level will have a decrease of 1.6 g/dL of effective hemoglobin, leading to an effective hemoglobin level of 6.4 g/L. With diminished reserve, the second patient will be more symptomatic than the first. Pulmonary and cardiac comorbidities and a host of other organ systems also diminish physiologic reserve.

Differential Diagnosis

There are multiple factors that can cause methemoglobinemia, mainly including the following:

1. Carbon monoxide poisoning
2. Pneumonia or other respiratory infection

3. Obstructive lung disease exacerbation
4. Volume overload from decompensated congestive heart failure
5. Pulmonary embolism
6. Anxiety attack
7. Sulfhemoglobinemia

Prognosis

The most important prognostic factors include methemoglobin level, time from symptom onset to treatment, chronicity of development, and underlying medical comorbidities.

Treatment

The decision to treat methemoglobinemia depends on symptoms and the methemoglobin level. Regardless of these two factors, the offending agent should typically be discontinued depending on a risk-vs-benefit analysis. Treatment is recommended for symptomatic patients and for patients with a methemoglobin level of greater than 20%. For patients with hereditary methemoglobinemia, treatment should be based on symptoms alone as these patients have elevated baseline methemoglobin levels.

First-line treatment is methylene blue, given 1–2 mg/kg intravenously. Repeating this dose after 30–60 min should be done if symptoms have not improved. Methylene blue is reduced to leucomethylene blue by NADPH-methemoglobin reductase using NADPH as a cofactor. Leucomethylene blue then reduces methemoglobin back to regular hemoglobin.

Other treatments include exchange transfusion and hyperbaric oxygen, but these treatments are rarely required because of the efficacy of methylene blue. High-dose vitamin C is an effective alternative treatment where methylene is not available or if the patient has a contraindication to methylene blue [4]. High-dose vitamin C may also be used to treat cosmetic cyanosis in patients with congenital methemoglobinemia.

Promising Clinical Studies (Potential Clinical Trials, Targeted Therapy, Gene Therapy)

NA

Caveats

- Patients with G6PD deficiency have reduced NADPH at baseline. Therefore, they are unable to reduce methylene blue as effectively to leucomethylene blue. Since methylene blue is an oxidizing agent before being reduced, excessive dosing of methylene blue among patients with G6PD deficiency can lead to methemoglobinemia.
- Methylene blue inhibits monoamine oxidase A, so it can precipitate serotonin syndrome among patients on selective serotonin reuptake inhibitors. The use of selective serotonin reuptake inhibitors is not a contraindication for methylene blue but must be administered with caution.

Board Question

1. A 64-year-old male who underwent transesophageal echocardiogram with topical benzocaine anesthetic 6 h previously gradually develops cyanosis and dyspnea. His oxygen saturation ranges from 94% to 96%; heart rate is 120 beats per minute; and blood pressure is 135/90 mmHg. Laboratory tests are drawn and show a stable hemoglobin of 14.5 g/L and CO_2 of 25. Despite starting maximal oxygen via nasal canula, his oxygen saturation does not improve. A computed tomographic angiogram of his chest demonstrates no pulmonary embolism or other pulmonary abnormality. What is the next best step in diagnosis?

   A. Arterial blood gas with co-oximetry
   B. Thoracic surgery consultation for evaluation of esophageal perforation
   C. Empiric chest tube placement for postoperative pneumothorax
   D. Intubation

Answers: the answer is A. The clinical presentation of cyanosis and dyspnea following the use of topical benzocaine anesthetic during a transesophageal echocardiogram (TEE), along with an oxygen saturation of 94–96%, suggests the possibility of methemoglobinemia. The next best step in the diagnosis would be to obtain a co-oximetry measurement to assess methemoglobin levels, as pulse oximetry may not accurately reflect oxygenation status in methemoglobinemia

2. A 54-year-old male dentist is evaluated in the emergency for cyanosis and dyspnea. On further questioning, he was inhaling nitric oxide earlier in the day. His initial oxygen saturation on the pulse oximeter is 95%, and an arterial blood gas with co-oximetry shows a methemoglobin level of 21%. Methylene blue is administered at 2 mg/kg, but the dentist's hemoglobin drops from 13.5 to 11.0 g/L, and his methemoglobin level increases to 35%. Haptoglobin is undetectable, and lactate dehydrogenase is 475 IU/L. The dentist is given hyperbaric oxygen and 10 mg of intravenous vitamin C, and he eventually recovers. Which of the following would explain his clinic course?

   A. Increased stabilization of Fe^{3+} in hemoglobin caused by α-chain mutation.
   B. Depleted baseline NADPH caused by mutation in RBC protein
   C. Abuse of additional dopaminergic toxin
   D. Mutation in the complement cascade

Answers: The answer is B. The drop in hemoglobin from 13.5 to 11.0 g/L following methylene blue administration in a patient with methemoglobinemia is concerning and warrants further investigation. Hemolysis is a known but rare side effect of methylene blue, especially in individuals with glucose-6-phosphate dehydrogenase (G6PD) deficiency. It is recommended to check for G6PD deficiency before administering methylene blue, as individuals with this deficiency are at increased risk for hemolysis when exposed to oxidative stress.

References

1. Ash-Bernal RMD, Wise R, Robert MD, Wright SM, Scott MMD. Acquired methemoglobinemia: a retrospective series of 138 cases at 2 teaching hospitals. Medicine. 2004;83(5):265–73.
2. Keohane EM, Otto CN, Walenga JM. Rodak's hematology: clinical principles and applications. 6th ed. St. Louis: Elsevier; 2020.
3. Chan ED, Chan MM, Chan MM. Pulse oximetry: understanding its basic principles facilitates appreciation of its limitations. Respir Med. 2013;107(6):789–99. https://doi.org/10.1016/j.rmed.2013.02.004. Epublished March 13, 2013 Mar 13. PMID.
4. Rino PB, Scolnik D, Fustiñana A, Mitelpunkt A, Glatstein M. Ascorbic acid for the treatment of methemoglobinemia: the experience of a large tertiary care pediatric hospital. Am J Ther. 2014;21(4):240–3. PMID: 24914501.

Extrinsic Non-immune Hemolysis

19

Caroline K. Hana and Atif M. Hussein

Introduction

Red blood cells (RBC) normally are destroyed and removed from the circulation after approximately 120 days. Hemolysis refers to the premature destruction of RBCs. Hemolysis can be classified into extrinsic vs intrinsic, intravascular (occurring in the circulation) vs extravascular (in the reticuloendothelial system), and immune (mediated by antibodies) vs non-immune. When the hemolysis is too severe to be compensated by the bone marrow's overproduction, hemolytic anemia develops.

The term "microangiopathic hemolytic anemia" (MAHA) is a descriptive term for the state of intravascular non-immune hemolysis resulting from microvascular abnormalities, e.g., in cases of thrombotic microangiopathies (TMA) or from intravascular devices. We focus on the extrinsic non-immune causes of hemolytic anemia in the chapter.

C. K. Hana (✉) · A. M. Hussein
Department of Hematology and Medical Oncology, Memorial Healthcare System, Hollywood, FL, USA
e-mail: chana@augusta.edu

L. Sokol, L. Zhang (eds.), *Non-Neoplastic Hematologic Disorders*,
https://doi.org/10.1007/978-3-031-62373-8_19

Pathogenesis

The pathogenesis of extrinsic non-immune hemolysis is complex that can be mediated via physical or chemical insults, or RBC membrane destruction, or MAHA. All are simplified in Fig. 19.1.

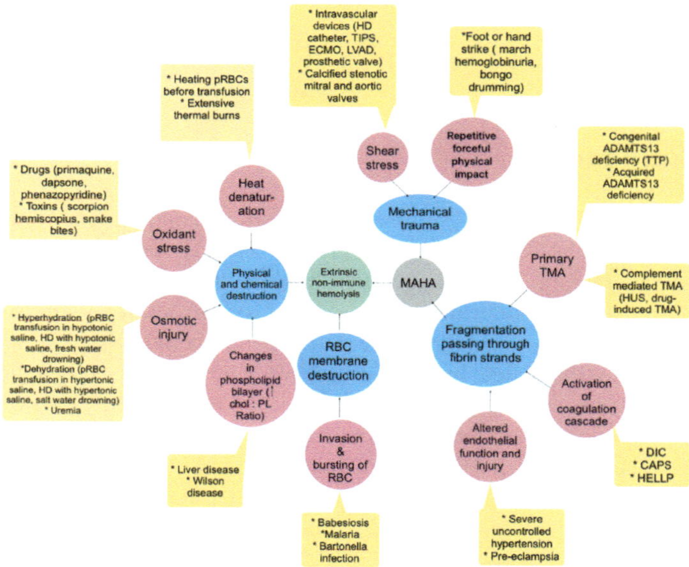

Fig. 19.1 The mechanisms of extrinsic non-immune hemolytic anemia. ADAMTS-13 a disintegrin and metalloproteinase with a thrombospodin type motif, member 13, CAPS catastrophic antiphospholipid syndrome, Chol:PL ratio cholesterol to phospholipid ratio, DIC disseminated intravascular coagulopathy, ECMO extracorporeal membrane oxygenation, HD hemodialysis, HELLP hemolysis, elevated liver enzymes and low platelet count syndrome, HUS hemolytic uremic syndrome, LVAD left ventricular assist device, TIPS transjugular intrahepatic portosystemic shunt, TMA thrombotic microangioplasty, TTP thrombotic thrombocytopenic purpura

Diagnosis

In general, the first step in diagnosis is to confirm the presence of hemolysis.

1. *Complete blood count (CBC):* It confirms the presence of normocytic normochromic anemia, with decreased hemoglobin and hematocrit levels.
2. *Laboratory findings to confirm hemolysis:*

   - Elevated reticulocytes count (because of bone marrow compensation and early release of premature RBC)
   - Elevated LDH (because of RBC break down)
   - Elevated indirect bilirubin (because of excessive heme breakdown and formation of indirect bilirubin beyond the liver's capacity for conjugation)
   - Decreased haptoglobin (because it binds to free circulating hemoglobin)
   - Hemoglobinemia and hemoglobinuria (indicators of intravascular hemolysis). Hemoglobinuria can occur despite of no visible RBCs on microscopic examination of the urine preparation.
   - Blood smear: It shows evidence of schistocytes (Fig. 19.2), helmet cells, bite cells (in case of oxidant stress), and poikilocytosis.

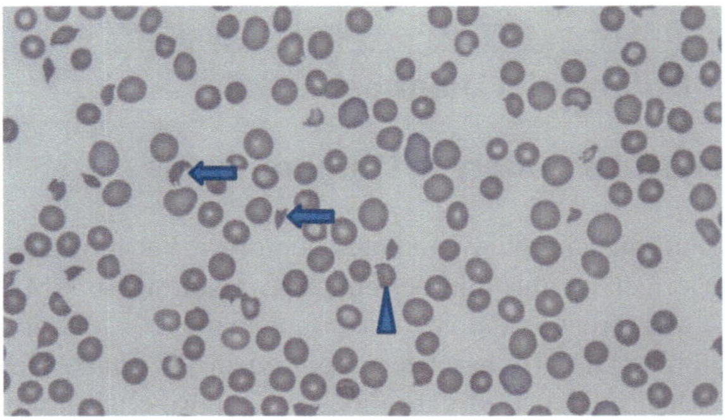

Fig. 19.2 Blood smear showing schistocytes (arrows) and helmet cells (arrowhead)

3. *Rule Out Immune-mediated Hemolytic Anemia*: It is done by performing the Coombs test. Non-immune hemolytic anemias are, by definition, Coombs negative.
4. *Identifying the Cause*

Certain information in the patient's history can guide towards the cause of hemolysis, e.g.,

- Recent drug exposure can be in case of drug-induced TMA (DITMA).
- Dietary ingestions of fava beans can lead to oxidative stress especially in patients with enzymopathies, e.g. G6PD deficiency.
- Patients with liver disease and splenomegaly could be experiencing hypersplenism.
- History of cardiac devices.
- Fever and recent infection ➔ direct lysis by pathogen.
  Laboratory findings that can help identify the cause include:
- Abnormal coagulation ➔ liver disease, DIC, TMA
- Abdominal ultrasound to check for splenomegaly in suspected hypersplenism
- Renal dysfunction ➔ complement mediated TMA or Shiga-toxin mediated HUS
- Flow cytometry if suspecting hematologic malignancy
- Blood smear: may show intracellular organisms like malaria, or babesiosis. Presence of bite cells in oxidant stress

Major Differential Diagnosis

Hemolysis Secondary to Drugs or Toxins

Drugs can cause immune-mediated hemolysis but can also induce a toxic effect on the microcirculation, resulting in TMA with MAHA or a direct oxidative toxic effect on the RBC membrane or hemoglobin. DITMA has been reported in 93 drugs. However, only 30 had evidence of causality. Cyclosporine, sirolimus, and tacrolimus are the most common culprits for DITMA. The mechanisms of DITMA included drug-dependent antibodies to platelets or other cells as in the case of quinine, oxaliplatin, and vancomycin, drug-induced ADAMTS-13 deficiency, complement-mediated damage, and a dose-dependent cumulative toxicity effect [1]. Some medications, such as dapsone, rasburicase, and methylene blue, induce hemoglobin oxidation, leading to methemoglobin production. This process eventually harms the RBC membrane by generating hemichromes and Heinz bodies, which either directly damage membrane function or oxidize its proteins and lipids. Intravenous immunoglobulin (IVIG) causes hemolysis via an immune-mediated mechanism; however, it has also been reported to cause complement-mediated hemolysis.

Wilson Disease (WD)

WD is a rare autosomal recessive inherited disease where a defect in the copper-transporting P-type ATPase, due to mutations in the *ATP7B* gene, causes impaired excretion of copper. NIHA is thought to be secondary to direct copper oxidant effects on hemoglobin, direct damage to membrane phospholipid or inhibition of glycolysis [2].

Infections

Some infections cause lysis of the RBCs through invasion and bursting or via toxic effect on the RBC membrane.

(a) Malaria: It is a mosquito-borne parasitic infection by *plasmodium* (p) *malariae*, *p. falciparum*, *p. vivax,* or *p. ovale*. The plasmodial merozoites invade RBC by means of its rhoptries which attach on RBC surface receptors, i.e., Duffy blood group antigen in case of *P. vivax*, and the Rh5-interacting protein in *P. Falciparum* [3]. It digests the hemoglobin and eventually bursts out of the RBC causing intravascular hemolysis. Extravascular hemolysis also occurs because of changes in the splenic microvasculature and activation of a monocyte-macrophage system.

(b) Babesiosis is another intraerythrocytic parasite transmitted by adult ticks on the West Coast, especially Washington and California, and in Bartonellosis or Carrión disease, a bacterial infection by bartonella bacilliformis via the bite of sandflies. Interestingly, prior splenectomy appeared to protect a patient from hemolysis during acute infection, an observation that highlights the role of the spleen in clearing the infected cells.

(c) Clostridial infection causes direct damage to the RBCs by releasing enzymes that acutely degrade the phospholipids and the structural proteins of the RBC membrane resulting in spherocytes that are extremely sensitive to osmotic lysis. It presents very abruptly, with profound hemolysis. Blood smear would show spherocytes but not necessarily schistocytes or helmet cells.

(d) Other infections that can cause hemolysis include *Hemophilus influenza B*, HIV, CMV, and visceral leishmaniasis.

Thrombotic Microangiopathies

Thrombotic Thrombocytopenic Purpura (TTP)

A lack of the enzyme ADAMTS-13 leads to the accumulation of large von Willebrand factor multimers. These multimers adhere to endothelial cells, prompting platelet aggregation and the formation of microvascular clots even without endothelial injury. This results in RBC destruction through physical damage. Diminished ADAMTS-13 activity can be caused by genetic mutations or acquired antibodies against it. TTP poses a serious risk and demands prompt recognition and intervention (see Chap. 28),

Disseminated Intravascular Coagulopathy (DIC)

DIC develops secondary to widespread coagulation activation within blood vessels, triggered by a variety of inflammatory cytokines that stimulate tissue factor mediated pathways, combined with a failure to regulate anticoagulant mechanisms, and enhanced suppression of fibrinolysis through plasminogen activator inhibitor 1 (see Chap. 34).

Hemolytic Uremic Syndrome (HUS)

HUS is characterized by MAHA with acute kidney injury, thrombocytopenia, and neurologic dysfunction 5–10 days following a diarrheal illness. It is mainly caused by Shiga toxin producing *Escherichia coli* and other organisms. Atypical HUS is the result of dysregulated complement system secondary to gene mutations coding for complement factor H (CFH), C3, factor B, factor I, and CD46. Cases with secondary HUS have also been described in patients with coexisting diseases, e.g., autoimmune diseases, transplantation, cancer, infection, pregnancy, or use of cytotoxic drugs [4]. (For details, see Chap. 28).

Tumor-Related TMA

The most common cancer associated with such condition include tumors of gastric or mammary origin.

Intravascular Devices

Changes to the laminar blood flow with very rapid acceleration or deceleration alter the physical integrity of the RBC membrane and can result in MAHA. This is often seen in patients with mitral prosthetic regurgitation who had peak shear stresses.

Hemolysis Associated with Liver Disease

Patients with liver disease have an increased RBC membrane cholesterol to the phospholipid ratio, which results in distorted RBCs, e.g., echinocytes and acanthocytes with the extreme forms called spur cells. These distorted RBCs are removed from the circulation by the spleen resulting in extravascular hemolytic anemia.

Hypersplenism

The classical criteria for hypersplenism include single or multilineage cytopenias, compensatory bone marrow hyperplasia, splenomegaly, and cytopenias will be corrected after splenectomy.

Hypersplenism can be primary or secondary. Primary hypersplenism is when the cause cannot be identified, e.g., primary splenic hyperplasia, non-tropical idiopathic splenomegaly, and primary splenic pancytopenia. Secondary hypersplenism is when a clear cause can be identified, e.g., liver cirrhosis, infections, granulomatous inflammation, malignancies, and lipid storage diseases, e.g., Gaucher's disease and Niemann-Pick disease.

A study showed an imbalance between upregulated and downregulated cytokines and genes, which plays an important role in macrophages activation and phagocytosis in hypersplenism [5].

Toxins Caused by Insect, Snake, or Spider Bites

This entity includes bee stings and spiders (mainly southern Black widow and the brown recluse) in the Southern US. Envenomation results in the cleavage of RBC glycophorins by its metalloproteases. In certain parts of the world, Cobra snake venom can cause intravascular hemolysis through its phospholipases.

Pregnancy Associated Hemolysis

- Pre-eclampsia syndrome entails severe hypertension with proteinuria and hyperuricemia. It can result in MAHA in a mechanism similar to uncontrolled hypertension causing endothelial injury and microangiopathy.
- HELLP syndrome, characterized by hemolytic anemia, elevated liver enzymes, and a low platelet count, can lead to severe complications such as liver rupture, vision loss, DIC, seizures, and heart failure. Urgent delivery of the baby is recommended to mitigate these risks. It is important to differentiate preeclampsia from HELLP syndrome. Hypertension and renal impairment are uncommon in HELLP while liver impairment is unusual in preeclampsia.

Treatment

Treatment of hemolytic anemia includes (1) treatment of the anemia with supportive care and (2) treatment of the underlying cause. Transfusion of packed RBCs may sometimes be necessary in severe cases. Patients can become iron and folate deficient because of the ongoing hemolysis; hence, supplementation with iron and folate may also be needed.

Special attention should be paid to medical emergencies as in case of TTP, HUS, DIC, HELLP, and preeclampsia.

Otherwise, treatment should be directed towards the cause of hemolysis, e.g.,

- *DITMA*: stop the offending medication and continue supportive care.
- *Methemoglobinemia secondary to oxidative stress*: use methylene blue. If methylene blue is contraindicated, ascorbic acid can be used.
- *Wilson disease*: for asymptomatic patients, zinc preparations are recommended. However, symptomatic patients should be treated with copper-chelating agents; D-penicillamine, or trientine. In cerebral Wilson disease, zinc in combination with tetrathiomolybdate or dimer-captosuccinic acid (DMSA) should be used first. In case of liver failure, plasmapheresis and hemofiltration can be used as bridge to transplant [6].
- *Malaria:* treatment depends on the type of malaria and the pattern of local resistance. It usually consists of chloroquine or an artemisinin combination therapy. In chloroquine resistant regions, primaquine or tafenoquine can be used. *P. Vivax* and *P. ovale* hypnozoite liver stage should be targeted with primaquine after the symptoms subside.
- *Clostridial infection:* Antibiotics must be started immediately. The patient should also be monitored for DIC.
- *TTP*: Assessment of ADAMTS13 enzyme activity is diagnostic for TTP but making a presumptive diagnosis and prompt initiation of exchange transfusion is important. Caplacizumab

is approved for acute aTTP plus plasma exchange and additional immunosuppressive therapy (e.g., steroids and rituximab) (see Chap. 28).

- HUS: supportive care with frequent monitoring of the renal function. For aHUS, plasma exchange has been the standard of care since 1980. In patients with significant disease and organ dysfunction, Eculizumab has been shown effective [7] (see Chap. 28).
- *Hypersplenism*: Treatment of its underlying cause is the primary goal. Splenic irradiation and radiofrequency ablation is optional in few cases with promising results. Splenectomy is performed to correct the effects of low blood cell and platelet counts [5].
- *Treatment after a spider bite*: corticosteroids may help. Hemolysis can be self-limited but might need RBC transfusion support.

Caveats

- Artesunate has replaced quinine as the recommended first-line treatment of severe malaria. Delayed hemolysis post artesunate has been reported in 7%–21% of patients 2–3 weeks after initiation of the treatment. Severe case may need transfusion.
- In treatment of methemoglobinemia, if methylene blue does not turn the chocolate color blood back to normal quickly, one must think of the presence of G6PD deficiency.

Promising Clinical Study

NA

Board Question

A 45-year-old male physician is referred to the hematology clinic for evaluation of anemia. The patient traveled on a medical mission to Nigeria 3 months ago. During his trip, he was taking prophylactic Atovaquone-proguanil for chemoprevention of malaria infection. Upon arrival to USA, he started developing cyclic fever. CBC showed hemoglobin 6.5 mg/dL, WBC 4.9 × 10^9/L, platelets 437 × 10 ^{9}/L, and ANC 3.7 × 10 ^{9}/L.

Blood smear review showed *plasmodium Vivax*.

The patient received blood transfusion and was started on Artesunate-mefloquine with significant improvement in his H/H and symptoms. Approximately 4 weeks later, the patient started to feel significant fatigue and malaise. He presented to the ED, and his CBC showed the following: hemoglobin 5.9 mg/dL, WBC 6.7 10^9/L, platelets 281 × 10^9/L and ANC 5.3 × 10^9/L.

What is the best next step?

A. Obtain blood smear
B. Transfuse pRBCs
C. Start primaquine treatment
D. Nothing

Correct answer: A

A blood smear should be obtained to differentiate a re-infection by hypnozoites from a drug-induced hemolysis by Artesunate, which can occur 2–3 weeks after the initiation of treatment. The patient should be transfused with matched pRBCs. Primaquine should always be administered for patients with *plasmodium vivax* or *ovale* infections, to eradicate the liver hypnozoites, however, at this point, a diagnosis should be made first.

References

1. Tsubota A, Shimada N, Abe H, Yoshizawa K, Agata R, Yumoto Y, et al. Several factors including ITPA polymorphism influence ribavirin-induced anemia in chronic hepatitis C. World J Gastroenterol. 2012;18(41):5879–88.
2. Rodriguez-Castro KI, Hevia-Urrutia FJ, Sturniolo GC. Wilson's disease: a review of what we have learned. World J Hepatol. 2015;7(29):2859–70.
3. Paul AS, Egan ES, Duraisingh MT. Host-parasite interactions that guide red blood cell invasion by malaria parasites. Curr Opin Hematol. 2015;22(3):220–6.

4. Jokiranta TS. HUS and atypical HUS. Blood. 2017;129(21):2847–56.
5. Lv Y, Lau WY, Li Y, Deng J, Han X, Gong X, et al. Hypersplenism: history and current status. Exp Ther Med. 2016;12(4):2377–82.
6. Li WJ, Chen C, You ZF, Yang RM, Wang XP. Current drug managements of Wilson's disease: from west to east. Curr Neuropharmacol. 2016;14(4):322–5.
7. Mentzer WC, Schrier SL, Editors. Extrinsic nonimmune hemolytic anemias. Hematology: Basic Principles and Practice, Chapter 47. 2018:663–72.

Pure Red Cell Aplasia

20

Nikolaos Papadantonakis
and Deniz Peker

Introduction

The hallmark of pure red cell aplasia (PRCA) is normocytic anemia coupled with the absence or marked reduction of erythroid progenitors (less than 1% erythroblasts on bone marrow exam or less than 5%, if proerythroblasts are included) and reticulocytopenia (reticulocytes less than 10,000/microliter). Leukocytes and platelets are usually normal in number.

PRCA is a rare condition, and the incidence is estimated to be 1–2 cases per million a year [1]. PRCA can be an inherited (Diamond-Blackfan Anemia [DBA]) or an acquired condition [2, 3].

In DBA, macrocytic or normochromic anemia manifests within the first 4–5 years of life and, in most cases, within the first few months after birth [4]. DBA may also manifest with mild leukopenia or thrombocytosis and, depending on the chromosomal aberra-

N. Papadantonakis (✉)
Department of Hematology and Medical Oncology, Winship Cancer Institute of Emory University, Atlanta, GA, USA
e-mail: Nikolaos.papadantonakis@emory.edu

D. Peker
Department of Pathology and Laboratory Medicine, Winship Cancer Institute of Emory University, Emory University School of Medicine, Atlanta, GA, USA
e-mail: Deniz.peker@emoryhealthcare.org

L. Sokol, L. Zhang (eds.), *Non-Neoplastic Hematologic Disorders*,
https://doi.org/10.1007/978-3-031-62373-8_20

tions, can be associated with skeletal and developmental manifestations. There is a near absence of erythroblasts, with a blockade of differentiation between the early stage burst forming unit erythroid (BFU-E) and late-stage colony forming unit erythroid (CFU-E).

Acquired PRCA includes idiopathic cases and cases secondary to other conditions such as thymoma [5], infections [6], erythropoiesis stimulating agent (ESA) use, medications, lymphoprolif-

Table 20.1 Secondary causes of pure red cell aplasia

Autoimmune/connective tissue disorders	
Rheumatoid arthritis Systemic lupus erythematosus	Crohn's disease Ulcerative colitis
Lymphoproliferative disorders	
Chronic lymphocytic leukemia Large granular lymphocytic leukemia Myeloma	Hodgkin lymphoma Non-Hodgkin lymphomas Castleman disease
Myelodysplastic and myeloproliferative neoplasms	
Myelodysplastic syndrome Chronic myeloid leukemia	Chronic myelomonocytic leukemia Primary myelofibrosis
Solid tumors	
Thymoma Breast cancer Gastrointestinal cancers	Lung cancer Thyroid cancer Renal cell carcinoma
Infections	
Parvovirus B19 HIV EBV CMV	Viral hepatitis Tuberculosis Sepsis
Drugs	
Azathioprine Diphenylhydantoin Recombinant human erythropoietin Isoniazid Rifampicin Valproic acid Carbamazepine Interpheron-alpha Ribavirin	Dapsone/pyrimethamine Chlorpropamide Chloroquine d-Penicillamine Fludarabine Leuprolide Sulfasalazine Sulindac Tacrolimus

erative diseases, pregnancy, and rheumatologic conditions etc [7]. (Table 20.1). Acquired PRCA can occur at any age. The median age reported in several studies is between the fifth and seventh decades of life. Some studies have reported a female predominance.

Pathogenesis

Congenital PRCA Ribosome abnormalities lead to apoptosis in inherited cases such as DBA. Approximately 50% of DBA cases follow autosomal dominant inheritance fashion, while a smaller percentage exhibit an autosomal recessive pattern. Approximately half of the patients have ribosomal mutations, and mutations affecting *GATA-1* gene are also reported, but infrequently. The most common ribosomal mutations affect RPS19, but other implicated genes are interspersed in more than 10 chromosomes. The mechanisms of ribosomal mutations are likely apoptotic. Haploinsufficiency is adequate to lead to pathogenic manifestations, but penetrance is variable.

Acquired PRCA In the acquired cases, the absence of the erythroid precursors can result from an autoimmune disorder, viral infection, hematologic malignancy, antibody-mediated destruction, T-cell cytotoxicity, or medication effect. Antibodies can target erythroblasts and lead to their destruction through antibody-mediated cytotoxic activity. Antibodies can also bind on erythropoietin or block erythropoietin signaling. Antibody generation could be secondary to infections, immune system dysregulation from autoimmune conditions, or malignancies. NK and T-cell disorders including large granular lymphocytic leukemia may cause cytotoxic destruction or growth inhibition of erythroblasts, leading to red cell aplasia.

Thymomas are rare tumors that could be associated with paraneoplastic phenomena. Relatively few cases of PRCA in patients with thymoma have been described. PRCA can present concomitantly with thymoma or develop several months after its diagnosis.

PRCA has been described in patients treated with erythropoiesis stimulating agents (ESA) [8]. The mechanism is antibody-mediated and hinders the interaction of erythropoietin with its receptor. A genetic predisposition based on specific HLA epitopes has been proposed as a potential explanation. The cases primarily involved epoetin-a [Eprex] preparations, but a few cases involving other formulations have been reported.

PRCA can also accompany solid tumors and lymphoproliferative disorders [9]. The association is quite rare, reported to be ~1% of 3945 chronic lymphocytic leukemia (CLL) patients at Mayo Clinic. Of note, a sizeable number of patients evaluated were positive for parvovirus B19. PRCA development timing in the setting of CLL was variable, with a median of 4.5 years.

PRCA after hemopoietic stem cell transplant has been reported rarely in the literature. Plasma cells secrete antibodies that recognize donor derived erythroid lineage cells. PRCA has been described in pregnant patients. Reports are very limited, but immune-mediated causes are suspected.

Many medications have been implicated in developing PRCA, including sulfa drugs, allopurinol, antimetabolites such as azathioprine, and penicillin antibiotics. The association is more established for a few medications.

Reports of molecular annotation of acquired PRCA are limited. In one of the most comprehensive reports, approximately 50% of the patients had mutations. Mutations were similar to the repertoire found in aplastic anemia and clonal hematopoiesis including *DNMT3A, ASXL1,* and *BCOR.*

Diagnosis

The diagnostic workup of PRCA involves a comprehensive history, physical exam focusing on lymphadenopathy, splenomegaly, and musculoskeletal deformities, laboratory studies including complete blood counts, autoimmune disease, and infectious profile. Especially in pediatric patients, the physical exam findings may raise suspicion or point more conclusively toward DBA. Nutritional and family history are also important components.

The complete blood count (CBC) analysis reveals decreased hemoglobin/hematocrit, mild leukopenia or thrombocytosis may accompany in rare cases, especially DBA. Despite anemia, the reticulocyte count is markedly decreased (less than 10,000/microliter) which is one of the critical laboratory findings. Polychromasia is absent in the peripheral smear, and dysplastic features are not observed (unless PRCA occurs in the context of myelodysplastic syndromes) (Fig. 20.1).

Erythropoietin levels are elevated, and at times, it can be markedly. The presence of blasts or left shifted hematopoiesis in the differential in the absence of infections points towards different etiologies. Direct antiglobulin test is typically negative, and if positive, the presence of microspherocytes, high reticulocyte count, and undetectable haptoglobin are indicative of hemolytic anemia.

The primary diagnostic modality is bone marrow biopsy. The marrow can be variably cellular (ranging between hypo- and hypercellular) with the near absence of erythroid lineage (Fig. 20.2). Erythroid precursors, by definition, are scant, resulting in markedly increased myeloid to erythroid ratio by bone marrow manual differential count. Next-generation sequencing analysis

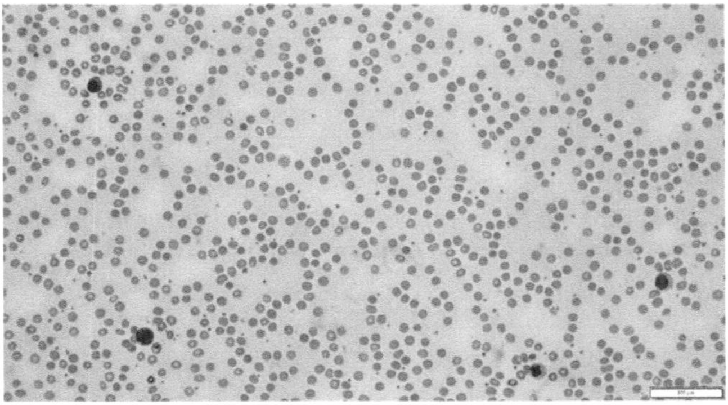

Fig. 20.1 Peripheral blood with moderate to severe anemia and unremarkable white cells and platelets (Wright stain, 200×). Polychromatic cells are not increased indicating low reticulocyte count

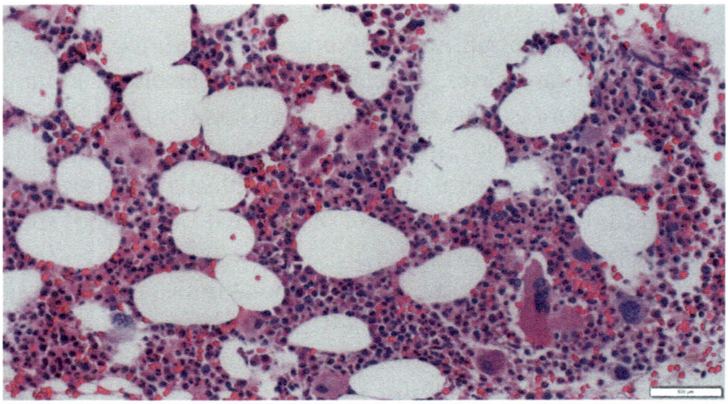

Fig. 20.2 Hypercellular marrow with markedly decreased erythropoiesis (Wright-Giemsa, 200×)

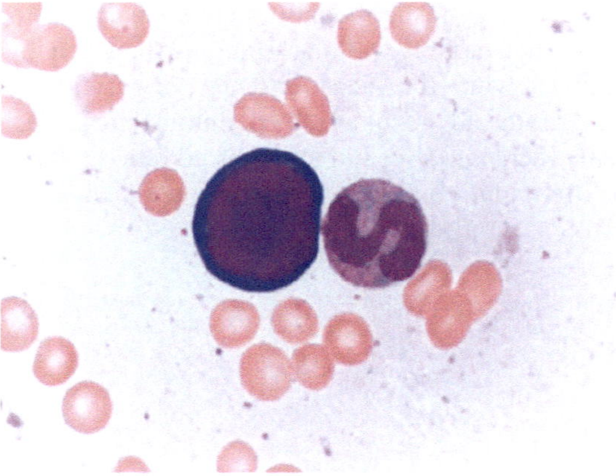

Fig. 20.3 Early erythroid precursors infected by Parvovirus displaying nuclear inclusion (bone marrow aspirate smear, Wright-Giemsa, 200×)

may reveal mutations found in clonal myeloid disorders, including clonal hematopoiesis of indeterminate significance.

In parvovirus B19 infection cases, eosinophilic intranuclear viral inclusions may be noted in early erythroid precursors (Fig. 20.3). Parvovirus PCR assay, immunohistochemical study, and in situ hybridization assay can be essential to establish the diagnosis.

Flow cytometry and immunohistochemistry are valuable tools for assessing light chain clonality and aberrant antigen expression, which helps exclude certain lymphoproliferative disorders. These techniques can also identify blast populations or granulocytic dysmaturation. Additionally, flow cytometry can be used to rule out paroxysmal nocturnal hemoglobinuria (PNH) by confirming a negative result for PNH testing, thus excluding the presence of a PNH clone.

Molecular testing should be employed to rule out T-cell clonality using polymerase chain reaction and *STAT3* and *STAT5B* mutations using gene sequencing methods, particularly if there is a suspicion for T-cell large granular lymphocytic leukemia or proliferation-related PRCA. Results of T-cell clonality should be interpreted in conjunction with morphological findings and flow cytometry analysis.

Differential Diagnoses

Congenital PRCA

Fanconi anemia (FA) is an inherited bone marrow failure syndrome accompanied by skeletal, skin, and developmental abnormalities. Anemia is usually not isolated, often accompanying with leukopenia and thrombocytopenia. DNA breakage analysis positivity is diagnostic of FA.

Pearson syndrome is a rare mitochondrial disorder with a hallmark of large-scale mitochondrial DNA deletions. Pearson syndrome can affect the hemopoietic system, and patients present with hypoproliferative anemia early in life. The bone marrow biopsy may indicate dysplastic features, ring sideroblasts, and vacuolization of erythroid precursors. Mitochondrial DNA analysis of blood/bone marrow cells can secure the diagnosis.

Acquired PRCA

Patients who present with anemia and low reticulocyte count can pose a diagnostic challenge. A thorough workup is required to exclude other etiologies with similar presentations, especially in children, including unstable hemoglobinopathies and congenital red blood cell membrane defects.

Aplastic anemia can present with anemia and reticulocytopenia and often accompanies with neutropenia and/or thrombocytopenia. Bone marrow biopsy usually demonstrates hypocellularity, and other lineages, including megakaryocytic, are affected. In addition, erythroid progenitors can represent more than 5% of cellularity.

Hemolytic anemia (idiopathic or secondary) can present with a profound decrease in hemoglobin. However, reticulocyte count is typically elevated, haptoglobin is undetectable, indirect bilirubin is elevated, and direct antiglobulin test is positive for IgG or complement. Bone marrow biopsy shows erythroid hyperplasia to compensate with the peripheral destruction of RBCs. In rare cases, the antibodies can also recognize erythroid progenitors leading to diminished reticulocytes. In these cases, reticulocytopenia defines concurrent PRCA and hemolytic anemia. The bone marrow biopsy is reported to be normocellular with diminished erythropoiesis.

Acute leukemias can manifest with hypoproliferative anemia. A peripheral blood smear may indicate the presence of blasts, and bone marrow biopsy reveals infiltration by blasts.

Acute blood loss can be initially accompanied by low reticulocytes, but within a brief period of time reticulocyte count increases to compensate for anemia.

Treatment

Treatment of PRCA relies on treating the cause and supportive therapy [10]. Potential offending medications should be discontinued, and recovery of hematopoiesis may require several weeks.

Transfusion support is initially utilized for life-threatening anemia.

Monitoring for transfusion requirements is essential to determine a program that mitigates complications of anemia and the potential of iron overload or other transfusion-related complications. Nutritional deficiencies such as vitamin B12 and folate should be corrected. Spontaneous remissions have been reported.

Surgical management of thymoma should be strongly considered.

PRCA associated with ESA administration has become less prevalent, as ESA formulations that were more strongly associated with PRCA are no longer available [11]. In associated PRCA cases, ESA should be discontinued, and blood transfusions need to be instituted. Immune suppression may be helpful.

PRCA associated with lymphoproliferative disorders is an indication for treatment. Rituximab has been successful in cases of B-cell lymphoproliferative disorders. In a Mayo clinic CLL associated with the PRCA series, treatment modalities included monotherapy with rituximab, immunosuppressants, steroids, or a combination of steroids and rituximab, immunosuppressants, or Intravenous Immunoglobulin (IVIG).

Idiopathic PRCA is treated with a combination of modalities in a stepwise approach [3, 12]. An initial course of steroids such as 1 mg/kg prednisone in the absence of contraindications is a common approach. Responses usually occur within a few weeks and are heralded by increased reticulocyte counts. Slow tapering of prednisone in responders may help to avoid relapses. Cyclosporine is commonly added to steroids or used as an initial combination. The median time to response for the combination is ~1 month. The cyclosporine levels must be carefully monitored, aiming for a level close to 200 ng/ml (reported target range in literature 150–250 ng/ml). After a response is achieved and maintained for several months, slow tapering of cyclosporine is crucial to prevent relapses.

An increase of cyclosporine or its reintroduction can be an effective salvage strategy. Cyclophosphamide is another agent that is used in relapsed or refractory settings. The cyclophosphamide dose is 50–100 mg oral daily with dose escalation to 150 mg daily if cytopenias do not ensue. Responses may require several weeks with a median time of response of ~3 months of treatment. Slow tapering is again recommended to avoid relapses.

Sirolimus is an alternative to cyclosporine or cyclophosphamide. With a median time to response of 4 months, responses to sirolimus may be slower than cyclosporine or cyclophosphamide.

Alemtuzumab, a monoclonal antibody targeting CD52, has been used in the setting of immune mediated PRCA in the relapsed/refractory setting. Alemtuzumab is not commercially available in the US, but it can be obtained through the manufacturer. The main complications are infections and cytomegalovirus viremia. Response rates have been variable; a weekly administration schema appears to be safe and effective. Parvovirus-mediated PRCA is often associated with solid organ transplantation in immunocompromised patients. Administration of IVIG is associated with the improvement of hematopoiesis in the overwhelming majority of patients. Utilized doses in the literature vary. However, relapses can occur within a few months, and close monitoring is warranted.

Bortezomib and eltrombopag use is infrequently reported in the context of PRCA. Bortezomib was used successfully in a case of PRCA following an ABO-mismatched hematopoietic transplant. A clinical trial utilizing bortezomib is ongoing.

Equine Antithymocyte Globulin (ATG) in combination with cyclosporine has been used in aplastic anemia for decades. In the setting of PRCA, this treatment approach is less commonly used. The dose and schedule of ATG are similar to that used in AA.

Refractory PRCA may require allogeneic hematopoietic stem cell transplant.

DBA treatment consists of supportive care with transfusions and steroids. Hematopoietic stem cell transplant may be required in some cases.

Promising Clinical Studies

Given the rarity of the condition, clinical trials are challenging to conduct. A clinical trial is currently recruiting (NCT04423367) that examines the role of bortezomib plus dexamethasone in PRCA.

Caveats

1. PRCA is a rare condition and requires extensive diagnostic workup.
2. Thymoma, lymphoproliferative disorders, and autoimmune conditions may accompany PRCA. It would be essential to exclude the presence of such conditions.
3. PRCA in early life may be secondary to DBA, a disease of ribosomal biogenesis.
4. Genetic testing may be required, and genetic counseling for parents should be considered.

Board Questions

1. A three-year-old boy is diagnosed with DBA. An initial course of steroids is pursued but remain transfusion dependent. Which treatment option is considered ineffective for this patient?

   A. Red cell transfusion and iron chelation
   B. Cyclosporine in combination with steroids
   C. Hemopoietic Stem cell transplantation
   D. Clinical trial

   Answer: B. Cyclosporine therapy in DBA has not shown benefit and may be associated with toxicities.

2. A 56-year-old woman with prior medical history of gastric bypass and using zinc supplements is seeking medical attention due to fatigue. She also reports myalgias/arthralgias. Labs reveal mild leukopenia, moderate macrocytic anemia, and moderate thrombocytopenia. Reticulocyte count is severely decreased. What is the best next approach?

   A. Bone marrow biopsy
   B. Vitamin/nutrient panel testing
   C. Parvovirus B19 testing
   D. Paraproteinemia work up.

Answer: B. patient is at increased risk for vitamin and mineral deficiencies secondary to gastric bypass. In addition, zinc use can aggravate copper deficiency. At times, severe nutritional deficiencies can lead to anemia with decreased reticulocytes. Before proceeding to bone marrow biopsy, it is essential to exclude deficiencies.

Acknowledgments We thank Andrea Wecker for language editing/proof reading of the manuscript.

References

1. Nakazawa H, Sakai K, Ohta A, et al. Incidence of acquired pure red cell aplasia: a nationwide epidemiologic analysis with 2 registry databases in Japan. Blood Adv. 2022;6(24):6282–90. PMID: 35522950.
2. Means RT Jr. Pure red cell aplasia. Blood. 2016;128(21):2504–9. https://doi.org/10.1182/blood-2016-05-717140.
3. Red P, Aplasia C. Update on pure red cell aplasia, etiology, diagnosis, and treatment. Clin Adv Hematol Oncol. 2022;20(1):18–21. PMID: 35060958.
4. Gallagher PG. Anemia in the pediatric patient. Blood. 2022;140(6):571–93. PMID: 35213686.
5. Yen CC, Huang WL, Li SS. Pure red cell aplasia and other haematological diseases associated with thymoma: a case series and systematic review. Frontiers in Medicine. 2021;8:759914. PMID: 34966753.
6. Chang HJ, Sinn DH, Cho SG, et. al. Pure red-cell aplasia and autoimmune hemolytic anemia in a patient with acute hepatitis A. Clin Mol Hepatol. 2014;20(2):204–7. PMID: 25032187
7. Lobbes H, Mahevas M, Alviset S. Pure red cell aplasia in systemic lupus erythematosus, a nationwide retrospective cohort and review of the literature. Rheumatology (Oxford). 2022;61(1):355–66. PMID: 33871586.
8. Panichi V, Ricchiuti G, Scatena A, et al. Pure red cell aplasia induced by epoetin zeta. Clin Kidney J. 2016;9(4):599–602. PMID: 27478604.
9. Vlachaki E, Diamantidis MD, Klonizakis P. Pure red cell aplasia and lymphoproliferative disorders: an infrequent association. Sci World J. 2012;2012:475313. PMID: 22593689.
10. Balasubramanian SK, Sadaps M, Thota S, et al. Rational management approach to pure red cell aplasia. Haematologica. 2018;103(2):221–30. PMID: 29217782.
11. Casadevall N. What is antibody-mediated pure red cell aplasia (PRCA)? Nephrol Dial Transplant. 2005;20(SUPPL. 4):3–8. PMID: 15827056.
12. Fisch P, Handgretinger R, Schaefer HE. Pure red cell aplasia. Br J Haematol. 2000;111(4):1010–22. PMID: 11167735.

Aplastic Anemia 21

Zaker Schwabkey, Yehuda Deutsch,
and David Sallman

Introduction

Aplastic anemia (AA) is a type of bone marrow failures characterized by pancytopenia caused by an insult to the hematopoietic stem cells (HSCs), leading to ineffective hematopoiesis. Therefore, the name "anemia" is a misnomer. AA can be divided into acquired or inherited, e.g., Fanconi anemia or Dyskeratosis Congenita. Given limited space, we only discuss about acquired AA in the chapter. The incidence of acquired AA is very low (<2 per million), However, it tends to be higher in Asia than Western countries. It is considered that patients living in the Asian countries with increased exposure to drugs and toxin and indigenous viruses might be the causes for the higher incidence. Almost half of the cases occur before the age of 40. The ratio of male to female is 1:1. For acquired AA, most commonly, the insult is autoimmune

Z. Schwabkey (✉)
Division of Hematology and Hematologic Malignancies, Huntsman Cancer Institute at University of Utah, Salt Lake City, UT, USA
e-mail: Zaker.Schwabkey@hci.utah.edu

Y. Deutsch
Department of Malignant Hematology and Cellular Therapy, Memorial Healthcare System, Moffitt Cancer Center, Pembroke Pines, FL, USA

D. Sallman
Department of Malignant Hematology, Moffitt Cancer Center, Tampa, FL, USA

L. Sokol, L. Zhang (eds.), *Non-Neoplastic Hematologic Disorders*,
https://doi.org/10.1007/978-3-031-62373-8_21

or idiopathic, and if untreated, it is almost universally fatal [1]. Clinically, it is challenging to identify an accurate etiology of the acquired AA and to perform differential diagnosis between AA and other AA mimickers, e.g., hypoplastic myelodysplastic syndrome/neoplasm (MDS), paroxysmal nocturnal hemoglobinuria (PNH), or T/NK-cell large granular lymphocytic leukemia not only because of overlapping bone marrow findings but also the coexistence of these diseases. An accurate diagnosis is critical for appropriate management and the majority of patients require consultation at a tertiary center both for treatment and consideration of allogeneic hematopoietic cell transplantation (allo-HCT).

Pathogenesis

The exact pathogenesis of acquired AA remains unclear; however, an immune attack on the hematopoietic stem cell is mostly accepted. Approximately 50% of acquired AA is idiopathic. But other etiologies such as toxins, drugs (e.g., antineoplastic drugs, antibiotics, quinacrine, penicillamine, antiseizure medication, and nonsteroidal antiinflammatory drugs), chemicals (e.g., benzene and pesticides, inorganic arsenic), pregnancy, irradiation, or viral infections (hepatitis viruses mostly in young men and human immunodeficiency virus, EBV, CMV) can also act directly or as an autoimmune sequalae to such insults. It is important to note that predictable cytopenias associated with these exposures are not considered AA.

Loss of marrow HSCs is the hallmark of AA pathogenesis. Interferon gamma (IFN gamma) was found to be a key contributor in the autoimmune process. In observational studies, the presence of IFN gamma-containing T cells predicts response to immunosuppressive therapy.

AA can coexist or rarely evolve into another hematological disease, commonly a myeloid neoplasm such as myelodysplastic syndrome (MDS) and acute myeloid leukemia (AML), in 10% and 7% respectively, at 10 years follow-up, or paroxysmal nocturnal hemoglobinuria (PNH). PNH roughly coexists with half of AA cases and should be suspected especially in the setting of hemolytic anemia and thrombosis. However, PNH clones are often very small, and in the majority of cases, it do not require therapy (i.e., focus on the AA management). Importantly, the clonal burden of PNH can be challenging in the hypocellular state and should be reevaluated after AA therapy.

Cytogenetic abnormalities commonly include abnormalities in chromosomes 6, 7, and 13. Common mutated genes in AA include *ASXL1, BCOR, BCORL1, DMNT3A,* and *PIGA* (implicated in PNH).

Diagnosis

Clinically AA can manifest with insidious onset of cytopenia-related symptoms and signs at variable degree including weakness, fatigue, petechiae, gingival bleeding, infection, upon the degree of decreased counts. The onset duration crosses over weeks or months after the patient have been exposed to toxin (e.g., benzene), virus, or certain medications. Acute onset of AA has also been reported. Severe AA could be life threatening, requiring immediate diagnosis and treatment. Aplastic anemia is a diagnosis of exclusion. A comprehensive investigation is necessary to make an accurate diagnosis following a proposed diagnostic algorithm (Fig. 21.1) [1–4],

A. Medical history and physical exam are very important as they often lead to the possible cause (exposure to drugs, recent viral infections, etc.).
B. Laboratory study: Complete blood count (CBC) reveals pancytopenia, and low reticulocyte count indicating decreased marrow hematopoiesis. If the patient is medically stable with reasonable blood counts, then observation is preferred prior to an extensive workup. Serum B12 and folate levels should be checked as deficiency of these nutrients can also cause pancytopenia. Also, to include serum chemistry, liver, and renal function tests to exclude potential etiologies leading to pancytopenia or concurrent with renal or liver malfunction.

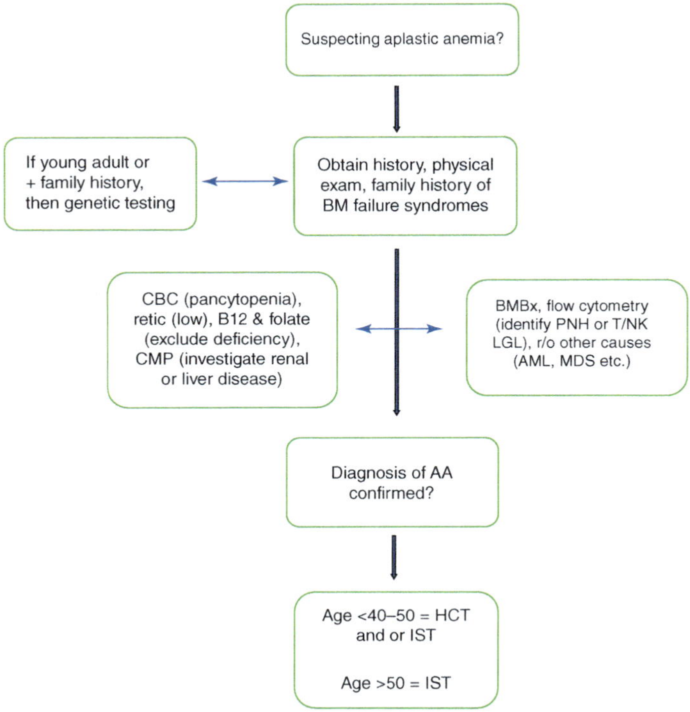

Fig. 21.1 Diagnostic algorithm for aplastic anemia

C. Bone marrow biopsy in conjunction with cytogenetics and molecular study is indicated for the patients highly suspicious for severe AA. Of note, AA cannot be distinguished from other causes of marrow hypoplasia only based on morphologic findings in a bone marrow biopsy.

Bone marrow aspiration and core biopsy from AA patients often reveals hypocellular marrow involving significant decrease in more than one or all hematopoietic cell lineages without significant megaloblastic, dysplastic (<10% if present), or fibrotic changes. CD34 positive blasts should not be increased. Cytogenetic and molecular studies are essential to investigate possible coexisting hematological disorders or alternative diagnoses. Interpretation of the presence of cytogenetic or molecular alteration should be of caution as certain genetic abnormalities (e.g., +6, +15, +8) or gene mutations (*CBL*) can also be observed in AA, which could result in a diagnostic challenging to distinguish from other clonal diseases.

D. Flow cytometry for PNH is guided by clinician's suspicion. Small clones of PNH may be present without evidence of hemolysis. Flow cytometry is also useful to identify T-/NK cell large granular lymphocytic leukemia.

E. Genetic testing for inherited AA is recommended for all children and selected cases in young adults, especially for those with positive family history or characteristic dysmorphia.

The AA is stratified into severe, very severe, and nonsevere (Table 21.1) [4]. Patients with AA often have a hypocellular marrow with <25% cellularity, especially those with severe form. AA is stratified into severe when two of the following peripheral CBC changes are present: absolute neutrophil count (ANC) $< 0.5 \times 10^9$/L, platelets count $<20 \times 10^9$/L, and reticulocyte count <60,000/μL. If ANC is $<0.2 \times 10^9$/L, then it is considered very severe AA. Notably, patients can have severe cytopenia of one lineage (e.g., thrombocytopenia) despite not meeting criteria for severe or very severe AA, which can create some treatment dilemmas. In general, we will treat these patients similar to severe or very severe AA patients.

Major Differential Diagnosis

Megaloblastic anemia, hypersplenism, MDS (especially hypoplastic MDS), AML, PNH, tumor marrow infiltration, or as part of inherited diseases such as Fanconi anemia, Shwachman-Diamond syndrome, and telomere diseases (Table 21.2). In addition to reversible marrow suppressions from various exposures.

Table 21.1 Definition of aplastic anemia with severity criteria [5]

	Bone marrow findings	ANC	ARC	Platelets	Criteria
Severe	<25% cellularity *	$<0.5 \times 10^9$/L	$<60 \times 10^9$/L	$<20 \times 10^9$/L	Meet bone marrow findings + any two of the three PB findings listed on the left
Very severe	<25% cellularity *	$<0.2 \times 10^9$/L	$<60 \times 10^9$/L	$<20 \times 10^9$/L	See above, but ANC must be $<0.2 \times 10^9$/L
Nonsevere	<25% cellularity *	$>0.5 \times 10^9$/L	$<60 \times 10^9$/L	$<20 \times 10^9$/L	

Or <50% of <30% of marrow is hematopoietic cells

AA aplastic anemia, *ANC* absolute neutrophil count, *ARC* absolute reticulocyte count

Table 21.2 Differential diagnoses of acquired AA

	Clinical and laboratory findings	Bone marrow findings	Cytogenetic findings	Molecular findings
Acquired				
Megaloblastic anemia	Decreased vitamin B12 and/or folate level, elevated MCV	Megaloblastic findings in myeloid and erythroid lineage	NA	NA
Hypersplenism	Enlarged spleen, associated with cytopenia	Unremarkable, or with mild megakaryocytic hyperplasia	None	None
Hypoplastic MDS	Pancytopenia	Hypoplasia, with overt morphologic dysplasia seen in megakaryocytic or granulocytic lineage, with or without increased blasts	MDS related cytogenetic abnormalities	Often associated with myeloid gene mutations, e.g., *SRSF2, TET2, SF3B1, ASXL*
AML	Circulating blasts	Increased blasts, with or without dysplasia	Recurrent cytogenetic abnormalities associated with AML or MDS	Often associated with myeloid gene mutations e.g., *IDH1/2, FLT3, NPM1, ASXL1, TP53*
PNH	Positive for PNH clone	Occasional dysplastic forms can be seen	Usually, normal karyotype	*PIAG, CBL1* gene mutations

(continued)

Table 21.2 (continued)

	Clinical and laboratory findings	Bone marrow findings	Cytogenetic findings	Molecular findings
T/NK-LGL leukemia	Predominantly neutropenia, or sometimes bi- or pancytopenia, increased T/NK cells	Erythroid hypoplasia, interstitial T-LGLs,	NA	*STAT3* mutation in 30–40% of CD8+T-/NK- LGL leukemia, STAT5b mutations in 22–55% of CD4+ T-LGL leukemia
Pure red cell aplasia	Anemia, parvovirus B19 test negative	Erythroid hypoplasia or aplasia, without excess blasts or dysplasia	NA	NA
Inherited				
Fanconi anemia	Pancytopenia and physical abnormalities (e.g., short stature, microcephaly, skin lesions)	Hypoplasia, and hypocellular same as AA in adults. In infants, can be normocellular	Abnormalities in chromosomes 1q, 3q and 7	*FANCA, FANCC, FANCG* gene mutations
Shwachman-Diamond syndrome	Intermittent neutropenia, pancytopenia, skeletal abnormalities, and exocrine pancreatic dysfunction	Nondiagnostic as it shows varying cellularity and dysplastic changes	Monosomy 7, isochromosome 7, del (7q) and del(20q)	*EIF6, TP53, PRPF8, CSNK1A1* and possible *DNMT3A, ASXL1 and TET2*

Dyskeratosis congenita	Anemia and thrombocytopenia, nail and skin findings, pulmonary fibrosis	NA	NA	Mutations in genes encoding components of the telomerase complex, e.g., *ACD, CTC1, DKC1*. Other telomere abnormalities include mutations in *TERT* or *TERC*
Abnormal thrombopoietin or its receptor	NA	NA	NA	Mutations in *TPO* or *MPL*

Prognosis

Untreated severe AA has a 1-year mortality of over 70%. With treatment, the 5-year survival is as high as 90%. Studies have shown that these factors are associated with favorable outcomes: younger age, less severe disease, higher absolute reticulocyte count, and higher absolute lymphocyte count. Both the trisomy 8 and deletion of 13q correspond to better response to the immunosuppressive agent antithymocyte globulin (ATG) [1].

Treatment

Treatment approaches include immunosuppressive therapy (IST) or allogeneic hematopoietic stem cell transplantation (allo-HCT) or both [4–8]. Urgency to treat generally depends on the disease severity and patient's age or medical fitness. Patients with severe or very severe AA need to be treated urgently. For medically fit patients who are <40 years old, although age cut-off varies by institution, it is generally recommended to proceed directly to allo-HCT if a matched related donor (MRD) is available. This is the preferred approach for this patient population as it rapidly normalizes blood counts and avoid any possible clonal evolution while on IST. Key questions in the field surround potential direct to allo-HSCT with matched unrelated donors and/or haploidentical donors, given incredible long-term survival even in the setting of alternative donor sources. However, most of the time, patients are started on IST because they are hospitalized with cytopenia-related complications, do not have a readily available MRD, or search process for a matched unrelated donor (MUD) can take weeks to months. For patients aged 40 years or older, treatment consists of triplet IST typically with equine antithymocyte globulin (ATG), cyclosporine, and eltrombopag. Triplet IST is superior to ATG plus cyclosporine in a randomized phase 3 study.

- ATG: Horse ATG leads to a superior response than rabbit ATG. ATG must be administered in an inpatient setting at a dose of 40 mg/kg intravenously daily for 4 days through a central line. The most common adverse events are infusion reactions which occur immediately. Serum sickness which can start days to weeks after initiating treatment is quite rare in the era of a corticosteroid taper over 3 weeks with therapy. It is recommended to stop beta-blockers prior to therapy and administer adequate fluids to allow for circulatory compensation in anticipation of possible infusion reaction.

- Cyclosporine: Initial dose is 6 mg/kg orally daily in two equally divided doses starting on day one of IST (or often initiated at the time of discharge from the hospital). Use of concurrent azole antifungal and altered baseline renal function need dose optimization. Cyclosporine is typically continued for total of 18–24 months. After initial 12 months of therapy, it can be slowly tapered over 6–12 months (about 10% per month). Alternatively, full dose can be administered for 6 months followed by a dose reduction for a trough level of 100–150 for 12–18 months. At any point during treatment, if blood counts drop, cyclosporine can be reinitiated at the full dose. Most common adverse events are hypertension, renal insufficiency, and magnesium wasting. Future research is required to understand the optimal tapering plan and whether gradual tapering vs rapid discontinuation leads to differential outcomes.
- Eltrombopag (EPAG): It is a nonpeptide thrombopoietin receptor (TPO-R) agonist. It is recommended that EPAG is started on day one of IST at a dose of 150 mg once daily orally and is continued for 6 months. Starting day 1 was superior to starting later in treatment from an efficacy perspective, although if severe transaminitis occurs with ATG, these can be delayed. Special attention must be given for concurrent use of magnesium or supplements such as zinc, calcium, or iron as they alter gastrointestinal absorption and must be separated by at least 4 h from EPAG dose. Most common adverse events are gastrointestinal such as nausea and diarrhea in addition to headache and elevated indirect bilirubin.
- Other agents: Romiplostim is mostly used in the refractory or relapsed AA. It is a TPO agonist with an initial dose of 10 mcg/

kg subcutaneously weekly. Dose can be up-titrated based on platelet count.

- Alemtuzumab, which is a CD52-targeted monoclonal antibody, can be given for patients as a salvage therapy. The most common regimen is a 10 mg daily for 10 days, preceded by a 1 mg test dose.

Monitoring for treatment response and adverse events should occur every 2–4 weeks for the first 6 months with transfusion support as needed. Bone marrow biopsy and aspirate can be considered at 3 and 6 months follow-up to check for improvement in marrow cellularity although count improvement is most critical and unclear data of the benefit of serial bone marrow evaluation if clinical improvement.

Hematological response is achieved with transfusion independency. Median time to this response is 3 months. Complete response is defined as hemoglobin >10 g/dL and platelets >50,000/μL.

- Allogeneic hematopoietic cell transplantation (Allo-HCT): HCT replaces the immune system responsible for depleting hematopoietic stem cells, can cure AA but with considerable side effects but outcomes in children and adolescents are historically superior to adults >40 years old. In general, for fit patients <40–50 years old, with severe AA or very severe AA, it is advisable to proceed to HCT directly if a donor is available. If the donor is not readily available, then IST can be used in the interim if the donor search may take long time. A matched related donor is superior to matched unrelated, but both options are acceptable. Transplant should be considered for all fit patients under the age of 75 years of age who have relapsed therapy.

Promising Clinical Studies

Sirolimus is being studied for use in patients with severe AA to prevent relapse after standard of care IST (Phase 2 clinical trial: NCT02979873). Additionally, ruxolitinib (JAK1/2 inhibitor) is being studied for relapsed/refractory immune bone marrow failure including AA (NCT05998408). A potential investigational drug under study is REGN7257, which is an Anti-Interleukin 2 Receptor Subunit Gamma [IL2RG] Monoclonal Antibody (NCT04409080).

Caveats

- Aplastic anemia is a bone marrow disorder, most commonly autoimmune in nature but can occur from other causes.
- Management begins with recognizing and avoiding any possible trigger, if exists, such as medications.
- The standard treatment is generally a triple IST (eltrombopag, cyclosporine, and antithymocyte globulin).

Board Question

Q1. A 29-year-old Caucasian woman presented to the hospital with fatigue and shortness of breath, she was found with pancytopenia (Hemoglobin of 7.8 g/dL, absolute neutrophils of 0.49×10^9/L and platelet count of <20×10^9/L). The bone marrow biopsy was diagnostic of aplastic anemia (AA) with 5% cellularity. The concurrent cytogenetics/molecular studies were normal. She is interested to be treated as soon as possible. She is currently stable and has required only a few transfusions since hospitalization. You explain that the most favorable treatment approach is:

A. Double-immunosuppressive therapy
B. ATG, cyclosporine and, eltrombopag
C. Send directly to allo-HCT if donor and pre-transplantation workup are readily available.
D. ATG, cyclosporine and, eltrombopag followed by allo-HCT

Answer: C. based on treatment guideline for AA, allogeneic hematopoietic transplant is indicated for patients younger than 40 with serve AA.

Q2. A 47-year-old man otherwise healthy presented 3 months ago to his primary care physician with symptoms of shortness of breath and fatigue, CBC revealed pancytopenia, and other laboratory tests including B12, folate and iron studies were normal, upon referral to hematology, he was eventually diagnosed with AA. Patient lost to follow up for 6 weeks due to relocating to another city. He established with a new hematologist who concurred with the diagnosis of aplastic anemia based on the records he received; however, a repeat bone marrow biopsy revealed increased blasts (19%), NGS revealed *NPM1* mutation and cytogenetics showed normal male karyotype. You recommend treatment with:

A. ATG, cyclosporine and, eltrombopag
B. 7 days of cytarabine and 3 days of anthracycline
C. Send directly to allo-HCT
D. ATG, cyclosporine and, eltrombopag followed by allo-HCT

Answer: B. The patient's disease has transformed to secondary acute myeloid leukemia. An immediate treatment should be intensive (7 days of cytarabine and 3 days of anthracycline).

References

1. Killick SB, Bown N, Cavenagh J, et al. Guidelines for the diagnosis and management of adult aplastic anaemia. Br J Haematol. 2016;172:187. PMID: 26568159.
2. Young NS. Aplastic Anemia. N Engl J Med. 2018;379:1643. PMID: 30354958.
3. DeZern AE, Symons HJ, Resar LS, et al. Detection of paroxysmal nocturnal hemoglobinuria clones to exclude inherited bone marrow failure syndromes. Eur J Haematol. 2014;92(6):467–70. https://doi.org/10.1111/ejh.12299.

4. Guinan EC. Diagnosis and management of aplastic anemia. Hematol Am Soc Hematol Educ Program. 2011;2011:76–81. PMID: 22160015
5. Tichelli A, Peffaultde Latour R, Passweg J, et al. Long-term outcome of a randomized controlled study in patients with newly diagnosed severe aplastic anemia treated with antithymocyte globulin and cyclosporine, with or without granulocyte colony-stimulating factor: a Severe Aplastic Anemia Working Party Trial from the European Group of Blood and Marrow Transplantation. Haematologica. 2020;105(5):1223–31.
6. Scheinberg P, Wu CO, Nunez O, Young NS. Predicting response to immunosuppressive therapy and survival in severe aplastic anaemia. Br J Haematol. 2009;144:206. PMID: 19036108.
7. Tichelli A, Socié G, Henry-Amar M, et al. Effectiveness of immunosuppressive therapy in older patients with aplastic anemia. European Group for Blood and Marrow Transplantation Severe Aplastic Anaemia Working Party. Ann Intern Med. 1999;130:193. PMID: 10049197.
8. Peffault de Latour R, Kulasekararaj A, Iacobelli S, Severe Aplastic Anemia Working Party of the European Society for Blood and Marrow Transplantation, et al. Eltrombopag added to immunosuppression in severe aplastic anemia. N Engl J Med. 2022;386(1):11–23.PMID: 34986284.

Porphyrias

22

Kai J. Rogers, Sabarish Ayyappan, and Prerna Rastogi

Introduction [1]

Porphyria is a cluster of rare metabolic disease resulting from genetic defects in heme synthesis, leading to abnormal accumulation and deposition of toxic intermediates in neurologic and/or cutaneous tissue. The heme biosynthetic pathway enzymes are most active in the bone marrow and liver, and the intermediates are excreted in the bile and urine (turn to be reddish-purple in color). Porphyrias can be classified as either erythropoietic or hepatic, based on the site of accumulation of excess heme synthetic pathway intermediates. Erythropoietic porphyrias arise from the excess intermediates during the heme synthesis pathway and accumulates in the erythroid cells of the bone marrow. These conditions typically manifest at birth or early childhood with sensitivity to light, except for Congenital Erythropoietic Porphyria (CEP), which may appear in utero as nonimmune hydrops.

K. J. Rogers · P. Rastogi (✉)
Department of Pathology, University of Iowa, Carver College of Medicine, Iowa City, IA, USA
e-mail: prerna-rastogi@uiowa.edu

S. Ayyappan
Department of Internal Medicine, University of Iowa, Carver College of Medicine, Iowa City, IA, USA

L. Sokol, L. Zhang (eds.), *Non-Neoplastic Hematologic Disorders*, https://doi.org/10.1007/978-3-031-62373-8_22

Of the nine major porphyrias, hepatic porphyrias are most common with overproduction and accumulation of porphyrin and precursors in the liver. Interestingly, a majority of the hepatic porphyrias primarily present after puberty, presumably due to the influence of various hormones that function as precipitating factors and reflecting distinct hepatic regulatory mechanisms for heme biosynthesis. This contrasts with ALA dehydratase deficiency porphyria (ADP), CEP, and erythropoietic protoporphyria (EPP) which manifest in infancy, and generally, they have a stable clinical course, making age of onset a useful clinical marker in making the diagnosis. Acute intermittent porphyria (AIP) and porphyria cutanea tarda (PCT) are the most common subtypes of acute and cutaneous porphyrias in the United States (US), respectively.

Each porphyria is secondary to abnormal (lacking or increased) activity of the heme synthesis pathway. The genetic sequences and chromosomal loci for the various genes affect the various steps in the heme synthesis, and this has helped identify the multiple disease-specific mutations that has been identified in each of the porphyrias, except for PCT which is an acquired type, secondary to an inhibitor that reduces the activity of the uroporphyrinogen decarboxylase (UROD) in the liver. Characteristic patterns of inheritance have been identified for diverse types of porphyrias, and this is reflected in severity of presentation and the influence of other factors necessary for manifestation. Porphyrias that are autosomal dominant display low penetrance, with symptoms often activated by a combination of other genetic factors, environmental exposures, and metabolic disturbances. Autosomal recessive inherited porphyrias are more dependent on the genetic derangements, as symptom severity correlates with the severity of the specific familial disease variant. The hepatic porphyrias commonly present with acute neurovisceral symptoms including AIP, HCP (hereditary coproporphyria), VP (variegate porphyria), and ADP while the erythropoietic porphyrias which consists of EPP, XLP (X-linked proptoporphyria), and CEP present with cutaneous manifestations because of phototoxicity. HCP and VP have clinical features overlapping in both the groups while the two hepatic porphyrias, PCT and HEP (hepatoerythropoietic porphyria), show cutaneous symptoms but without acute neural presentation. As an overview, a simplified summary of the various porphyrias divided by the predominant presenting symptom is provided in Table 22.1.

Table 22.1 Summary table. General characteristics of the porphyrias. Approximate incidence based on US population, except for VP which is found at 1 in 300 in South Africa and 1 in 75,000 in Northern Europe. Screening test results are simplified to focus on the defining intermediate and are not comprehensive

	Disease	Abbreviation	Enzyme deficiency	Inheritance	Incidence	screening	Confirmation
Acute	ALA dehydratase deficiency porphyria	ADP	Aminolevulinate dehydratase	AR	<10 reported	*Urine*: PBG Negative	*Blood*: ↑ ALA
	Acute intermittent porphyria	AIP	Hydroxymethylbilane synthase	AD	1 in 10,000	*Urine*: ↑ PBG *Feces*: Negative	*Blood*: HMB Synthase activity
	Hereditary coproporphyria	HCP	Coproporphyrinogen oxidase	AD	1 in 500,000	*Urine*: ↑ PBG *Feces*: Coproporphyrin only	*Serum*: ↑ Coproporphyrin
	Variegate porphyria	VP	Protoporphyrinogen oxidase	AD	Variable	*Urine*: ↑ PBG *Feces*: ↑ Porphyrins	*Serum*: ↑ Porphyrins
Skin	Porphyria cutanea tarda	PCT	Uroporphyrinogen decarboxylase	Sporadic (20% AD)	1 in 10,000	*Urine/serum*: 7-Carboxyporphyin	Molecular
	Hepatoerythropoietic porphyria	HEP	Uroporphyrinogen decarboxylase	AR	<50 reported	*Urine/serum*: 7-Carboxyporphyrin	Molecular
	Congenital erythropoietic porphyria	CEP	Uroporphyrinogen synthase	AR	1 in 1,000,000	*Urine/serum/feces*: Coproporphyrin	Molecular
	Erythropoietic protoporphyria	EPP	Ferrochelatase	AR	1 in 100,000	*Blood*: ↑ Erythrocyte protoporphyrin	Molecular
	X-linked protoporphyria	XLP	Aminolevulinate synthase	X-linked dominant	1 in 1,000,000	*Blood*: ↑ Erythrocyte protoporphyrin	Molecular

Progress has been made in understanding the heme synthesis pathway and identifying the housekeeping and erythroid specific transcripts regulating the heme synthesis. Identifying the genetic perturbations and understanding the various interactions holds promise for discovering novel therapies for management.

Pathogenesis [2, 3]

The porphyrias are characterized by deficiencies, either hereditary or acquired, in key enzymes in the heme biosynthesis pathway (Fig. 22.1). Heme synthesis occurs primarily in two sites, the bone marrow, which is vital to produce mature erythrocytes, and the liver, which serves as a key cofactor for the cytochrome P450 enzymes (CYPs) which play a key role in metabolism. When the individual steps in this process function suboptimally, intermediates in this pathway accumulate and exert toxic effects, leading to the clinical manifestations associated with porphyria. Broadly, these are classified into two major groups, those manifesting with primarily neurologic findings (the "acute" porphyrias) and those presenting as severe photosensitivity and blistering disorders (the "cutaneous" porphyrias).

While the precise mechanisms underlying these clinical presentations are incompletely understood, it is thought that porphyrin precursors, specifically aminolevulinic acid (ALA) and porphobilinogen (PBG), are neurotoxic at high levels, whereas porphyrins (protoporphyrin, uroporphyrin, and coproporphyrin) are deposited in the skin where they produce free radicals in response to photoexcitation that subsequently cause oxidative stress and cellular damage. It is important to note that environmental factors also contribute to the manifestation and severity of disease as penetrance is incomplete and acute attacks are frequently precipitated by an exposure, frequently drugs, given the role of heme in CYP function, but also infections, diet, stress, alcohol use, and many others. A comprehensive drug safety database for patients with porphyria can be found at https://porphyriafoundation.org/drugdatabase/drug-safety-database-search/.

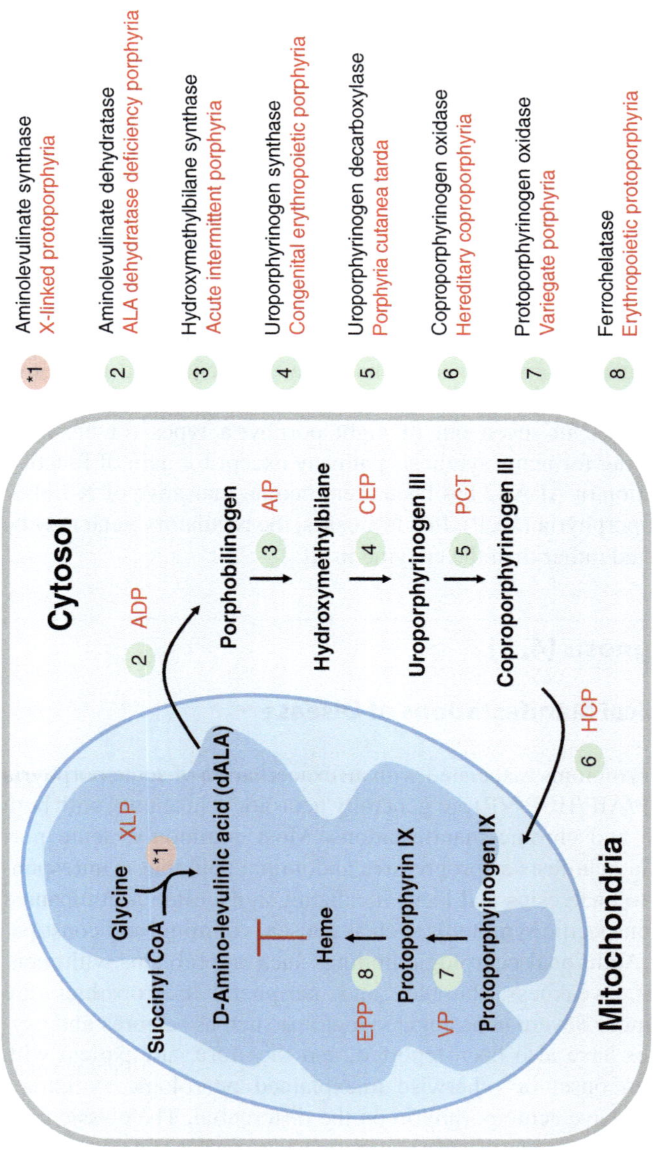

Fig. 22.1 Pathogenesis of porphyrias. The heme biosynthesis pathway is shown with key enzymes (numbered circles) and the porphyria (red text) associated with their deficiency. * indicates the rate-limiting step in heme biosynthesis and indicates negative feedback

Heme biosynthesis is regulated through multiple mechanisms with the ALA-synthase (ALAS) enzyme playing a significant role. This has two isoforms such as ubiquitously expressed ALAS1 encoded by a gene in chromosome 3 and erythrocyte specific ALAS2 encoded by a gene located on X-chromosome. ALAS1 gene expression can be influenced by multiple factors like stress and nutritional status, drugs, and cytochrome P 450 inducers in the liver while heme itself has negative feedback on the ALAS1 activity. ALAS2 expression is regulated by erythroid-specific transcription factors such as GATA1, along with the body's iron reserves and various iron metabolism and transport regulators. In majority of inherited cases of porphyria, the causative genetic mutation influences the gene encoding the corresponding heme synthesis enzyme. There is loss of function mutations, in seven out of eight porphyria types for enzymes encoding for heme synthesis pathway except for gain of function mutation of ALAS2 has been identified, as causative of X-linked protoporphyria (XLP). In a few cases, the regulatory gene may be affected rather than the enzyme itself.

Diagnosis [4, 5]

Clinical Manifestations of Disease

The symptoms associated with an exacerbation of acute porphyria (ADP/AIP/HCP/VP) are generally neurologic in nature, with both acute and chronic manifestations. Most commonly, acute porphyria manifests as progressive abdominal pain that is unresponsive to analgesics and lacks localizing signs, often accompanied by nonspecific symptoms such as nausea, vomiting, and constipation. Additional neurologic findings such as problems with mentation, weakness, fatigue, and peripheral neuropathies are common. Severe neurologic symptoms such as seizures and psychoses have also been reported, and therefore, any patient with sudden onset or otherwise unexplained neurologic symptoms should have acute porphyria on the differential. The classic triad of clinical symptoms with abdominal pain, peripheral neuropathy, and central nervous system abnormalities should prompt a workup for acute porphyria. Cases of homozygous AIP, HCP, and VP manifesting with a distinct phenotype and increased levels of erythrocyte zinc protoporphyrin have been documented, though they are rare. Clinical presentation includes impaired neurologic development and chronic skin blisters occurring in early childhood; however, no acute porphyria attacks noted. In contrast, cutaneous porphyrias (CEP/PCT/EPP/XLP) manifest as severe photosensitivity that can be either acute, resulting in immediate stinging/burning pain, or delayed, resulting in blister formation in sun exposed areas. Chronic sun damage in photosensitive areas can result in scarring and hyperpigmentation that can be disfiguring. While it is convenient to separate the porphyrias by the predominant symptomatology, it is important to note that significant overlap can occur. To this point, HCP and VP can also manifest as blistering disorders between acute attacks and should be considered even in the absence of a history of acute attacks. Although AIP is not included among cutaneous porphyria, blistering skin lesions have been noted with individuals with AIP and chronic kidney disease secondary to elevated plasma porphyrin levels.

Laboratory Diagnosis

The laboratory diagnosis of porphyria is generally divided into two steps, screening based on the detection of intermediates in heme synthesis, followed by confirmation with enzymatic tests or expanded biochemical panels and finally molecular testing for specific variant analysis if desired or in the case of indeterminate results.

Screening

There are numerous laboratory assays available for screening for porphyria. The most common approach is to first perform a qualitative screen for heme intermediates. This can be done by testing the urine for the presence of PBG as this intermediate is produced early in heme biosynthesis and is thus increased to at least 10× the upper limit of normal in many forms of acute porphyria (AIP, HCP, and VP) especially during an acute attack. For patients presenting primarily with cutaneous symptoms, an alternative approach is to perform fractionation and quantitation of porphyrins in the urine as cutaneous porphyrias result in increased excretion of heme intermediates. Additionally, for patients presenting with immediate photosensitivity (itching, burning, and pain), erythrocyte porphyrins can be measured directly. This is possible as erythrocytes retain some elements of the heme biosynthetic pathway, making the measurement of porphyrins useful, particularly in the diagnosis of EPP and XLP.

Confirmation

In the case of a positive screening test, additional testing is warranted. Biochemical analysis of feces is a commonly utilized approach as individual porphyrias have well-defined biochemical profiles in feces, and thus, this testing is especially helpful in distinguishing AIP, VP, and HCP as they have increased excretion in the feces. Additionally, in the case of cutaneous porphyrias, it can be useful to assess levels of porphyrins in the serum qualitatively or quantitatively through fluorometric assays. A more definitive diagnosis can be made by testing levels of enzymatic activity (both hydroxymethylbilane synthase and aminolevulinate dehydratase can be tested directly) or through molecular analysis. Of note, molecular analysis presents its own set of challenges as mutations effecting regulatory genes may be disease causing but not readily identified. The approach to testing and expected results in various porphyrias are summarized in Fig. 22.2.

Genetic testing is available and can help diagnosis asymptomatic individuals with elevated porphyrin can be identified, and this can help confirm diagnosis if clinical findings or biochemical test findings are atypical. Genetic counselling may be warranted for first-degree relatives screening and preconceptual counselling.

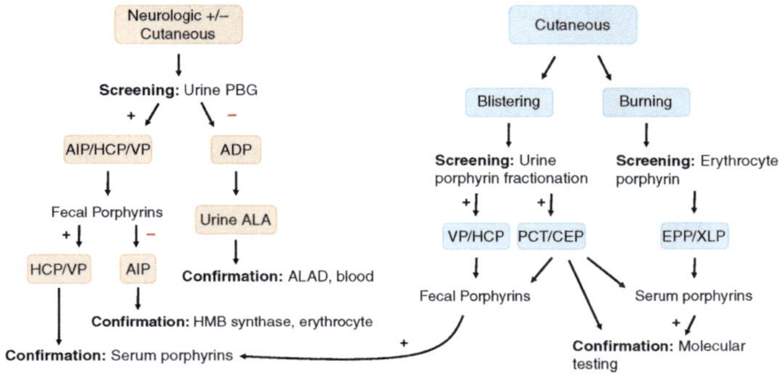

Fig. 22.2 Approach to testing for porphyrias - General approach to testing for porphyrias divided by the primary clinical presentation. Algorithm is modified from ARUP testing algorithm (https://arupconsult.com/algorithm/porphyrias-testing-algorithm)

Major Differential Diagnosis

Cutaneous porphyrias (CEP/PCT/EPP/XLP)

- Pseudoporphyria
- Autoimmune blistering disorders
- Infection
- Photosensitivity (chemicals, drugs, sunburn, and allergic)

Acute porphyrias (ADP/AIP/HCP/VP)

- Abdominal pain
- Neurologic disorders
- Liver disease
- Lead poisoning

Prognosis

Prognosis varies significantly among the porphyrias and is further variable among individuals with the same disease, given the range in severity that is observed. Generally, the prognosis has improved as diagnostic advances allow us to identify at-risk individuals and minimize exposure to precipitating factors, thereby reducing the frequency and severity of acute attacks while also starting the appropriate targeted therapies, advances in which have reduced the morbidity and mortality associated with disease. Notably, it is recommended that genetic counseling be performed in all cases of porphyria.

Treatment

Porphyrias with their varied age of presentation, diverse phenotype, and chronic disability have treatment options focusing on symptom control and improving quality of life. Curative options are limited to liver and hematopoietic transplantation for severe cases with complications as discussed below. The treatment for the porphyrias is dependent on the type, severity, and chronicity of clinical presentation. An acute porphyria attack needs to be identified rapidly, and if diagnosis work up is ongoing, the testing is expedited, so that appropriate treatment can be instituted to abate the acute symptoms and preventing further progression. It is important to provide supportive care including pain control, hydration, and hospitalization may be required for monitoring of neurologic symptoms, respiratory symptoms, and correction of electrolytes. In individuals suspected of acute porphyria or with established diagnosis, intravenous hemin, and carbohydrate (glucose) loading can quell the attack. These therapies downregulate hepatic ALAS-1 and reduce ALA, PBG and porphyrin-metabolites formation. Hemin with a more potent activity can be used for severe attacks while glucose loading can be utilized for milder attacks or when hemin is unavailable. During acute attacks, three to four IV hemin infusions are necessary to control attacks to reduce ALA and PBG levels and those with frequent attacks may benefit from weekly or monthly prophylactic infusions. Symptomatic therapy for pain, nausea, and treatment of life-threatening complications like paralysis, seizures can be commenced before a diagnosis of porphyria is confirmed. Exacerbating factors that contribute to the attack needs to be corrected like carbohydrate repletion, treatment of infection, avoidance of offending drugs is important to prevent further progression. Givosiran is a small interfering RNA, that targets and downregulates hepatic ALAS1, the gene that is induced in individuals with active AIP. Givosiran is FDA approved for management of acute porphyrias and has shown to reduce the frequency of attacks. Weekly hemin administration can be used for prophylaxis to prevent attacks, and if unsuccessful, Givosiran is used to reduce the chronicity. Liver transplantation in recommended in patients with liver damage or those with hepatocellular carcinoma secondary to recurrent AIP attacks.

The management of cutaneous porphyrias is chronic, and immediate therapy is often not required. Avoidance of sunlight is advised to prevent blistering and adequate skin care and preventing skin infections is more important once blisters have formed. PCT is the prototype for treatable porphyria and responds well to iron reduction strategies like phlebotomy and low dose hydroxychloroquine that carries porphyrins from the liver. The other blistering cutaneous poprhyrias do not respond to iron reduction strategies and treatment is individualized to subtype. PCT is a chronic disease that can relapse over time and control of exacerbating factors like avoidance of alcohol, suppression of HCV infection can reduce the relapses. Once remission is achieved, periodic monitoring of urine and plasma porphyrin levels can help detect a relapse and treatment can be reinstituted. For CEP, mainstay of treatment is avoidance of sunlight exposure to skin and eyes, and in severe cases, allogenic stem cell transplantation could be considered. Routine vitamin D supplementation is advised to prevent concomitant vitamin D deficiency from poor sunlight exposure.

The cornerstone of management of nonblistering cutaneous protoporphyrias like EPP, XLP involves sun avoidance, and this often is difficult as it impairs quality of life and warrants daily life change. Use of long clothing and hats outdoors and broad-spectrum sunscreen preparations with high sun protection factor (SPF) may be beneficial. Beta-carotene available as over-the-counter oral supplement, was originally developed for EPP, can improve sunlight tolerance. Afamelanotide, FDA approved synthetic analogue of human alpha melanocyte stimulating hormone, increases cutaneous pigmentation by enhancing melanin production and increases sunlight tolerance in protoporphyria patients. They function by the reduction of free radical production and cytokine formation and does not affect porphyrin production or alter the underlying disease process. Liver transplantation could be considered in a patient with cirrhosis or severe hepatopathy related to protoporphyria. Hematopoietic stem cell transplantation if a suitable donor is available could be considered in a patient with allograft liver or one who has recovered from severe hepatopathy to essentially cure of EPP or XLP to prevent a recurrent liver complication.

Promising Clinical Studies [6]

Dersimelagon (MT-7117) is a synthetic melanocortin-1 receptor agonist currently in Phase 3 clinical trials (NCT05005975) for patients with EPP or XLP. Mechanistically, Dersimelagon stimulates melanin production with the goal of reducing photosensitivity in patients, as demonstrated in the ENDEAVOR trial (NCT03520036). Bitopertin (DISC-1459) is a small molecule inhibitor of glycine transporter 1 (GlyT1) that is currently in Phase 2 clinical trials (NCT05308472) for patients with erythropoietic porphyrias (EPP, XLP, CEP). By preventing glycine transport, the first step of heme biosynthesis is inhibited, resulting in decreased levels of toxic metabolites that accumulate in patients with porphyrias. Gene therapy, gene editing targeting culprit genes and novel vector-based drug delivery are being investigated and holds promise for future therapy.

Caveats

1. Porphyrias are often misdiagnosed and can be missed unless this is considered in differential.
2. Initial diagnosis of porphyria is made by biochemical testing, but the diagnosis is confirmed by specific genetic mutation.
3. Photosensitive dermatoses should be evaluated with detailed history, physical exam, phototesting, and photopatch testing.

In patients with photosensitivity and bullous lesions, dermatologic conditions as detailed above needs to be kept in mind.

Board Question

1. A 30-year-old woman, emigrant from South Africa has been referred for evaluation with suspicion for porphyria. She has had multiple hospitalizations for chronic abdominal pain and cramping in her adulthood, and she had no medical problems growing up. She has completed thorough gastrointestinal exam and recent exploratory laparotomy was negative. She has a family history of multiple family members with chronic blistering skin conditions, psychiatric illness, and abdominal pain. Patient is otherwise healthy and is on chronic pain medications. Physical exam reveals new blisters on the dorsal surface of her hands and diffuse abdominal tenderness to palpation. Blood work shows normal white cell count, hemoglobin, hepatic liver enzymes, but elevated 24-h urine porphobilinogen. What is the most likely diagnosis for this patient?

   A. Acute intermittent porphyria
   B. Congenital Erythropoietic porphyria
   C. Porphyria Cutanea Tarda
   D. Variegate porphyria

   Answer: D. AIP and VP present with acute symptoms and CEP and PCT present with cutaneous symptoms. VP can have features of acute neurovisceral or cutaneous blisters or both at presentation. VP is a hepatic porphyria, autosomal dominant type caused by a deficiency of protoporphyrinogen oxidase and has been described to have higher prevalence in South Africa and Finland. The acute symptoms can be similar to AIP and biochemical test reveal elevated urine ALA, PBG and porphyrins.

2. A 34-year-old female presents to her local emergency department with a chief complaint of severe abdominal pain. She is unable to communicate clearly with staff and her partner notes

that she has not been "acting like herself" since starting treatment for a UTI. A battery of testing is performed and urine porphobilinogen is found to be elevated. Further testing, revealed negative plasma, urine and fecal porphyrins. Given this finding and the overall clinical picture, which of the following enzymes is most likely to be deficient in this patient?

A. aminolevulinate synthase
B. coproporphyrinogen oxidase
C. protoporphyrinogen oxidase
D. hydroxymethylbilane synthase
E. ferrochelatase

Answer: D hydroxymethylbilane synthase. AIP- Most common acute porphyria in the US, presents with elevated PBG, caused by deficiency in hydroxymethylbilane synthase. HCP and VP have been ruled out with negative fecal porphyrin testing and absence of cutaneous lesions.

References

1. American porphyria foundation. Updated 2022. https://porphyriafoundation.org/. Accessed 20 Dec 2022.
2. Kakoullis L, Louppides S, Papachristodoulou E, Panos G. Porphyrias and photosensitivity: pathophysiology for the clinician. Postgrad Med. 2018;130(8):673–86. https://doi.org/10.1080/00325481.2018.1533380.
3. Bissell DM, Anderson KE, Bonkovsky HL. Porphyria. N Engl J Med. 2017;377(9):862–72. https://doi.org/10.1056/NEJMra1608634.
4. Di Pierro E, De Canio M, Mercadante R, et al. Laboratory diagnosis of porphyria. Diagnostics (Basel). 2021;11(8):1343. https://doi.org/10.3390/diagnostics11081343.
5. Frank EL. ARUP consult porphyrias. Updated May 2020. https://arupconsult.com/content/porphyrias. Accessed 20 Dec 2022.
6. Clinical Trials. National Institutes of Health (NIH). Updated 2022. https://clinicaltrials.gov/. Accessed 20 Dec 2022.

Hereditary and Acquired Iron Overload Disorder

23

Sushmita Khadka and Lubomir Sokol

Introduction

Iron overload disorders are the clinical conditions where there is deposition of iron in the body tissue or organ leading to organ damage. Iron overload disorder could be primary or secondary. Primary iron overload is caused by congenital disorder known as hereditary hemochromatosis whereas secondary iron overload is the acquired disorder from excess blood transfusion, conditions leading to ineffective hematopoiesis and from liver diseases.

A iron homeostasis pathway is a highly regulated complex process, requiring several proteins. Of them, hepcidin, a peptide hormone synthesized by liver, is the key regulator in response to erythropoiesis, ongoing inflammation, and daily supplies of iron. Factors that could suppress or stimulate hepcidin, such as cytokine, hormones, erythropoietin, also play critical roles in iron

S. Khadka (✉) · L. Sokol
Moffitt Cancer Center, Tampa, FL, USA
e-mail: sushmita.khadka@moffitt.org

L. Sokol, L. Zhang (eds.), *Non-Neoplastic Hematologic Disorders*,
https://doi.org/10.1007/978-3-031-62373-8_23

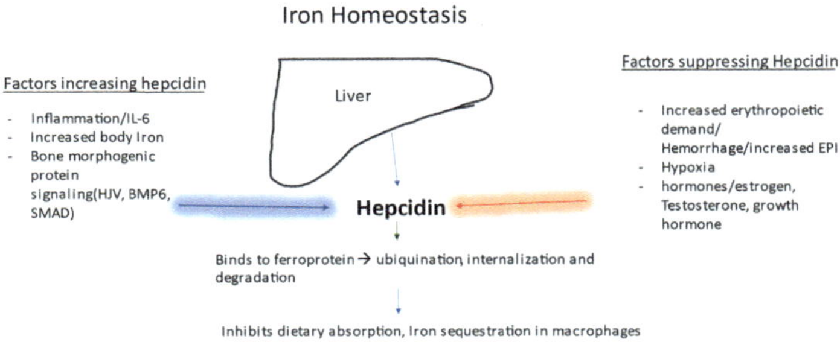

Fig. 23.1 Iron homeostasis

homeostasis (Fig. 23.1). Total body content of iron is 3.0–4.0 g. We consume (15–25 mg/day) out of all dietary supply, of which 1.0–2.0 mg is absorbed through the gastrointestinal (GI) tract and 1.0–2.0 mg are lost through GI epithelial cells and menstruation [1].

Pathogenesis, Diagnosis, and Treatment

The pathogenesis, clinical presentation, diagnosis, treatment, and prognosis will be discussed individual according to primary or secondary hemochromatosis and their variants.

Hereditary Hemochromatosis

Hereditary hemochromatosis is a disorder marked by genetic variability, leading to iron accumulation due to mutations in genes that control the hepcidin/ferroportin axis, which increases iron absorption in the gastrointestinal tract [2], see Table 23.1.

Table 23.1 The types of hereditary hemochromatosis

Name	Mutation involved	Mode of inheritance
1. HFE hemochromatosis	*HFE* gene	AR
2. Juvenile hemochromatosis		AR
HJV hemochromatosis	*HJV* gene	
Hepcidin/HAMP hemochromatosis	*HAMP* gene	
3. TFR2 hemochromatosis	*TFR2* gene	AR
4. Ferroprotein disease	*SLC40A1* gene	AD
5. Congenital aceruloplasminemia	*CP* gene	AR
6. Congenital atransferrinemia	*TF* gene	AR

AR autosomal recessive, *AD* autosomal dominant, *HFE* high Fe (iron)

HFE Hemochromatosis

HFE Hemochromatosis is the most common inherited type of hemochromatosis, predominantly seen in individuals of the European descent. It is extremely rare in the population of East Asia. It is transmitted in autosomal recessive fashion. The HFE (high Fe) gene is in the short arm chromosome −6. Low HFE protein causes inappropriately low hepcidin and decreased response of hepcidin to body iron.

Pathogenesis Homozygous *C282Y* mutation is the common associated mutation accounting for up to 90% of cases. Compound heterozygotes C282Y/H63D account for the rest of the cases. Clinical penetrance of C282 mutation is approximately 30% in male and 1% in female. The sequelae of HFE gene mutation include inappropriately high absorption of iron from the small intestine, even when dietary iron supply is within normal range, increased iron storage, and ultimately target organ damage and failure.

Clinical Presentation

The affected patients typically present between the age of 40 and 60, with a higher prevalence in men. Clinical symptoms vary from nonspecific to specific symptoms related to iron deposition in organs or tissues. Early symptoms are related to fatigue, weight loss, arthralgias, and abdominal pain, and at late-stage patients often manifest with symptoms or signs secondary to liver cirrhosis, arthritis, skin pigmentation, and/or multiple endocrine abnormalities (diabetes, hypothyroidism, and erectile dysfunction), cardiac symptoms with conduction defects, and restrictive heart disease.

Diagnosis

Please refer to "an objective and practical set of recommendations for treatment of persons with hemochromatosis and p.Cys282Tyr homozygosity" recommended in the 2017 Hemochromatosis International meeting [PMID: 29589198].

A. Iron studies are the initial part of workup. Elevated transferrin saturation (> 50% in male/ >45% in female) and ferritin >150 ng/ml are suspicious of iron overload. Transferrin saturation is a more reliable indicator when elevated to 60% (men) and 50% (women), while ferritin is nonspecific.
B. Liver biopsy is gold standard and helps to assess extent of fibrosis and cirrhosis. It is indicated in patients with ferritin >1000 ng/ml or in patient to rule out other etiologies of liver failure.
C. Noninvasive diagnostic tools like MRI of liver/heart can estimate body iron stores and is commonly done.
D. PCR testing for variants of C282Y and H63D is recommended for individuals with iron overload or in first-degree relative with hereditary hemochromatosis.

Treatment

Therapeutic phlebotomy is considered as mainstay treatment. Phlebotomy of 1 U of blood is able to eliminate 250 mg of iron. The frequency of phlebotomy is tapered from every 1–2 week with a goal to keep ferritin of 50 ng/ml and hematocrit >33–35%. Iron chelation therapy seems not helpful. Therapeutic replacement of hepcidin which could provide cure is currently investigational [3, 4].

Prognosis

Prognosis of hereditary hemochromatosis depends on the degree of organ damage. Some patients may have a normal life expectancy in case of no evidence of end-organ damage, while in others, the condition can be lethal due to liver cirrhosis, diabetes mellites, heart failure, or malignancy (hepatocellular carcinoma).

Caveats

1. The mechanisms of hemochromatosis are heterogenous, primary, or secondary. Hepcidin is the key regulator of iron hemostasis.
2. The severity of disease depends upon the degree of organ damage or failure.
3. Elevated serum ferritin alone is not specific for iron overload as it is an acute-phase reactant that can be elevated in inflammatory or neoplastic disorders.
4. Iron chelation therapy is not indicated in hereditary hemochromatosis.

Juvenile Hemochromatosis

Juvenile hemochromatosis is a group of hereditary hemochromatosis with clinical presentation of iron overload in late teens to early adulthood. There are two types of Juvenile hemochromatosis. Inheritance of loss-of-function mutations in an autosomal recessive fashion in the HJV gene causes type 1 juvenile hemochromatosis, while mutations in the hepcidin (HAMP) gene are responsible for type 2 juvenile hemochromatosis. Clinical presentation varies in accordance with the degree of organ iron deposition and damage. The diagnosis hinges on evaluating the patient's medical history and identifying mutations in either the HJV or HAMP gene. Treatment is similar to HFE hereditary hemochromatosis.

TFR2 Hemochromatosis

It is an autosomal recessive hereditary hemochromatosis caused by the inactivation of TRF2 gene encoding transferrin receptor-2 (TFR2). These mutations have almost complete penetrance and clinically similar to HFE hemochromatosis.

Ferroportin Disease

Ferroportin disease is an autosomal dominant hereditary hemochromatosis. It is caused by mutation in *SLC40A1* gene encoding FPN1/ferroprotein protein. Ferroportin protein functions as an iron exporter helping to transport the iron out of the storage tissue to bloodstream. Partial loss-of-function or gain-of-function mutation in *FPN1* causes classical ferroprotein disease. There is also nonclassical ferroprotein disease with gain of function mutation in FPN1 protein. Hepcidin resistance with inability to cause internalization and degradation of ferroportin protein is the hallmark of the disease.

Congenital Aceruloplasminemia

It is a rare autosomal recessive form of hereditary hemochromatosis. There is a mutation in ceruloplasmin (CP) gene that leads to a loss of expression in ceruloplasmin protein. It leads to inability to convert ferrous iron to ferric form, ultimately leading to low transferrin saturation and iron deposition in cells and visceral organs [5]. They tend to have significant features of iron deposition in the brain, leading to neurodegenerative symptoms.

Congenital Atransferrinemia

It is an extremely rare autosomal recessive hereditary hemochromatosis caused by mutations in transferrin (*TF*) gene leading to complete absence of transferrin. It causes inability to transport iron into circulation causing severe iron deficiency and the deposition of iron in visceral organs. Symptoms appear in infancy and include anemia, growth retardation, liver disease and cardiomyopathy. Increased erythropoietic demand causes low hepcidin. Transferrin levels are low with high saturation in residual transferrin.

Treatment involves replenishing plasma with apo-transferrin rich plasma combined with therapies to remove excess iron.

Acquired Iron Overload Disorder

Acquired iron overload disorder is also known as secondary hemochromatosis where iron accumulates in the body due to factors other than genetic mutations. Common causes of acquired iron overload are summarized in Table 23.2.

Table 23.2 Common etiologies of acquired iron overload

1. Clinical condition with ineffective erythropoiesis and requiring regular blood transfusion. Thalassemias Sickle cell anemia Aplastic anemia MDS Hematological malignancies/Hematologic stem cell transplantation
2. Chronic liver diseases Alcoholic liver disease Nonalcoholic fatty liver disease Hepatitis B Hepatitis C Porphyria cutanea tarda
3. Hemolytic anemias
4. Chronic kidney disease/end-stage renal disease
5. Iatrogenic/inappropriate iron supplementation

Treatment

Treatment of secondary iron overload is usually challenging with coexisting anemia. Management of underlying causes of iron overload should be the primary focus to prevent further complications. Splenectomy might be helpful in some forms of anemia to reduce the transfusion requirement causing iron overload.

Phlebotomy could be impractical and harmful in certain circumstances.

Iron chelation therapy is the key treatment for patient intolerant to phlebotomy. In patients with hemoglobinopathies iron chelation therapy prevents and reverses the end organ damage from iron deposition. It is recommended in patients requiring regular transfusion for >2 years or requiring more than10 PRBC transfusion or if the serum ferritin is >1000 ng/ml.

There are three commonly available iron chelators for use. The administration methods and side effects are summarized in Table 23.3.

Table 23.3 Iron chelators

Name of drug	Route	Dosage	Indication	Side effects
Deferoxamine	IV or SC	20-60 mg/kg/day over 8–24 h given for 5 days/week	Chronic or acute iron overload	injection site reaction, Auditory and ophthalmic toxicity.
Deferiprone-	PO	75–100 mg/kg/day divided in three doses	Anemia due to thalassemia syndromes	neutropenia requiring CBC monitoring, arthralgias and transaminitis
Deferasirox	PO	20–40 mg/kg/day	Transfusional hemosiderosis	renal failure, transaminitis, GI disturbances

CBC complete blood count, *PO* per oral, *SC* subcutaneous, *IV* intravenous, *GI* gastrointestinal

Promising Clinical Studies

There are various promising studies suggesting potential for new treatment of hemochromatosis.

- Study targeting the hepcidin protein as an approach to treat hemochromatosis. In the mice study it was possible to reduce iron accumulation by increasing hepcidin level [6].
- There are also in vitro studies looking into gene therapy to deliver a normal copy of *HFE* gene through virus to liver cells restoring normal iron metabolism in animal model with hemochromatosis.
- There are also ongoing trials exploring hepcidin mimics.

Caveats

- Although genetic testing is crucial for diagnosis of Hereditary Hemochromatosis, only presence of specific gene mutations is diagnostic.

- Hemochromatosis is usually diagnosed later after the symptoms have already developed; it can make the treatment less effective.
- Phlebotomy, a mainstay of treatment, can lead to anemia, hypotension, and fatigue. It might worsen underlying anemia in patients with secondary iron overload.
- Multiple organs like liver, heart, and pancreas can be involved in iron overload. It requires a multidisciplinary approach with multiple specialties involved.

Board Question

1. A 55-Year-old man is brought by his wife with new onset of mental status changes. He was diagnosed with diabetes 1 year back. He has been drinking alcohol regularly. Family history is positive for liver cirrhosis in his brother at the age of 50 and his father died of liver cirrhosis at age of 65 years. On examination vitals are normal. He has icterus, distended abdomen with fluid thrill. He has hemoglobin of 9.5 g/dl. Ferritin of 5000 ng/ml and transferrin saturation 60%. What is the next best step for management?

   A. T2 weighted MRI showing severe iron overload.
   B. Genetic testing showing C282Y/C282Y in HFE.
   C. Bone marrow biopsy to evaluate anemia.
   D. Getting the medical records of his brother.

   Answer: A. it is important to assess any organ damage using imaging study for the patient who has positive family history of possible hemochromatosis, and recently present with diabetes.

2. What is the most common mode of inheritance of hereditary hemochromatosis?

   A. Autosomal Dominant
   B. Autosomal Recessive

C. X- linked disease
D. All of the above

Answer: B. Autosomal recessive is the most common inheritance mode of hereditary hemochromatosis.

References

1. Camaschella C, Nai A, Silvestri L. Iron metabolism and iron disorders revisited in the hepcidin era. Haematologica. 2020;105(2):260–72. https://doi.org/10.3324/haematol.2019.232124. Ferrata Storti Foundation.
2. Pantopoulos K. inherited disorders of iron overload. Front Nutr. 2018;5:103. https://doi.org/10.3389/fnut.2018.00103.
3. Kowdley KV, Brown KE, Ahn J, Sundaram V. ACG clinical guideline: hereditary hemochromatosis. Am J Gastroenterol. 2019;114(8):1202–18. https://doi.org/10.14309/ajg.0000000000000315.
4. Sivakumar M, Powell LW. Management of human factors engineering-associated hemochromatosis: a 2015 update. World J Hepatol. 2016;8(8):395–400. https://doi.org/10.4254/wjh.v8.i8.395. Baishideng Publishing Group Co.
5. Yoshida K, et al. A mutation in the ceruloplasmin gene is associated with systemic hemosiderosis in humans. Nat Genet. 1995;9(3):267–72. https://doi.org/10.1038/ng0395-267.
6. Sebastiani G, Wilkinson N, Pantopoulos K. Pharmacological targeting of the hepcidin/ferroportin axis. Front Pharmacol. 2016;7:160. https://doi.org/10.3389/fphar.2016.00160. Frontiers Media S.A.

Polycythemia/ Erythrocytosis

24

Aryanna Jordan, Lubomir Sokol, and Ling Zhang

Introduction

The terms of erythrocytosis or polycythemia refer to an absolute increase in red cell mass (RCM) (volume) that is defined in clinical practice as follows:

- Hemoglobin concentration >16.5 g/dL among men or >16.0 g/dL among women
- Hematocrit concentration >49% among men or >48% among women

In the past, red blood cell (RBC) mass was measured by Cr^{51} radiolabeled autologous RBCs. The normal range is 36 ml/kg among males and 32 ml/kg among females. The measurement of RBC mass was used to differentiate absolute (true) polycythemia from relative (spurious) polycythemia caused by plasma-volume contraction. However, this test is no longer in daily clinical

A. Jordan (✉) · L. Sokol
Department of Malignant Hematology, H. Lee Moffitt Cancer Center and Research Institute, Tampa, FL, USA
e-mail: Aryanna.Jordan@moffitt.org

L. Zhang
Department of Hematopathology, H. Lee Moffitt Cancer Center and Research Institute, Tampa, FL, USA

L. Sokol, L. Zhang (eds.), *Non-Neoplastic Hematologic Disorders*, https://doi.org/10.1007/978-3-031-62373-8_24

practice because of limited diagnostic utility, cost, and exposure of laboratory personnel to a radioactive compound. The simplified serum erythropoietin (EPO)-level measurements and genetic testing significantly refined our differential diagnosis of polycythemias.

Polycythemias can be stratified according to pathogenic mechanisms into primary and secondary or acquired and familial. Primary polycythemias are diseases of bone marrow hematopoietic stem cells or progenitor cells, in contrast to secondary polycythemias, resulting from pathogenic mechanisms external to bone marrow cells.

Polycythemia vera (PV) is an acquired, clonal disorder or a hematopoietic stem cell caused by somatic mutation JAK2 V617F in exon 14 or mutations in JAK2 exon 12, which altogether comprise >99% of patients with PV.

Primary familial and congenital polycythemias (PFCP) is very rare disease caused by germinal gain-of-function mutations in the erythropoietin-receptor gene, resulting in increased sensitivity of erythroid progenitor cells to a low dose of erythropoietin.

In contrast to primary polycythemias, secondary polycythemias are a more heterogeneous group of hematologic disorders, most frequently resulting from elevated erythropoietin levels. Increased RCM and development of polycythemia can be appropriate because of a compensatory mechanism of chronic hypoxemia, resulting in tissue hypoxia, which leads to increased production of erythropoietin in kidneys. Inappropriate increase of RCM occurs under tissue normoxia, for instance, secondary to increased production of erythropoietin in patients with paraneoplastic syndromes. Familial secondary polycythemia is caused by mutations in several distinct genes, such as genes coding for hemoglobins, resulting in high-affinity Hb or genes implicated in oxygen-sensing pathways. The prevalence of secondary polycythemia is less known in contrast to PV, with an estimated incidence rate of 22/100 000 individuals). Clinically, patients with secondary polycythemias have a lower risk of thrombotic events caused by hyperviscosity, in contrast to patients with PV. Transformation into secondary myelofibrosis or acute myeloid leukemia can be observed only in patients with PV. This chapter will focus only on polyclonal polycythemias (erythrocytosis) and discuss the potential etiology, pathogenesis, and treatment of each polycythemia subtype.

Pathogenesis

Primary familial and congenital polycythemias are caused by gain-of-function mutations in the erythropoietin-receptor gene, resulting in an increased sensitivity of erythroid progenitors (BFU-E/CFU-E) to low doses of erythropoietin. Secondary polycythemias are caused by increased levels of erythropoietin in a majority of subjects. Appropriate increase in RCM in secondary polycythemias is caused by tissue hypoxia. Numerous acquired or genetic pathogenic mechanisms, such as lung disease, heart disease with right-to-left shunt, chronic smoking, mutations in hemoglobin gene resulting in high-affinity Hb, or methemoglobinemia, have been identified in this group of secondary polycythemias. Inappropriate increase in RCM can be observed among patients under tissue normoxia, such as paraneoplastic production of EPO by several malignant or benign tumors, such as hepatoma, hemangioblastoma, uterine fibroids, and pheochromocytoma.

PFCP is inherited in autosomal-dominant fashion. Erythropoietin serum level is low, and patients can suffer from vascular (venous or arterial) events despite phlebotomies. Because of the rarity of this disease, there is no established standard therapy, but patients with symptoms of hyperviscosity caused by polycythemia can be treated with phlebotomies. Cytoreductive therapy used for patients with PV is not recommended for this disease [1].

Diagnosis

Diagnostic approaches of polycythemia should start with history, physical exam, laboratory testing, and imaging studies. Bone marrow biopsy can be useful if there is a suspicion for evolving PV (Fig. 24.1).

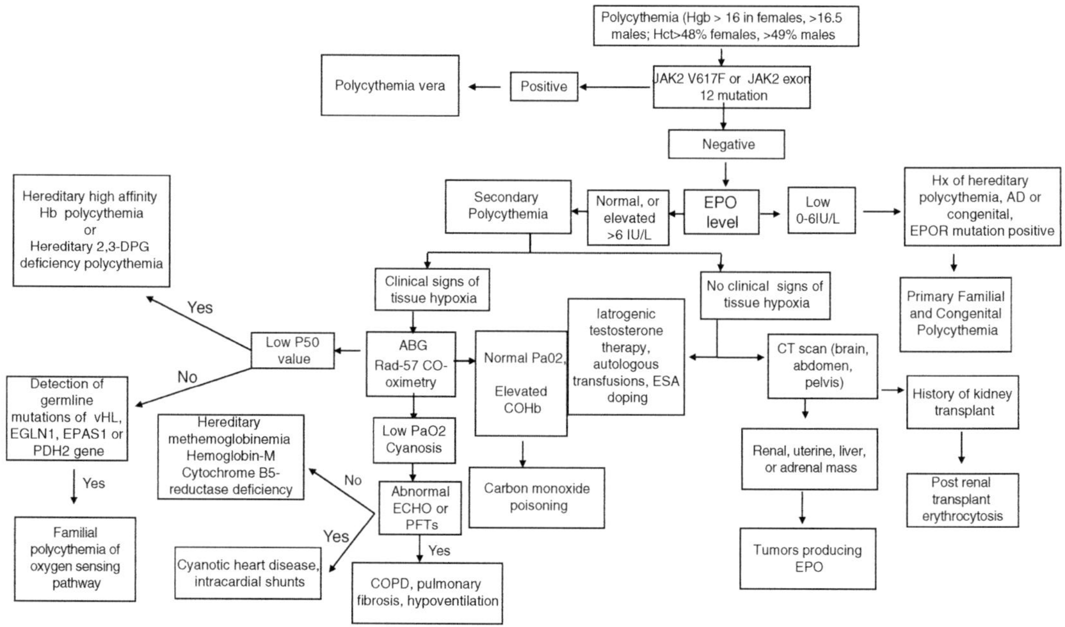

Fig. 24.1 Diagnostic/treatment algorithm for polycythemia. ABG arterial blood gas, AD autosomal dominant, COHb carboxyhemoglobin, COPD chronic obstructive pulmonary disease, EPO erythropoietin, ESA erythropoietin stimulating agent, Hct hematocrit, Hgb hemoglobin, Hx history, PFT pulmonary function tests

1. Laboratory investigation
   (a) Complete blood count, comprehensive metabolic panel (CMP), blood smear, serum EPO level, mutational analysis searching for JAK2 V617V and exon 12 mutations, and genetic testing should be considered to search for germline mutations (Table 24.1). A low EPO level and positive test for JAK2 mutation confirms diagnosis of PV. An MRI of brain and CT scan of abdomen and pelvis can uncover tumor-producing erythropoietin. Arterial blood gas analysis can yield p50 values and illustrate the hemoglobin dissociation curve, both of which are essential for determining the affinity of Hb for oxygen. Co-oximetry is used to measure the different forms of hemoglobin in blood such as oxyhemoglobin, deoxyhemoglobin, carboxyhemoglobin and methemoglobin by spectroscopic analysis.
2. Symptoms and signs
   (a) Symptoms of hyperviscosity such as headaches, fatigue, hypertension, and blurry vision
   (b) Arterial and venous thrombosis
3. Physical examination: plethoric facial appearance and splenomegaly
4. Imaging study: organomegaly, COPD, renal cysts, renal, hepatic, and uterine and cerebellar tumors
5. Family history: any myeloid neoplasm and germline mutations
6. Social history
   (a) Smoking
   (b) Carbon monoxide exposure (working with combustion engines, fireplaces)
   (c) Use of anabolic steroids, cobalt, manganese, or history of transfusions
7. Medical history
   (a) History of diarrhea, volume loss, and cardiopulmonary disease

Table 24.1 Genetic alteration associated with hereditary polycythemia

Hereditary polycythemia	Gene alteration	Key features
Primary familial and congenital polycythemia	Gain-of-function EPO receptor mutation	AD Mutated *EPOR* causes increased sensitivity of erythroid progenitors to low-dose EPO because of absence of negative regulatory domain or EPOR. PFCP comprise about 15% of cases with idiopathic erythrocytosis. Dx: isolated erythrocytosis in a patient with a normal spleen and absence of secondary causes of polycythemia, positive family history
High-affinity hemoglobin polycythemia	AD 100 high-oxygen affinity variants have been described with both α and β globin genes resulting in unstable and stable Hb	High-affinity hemoglobin resulting in low p50 and left shifted oxygen dissociation curve, results in relative hypoxia in kidney tissue causing excess EPO production. Dx: high-affinity hemoglobin, lower P50 value. Some variants can be detected by hemoglobin electrophoresis, others require direct sequencing of globin genes
2,3 BPG-deficiency polycythemia	*BPGM* gene	AR or AD. Binding 2,3 BPG converts Hb molecule to low oxygen affinity state which shifts the affinity curve to the right, absence of 2,3 BPG shifts the curve to the left causing relative hypoxia and an increase in EPO production. Dx: a low P50 (partial pressure of oxygen at which 50% of hemoglobin is saturated) level, normal hemoglobin structure, and decreased BPGM activity

(continued)

Table 24.1 (continued)

Hereditary polycythemia	Gene alteration	Key features
Congenital methemoglobinemia	Cytochrome b5-reductase gene mutation	Inability of Hb to bind and carry oxygen which shifts the oxygen dissociation curve to the left which results in decreased oxygen delivery to tissues. *Type 1:* deficiency in cytochrome b5 reductase in RBC, increased methemoglobinemia, asymptomatic until later in life or when patients are exposed to oxidizing agents. *Type 2:* cytochrome b5-reductase deficiency in all cells and not just RBCs. Tends to develop symptoms early in life and most die in infancy. Dx: decreased cytochrome b5 reductase activity. Observation of appearance of blood (chocolate brown)
Chuvash polycythemia	*VHL* gene mutation, mutation in oxygen-sensing pathway	Homozygous 598 C > T/598 C > T (R200W) germline mutation in *VHL* gene. VHL homozygotes have elevated levels of hypoxia inducible factor (HIF-1 alpha) leading to increased EPO level and increased RBC mass. Endemic in the Chuvash Republic of the Russian Federation (an incidence of 200 in 1.5 million). Dx: NGS

(continued)

Table 24.1 (continued)

Hereditary polycythemia	Gene alteration	Key features
Proline hydroxylase mutation (PDH2)	*EGNL-1* gene mutation, encodes proline hydroxylase leading to increased EPO levels, mutation in oxygen sensing pathway	*EGLN1* mutations reduce PHD2 protein stability and prolyl hydroxylase activity leading to an increase in HIF-1a protein levels, causing an increase in EPO level and RBC mass. A heterozygous missense mutation [2, 3] Dx: NGS
HIF- 2 alpha mutation	Heterozygous *EPAS-1* gene mutation, encodes transcription factor HIF-2 alpha, leading to increased EPO levels	Mutation results in impairment of hydroxylation of HIF-2 alpha and binding to *VHL* leading increase in EPO levels and erythrocytosis. Mutations link to malignancy such as paragangliomas and somatostatinomas [4]. Dx: NGS
Gain-of-function mutation in EPO in familial erythrocytosis	Heterozygous single-base deletion in exon 2 of EPO	Single nucleotide deletion of c.32delG causes a frameshift mutation in exon 2 and introduces a frameshift mutation causing a noncoding mRNA transcribed from a region inside EPO intron 1 into a mRNA that produces a functional erythropoietin protein. This leads to increased EPO levels [5]. Dx: positive family history, genetic sequencing

AD autosomal dominant, *AR* autosomal recessive, *BPGM* bisphospholgycerate mutase, *Dx* diagnosis, *Hb* hemoglobin, *EPOR* erythropoietin receptor, *mRNA* messenger RNA, *NGS* next-generation sequencing, *PFCP* primary and congenital polycythemia, *RBC* red blood cell

Differential Diagnosis

It is critical to differentiate PV from other types of polycythemias. PV is a hematologic malignancy with the highest risk of vascular events among all polycythemias, which can be prevented or significantly decreased with phlebotomies, low-dose aspirin, cytoreductive therapy with hydroxyurea, interferon, or JAK-2 inhibitors. It is also important to diagnose secondary polycythemia caused by malignancy-producing erythropoietin because early diagnosis of malignancy can result in a better overall prognosis.

Primary Polycythemia

Hereditary

Primary familial and congenital polycythemia is a rare familial or congenital disease inherited in autosomal-dominant fashion because of a gain-of-function erythropoietin receptor mutation (EPOR). The mutations in EPOR most frequently result in truncation of cytoplasmic-negative regulatory domain. Erythroid progenitors in this disease demonstrate increased sensitivity to low erythropoietin levels in in vitro studies. The erythropoietin level is usually very low, <5 in affected subjects, similarly in patients with PV. PFCP caused by EPOR mutations comprise only 15% of cases with idiopathic polycythemias. Clinically, patients usually manifest with isolated erythrocytosis and normal spleen size. A family history of polycythemia inherited in autosomal-dominant fashion supports this diagnosis [5, 6].

Acquired

Primary Polycythemia PV will not be discussed in this chapter.

Secondary Polycythemias

Secondary polycythemias include a spectrum of hereditary and acquired disorders. It is characterized with elevated RBC mass caused by an increased level of EPO caused by appropriate response to hypoxia/hypoxemia or inappropriate EPO production in subjects with normoxia.

Hereditary

I. Chuvash polycythemia: Von Hippel-Lindau (VHL) syndrome gene mutation (compound heterozygotes of C598T) [7]
II. EGLN1: loss of function mutation of EGLN1 (encodes proline hydroxylase 2)
III. EPAS1: gain-of-function mutation of EPAS1 (encoding HIF-2 alpha)
IV. 2,3-bisphosphoglycerate mutase deficiency (BPGM deficiency)
V. High-affinity hemoglobin polycythemia (low p50)
VI. Congenital methemoglobinemia: (i) cytochrome b5 reductase (CYB5R) deficiency (autosomal recessive); (ii) globin gene mutations or hemoglobin-M (autosomal dominant)

Acquired

1. Appropriate secondary polycythemia (presence of tissue hypoxia)

   (a) Secondary polycythemia caused by high altitude
   An increased number of erythrocytes has been observed in normal subjects who dwell at high altitude compared to those at sea level. Patients were found to have polycythemia, cyanosis, hypertension, and right heart failure caused by decreased oxygen saturation. Chronic mountain sickness usually occurs in those who live long term at 3200 m above sea level. Treatment with angiotensin-converting enzyme (ACE)-inhibitors can improve the above symptoms.

   (b) Secondary polycythemia caused by lung disorders
   Lung disorders, such as chronic obstructive pulmonary disease (COPD), alveolar hypoventilation, chronic lung infections, and fibrosis, lead to compensatory erythrocytosis caused by chronic hypoxemia resulting in tissue hypoxia. Diagnosis can be made by elevated hemoglobin/hematocrit, hypoxemia on pulse oximetry, and elevated EPO levels. Patients may have symptoms of hyperviscos-

ity. Even though treatment with regular phlebotomies is not recommended, patients with Hct >0.55 can benefit from phlebotomies.

(c) Secondary polycythemia caused by cardiovascular disorders
Patients who have cyanotic heart disease (right-to-left shunts, cor pulmonale) are at risk for development of secondary polycythemia caused by chronic tissue hypoxia. Diagnosis is based on 2D echocardiogram, pulse oximetry, and high EPO levels.

(d) Secondary polycythemia caused by exposure to cobalt and carbon monoxide.
Smoking is the most common cause. Increased levels of carboxyl hemoglobin not only reduce Hb oxygen-carrying capacity but also shift Hb dissociation curve to the left, resulting in tissue hypoxia. Smoking discontinuation usually results in polycythemia resolution. Cobalt chloride has been used in the past to promote erythropoiesis, but the exact mechanism is not well understood. Recently, it has been suggested that the inhibition of prolyl hydroxylases and upregulation of HIF-1 alpha leads to increased EPO production. Diagnosis is made by history, and treatment involves avoidance of cobalt ingestion.

2. Inappropriate secondary polycythemia (absence of hypoxia)

(a) Renal disorders

(i) Renal cysts
Patients with autosomal-dominant polycystic kidney disease were found to have elevated EPO levels as well as those patients with unilateral renal cysts. Further investigation found that cells within proximal tubules are thought to be a source of excess EPO. Diagnosis is made by CBC, CT scan of abdomen/pelvis, or renal ultrasound, showing renal cysts and absence of other secondary causes of polycythemia.

(ii) Renal tumors
Paraneoplastic syndromes have been reported in renal cell carcinoma. A search for genetic mutations, such as those associated with VHL syndrome, have been

shown to be related to renal cell carcinoma, loss-of-function mutations in the *VHL* gene result in upregulation of HIF-1 alpha transcription factor and increased production of EPO.

(iii) Postrenal transplant polycythemia

Persistent EPO secretion from the diseased kidneys or chronically ischemic kidneys does not respond to feedback inhibitory mechanism. It occurs in 10–15% of transplant recipients and usually develops within 2 years after engraftment. Patients present with symptoms of polycythemia and hyperviscosity. EPO levels in most patients remain normal. It is thought that the erythrocytosis is caused by production of growth factors, such as angiotensin II or IGF-1. Angiotensin-II receptors are expressed by erythroid progenitor cells. Treatment with ACE-inhibitors can correct polycythemia.

(b) Secondary polycythemia caused by EPO-producing tumors (paraneoplastic polycythemia).

(i) Renal tumors
(ii) Cerebellar hemangioblastoma
(iii) Hepatocellular carcinoma
(iv) Uterine leiomyoma
(v) Pheochromocytoma

The above tumors cause polycythemia by producing ectopic EPO; treatment involves resection of the tumor.

(c) Secondary polycythemia caused by adrenal disorders

(i) Cushing syndrome

Polycythemia has been documented as one of the first symptoms of Cushing syndrome. Diagnosis is made by confirmation of Cushing syndrome by adrenocorticotropic hormone (ACTH) suppression test, imaging with MRI of brain to evaluate for pituitary tumors, or CT of abdomen searching for adrenal tumors.

(d) Secondary polycythemia caused by Iatrogenic/doping administration

(i) Androgens

Exogenous testosterone supplementation has been associated with erythrocytosis, which was used as a treatment for anemia in the past. Testosterone leads to increased EPO by increasing the availability of iron by reducing hepcidin levels. Testosterone should not be used in patients with hematocrit levels >50% or in male patients with increased risk of prostate cancer.

(ii) Autotransfusion

Autologous blood transfusions (blood doping) have been used as performance enhancement for top athletes. It has been suggested that athletic performance could increase by 4% after reinfusion of whole blood, but the blood transfusions are associated with health risks, such as transfusion reactions and thrombotic events caused by increased blood viscosity secondary to iatrogenic erythrocytosis enhanced with dehydration, especially seen in long-distance runners.

(iii) Erythropoietin-stimulating agents (ESA)

ESA are often used in patients with chronic kidney disease and myelodysplastic syndromes that lead to anemia. Inappropriate use of ESA in athletes can lead to polycythemia with symptoms of hyperviscosity and development of thrombotic events.

Treatment

There are no evidence-based guidelines for therapy of patients with diagnosis of primary familial and congenital polycythemia. Based on case reports and small case series, phlebotomies are usually recommended for patients with symptoms of hyperviscosity, but the impact of this approach on prevention of vascular events is not known. In some reports, patients with PFCP developed vascular complications despite having controlled Hb/Hct with phlebotomies.

The treatment of choice for patients with a majority of secondary polycythemias is focused on elimination or correction of the factor implicated in increased EPO production.

Phlebotomy is usually used in patients with hyperviscosity symptoms. Regular phlebotomies to keep hematocrit <45% as recommended for patients with PV are rarely indicated. Even though a low-dose aspirin has not been evaluated in prospective studies in conjunction with phlebotomies in patients with PFCP or secondary polycythemias as a preventive measure of vascular events, it is sometimes recommended in the literature for selected patients based on retrospective studies.

For patients with lung or heart disease who develop erythrocytosis as a compensatory mechanism for hypoxemia and tissue hypoxia, regular phlebotomies are indicated only for patients with hyperviscosity symptoms or very high Hct levels, such as >0.55. Under very high Hct states, the hyperviscosity usually limits blood circulation through small blood vessels and oxygen delivery to tissues. For selected patients with secondary polycythemias associated with right heart failure, careful use of phlebotomies can decrease preload and improve cardiac function.

Prognosis

In contrast to patients with PV, polyclonal polycythemias have been called benign erythrocytosis in the past because of a lower incidence of vascular events and absence of evolution into secondary myelofibrosis or acute myeloid leukemia. However, with better molecular characterization of primary and secondary polycythemias and longer follow-up, increased risk of vascular events has been reported, for instance, among patients with Chuvash polycythemia and PFCP [6, 7]. Symptoms of hyperviscosity can be observed in all patients with polyclonal polycythemias, and selected patients can benefit from phlebotomies.

Promising Clinical Studies

Because of the rarity of acquired and hereditary polyclonal polycythemias, it is difficult to conduct prospective clinical studies. Some agents, such as HIF-1 alpha or JAK2 inhibitors, could be used in the future in Chuvash polycythemia patients.

Caveats

1. The most important goal of differential diagnosis is to identify patients with PV and paraneoplastic secondary polycythemias, because early diagnosis and interventions in these diseases can result in significantly improved prognosis and outcomes.
2. For patients with idiopathic erythrocytosis, despite extensive clinical and laboratory examinations, a search for rare gene mutations associated with familial or congenital polycythemias is indicated.

Board Questions

1. A 27-year-old male patient, a professional cyclist, presents with an Hb of 19 g/dL, a white blood cell counts of 5.6×10^9/L, and a platelet count of 235×10^9/L. The differential count is within normal limits. His medical history is negative. His father has been treated with phlebotomies since young adulthood. *JAK2* exons 12 and 14 mutational analysis is negative. Serum erythropoietin level is 3 mU/mL. Ultrasound of abdomen showed normal sizes of liver and spleen.

What is his most probable diagnosis?

A. Chuvash polycythemia
B. VHL syndrome
C. PFCP
D. Parenteral erythropoietin-induced polycythemia
E. Spurious polycythemia

Correct answer: C. PFCP
Explanation: Chuvash polycythemia and VHL syndrome are hereditary disorders associated with secondary polycythemia caused by mutations in VHL genes regulating oxygen sensing pathway; Chuvash polycythemia is autosomal recessive disease caused by loss-of-function mutations in VHL gene. vHL syndrome is an autosomal dominant disorder caused by loss-of-function mutations in vHL gene. This syndrome is associated with develop-

ment of several distinct malignancies. This patient has very low EPO level, which makes diagnosis of secondary polycythemia unlikely. Parenteral use of erythropoiesis-stimulating agents would also be unlikely in this patient with a positive family history. Spurious polycythemia is caused by volume contraction, such as dehydration, which is not consistent with the clinical picture.

2. Which disease has not been associated with polycythemia/erythrocytosis?

   A. VHL syndrome
   B. COPD
   C. Eisenmenger complex
   D. TEMPI
   E. Bing-Neel syndrome

   Correct answer: E
   Explanation: All diseases but Bing-Neel syndrome have been associated with development of polycythemia. vHL syndrome, COPD, Eisenmenger complex and TEMPI are diseases associated with secondary polycythemia due to elevated erythropoietin level. Bing-Neel syndrome is caused by infiltration of central nervous system with lymphoplasmacytic cells in patients with diagnosis of Waldenström macroglobulinemia. It has not been associated with polycythemia.

References

1. McMullin MF, Bareford D, Campbell P, Green AR, Harrison C, Hunt B. Guidelines for the diagnosis, investigation, and management of polycythaemia/erythrocytosis. Br J Haematol. 2005;130:174–95.
2. Percy MJ, Zhao Q, et al. A family with erythrocytosis establishes a role for prolyl hydroxylase domain protein 2 in oxygen homeostasis. Proc Natl Acad Sci USA. 2006;103:654–9.

3. Gaspersic J, Kristan A, Kunej T, Zupan IP, Debeljak N. Erythrocytosis genes and pathways involved in disease development. Blood Transfus. 2021;19:518–32.
4. Percy MJ, Furlow PW, et al. A gain-of-function mutation in the HIF2A gene in familial erythrocytosis. N Engl J Med. 2008;358:162–8.
5. Zmajkovic J, Lunberg P, et al. A gain-of function mutation in EPO in familial erythrocytosis. N Engl J Med. 2018;378:924–30.
6. Sokol L, Luhovy M, Guan Y, Prchal JF, Semenza GL, Prchal JT. Primary familial polycythemia: a frameshift mutation in the erythropoietin receptor gene and increased sensitivity of erythroid progenitors to erythropoietin. Blood. 1995;86:15–22.
7. Ang SO, Chen H, Hirota K, Gordeuk VR, Jelinek J, Guan Y. Disruption of oxygen homeostasis underlies congenital Chuvash polycythemia. Nat Genet. 2002;32:614–21.

Part III

Disorders of Platelets

Congenital Platelet Disorders

25

Ahmed Arfa and Loveleen C. Kang

Introduction

Congenital platelet disorders are a group of diseases that have a low prevalence rate in general population; however, some diseases have autosomal dominant (AD) inherence pattern. These diseases may present in the first few days in newborns or may only present later in life as mild mucocutaneous bleeding. Life-threatening bleeding can occur in some severe cases. The pathogenesis includes, but not limited to, abnormalities in the platelet cell membrane receptor (Bernard-Soulier syndrome and Glanzmann's disease), an abnormality in the platelet dense or alpha granules or lysozyme (Gray platelet syndrome, Chediak-Higashi syndrome, and Hermansky-Pudlak syndrome), or secondary to gene mutation. The diagnosis requires careful review of the family history, bleeding history, complete blood count, platelet aggregation studies, and molecular studies. The management is mainly prevention by educating the patient and parents to avoid

A. Arfa
Department of Pathology, Medical College of Georgia, Augusta University, Augusta, GA, USA

L. C. Kang (✉)
Department of Pathology and Laboratory Medicine, James A. Haley, Veterans' Hospital, Tampa, FL, USA
e-mail: loveleen.kang@va.gov

L. Sokol, L. Zhang (eds.), *Non-Neoplastic Hematologic Disorders*,
https://doi.org/10.1007/978-3-031-62373-8_25

possible accidents and trauma with bleeding risk. In case of moderate to severe bleeding, hemostatic measures including platelet transfusions may be warranted. Additionally, hematopoietic stem cell transplantation may be useful in some cases.

Pathogenesis

Platelets are the final product of megakaryocytes; they are responsible for primary hemostasis after any vascular injury through the following five steps (Fig. 25.1). Congenital defects can have impact on any of the following pathways.

1. *Platelet adhesion*: Adhesion of the platelets (through Gb1b receptors) to the injured blood vessel in the presence of Von Willebrand factor.

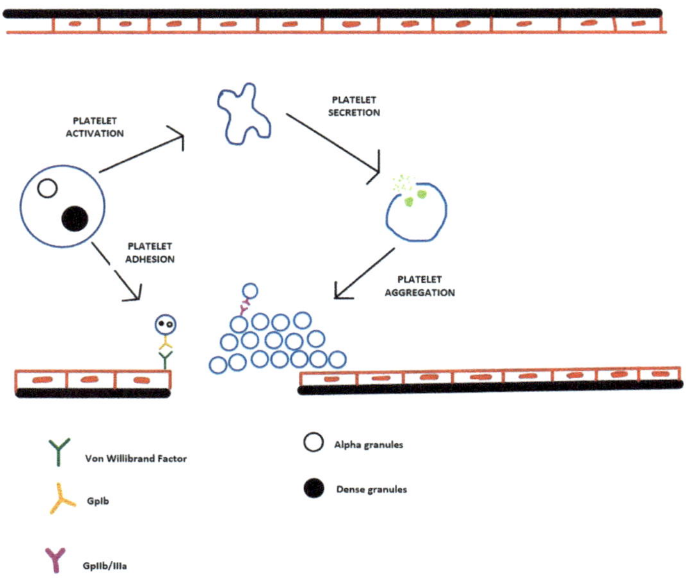

Fig. 25.1 Normal platelet function (primary hemostasis): platelet adhesion → platelet activation → platelet secretion → platelet aggregation

2. *Platelet activation*: Three subtypes of ADP receptors (it is an activator of adhesiveness and platelet aggregation. Also, it has a paracrine function):

    - *P2Y12 receptor* responsible for ADP-dependent amplification of the response with sustained and stabilized platelet aggregation.
    - *P2Y1 receptor* causes mobilization of internal calcium stores leading to initial reversible and transient platelet aggregation.
    - *P2X receptor* is not fully understood.

3. *Platelet aggregation*: Binding of the platelets to each-others via GPIIb/GPIIIa receptors.
4. *Platelet secretion*:

    - *α-granules* (contain fibronectin, factor V, vWF, P-selectin, & platelet factor 4).
    - *Dense granules* (contain ADP and serotonin)
    - *Lysosomes* (containing hydrolases to dissolve platelet aggregates into the circulating blood)

5. *Expression of Procoagulant Activity:*

    - Platelets activate in two pathways, both dependent on calcium, resulting in formation of factor Xa and then conversion of the prothrombin activation to thrombin.
    - Phosphatidylserine (PS) and phosphatidylethanolamine (PE)

        (i) Optimal exposure of (PS & PE) → interaction with the coagulation factors → promote assembly and catalysis of the tenase complex (FVIIIa, IXa, X) and prothrombinase complex (FVa, Xa, prothrombin) → to enhance thrombin formation.
        (ii) It is also critical for the anticoagulant activity of activated protein C.

Pathogenesis and Clinical Presentations

Congenital platelet disorders are uncommon and characterized by mild to moderate mucocutaneous bleeding after immediate injury congenital platelet disorders:clinical presentations, but in some cases, the bleeding could be severe and even life threatening. It can be classified into two types: thrombocytopenia (decreased number of platelets) and thrombocytopathies (platelet function defects) (Tables 25.1 and 25.2).

Table 25.1 Pathogenesis of common congenital thrombocytopathy

Defected function	Affected proteins/gene	Disease
Platelet adhesion	GP1b/GPIXIV	Bernard-Soulier syndrome (BSS) VWD platelet type
Platelet activation	ADP receptor	
Platelet aggregation	GPIIb/GPIIIa	Glanzmann's disease
Platelet secretion (storage pool disease)	GATA1 missense mutation → α-granules	Gray platelet syndrome
	Increased platelet stores of UPA	Quebec platelet disorder
	7 genes of *HPS* (1–7)	Hermansky-Pudlak syndrome
	CHS1/LYST	Chediak-Higashi syndrome
Pro-coagulant activity	*ANO6* (*TMEM16F*) gene	Scott syndrome

VWD Von Willebrand disease, *UPA* urokinase-type plasminogen activator

Table 25.2 Pathogenesis of common congenital thrombocytopenia

Platelet size	Defected gene	Disease	Clinical and laboratory features	Inheritance
Macrothrombocytopenia	Del(22q)	Velocardiofacial (*DiGeorge*) syndrome	Right heart defect, T cell immune deficiency, Evans syndrome, Palate defects	AD
	GP1ba	Mediterranean macrothrombocytopenia Von Willebrand disease-platelet type	Platelet clumping. Abnormal (hyperreactive) ristocetin-induced platelet agglutination	
	MYH9	Epstein syndrome Fechtner syndrome May-Hegglin anomaly Sebastian syndrome	Neutrophil inclusions ± cataract ± renal defect ± hearing loss. Giant platelets	
Normal size platelets	*CMPL*	Congenital amegakaryocytic thrombocytopenia (CAMT)	Hypo-megakaryocytic thrombocytopenia→ Progressing to bone marrow aplasia	AR & AD
	HOXA11	Thrombocytopenia-absent radius (TAR)	Reduced-absent megakaryocytes, with radio-ulnar synostosis ± other malformations. Possible sensorineural hearing loss	
Microthrombocytopenia	*WAS*	Wiskott-Aldrich syndrome X-linked thrombocytopenia	Severe immunodeficiency, eczema, and defective WAS protein	X-linked

AD autosomal dominant, *AR* autosomal recessive

Congenital Thrombocytopenia

It may present with severe bleeding in the first to second month of life, or it may remain undetected even in adulthood.

Macrothrombocytopenia

1. *Velocardiofacial (DiGeorge) syndrome:*
    - *Pathogenesis:* Deletion of a portion of long arm of chromosome 22 (22q11.2), often associated with organ abnormality and immunodeficiency.
2. *Mediterranean macrothrombocytopenia*:
    - *Pathogenesis:* Heterozygous mutations in *GP1BA* or *GP1BB* genes (*GP1BA* missense mutation is the most common genotypic abnormality → substitution of (Val156Ala), known as the Bolzano variant).
    - It manifests with mild macrothrombocytopenia, normal platelet functions, and a normal number of megakaryocytes, and no significant bleeding.
3. *Pseudo von Willebrand disease (pseudo-vWD)*
    - *Pathogenesis:* Gain-of-function in the mutations in the *GPIBA* gene → conformational change of carboxy-terminal of GPIbα→ increased affinity of VWF for the GPIb/IX/V complex ligand→ increased removal of VWF multimers and platelets from the circulation → bleeding diathesis.
    - It presents with giant platelets and mild thrombocytopenia, as seen in type 2 VWD.
4. *MYH9-related disorders*: A group of autosomal dominant disorders includes *Epstein syndrome* (ES), *Fechtner syndrome* (FTNS). *May-Hegglin anomaly* (MHA), and *Sebastian syndrome* (SBS).
    - *Pathogenesis:* Mutations in the myosin heavy chain 9 (*MYH9)* gene on chromosome 22 (22q12–13) which

encodes nonmuscle myosin heavy chain peptide (NMMHC)-IIA. NMMHC-IIA is expressed in many organs/tissues including platelets, renal parenchyma, and leukocytes and is responsible for cell motility.
- Characterized by macrothrombocytopenia, Döhle-like bodies in leukocytes, and for some of these patients, this disease is associated with nephritis and sensorineural deafness.

Thrombocytopenia with Normal Platelet Size

1. *Congenital amegakaryocytic thrombocytopenia (CAMT)*:
   - *Pathogenesis: CMPL* gene defect which encodes the cmpl receptor (the ligand for thrombopoietin (TPO)). The disease severity depends on the type of the mutation (nonsense or frameshift is more severe than the miss-sense mutation)
   - Isolated severe thrombocytopenia ($<10 \times 10^9$/L), elevated serum TPO levels, and bone marrow absence of megakaryocytes. 10–30% may have neurologic or orthopedic abnormalities or intracranial hemorrhage (could be lethal).
2. *Thrombocytopenia-absent radius (TAR):*
   - *Pathogenesis:* The pathogenesis is still elusive. Recent studies have signaled a role in regulation of home-box genes (*HOXA10, HOXA11* and *HOXD11).*
   - Clinical and laboratory manifestation with hypo-megakaryocytic thrombocytopenia with severe bleeding during infancy, and bilateral absence of the radii or ulna defect, some with cardiac and renal malformations.

Microthrombocytopenia

- *Wiskott-Aldrich syndrome*
  - *Pathogenesis*: X-linked defect in WAS protein (which may play important role for hematopoietic cell lineage activa-

tion, progression of cell motility through the cytoskeleton actin filaments).
- Young boy presenting with mild bleeding diathesis, marked thrombocytopenia and small platelets. Other features include T-cell abnormalities, IgM deficiency and eczema.

Congenital Thrombocytopathies

Defective Platelet Adhesion Function

- *Bernard-Soulier syndrome (BSS):*
  - *Pathogenesis:* Quantitative or qualitative defects of the GPIbIX/V complex on the surface of platelets, GPIbIX/V is the main receptor for VWF and plays a role in platelet adhesion.
  - It can present with mild to severe bleeding, the platelets appear giant, it usually ranges from less than 30,000–200,000/μL. Flow cytometry with loss of CD42. Platelet aggregation studies show no aggregation when exposed to ristocetin. The lack of aggregation cannot be rescued by adding normal plasma, which discerns BSS from VWD.

Defective Platelet Activation Function (ADP Receptor Defects)

- *Pathogenesis:* ADP receptors defects are not common
  - P2Y12 deficiency: AR disease reported in a few families, it presents with moderate to severe mucocutaneous bleeding (only a family has AD inheritance and has with severe hemorrhage).

Defective Platelet Aggregation Function

- *Glanzmann disease:*
  - *Pathogenesis:* Mutations in platelet surface receptors the *GP2B* (*ITGA2B*) or *GP3A* (*ITGB3*) gene lead to either qualitative and/or quantitative deficiency of the platelet GPIIb/GPIIIa complex (CD41a, CD61) which have key binding sites for certain ligands such as fibrinogen, VWF, fibronectin, and vitronectin. There are three phenotypic subtypes (1–3, with variable degree of receptor deficiency, severe to mild).
  - Laboratory tests show prolonged bleeding time, and decreased aggregation in response to platelet agonists, e.g., ADP, collagen, epinephrine, serotonin, and thrombin, normal platelet agglutination to ristocetin and diminished or absent clot retraction. Flow cytometry shows loss of CD41a, CD61 expressions. However, platelet count remains normal.

Defective Platelet Secretion Function (Storage Pool Disease)

- Very rare and presents with mild to moderate mucocutaneous bleeding. It is challenging to diagnose as it has a significant inconsistency in various laboratory testing, for example, abnormal aggregation in response to different agonists, and impaired platelet secretion induced by various platelet agonists.

1. *Gray platelet syndrome (GPS):*
   - *Pathogenesis:* Deficiency of the α-granules.
   - Moderate macrothrombocytopenia with pale staining/greyish platelets by morphology platelet aggregation may be only moderately affected.
2. *Quebec platelet disorder (QPD):*
   - *Pathogenesis:* AD disorder, characterized by increased expression and storage of urokinase-type plasminogen

activator in platelets → intraplatelet generation of plasmin → degradation of many α-granule proteins stored in platelets.

- It presents with moderate to severe delayed bleeding (usually happens 12–24 h after surgery or trauma), due to increased lysis of clots, low platelet count, absent platelet aggregation in response to epinephrine, and variable (normal to abnormal) aggregation in response to collagen and ADP.

3. *Hermansky-Pudlak syndrome (HPS):*

   - *Pathogenesis:* AR disorder due to mutations in one of the seven orthologous genes (*HPS1, HPS2, HPS3, HPS4, HPS5, HPS6,* and *HPS7*) →abnormal formation of intracellular vesicles and impaired function of specific lysosomal organelles and vesicles.
   - Patients from Puerto Rico or Japan with albinism, pulmonary fibrosis, platelet dysfunction, prolonged bleeding, absence of platelet dense granules, lysosomal ceroid lipofuscin storage, congenital neutropenia, and granulomatous colitis.

4. *Chediak-Higashi syndrome (CHS):*

   - *Pathogenesis:* Autosomal recessive disorder due to mutation in *CHS1/LYST (lysosomal trafficking regulator)* gene which affects dense granules in all granules containing cells including granulocytes, lymphocytes, melanocytes, and neurons leading to giant lysosomal granules which cannot fuse with phagosomes, so ingested bacteria cannot be lysed normally.
   - Hypopigmentation, recurrent infections, lack of natural killer cell function, severe immunological deficiency, mild coagulation defects, and neuropathy.

Defective Platelet Procoagulant Function

Scott syndrome:

- *Introduction:* AR bleeding disorder due to *ANO6 gene mutation.*
- *Pathogenesis:* Impaired exposure of phosphatidylserine (PS) and phosphatidylethanolamine (PE) on the platelet membrane and thus failure to stimulate prothrombinase and tenase activity, resulting in decrease thrombin generation.
- It is an extremely rare disease, usually presents with posttraumatic/surgery bleeding or severe spontaneous mucocutaneous bleeding. Laboratory tests show elevated residual levels of prothrombin in serum and reduced platelet coagulation activity. The number, morphology, and function (adhesion, secretion, and aggregation) of platelet are not altered.

Diagnosis

The diagnostic algorithm is proposed in Fig. 25.2.

- Platelet count: Performed on automated cell counters as part of CBC.
- Slide or tube platelet aggregation studies: Performed on platelet rich plasma using aggregometry reagent.
- Platelet function test: It measures time taken for whole blood to plug fine capillary with internal surface coated with collagen and epinephrine (CEPI) or collagen and ADP (CADP). This is called the closure time (CT) and is measured in seconds. Normally, CT for CEPI is 80–192 and CT for ADP is 60–112 s. Prolongation of CT indicates low platelet function.

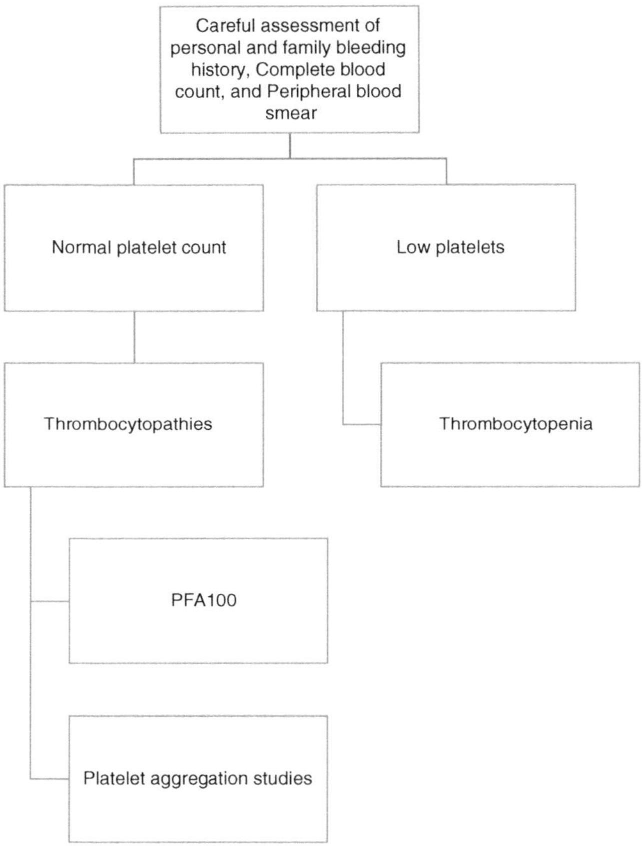

Fig. 25.2 Diagnostic algorithm

Differential Diagnosis A variety of secondary bleeding disorders are more common than congenital platelet disorders. These disorders may be related to:

- Decrease synthesis (aplastic anemia, chemotherapy and bone marrow fibrosis or infiltration by leukemia/lymphoma or carcinoma).

- Increase degradation (idiopathetically thrombocytopenic purpura (ITP), thrombotic thrombocytopenic purpura (TTP), hemolytic uremic syndrome (HUS), disseminated intravascular coagulopathy (DIC), paroxysmal nocturnal hemoglobinuria, heparin induced thrombocytopenia, and HELLP) for differential diagnoses.
- Sequestration (hypersplenism).

Careful history including (family history, bleeding history) and coagulation testing is the key to make the diagnosis.

Treatment

- General education of the parents and the patients about the disease including (good oral hygiene, avoid contact sports, avoid trauma, and avoid antiplatelet drugs like aspirin)
- In case of active bleeding:
  - Use a localized measurements to stop the bleeding form accessible sites (in epistaxis → compression as well as local application of tranexamic acid can help stop bleeding).
  - Platelets transfusion is the most effective treatment to stop bleeding in individuals with inherited thrombocytopenia. However, it might not be helpful for patients with severe bleeding that cannot be controlled with local interventions, or life-threatening hemorrhages, or bleeding at critical sites, e.g., CNS system.
  - Given possible clot formation, systemic administration of tranexamic acid, however, is avoided in hematuria as it may lead to blockage of the urinary tract.
  - Some studies recommend the use of platelet transfusion or short term of thrombopoietin receptor agonists prior to elective surgeries or baby delivery.
- For patients who have CAMT or WAS syndrome, hematopoietic stem cell transplantation is the treatment of choice.
- Alternatively, autologous hematopoietic stem cell gene therapy can be performed instead of HSCT.

Board Related Questions

1. A 2-year-old boy with history of easy bruising and frequent nose bleeds is referred to hematology for evaluation of possible inherited bleeding disorder. The patient has normal platelet count and unremarkable platelet morphology on peripheral blood smear. The bleeding time is increased. Platelet function studies show no secondary aggregation to ADP, collagen, and epinephrine with normal aggregation to ristocetin. The likely diagnosis is:

   A. von Willebrand Disease
   B. Platelet-type (pseudo) von Willebrand Disease
   C. Bernard-Soulier syndrome
   D. Glanzmann thrombasthenia
   E. Grey platelet syndrome

   Answer: D. Glanzmann thrombasthenia shows primary wave but lack secondary aggregation to ADP, collagen and epinephrine, due to qualitative and/or quantitative alteration of the platelet GPIIb/GPIIIa complex.

2. Peripheral blood smear from a patient with gray platelet syndrome show deficiency/ absence of which of the component?

   A. Platelet Factor 4
   B. Adenosine diphosphate
   C. Adenosine triphosphate
   D. Glycoprotein IIb/IIIa
   E. Glycoprotein Ib/IX

   Answer: A. Loss of platelet factor 4 is seen in gray platelet syndrome.

Further Reading

1. Balduini CL. Treatment of inherited thrombocytopenias. Haematologica. 2022;107(6):1278. https://doi.org/10.3324/haematol.2022.280856.
2. Cines DB, Bussel JB, McMillan RB, Zehnder JL. Congenital and acquired thrombocytopenia. ASH Educ Program Book. 2004;2004(1):390–406. https://doi.org/10.1182/asheducation-2004.1.390.
3. D'Andrea G, Chetta M, Margaglione M. Inherited platelet disorders: thrombocytopenias and thrombocytopathies. Blood Transfus. 2009;7(4):278. https://doi.org/10.2450/2009.0078-08.
4. Hayward CPM, Rao AK, Cattaneo M. Congenital platelet disorders: overview of their mechanisms, diagnostic evaluation, and treatment. Haemophilia. 2006;12:128–36. https://doi.org/10.1111/j.1365-2516.2006.01270.x.
5. Nurden P, Stritt S, Favier R, Nurden AT. Inherited platelet diseases with normal platelet count: phenotypes, genotypes, and diagnostic strategy. Haematologica. 2021;106(2):337. https://doi.org/10.3324/haematol.2020.248153.

26 Acquired Platelet Defects

Tauseef Ur Rehman, Elizabeth Rubin, Caroline K. Hana, and Atif Hussein

Introduction

Acquired defects in platelet function are the conditions that prevent blood clotting due to extrinsic factors. They are commonly seen in clinical practice and associated with a wide variety of etiologies, e.g., medication induced, procedures, or arise from a wide range of hematological or nonhematologic diseases. The degree to which the exact underlying mechanisms are understood remains variable. These platelet defects can often present with normal laboratory parameters, and hence, the diagnosis requires an astute review of patient's history and clinical presentation. Recognition of these qualitative defects in platelet function is very important to minimize the risk of bleeding, which can be devastating especially in the invasive procedural setting. However, in some of these diseases, patients can present with both qualitative and quantitative platelet abnormalities such as in DIC (disseminated intravascular coagulation), liver diseases or hematologic malignancies.

T. U. Rehman (✉) · E. Rubin · C. K. Hana · A. Hussein
Memorial Healthcare System, Pembroke Pines, FL, USA
e-mail: TRehman@mhs.net

L. Sokol, L. Zhang (eds.), *Non-Neoplastic Hematologic Disorders*,
https://doi.org/10.1007/978-3-031-62373-8_26

Clinically, these qualitative defects usually present with mucocutaneous bleeding such as epistaxis and skin ecchymosis. However, more severe visceral bleeding can be seen in some cases especially with invasive procedures. The diagnosis of qualitative defects can be challenging as there is a direct relationship between bleeding tendencies and laboratory testing including platelet aggregation studies. Hence, mitigation of the risk of bleeding requires close attention to the patient's medical history, along with a high index of suspicion. Treatment of the underlying disorder or removal of offending agents are often the most important steps in the management. In this chapter, we focus on the common causes of acquired defects in platelet function and briefly review some etiologies that present with quantitative defects as well.

Etiology and Pathogenesis

The most common etiologies of these defects can be broadly divided into systemic disorders, hematological disorders, and medications (Table 26.1).

Table 26.1 Common etiologies of acquired defects in platelet function

Category	Cause	Possible mechanism	Frequently used therapeutic interventions[a]
Systemic disorders	Uremia (chronic renal failure)	Platelets adhesion defect Acquired storage pool defect (decreased ADP, serotonin, TXA2) Defect in Integrin αIIbβ3 signaling Anemia	Correction of anemia (using transfusions, erythropoietin stimulating agents as indicated) Correction of uremia Desmopressin (DDAVP)
	Liver disease	Storage pool deficiency Defects in TXA2 GpIb abnormalities	Correction of coagulopathy (for example using fresh frozen plasma) Correction of nutritional deficiencies (Vitamin K)
	DIC	Dysfibrinogenemia	Cryoprecipitate
	Sepsis	Dysfibrinogenemia	Treatment of underlying medical trigger and source of sepsis
	Cardiopulmonary bypass and extraporeal membrance oxygenation	Acquired storage pool defect Acquired vWD	Platelet transfusions Anti-fibrinolytics DDAVP

(continued)

Table 26.1 (continued)

Category	Cause	Possible mechanism	Frequently used therapeutic interventions[a]
Hematologic disorders	Multiple myeloma	Paraproteinemia	Correction of factor X deficiency
	Waldenström macroglobulinemia	Paraproteinemia	
	Non-Hodgkin lymphomas	Acquired vWD	Correction of vWD deficiency (DDAVP, vWF concentrate)
	Myeloproliferative neoplasms (MPN)	Acquired vWD	
	Acute myeloid leukemia	Dysfibrinogenemia	Cryoprecipitate Fresh frozen plasma
	Myelodysplasia	Decreased thrombopoiesis	Thrombopoietin receptor agonists
Drug-induced platelets dysfunction	Aspirin	Irreversible inhibition of COX-1 Decreased TXA2	PFA-100 Platelet aggregation assays Stop exposure to offending agent as soon as safe and feasible Hold the medication prior to any planned surgery/procedure Platelet transfusion can be considered for life threatening or serious bleeding
	NSAIDs	Reversible inhibition of COX-1/COX-2	
	Ticlopidine, clopidogrel, prasugrel	Irreversible P2Y12 antagonists	
	Ticagrelor, cangrelor	Reversible P2Y12 antagonists	
	Abciximab, eptifibatide, tirofiban	Integrin $\alpha IIb\beta 3$ receptor blockers	
	Phosphodiesterase inhibitors	Increased platelets cAMP	
Drug-related platelets dysfunction as an adverse event	SSRIs	Abnormal aggregation and secretion in response to ADP, collagen, epinephrine, or thrombin	
	Antibiotics, especially β-lactam type	Inhibited interaction of agonists and vWF Modified platelet receptors chemically	
	Bruton tyrosine kinase inhibitors, e.g., Ibrutinib	Abnormal platelets adhesion to vWF Inhibited platelets aggregation	

(continued)

Table 26.1 (continued)

Category	Cause	Possible mechanism	Frequently used therapeutic interventions[a]
Certain herbs or foods	e.g.,Ginkgo (Ginkgo biloba) Garlic (Allium sativum) Ginger (Zingiber officinale) Asian, Siberian, or American ginseng Meadowsweet	Unclear	Stop the offending supplement particularly if other risk factors present for bleeding

ADP adenosine diphosphate, *cAMP* cyclic adenosine monophosphate, *COX* Cyclo-oxygenase, *DIC* disseminated intravascular coagulopathy, *DDAVP* Desmopressin, *GpIb* Glycoprotein Ib, *NSAIDs* non-steroidal anti-inflammatory drugs, *SSRI* selective serotonin reuptake inhibitor, *TXA2* thromboxane A2, *vWD* von Willebrand disease, *vWF* von Willebrand factor
[a]Treatment of the underlying disease process is the key in all the pathologies

Systemic Disorders

Renal Failure

Patients with uremia and renal failure are at high risk of bleeding complications, which is caused in large part due to platelet dysfunction. Varying degree of even mild renal insufficiency can increase the risk of bleeding in comparative terms. Patients with end-stage renal disease (ESRD) on dialysis and stage V chronic kidney disease (CKD) with eGFR less than 15 ml/min/1.73 m^2 are especially at higher risk. The exact mechanism of this dysfunction is not entirely understood but it is indeed a multifactorial phenomenon.

- The presence of a number of uremic toxins in blood has long been thought to have an effect on platelet function as supported by mixing of plasma from uremic patients with normal platelets [1]. Urea, methylguanidine, phenol and phenolic acids, and guanidinosuccinic acid have all been implicated as possible culprits.

- There appears to be more evidence that an important source of platelet dysfunction in renal failure is not intrinsic to platelets, but rather due to anemia. Anemia inducing elevated levels of cyclic adenosine monophosphate (AMP) and cyclic guanosine monophosphate (GMP) also lead to increased release of these inhibitors from endothelial cells. Increased hemoglobin in patients with uremia can also improve hemostasis secondary to changes in hemorheology. Thus, treatment of anemia with RBC transfusion and erythropoiesis-stimulating agents (ESA) will improve bleeding time in these patients [2].
- Further compounding factors include reduction in dense granule content, reduced synthesis of thromboxane A2 (TXA2) and impaired interaction with platelet surface glycoproteins in uremic status and additional antiplatelet or anticoagulation therapy for concurrent CAD [3].

Liver Disease

Similar to patients with CKD, dysfunction can be seen at multiple levels of primary and secondary homeostasis system leading to hemorrhagic complications in cirrhosis. Thrombocytopenia and prolongation of prothrombin time (PT) are commonly seen in liver disease. It is believed that qualitative platelet function worsens with increasing severity of cirrhosis. However, cirrhosis is now also increasingly recognized as a hypercoagulable state, which leads to further complexity to understand this condition.

- In the initial stages of cirrhosis, secretion of hypercoagulable particles by platelets and increased circulating von Willebrand factor (VWF) levels can compensate for a milder degree of thrombocytopenia. Naturally, it is evident that this does not protect from the severe bleeding complications seen commonly in acute and chronic liver disease. The platelet dysfunction seen in advanced liver disease represents a complex interplay of different factors including direct toxic effect of alcohol, deficiency of dense granules, decreased access to arachidonic acid (AA), and elevated levels of fibrin split products/dysfibrinogenemia [4].

Hematological Disorders

Paraproteinemia

Paraproteinemia blends into the interaction of primary homeostasis system with the coagulation pathway and can cause abnormalities of multiple coagulation studies including thrombin time, PT and occasionally aPTT as well. However, the pathway is most severe and thrombin time is often affected. This is hypothesized due to the inhibition of fibrin polymerization by the high paraprotein levels. Paraproteins can interact with platelet surface membranes glycoproteins leading to impaired platelet activation, aggregation, and clot retraction Therefore, platelet transfusions are not as effective in treating the bleeding complications. Symptomatic hyperviscosity and associated bleeding diathesis and thrombotic complication in WM is a medical emergency and requires prompt attention, with plasmapheresis being indicated in cases presenting with neurological dysfunction. Acquired von Willebrand disease (aVWD) should be carefully considered in patients with new onset of bleeding and underlying plasma cell dyscrasias. It is also seen in a variety of other hematological disorders as well including non-Hodgkin lymphomas, chronic lymphocytic leukemia, hairy cell leukemia, and frequently in the myeloproliferative disorders. While prolongation of aPTT can hint towards aVWD, normal aPTT does not rule out aVWD in this setting, as the factor VIII level can be near normal and the defect in platelet function is mostly due to loss of high molecular weight (HMW) VWF multimers. For more definitive evaluation, tests for VWF function with ristocetin cofactor activity should be obtained although now more sensitive assays are available for functional testing. Because aVWD can present like type 2 VWD, multimeric analysis may also be required (please refer to Chap. 40: Von Willebrand Disease for further details).

- Another important etiology for bleeding in patients with associated amyloidosis is deficiency of vitamin K-dependent factors. The deficiency of factor X is unique as it can happen independent of liver impairment and has been shown to be related to sequestration caused by adsorption to amyloid fibrils [5].

- The most effective treatment of paraproteinemia-related bleeding diathesis is removal of the abnormal paraproteins. Desmopressin (DDAVP) or VWF factor concentrates can be used depending on the severity of bleeding, until disease directed therapy can be started.

Myeloproliferative Disorders (MPDs)

MPDs can lead to increase in bleeding episodes which are usually mild in nature such as gingival hemorrhage, epistaxis, and bruising. More severe hemorrhagic complications can be seen with the use of high dose aspirin for preventing from thrombosis in patients with polycythemia vera and essential thrombocytosis. Spontaneous bleeding, on the other hand, is witnessed more frequently in patients with very high platelet counts, typically more than 1 million per cu mm causing aVWD. At such high levels, there is spontaneous biding of platelets and clearance of HMW VWF multimers from the circulation leading a defect in primary homeostasis. Another common finding is impairment in response to epinephrine and adenosine diphosphate-induced aggregation, which leads to poor platelet aggregation [6]. Bleeding risk in MPN cannot be predicted alone by the degree of thrombocytosis, bleeding time abnormalities, or platelet function testing.

Myelodysplasia

In contrast to MPDs, the bleeding seen in myelodysplasia is more often due to thrombocytopenia and dysfunctional platelets because of impairment in the hematopoietic process. Due to the impairment in thrombopoiesis, the platelets are already reduced and may contain fewer alpha granules and have aberrations in the dense tubular system, which have a negative impact on homeostasis.

Drug-Related Platelet Dysfunction

Platelet aggregation is stimulated in the circulation by certain agonists including collagen, thrombin, ADP, 5-hydroxytryptamine, and TXA2. Besides, agents that increase intracellular cyclic AMP or cyclic GMP may also impair the platelet function. Medications targeting these pathways can have an inhibitory effect on platelets causing increased risk of bleeding or a stimulatory effect causing a prothrombotic state.

Drugs are the most common cause of platelet dysfunction in elderly population. Certain drugs are used for its therapeutic effect of platelets function inhibition while others cause this inhibition as a side effect. These drugs can further increase the risk of bleeding, particularly in certain clinical situations (sepsis, disseminated intravascular coagulation), or iatrogenic scenarios (cardiopulmonary bypass surgery, liver transplantation), as discussed earlier.

Drugs Used for Their Direct Antiplatelet Effect

- Aspirin and other nonsteroidal antiinflammatory drugs (NSAIDs) inhibit cyclooxygenase I (COX-1) resulting in impaired TXA2 production, a stimulator of platelet aggregation. The effect of aspirin on COX-1 is irreversible, and so, its effects last 7–10 days which is the life span of the platelets [4, 7].
- Other antiplatelets medications include the P2Y12 inhibitors, e.g., clopidogrel and prasugrel, which can be activated to antagonize the ADP receptor P2Y12. Similarly, cangrelor and ticagrelor are direct reversible P2Y12 antagonists.
- The inhibition of TXA2 formation or antagonism of the ADP receptor P2Y12 stops positive feedback loops required for sustained platelet activation [4, 7].
- Integrin αIIbβ3 (GPIIb-IIIa) receptor blockers (e.g., abciximab, eptifibatide, and tirofiban) block platelet aggregation by binding nonselectively to GPIIb-IIIa receptors and preventing fibrinogen binding to the integrin.

- Phosphodiesterase inhibitors (such as cilostazol and dipyridamole) are known to affect platelet function by preventing the degranulation of cyclic AMP (cAMP), thus increasing platelet cyclic AMP levels.

Drugs with Antiplatelet Effect as an Adverse Effect

- Selective serotonin reuptake inhibitors (SSRIs), specifically fluoxetine, paroxetine, and sertraline, are associated more frequently with spontaneous hemorrhagic events. Some abnormal laboratory tests, including abnormal bleeding time, prolongation of closure times (PFA-100), and alteration in aggregation and secretion in response to ADP, collagen, epinephrine, or thrombin, may be seen in patients using SSRIs [7].
- Antibiotics, especially those of the β-lactam type such as penicillins and cephalosporins, can prolong the bleeding time even in normal volunteers. The exact mechanism of impaired platelet function by these antibiotics is currently unclear, although it has been hypothesized that they bind to the platelet membrane and inhibit the interaction of agonists and vWF or modify platelet receptors chemically [7].
- Bruton tyrosine kinase (BTK) inhibitors like Ibrutinib also affect other platelet kinases in addition to BTK. It has also been shown that ibrutinib causes inhibition of collagen and CRP-induced aggregation. These side effects are less observed with the second-generation BTK inhibitor acalabrutinib [8].
- Caplacizumab, a medication prescribed for treatment of acquired thrombotic thrombocytopenic purpura, inhibits platelet thrombi formation by binding with high affinity to the A1 domain of vWF and thus inhibiting the interaction of platelet GPIbα receptor with vWF [8].
- It has been reported that certain foods and dietary supplements cause platelets dysfunction and increased bleeding tendency. Garlic is among the more studied one, which has shown interference with platelets function both in vitro and in vivo. Other

reported substances include omega-3 polyunsaturated fatty acids, onions, ginkgo biloba, ginseng, Chinese cinnamon, black tree fungus, and others [8].

Quantitative Platelet Defects

Most laboratories define thrombocytopenia (in adults) as a platelet count of less than 150,000/mm^3. It is a commonly encountered condition in clinical practice, and its etiologies can be divided into three main categories.

(a) Decreased platelet production. This can be due to megakaryocytic hypoplasia as seen in certain infections, drugs, and bone marrow disorders such as aplastic anemia and myelodysplasia. It can also be caused by ineffective thrombopoiesis due to vitamin deficiencies such as B12, folate.
(b) Abnormal distribution. This can be caused by splenic sequestration due to splenomegaly and commonly seen in conditions such as liver cirrhosis and myelofibrosis.
(c) Increase in peripheral destruction. A wide spectrum of conditions falls under this category and can be further subdivided into immunologic and nonimmunologic destruction. Common immunological conditions include autoimmune destruction such as immune thrombocytopenic purpura (ITP), alloimmune destruction (posttransfusion purpura, neonatal), drug-induced and heparin-induced thrombocytopenia (HIT). Nonimmunological conditions include the thrombotic microangiopathic (TMA) syndromes, thrombotic thrombocytopenic purpura (TTP), hemolytic uremic syndrome (HUS), and disseminated intravascular coagulation (DIC). Peripartum patients are at the unique risk for TMA related to HELLP syndrome (hemolysis, elevated liver enzymes, and low platelet count).

Thrombocytopenia is a common question seen in consultative hematology. In clinical practice, it is helpful to rule out the most catastrophic etiologies (such as TTP, DIC, HIT, and HELLP) first and once these are ruled out, follow a stepwise algorithm to evaluate the other causes. Several conditions which cause qualitative defect in platelet function that we discussed above can also cause quantitative defects. For example, thrombocytopenia is a hallmark of cirrhosis, with a multifactorial etiology behind it. This includes splenomegaly, liver dysfunction, and nutritional deficiencies. Alcohol use is a common cause of cirrhosis, which can cause direct toxicity to the bone marrow and suppression of its function. Similarly, myelodysplasia and hematological malignancies often present with profound and severe thrombocytopenia. On the other hand, quantitative defects in platelet number may not be seen in plasma cell disorders depending on the degree of bone marrow infiltration and disruption of the normal hematopoiesis. Once again, these patients do remain at higher risk of bleeding due to a few reasons including qualitative platelet dysfunction and careful examination of bleeding risk is paramount.

Diagnosis

Adequate collection of clinical and medication history is important. Baseline laboratory workup includes CBC, review of peripheral blood smear, renal and liver function tests, PT, and aPTL Stepwise analysis following diagnostic algorithm (Fig. 26.1) that is helpful. Looking for a potential systemic disease that would lead to platelet dysfunction is fundamental for having better understanding disease pathogenesis and solving the bleeding disorder.

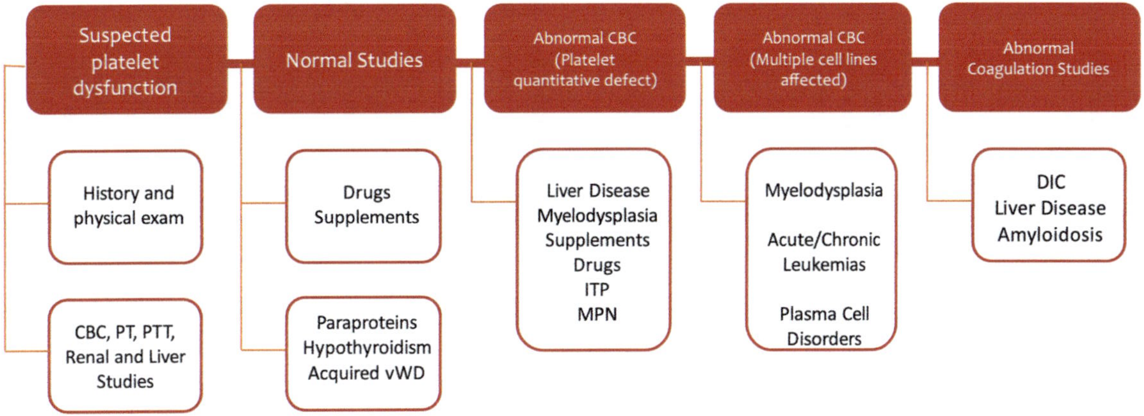

Fig. 26.1 Evaluation of suspected platelet function defect. CBC complete blood count, PT prothrombin time, PTT partial thromboplastin time, vWD Von willebrand disease, ITP immune thrombocytopenic purpura, MPN myeloproliferative neoplasm, DIC disseminated intravascular coagulation

Major Differential Diagnosis

Congenital platelet defects are included for main differential diagnoses. For details, see separate book chapter.

Prognosis

It varies upon the cause and degree of platelet defects. Patients with severe liver, or renal dysfunction, hematologic malignancy, or over dosage of platelet inhibitory medication have a tendency of severe visceral bleeding, especially those undergoing an invasive procedure.

Treatment

Acquired platelet defects represent a heterogenous group of disorders where treatment of the bleeding depends on individual patient specific factors. Treatment of the underlying disease process and control of the bleeding source, if feasible, remains the cornerstone of therapy. In general, platelet transfusions are not helpful to correct the platelet dysfunction alone, in the absence of a different indication. The transfused platelets will be again exposed to the systemic disorder or medication which caused platelet dysfunction in the first place, although they might be more useful for post-operative or procedural bleeding. Cryoprecipitate can be used in the setting with low or borderline fibrinogen levels; otherwise, it has a limited role. DDAVP is often cited in the treatment of platelet dysfunction bleeding particularly uremia although its clinical benefit remains uncertain. It causes release of vWF and Factor VIII from endothelial cells and may counter the effect of other deregulatory mechanisms in renal failure and can be used either for treatment or prevention (given 30–60 min before an invasive procedure). It is rapidly effective in the treatment of aVWD, where it causes release of the very high molecular weight VWF multimers from platelets which are effective for homeostasis. Its use is limited to 1–2 days and carries risk of thrombosis and tachyphylaxis. Electrolytes should be closely monitored during this time with limitation of free water intake.

Caveats

- There is a wide spectrum of etiology of acquired platelet defects. A systemic review of clinical history, in conjunction with a stepwise analysis of laboratory findings, is crucial, especially when patients do not have an overt systemic disease.
- Be aware that there is a long list of medications that could induce platelet dysfunction.
- Treatment of the underlying disease and control of the bleeding source, if feasible, remains the cornerstone of therapy.

Board Review Question

A 10-year-old child is referred to a hematologist for epistaxis. The patient has no past medical history of bleeding. The ENT specialist ordered a PFA-100 test. The results show prolonged PFA closure time with epinephrine, but not with ADP (adenosine diphosphate). Based on these results the hematologist suspects that the patient has recently taken aspirin. How does aspirin intake effect platelet function?

A. Inhibition of the glycoprotein IIb/IIIa receptor
B. Increased release of prostacyclin
C. Reversible inhibition of cyclooxygenase 1 (COX1)
D. Irreversible inhibition of cyclooxygenase 1 (COX1)
E. Irreversible inhibition adenosine diphosphate receptors

Answer: D. Irreversible cyclooxygenase-1 (COX-1) inhibitors including aspirin, and ADP receptor antagonists (clopidogrel and ticagrelor) are the drugs often used for anti-platelet therapy.

References

1. Evans EP, Branch RA, Bloom AL. A clinical and experimental study of platelet function in chronic renal failure. J Clin Pathol. 1972;25(9):745–53.
2. Cases A, Escolar G, Reverter JC, Ordinas A, Lopez-Pedret J, Revert L, et al. Recombinant human erythropoietin treatment improves platelet function in uremic patients. Kidney Int. 1992;42(3):668–72.
3. Kaw D, Malhotra D. Platelet dysfunction and end-stage renal disease. Semin Dial. 2006;19(4):317–22.
4. Scharf RE. 49—Acquired disorders of platelet function. In: Michelson AD, editor. Platelets. 4th ed. Academic; 2019. p. 905–20.
5. Choufani EB, Sanchorawala V, Ernst T, Quillen K, Skinner M, Wright DG, et al. Acquired factor X deficiency in patients with amyloid light-chain amyloidosis: incidence, bleeding manifestations, and response to high-dose chemotherapy. Blood. 2001;97(6):1885–7.
6. Papadakis E, Hoffman R, Brenner B. Thrombohemorrhagic complications of myeloproliferative disorders. Blood Rev. 2010;24(6):227–32.
7. Konkle BA. Acquired disorders of platelet function. Hematology Am Soc Hematol Educ Program. 2011;2011:391–6.
8. Brennan Y, Levade M, Ward CM. Acquired platelet function disorders. Thromb Res. 2020;196:561–8.

Heparin-Induced Thrombocytopenia (HIT)

27

Shrinjaya Thapa, Akriti G. Jain, and Loveleen Kang

Introduction

Heparin-induced thrombocytopenia (HIT) is a syndrome of antibody-mediated thrombocytopenia that paradoxically is often associated with thrombosis and high morbidity and mortality. It is a clinicopathological entity, where thrombocytopenia develops at least 5 days after immunizing exposure to heparin with detectable activating IgG class antibodies against factor 4 (PF4) and heparin (or other polyanion) complexes [1].

Variants of HIT

The incidence of HIT is approximately 0.2–5% of heparin-treated adults. Risk factors can be divided as heparin related and host related [2].

S. Thapa · A. G. Jain
H. Lee Moffitt Cancer and Research Center, Tampa, FL, USA

L. Kang (✉)
James A Haley VA, Tampa, FL, USA
e-mail: loveleen.kang@va.gov

L. Sokol, L. Zhang (eds.), *Non-Neoplastic Hematologic Disorders*, https://doi.org/10.1007/978-3-031-62373-8_27

1. Heparin related:
   (a) Type of heparin: unfractionated heparin (UFH) has fivefold to tenfold higher risk to develop HIT than low molecular heparin (LMWH). This may be explained by smaller molecules generating less charged anion. There is even smaller, maybe negligible risk with fondaparinux.
   (b) Longer courses of heparin are associated with higher risk.
   (c) Therapeutic dose of heparin has higher chances than prophylactic dose.

2. Host related:
   (a) Age: Middle age and older individuals are at significantly higher risk than children and young adults.
   (b) Sex: Female patients are at higher risk than men [3].
   (c) Surgical patients have threefold higher risk of HIT than medical patients [3].

Pathogenesis

Platelet factor 4 (PF4) is a highly positively charged tetrameric protein which is normally found in alpha granules of platelets. It binds heparin with high affinity and neutralizes it. The binding of polysaccharides to PF4 is dependent on the chain length; hence, LMWH (low molecular weight heparin) binds weakly to PF4 compared to UFH (unfractionated heparin) causing HIT less frequently [5].

The binding of heparin with PF4 results in a conformational change in PF4, generating neoantigens. This results in the rapid (within days) generation of IgG antibodies, without a primary IgM antibody response. Other negatively charged molecules like heparan sulphate can also induce similar responses.

The HIT IgG antibodies now form heparin -PF4- HIT antibody complexes which bind to platelets via their Fc receptor (FcyRIIa) in turn leading to platelet activation by a cascade of intracellular events leading to release of platelet granules, microparticles, and thromboxane biosynthesis [6]. PF4 released from platelet alpha granules leads to formation of more complexes with heparin and HIT antibody leading to further platelet activation. HIT antibodies also activate monocytes and bind heparin sulphate on endothelial surfaces leading to endothelial cell activation and injury, triggering release of tissue factor and thrombin generation. Neutrophil activation via the FcRIIa receptors and NETosis have lately been identified as key drives of thrombosis in HIT [7].

Thrombocytopenia in HIT is secondary to the removal of IgG coated platelets by macrophages of the reticuloendothelial system, like other drug-induced thrombocytopenia. The difference however with other drug-induced thrombocytopenia is the platelet activation and thrombosis with lesser degree of thrombocytopenia in HIT.

In most cases, patients have undergone a proximate immunizing exposure to heparin or certain other PF4-binding polyanions [1]. The mechanism of HIT formation is summarized in Fig. 27.1.

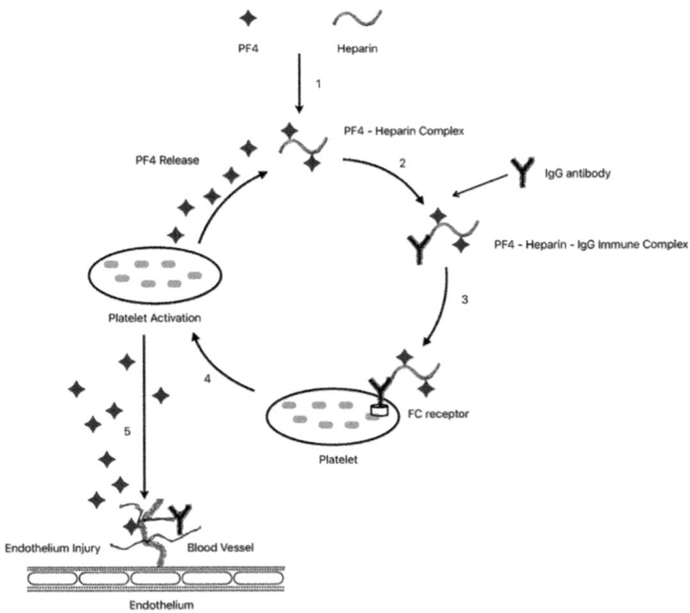

Fig. 27.1 Pathophysiology of HIT. 1: Heparin binds with PF4 and functions as immunogens. 2: IgG antibody produced forms PF4–heparin–IgG complex. 3: The complex then binds through Fc receptor to platelets and activates the platelets. 4: Activated platelet secrets additional PF4 and other granules. 5: Immune complex interacts with endothelial cells and enhances immune-mediated endothelial damage [4]

Clinical Features

HIT can be subcategorized into five variants in accordance with onset pattern and triggers.

1. Rapid onset HIT: Abrupt onset of thrombocytopenia, within one day of reintroduction of heparin, in an individual with recent exposure (within 100 days) to heparin.
2. Delayed onset HIT: Thrombocytopenia and/or thrombosis occurring 5 or more days after heparin has been stopped. It is considered a type of autoimmune HIT.
3. Spontaneous HIT: Development of HIT in an individual with no prior exposure to heparin. It is often associated with an infection or major surgical procedure. This is also considered a type of autoimmune HIT.
4. Type I HIT: Mild thrombocytopenia (platelet count is usually above 100,000/mL) with onset within first 2 days of exposure to heparin. Type I HIT is considered to be a direct effect of heparin on platelet causing nonimmune platelet aggregation. There is no risk of thrombosis.
5. Vaccine-induced immune thrombotic thrombocytopenia (VITT): Rare complication of adenoviral vectored COVID-19 vaccine with detectable PF4 antibodies causing platelet activation but are not heparin dependent.

Primarily, there are two main presentations of HIT such as thrombocytopenia and thrombosis.

Thrombocytopenia

- There is a temporal relationship between thrombocytopenia and exposure to heparin. Thrombocytopenia usually occurs 5–10 days after initiation of heparin in a typical onset HIT, irrespective of previous exposure to HIT.
- Degree of thrombocytopenia is usually a drop in platelet count of $<150 \times 10^9$/L or a relative 30–50% decline from baseline

platelet count, baseline being the highest platelet count that precedes the HIT related event [8]. This accounts for postoperative thrombocytosis seen in some patients after surgery, where the absolute count may still be normal but with a greater than 30–50% decrease compared to baseline platelet count.

- HIT usually presents with moderate thrombocytopenia, with a median platelet count of 55×10^9/L [8]. The range of thrombocytopenia is usually 55, 70×10^9/L with rare presentation with platelet count $<20 \times 10^9$/L.
- Thrombosis: recent study showed thrombocytosis occur between 20% and 64% of patients who was diagnosed with HIT [PMID: 28388835, PMID: 31350937, PMID: 33267665].
  - Venous thrombosis (~50%) is far more common than arterial thrombosis with pulmonary embolism being the most common cause of death, occurring in about 25% patients [12]. Lower limb thrombosis is the most common HIT associated thrombosis. Rare but well-described presentations include cerebral sinus thrombosis, mesenteric/portal thrombosis, and adrenal vein thrombosis causing adrenal hemorrhage [8].
  - Arterial thrombosis (10–15%) most commonly involves large lower limb arteries, with less often thrombotic stroke and myocardial infarction [8].
  - Heparin induced skin lesions, although rare, can occur at the site of heparin injection ranging from erythematous plaques to skin necrosis [8].

Acute systemic anaphylactic reactions have been described in patients with HIT which can be fatal.

Diagnosis

HIT being a clinicopathological entity requires both a compatible clinical picture and the presence of platelet activating antibodies. Any patient on heparin with thrombocytopenia should be evaluated for HIT, but confirmation with platelet activating assays is important to prevent overdiagnosis.

The first step to diagnosing HIT is assessing the pretest probability using different clinical scoring criteria, 4T score being the most widely used (Table 27.1) [9]. Another scoring system commonly used is the HIT Expert Probability (HEP) score which is a pretest probability model. These scoring systems have been useful in ruling out the diagnosis of HIT (high negative predictive value), because a low score indicates a <2% probability of having a positive platelet activation assay and this group does not need any further testing. However, if the probability of HIT is deemed

Table 27.1 Estimating the pretest probability of HIT: the "Four T's" (PMID: 31400811)

4T Score			
	2 points	1 point	0 point
Thrombocytopenia	>50% fall, or a nadir >= 20 × 10^9/L	>50% fall, or a nadir 10–19 × 10^9/L	<30% fall, or a nadir <10 × 10^9/L
Timing[a] of onset of platelet fall (or other sequelae of HIT)	Clear onset between days 5–10 OR platelet fall <=1 day with recent heparin within 30 days	>10 days, or timing unclear or < =1 day with recent heparin exposure within 30–100 days	<4 days without recent heparin
Thrombosis or other sequelae	Proven new thrombosis OR skin necrosis; acute systemic reaction post-IV UFH bolus	Progressive or recurrent thrombosis, non-necrotizing skin lesions, suspected thrombosis (not proven)	None
Other causes of thrombocytopenia	None evidence	Possible	Definite

According to the score, a higher 4T score is associated with a higher probability risk of an acute HIT reaction: 0–3 points: low probability of HIT (<1%); 4–5 points: moderate probability of HIT (~10%); 6–8 points: high probability of HIT (~50%); Maximal possible score = 8

[a]The first day immunizing heparin exposure is considered "0"

"high," only ~ 50% of patients have a positive confirmatory platelet activation assay and need further confirmation testing [10].

All patients with intermediate/high pretest probability are followed by laboratory testing. There are two main categories of laboratory testing for HIT:

1. Immunologic assays: Polyspecific enzyme-linked immunoassay which identifies circulating anti-PF4/heparin antibodies and is not dependent on detection of capacity of the antibodies to activate platelets. Their sensitivity is over 95% with a specificity of 50–89%, which makes them a good initial test but needs to be followed by a functional assay due to their poor positive predictive value [2].
2. Functional assays: There are the ^{14}C-serotonin release assay (SRA) and heparin-induced platelet activation assay (HIPA). They detect patient antibodies that induce heparin-dependent platelet activation. Their sensitivity and specificity are over 90% and used a confirmatory testing [2].

The algorithm proposed by Cuker et al. in Fig. 27.2 incorporates the clinical and laboratory data for initial management strategy [2].

Along with the laboratory confirmation of HIT, all patients should have lower extremity venous duplex done as they are the most common type of thromboses in HIT. If they have a central line catheter, upper extremity venous duplex should also be performed.

Based on the platelet count, immunoassay and functional assay, HIT can be divided into five phases [11] (Table 27.2):

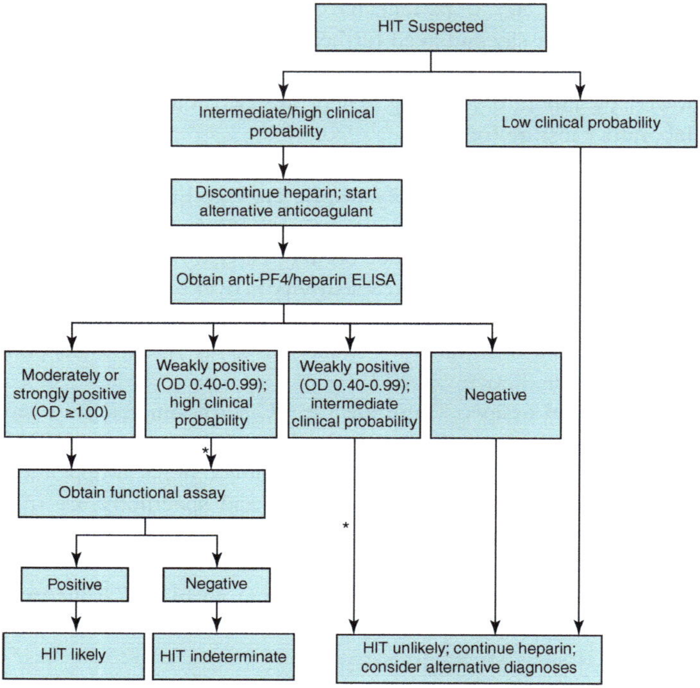

Fig. 27.2 Diagnostic approaches and initial management of patients with suspected HIT. *Estimates of the clinical probability of HIT in an individual patient may change over time. Thus, it is recommended to often reevaluate patients with questionable diagnosis and to adjust treatment accordingly [2]

Table 27.2 Five phases of HIT

Phase	Platelet count	Functional assay	Immunoassay
Suspected HIT	Decreased	Pending	Pending
Acute HIT	Decreased	Positive	Positive
Subacute HIT A	Normal	Positive	Positive
Subacute HIT B	Normal	Negative	Positive
Remote HIT	Normal	Negative	Negative

Differential Diagnosis

While the causes of thrombocytopenia can be vast, the main differential diagnosis of HIT can be listed as follows:

- Disseminated intravascular coagulation: abnormal DIC profile.
- Thrombotic microangiopathies: schistocytes, he pentad of fever, hemolytic anemia, thrombocytopenia, and renal and neurologic dysfunction, abnormal ADAMTS 13 assay.
- Immune thrombocytopenia: no hx of heparin use, thrombocytopenia, no thrombotic events, PF4 (-).
- Post transfusion purpura: profound thrombocytopenia developing within 2 weeks of transfusion, no history of heparin use.
- Drug-induced thrombocytopenia. No hx of heparin use, often associated with medication for cytoreduction/chemotherapy, no thrombotic episode.
- Venous thromboembolism unrelated to heparin causing consumption thrombocytopenia.
- Systemic lupus erythematosus and/or antiphospholipid antibody syndrome: prolonged aPTT, not corrected by mixed study.
- Use of any of the following intravascular devices such as extracorporeal circuits, balloon pumps, ventricular assist devices.

Treatment

Two most important steps in the management of HIT are to stop all heparin containing products, including flushes AND switch to a nonheparin anticoagulant. This should be instituted immediately when there is high clinical suspicion (see Fig. 27.2) while awaiting confirmatory laboratory testing.

Parenteral Anticoagulants

Nonheparin parenteral agents are typically used first, as anticoagulation can rapidly be achieved. This includes direct thrombin inhibitor (Argatroban and Bivalirudin) and indirect Factor Xa inhibitor (Danaparoid and Fondaparinux). These agents are summarized in Table 27.3.

Oral Anticoagulation

Direct oral anticoagulants can be used in acute HIT (see Table 27.2); however, warfarin is contraindicated in acute HIT. It has potential to cause a hypercoagulable state due to relative protein C deficiency with unopposed thrombin leading to venous limb gangrene. If a patient has been receiving warfarin at the time of diagnosis with HIT, urgent reversal with Vitamin K (intravenous preferred) is needed. Warfarin should only be started when a patient has been stably anticoagulated with nonheparin product and platelet count has recovered to normal levels (>150 × 10^9/L). Overlapping of parental anticoagulation for a minimum of 5 days until INR is therapeutic and avoiding high (>5 mg/day) initial doses of warfarin are other important considerations. If Argatroban is used as a parenteral anticoagulation, false elevation of INR should be accounted for while aiming for a therapeutic range on warfarin (Table 27.3).

Other Treatments

Intravenous Immunoglobulin (IVIG) may be used in autoimmune HIT along with standard approach as mentioned above.

Table 27.3 Guidance on selecting anticoagulant [11]

Drug	Mechanism of action	Route	Elimination (half-life)	Dosing	Laboratory monitoring
Argatroban	Direct thrombin inhibitor	IV	Hepatobiliary (40–50 min)	*Bolus:* None *Continuous infusion:* Normal organ function → 2 mg/kg/min When bilirubin >1.5 mg/dL (abnormal liver function → 0.5–1.2 mg/kg/min) Cardiac failure, anasarca, postcardiac surgery → 0.5–1.2 mg/kg/min	Adjust to APTT 1.5–3.0 times baseline
Bivalirudin	Direct thrombin inhibitor	IV	Enzymatic (25 min)	*Bolus:* None *Continuous infusion:* Normal organ function → 0.15 mg/kg/h Renal failure or abnormal liver function → dose reduction may be appropriate	Adjust to APTT 1.5–2.5 times baseline
Danaparoid	Indirect factor Xa inhibitor	IV	Renal (24 h)	*Bolus based on body weights:* >60 kg, 1500 units 60–75 kg, 2250 units 75–90 kg, 3000 units >90 kg, 3750 units Accelerated initial infusion: 400 units/h 3 4 h, then 300 units/h 3 4 h *Maintenance infusion:* Normal renal function → 200 units/h Renal failure → 150 units/h	Adjust to danaparoid-specific Anti-Xa activity of 0.5–0.8 units/mL

(continued)

Table 27.3 (continued)

Drug	Mechanism of action	Route	Elimination (half-life)	Dosing	Laboratory monitoring
Fondaparinux	Indirect factor Xa inhibitor	SC	Renal (17–24 h)	>50 kg → 5 mg × 1 per day 50–100 kg → 7.5 mg × 1 per day >100 kg → 10 mg × 1 per day	None
Apixaban[a]	Direct factor Xa inhibitor	PO	Hepatic (8–15 h)	*HITT:* 10 mg × 2 per day, ×1 week, then 5 mg × 2 per day *Isolated HIT:* 5 mg × 2 per day until platelet count normalized	None
Dabigatran[a]	Direct thrombin inhibitor	PO	Renal (12–17 h)	*HITT:* 150 mg × 2 per day, after >5 days of treatment with a parenteral nonheparin anticoagulant *Isolated HIT:* 150 mg × 2 per day until platelet count normalized	None

Rivaroxaban[a]	Direct factor Xa inhibitor	PO	Renal (5–9 h)	*HITT:* 15 mg × 2 per day × 3 weeks, then 20 mg × 1 per day *Isolated HIT:* 15 mg × 2 per day until platelet count normalized	None

HITT acute HIT complicated by thrombosis, *Isolated HIT* acute HIT without thrombosis

[a]Dosing for treatment of acute HIT is not well established. Suggested dosing is extrapolated from venous thromboembolism and based on limited published experience in HIT

Cardiovascular Surgery

In patients with acute or subacute HIT, a feasible cardiovascular surgery should be postponed until HIT antibodies are undetectable. However, if delaying surgery is not feasible, multiple approaches have been proposed. Heparin should be avoided preoperative and postoperatively, while intraoperatively the following options can be considered:

- Perform plasmapheresis preoperatively and use heparin intraoperatively.
- Administer high-dose IVIG preoperatively and use heparin intraoperatively.
- Use nonheparin agent such as bivalirudin intraoperatively.
- Coadminister epoprostenol with heparin intraoperatively.

In patients with remote history of HIT who require cardiovascular surgery, the American Society of Hematology panel recommends use of intraoperative anticoagulation with heparin rather than a nonheparin anticoagulation [8, 11]. Exposure, however, needs to be limited to intraoperative period, and close monitoring of platelet count following surgery is important.

Duration of Anticoagulation

In patients with acute HIT associated with thrombosis, a minimum of 3 months of anticoagulation with nonheparin anticoagulant is recommended. However, duration of anticoagulant use is unclear in patients with isolated HIT without thrombosis. Continuation of anticoagulants until normalization of platelet count (above 150×10^9/L) or 30 days after exposure to heparin is most recommended if risk factors for thrombosis are present [2, 11].

Reexposure to Heparin

Risk of thrombosis is highest within first 3 months of diagnosis of HIT; hence, heparin containing products should be strongly avoided during this period. In cases of remote HIT, heparin containing products are still recommended to be avoided, even if the risk of HIT is similar to heparin naïve patient, recurrence of HIT remains a possibility [1].

Caveats

- Any patient on heparin or recent exposure to heparin with thrombocytopenia should be evaluated for HIT, but confirmation with platelet activating assays is important to prevent overdiagnosis.
- Scoring system such as 4T score is used to calculate the pretest probability of HIT. Intermediate/high probability of HIT should be followed by immunoassay, which when positive is confirmed by functional assay.
- Prompt treatment should be initiated when there is intermediate or high probability of HIT while awaiting laboratory results.
- Two main steps in management are holding all heparin containing products and starting nonheparin anticoagulant.

Questions

1. 70-year-old man is being evaluated in the hospital for new onset thrombocytopenia. He was admitted to the same hospital 3 weeks ago for *coronary artery bypass graft surgery* following which he was discharged home. 30 h ago he presented to the ER for new onset chest pain, CT angiography confirmed right segmental pulmonary embolism. He was immediately started on therapeutic dose low molecular weight heparin. His other medications include aspirin, clopidogrel, metoprolol, lisinopril, furosemide and atorvastatin.

On examination he appears comfortable, on room air. Sternotomy scar is healing well. CBC today showed Hb 10.8 g/dl (11 g/dl on arrival), WBC count 12×10^9/L (10×10^9/L on arrival) and platelet count 90×10^9/L (250×10^9/L on arrival). Renal and hepatic function are within normal limits.

Peripheral smear appears normal. 4-T score is 5, consistent with intermediate risk for HIT. Immunoassay for PF4 antibodies have been ordered.

Which of the following would you like to do next?

A. Stop LMWH and start Rivaroxaban!
B. Stop LMWH, start Argatroban and coumadin.
C. Continue LMWH until the results of immunoassay for PF4/heparin antibody is back.
D. Stop LMWH and insert inferior vena cava filter.
E. Discontinue LMWH, aspirin and clopidogrel.

Answer: A.

2. 62-year-old female comes to your office for follow up after being diagnosed with HIT following right knee arthroplasty 1 month ago.

   During her hospitalization, she was found to have new onset thrombocytopenia 7 days after her surgery, consulting hematology team ordered PF4/heparin antibodies which were positive with an OD of 1.8. Subsequently serotonin release assay was also positive confirming HIT. Screening lower extremity venous duplex showed a right popliteal DVT. She was initially started on Argatroban during the hospitalization and switched to rivaroxaban at discharge.

   She has recovered well from her surgery, with minimal pain. On physical examination she has a well healed scar in the right knee with no lower extremity edema.

   She has been compliant with rivaroxaban. You repeat immunoassay for PF4/heparin antibody, and it is negative. She is eager to know how long she needs to be on rivaroxaban. Your answer would be:

A. Lifelong anticoagulation
B. She can stop now since the immunoassay was negative.
C. 3 months total anticoagulation
D. observation

Answer: C.

References

1. Warkentin TE. HIT paradigms and paradoxes. J Thromb Haemost. 2011;9(Suppl1):105–17.https://doi.org/10.1111/j.1538-7836.2011.04322.x. PMID: 21781246.
2. Cuker A, Cines DB. How I treat heparin-induced thrombocytopenia. Blood. 2012;119(10):2209–18. Epub 2012 Jan 13. PMID: 22246036.
3. Warkentin TE, Sheppard JA, Sigouin CS, Kohlmann T, Eichler P, Greinacher A. Gender imbalance and risk factor interactions in heparin-induced thrombocytopenia. Blood. 2006;108(9):2937–41. Epub 2006 Jul 20. PMID: 16857993.
4. Ahmed I, Majeed A, Powell R. Heparin induced thrombocytopenia: diagnosis and management update. Postgrad Med J. 2007;83(983):575–82. PMID: 17823223; PMCID: PMC2600013.
5. Chong BH. Heparin-induced thrombocytopenia. J Thromb Haemost. 2003;1(7):1471–8. PMID: 12871282.
6. Chong BH, Grace CS, Rosenberg MC. Heparin-induced thrombocytopenia: effects of heparin platelet antibody on platelets. Br J Haem. 1981;49:531–40.
7. Perdomo J, Leung HHL, Ahmadi Z, Yan F, Chong JJH, Passam FH, Chong BH. Neutrophil activation and NETosis are the major drivers of thrombosis in heparin-induced thrombocytopenia. Nat Commun. 2019;10(1):1322. PMID: 30899022; PMCID: PMC6428879.
8. Warkentin TE. Heparin-induced thrombocytopenia: pathogenesis and management. Br J Haematol. 2003;121(4):535–55. PMID: 12752095.
9. Lo GK, Juhl D, Warkentin TE, Sigouin CS, Eichler P, Greinacher A. Evaluation of pretest clinical score (4 T's) for the diagnosis of heparin-induced thrombocytopenia in two clinical settings. J Thromb Haemost. 2006;4(4):759–65. PMID: 16634744.

10. Warkentin TE. How I diagnose and manage HIT. Hematology Am Soc Hematol Educ Program. 2011;2011:143–9. PMID: 22160026.
11. Cuker A, Arepally GM, Chong BH, Cines DB, Greinacher A, Gruel Y, Linkins LA, Rodner SB, Selleng S, Warkentin TE, Wex A, Mustafa RA, Morgan RL, Santesso N. American Society of Hematology 2018 guidelines for management of venous thromboembolism: heparin-induced thrombocytopenia. Blood Adv. 2018;2(22):3360–92. PMID: 30482768; PMCID: PMC6258919.
12. Warkentin TE, Kelton JG. A 14-year study of heparin-induced thrombocytopenia. Am J Med. 1996;101(5):502–7. PMID: 8948273.

Thrombotic Thrombocytopenic Purpura/ Hemolytic-Uremic Syndrome/Atypical Hemolytic-Uremic Syndrome

28

Humaira Sarfraz, Akriti Jain,
and Loveleen Kang

Thrombotic Thrombocytopenic Purpura

Introduction

Thrombotic thrombocytopenic purpura (TTP) is a potentially fatal disorder characterized by acute episodes of systemic microvascular thrombosis and is associated with the presence of a severe deficiency of a disintegrin and metalloproteinase with thrombospondin motif member 13 (ADAMTS13) (activity <10%). ADAMTS13 deficiency is the only specific marker for TTP which can be acquired when autoantibodies to ADAMTS13, as demonstrated by positive anti-ADAMTS13 IgG identified in

H. Sarfraz (✉) · A. Jain
Department of Hematology/Oncology, Moffitt Cancer Center/University of South Florida, Tampa, FL, USA
e-mail: humaira.sarfraz@moffitt.org

L. Kang
Department of Pathology and Laboratory Medicine, James A. Haley, Veterans' Hospital, Tampa, FL, USA

L. Sokol, L. Zhang (eds.), *Non-Neoplastic Hematologic Disorders*,
https://doi.org/10.1007/978-3-031-62373-8_28

~75% of acute phase TTP or inherited (Upshaw-Schulman syndrome [USS]) [1]. The annual prevalence of TTP is ~10 cases/million people and an annual incidence of ~1–13 new case/million people [1]. Peak incidence is between 30 and 50 years for acquired form. Congenital forms are seen in children. Predisposing factors include higher rates in women and African American race, HLA DR1*11, and obesity [1]. Precipitating factors to increase Von Willebrand Factor (VWF) levels are inflammation, pregnancy, infections [1].

Clinical Findings

1. Microangiopathic hemolytic anemia with thrombocytopenia (platelets <30k classically) is noted.
2. Patients often present with petechias, weakness, and dyspnea or symptoms related to organ ischemia/infarction. In patients with brain infarction, they have neurologic symptoms at presentation, ranging from headache and confusion to seizures, stroke, and coma. Patients with myocardial ischemia or mesenteric ischemia attack may manifest with abdominal pain and sometimes diarrhea
3. ADAMTS13 deficiency with levels <10%.
4. Patients with acquired TTP show either an inhibitor to ADAMTS13 or ADAMTS13 immunoglobulin G (IgG) autoantibody.

Pathogenesis

Normally, the ultralarge multimers of VWF secreted from endothelial cells are cleaved by ADAMTS13 and then circulate as normal sized multimers in the blood. However, in TTP, due to the deficiency of ADAMTS13, the ultralarge multimers of VWF secreted from endothelial cells are not broken down and aggregate with platelets to cause microvascular thrombosis. This subsequently leads to the appearance of schistocytes in the peripheral blood and tissue ischemia.

Diagnosis

TTP is one of the hematological emergencies requiring prompt diagnosis and management to prevent complications and mortality. Diagnostic algorithm is proposed in Fig. 28.1.

Key lab findings:

I. Complete blood differential with normocytic/macrocytic anemia with markers consistent with hemolysis including high LDH, indirect bilirubin, AST, low haptoglobin, and high reticulocyte count. Peripheral smear with schistocytes more than or equal to 2 per high power field.
II. Thrombocytopenia with platelet count typically less than 30×10^9/L.
III. Coagulation profile usually shows normal INR, PTT, and fibrinogen levels.
IV. Kidney function is usually not impaired. If serum creatinine >2 mg/dl, aHUS should be considered; however, it must be

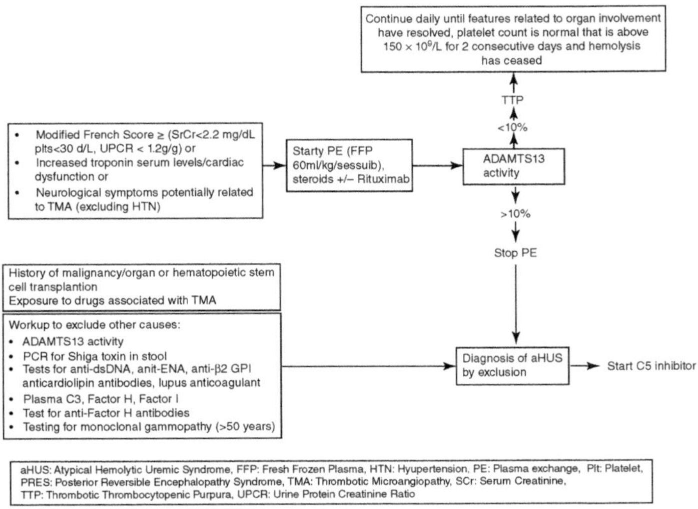

Fig. 28.1 Diagnostic algorithm for TTP

noted that acute renal failure does not exclude TTP as a diagnosis as acute kidney injury can occur in about 10–27% of patients with severe TTP (laboratory study confirmed ADAMTS13 activity <10%)

V. Evaluate for secondary etiologies as mentioned in potential differentials below.

VI. Deficiency of ADAMTS13 with levels less than 10% are confirmatory for TTP. While this test must be sent prior to initiation of treatment, we do not wait for the results to initiate empiric treatment.

VII. Patients with acquired TTP can show either an ADAMTS13 inhibitor or ADAMTS13 immunoglobulin G (IgG) autoantibody.

Table 28.1 (French score) and Table 28.2 (PASMIC score) reviewed were devised to predict the likelihood of ADAMTS13 activity ≤10% (to help estimate the pretest probability and support the diagnosis of TTP) in adults with features of thrombotic microangiopathy (TMA).

Major Differential Diagnosis

1. Atypical hemolytic uremic syndrome (aHUS).
2. Shiga toxin producing E. coli HUS (STEC-HUS).
3. Drug-induced TMA:
   (a) Immune mediated mechanism: Quinine, gemcitabine, oxaliplatin, and quetiapine

Table 28.1 French score

Platelet count $<30 \times 10^9$/L	1 point
Creatinine <2.26 mg/dl	1 point
Positive ANA	1 point

Score 1 or higher sensitivity of 98.8%. However, older patients may present with higher creatinine and less profound cytopenias to 60% at age > 60 years [2]. *ANA* antinuclear antibody

Table 28.2 PLASMIC score

	Score
Platelet count <30k	1
Hemolysis (Reticulocyte>2.5%, haptoglobin undetectable or indirect bilirubin>2 mg/dL	1
Active cancer	1
History of solid organ or stem cell transplant	1
MCV < 90 fL	1
INR < 1.5	1
Creatinine<2	1

Low risk (PLASMIC Scores ≤4): Consider alternative diagnoses [3]. Intermediate risk (PLASMIC Score 5): send ADAMTS-13 testing, keep close observation, obtain expert consultation, consider plasma exchange if no other cause identified. High risk (PLASMIC Scores ≥6): send for ADAMTS-13 testing, obtain expert consultation, immediate plasma exchange

(b) Nonimmune mediated mechanism: Gemcitabine, mitomycin, vincristine, proteosome inhibitors, vascular endothelial growth factor (VEGF) inhibitors such as bevacizumab, sunitinib; hematopoietic stem cell transplantation, cyclosporine, tacrolimus, sirolimus, intravenous use of oxymorphone or oxycodone, cocaine.

4. Transplant associated TMA.
5. Coagulation mediated TMA.
6. Disseminated Intravascular coagulation (DIC)
7. Systemic cancer
8. Severe hypertension
9. Severe Vitamin B12 deficiency
10. Severe preeclampsia, eclampsia, HELP (hemolysis, elevated liver enzymes, low platelets) syndrome (may be complement mediated TMA)
11. Antiphospholipid syndrome (may be complement mediated TMA)

Specific Subtypes of TTP Cases

Obstetric TTP

Pregnancy-associated TTP is commonly seen during the second and third trimester of pregnancy. Studies show a high rate of fetal loss at approximately 40%; however, the studies are predominantly retrospective and might include a high proportion of women misdiagnosed and receiving delayed therapy for TTP. This is different when compared to obstetrical TMA (preeclampsia or hemolysis elevated liver enzymes low platelet count syndrome: HELLP syndrome). In obstetric TTP, fetal extraction does not correct TTP symptoms; thus, if fetus is normal, the pregnancy should not be interrupted, and the mother should be managed in accordance with the usual recommendations.

Idiopathic TTP Associated with Other Autoimmune Conditions

Idiopathic TTP forms have two main common features indicating the strong autoimmune background of TTP: (1) a female predominance and approximately 90% of patients positive ADAMTS13 autoantibodies during acute TTP events and (2) ~10% of such patients develop other autoantibodies (e.g., anti-dsDNA) or clinical symptoms associated with another autoimmune disease such as systemic lupus erythematosus).

HIV Associated TTP

TTP may reveal a HIV infection that needs to be promptly identified. Management is usually standard measures in TTP management along with highly active antiretroviral therapy.

Cancer and Organ Transplantation Associated TTP

In patients with malignancy, hematopoietic stem cell transplantation, or organ transplantation, where there is TMA suspicion majority of them with detectable ADAMTS13 activity at presentation. These forms of TTP are commonly seen in older individuals, no gender predilection, not the result of an immune-mediated ADAMTS13 deficiency, and pose a worse prognosis in comparison with other forms of TTP. Cancer and organ transplantation associated TTP respond poorly to plasma exchange.

Prognosis

- TTP responds to plasma exchange but is rapidly fatal if untreated.
- Mortality is 90% for untreated patients and 10–20% with treatment.
- TTP is not just an acute disease, survivors are at risk for neurocognitive deficits, cardiovascular disease including hypertension, stroke, obesity, lupus, depression, posttraumatic stress disorder, and death.

Treatment

A durable treatment response lasts at least 30 days after the discontinuation of plasma exchange. An exacerbation is defined when disease is recurrent within 30 days after treatment response has been reached, and a relapse is considered when disease is recurrent 30 days or longer after treatment response has been achieved. A refractory disease is defined when there is no treatment response by day 30 and/or no durable treatment response by day 60.

1. Plasma exchange: This should be initiated as soon as the diagnosis of TTP is suspected or established. This is performed with 1–1.5 times plasma volume daily until features related to organ involvement have resolved, platelet count is normal that is above 150×10^9/L for two consecutive days and hemolysis has ceased.
2. Administration of methylprednisolone (high dose, 10 mg/kg/day for 3 days and then 2.5 mg/kg/day) appear to be more efficacious than standard-dose treatment (1 mg/kg/day) as an adjunctive treatment to TPE in patients with newly diagnosed TTP. Subsequently, treatment with glucocorticoids could be

tapered within 30 days after the last plasma exchange. The rationale for utilization of steroids in the treatment of acquired TTP is based on the autoimmune nature of disease; however, proof regarding efficacy remains quite low.

3. Rituximab: Depletes B cells that produce antibodies: Anti-ADAMTS13 antibodies disappear, and ADAMTS13 activity levels improve by 3 months. Used in de novo TTP (upfront therapy reduces relapse rate, reduced inpatient stay). This may also be used with refractory/relapsed TTP, during remission with low ADAMTS13. Dosing: 375 mg/m^2 weekly for 4 doses but some data support lower doses or biweekly dosing.

   In patients with refractory/relapsed TTP, 80%–100% response rate noted with Rituximab.

   Low ADAMTS13 (<10%) in remission predicts relapse. Preemptive Rituximab is effective in lowering relapse rate [4].
4. Caplacizumab: nanobody that binds to A1 domain of VWF and blocks VWF-platelet interaction. Faster resolution of thrombocytopenia reduces TTP recurrence, TTP related mortality, prevents thrombotic events were noted in patients who received caplacizumab in addition to standard therapy with plasma exchange, steroids +/− immunosuppressive treatment such as Rituximab.

   Mild mucocutaneous bleeding is the major side effect (causes a VWD type phenotype).

   Attention must be paid that there was a high rate of relapse after stopping caplacizumab 30 days after the last TPE session because caplacizumab does not treat the underlying autoimmune state [5].
5. Fresh frozen plasma (FFP): For inherited TTP, Upshaw-Shulman syndrome (USS), plasma infusions can usually control clinical features. Only a small subset of patients with USS may rely on regular plasma infusions every 2–3 weeks.
6. Refractory TTP: Rituximab, immunosuppression ([IS] corticosteroids, cyclosporine, vincristine, cyclophosphamide), splenectomy.

Promising Clinical Studies

N-acetylcysteine is adopted to inhibit platelet adherence to endothelial cell-anchored soluble ultra large VWF multimers via reducing their size,

Bortezomib, a proteasome inhibitor, is used aiming to plasma cell depletion

recombinant ADAMTS13 (BAX930) is also underway (ClinicalTrials.gov identifier: NCT02216084).

Caveats

- If high clinical suspicion with high PLASMIC score, initiate PLEX promptly. Plasma exchange has drastically reduced TTP mortality from >90% to <10–20%.
- Targeted therapies such as Rituximab and Caplacizumab will further improve outcomes of acute TTP.
- ADAMTS13 in remission predicts relapse. Rituximab is effective in targeting ADAMTS13 in remission.
- TTP is not just an acute disease–survivors are at risk for neurocognitive deficits, cardiovascular disease, depression, and death.

Hemolytic-Uremic Syndrome

Clinically, there are mainly five subtypes of HUS, including typical shiga toxin-producing Escherichia coli-associated (STEC) HUS, atypical HUS due to dysregulated complements, Streptococcal pneumonia associated HUS (Sp HUS), and lastly metabolic causes of HUS.

Typical Hemolytic-Uremic Syndrome

Introduction

Typical HUS is a TMA due to Shiga toxin–producing organisms (most commonly *Escherichia coli* and *Shigella dysenteriae*). Many HUS patients usually bloody present with diarrhea, and the disease is more common in children. The greatest burden of hemolytic uremic syndrome (HUS) occurs in children <5 years of age, followed by adults >60 years old. Almost one-third of *E. coli* O157:H7 infections occur in patients 20–59 years old.

Etiology

Shiga toxin–producing organisms (most commonly *Escherichia coli* and *Shigella dysenteriae).*

Clinical findings

1. The presence of "bloody diarrhea" has historically been associated with the diagnosis of typical HUS.. The terms diarrhea "positive" or "negative" HUS have also been used historically to differentiate typical HUS and aHUS. Nonetheless, as gastrointestinal symptoms can commonly be present in patients with both aHUS and acquired TTP, in basis of clinical gastrointestinal symptoms to differentiate these two conditions is limited.
2. Hemolytic anemia with thrombocytopenia.
3. ADAMTS13 > 10% levels.

Diagnosis

Selective culture for *E. coli* O157:H7 and Shiga toxin testing, either by immunoassay following overnight broth culture or by molecular technology vs molecular testing with nucleic acid amplification testing.

Prognosis

The hematologic manifestations of STEC-HUS (typical) completely resolve usually within 1–2 weeks. The patients with recovery of renal function have favorable clinical outcome, clinical symptoms starts to resolve after hematologic improvement. The mortality rate is less than 5%, but another 5% of patients have very adverse outcome (e.g., stroke or end-stage renal disease).

Treatment

1. Aggressive fluid resuscitation.
2. Consensus recommendations against treating confirmed or suspected STEC infections (either *E. coli* O157:H7 or non-O157:H7) with antibiotics.

Atypical Hemolytic-Uremic Syndrome

Introduction

aHUS is characterized by thrombotic microangiopathy (TMA) that is associated with the dysregulation of the alternative pathway of complement secondary to complement gene mutations or dCFH (Complement Factor H) autoantibodies predominantly involving the kidney [6]. Age at diagnosis is 0.1–79.7 years with median age of diagnosis 29.3 years with female predominance.

Etiology

aHUS is likely thought to be due to the combination of rare and common complement gene mutations, also namely complement genes haplotypes, mainly homozygous *CFH-H3* and/or *CD46* GGAAC haplotypes (found in ~5% of healthy individuals), and presence of some triggers (e.g., pregnancy or infection).

Novel Findings

Atypical hemolytic uremic syndrome has pleomorphic manifestations including:

I. Microangiopathic hemolytic anemia, hemolytic anemia with thrombocytopenia and/orvenous thromboembolism.
II. CNS manifestations including stroke, seizures, vision problems, confusion, and headache.
III. Cardiovascular manifestations including malignant hypertension, myocardial infarction, peripheral ischemia, and cardiomyopathy. Hypertensive emergency complicates half of the aHUS cases. Table 28.3 reviews distinguishing features for aHUS in comparison to other hypertensive emergencies.
IV. GI manifestations including diarrhea, colitis, GI bleeding, transaminitis, and pancreatitis.
V. Pulmonary manifestations including pulmonary hemorrhage and pulmonary edema.

Table 28.3 Proposed features with variable weighting that help distinguish aHUS from other causes of hypertensive emergencies. These features may be used to calculate a score; the higher the score, the higher the probability of aHUS. The higher the score, the higher the probability of aHUS complicated by hypertensive emergency [6]

Features selected to distinguish aHUS from other etiologies of hypertensive emergency	Score
At diagnosis	
Female	+1
Age < 45 years	+1
Family history of atypical aHUS	+4
Absence of hypertension or of anti-hypertensive drug use(cessation)	+1
Absence of left ventricular hypertrophy. Requirement for dialysis	+1
Rapid (<48 h) resolution of hematological TMA after strict BP control	−2
Low C3 plasma level	+2
During follow up	
Free of thrombi in glomeruli in kidney biopsy	−2
Persistent low C3, factor H and/or factor I plasma levels	+3

VI. Renal complications with acute kidney injury with 50–75% patients requiring acute dialysis.
VII. ADAMTS13 > 10% levels

Pathogenesis

Triggers for atypical HUS include inflammation, surgery, pregnancy, and autoimmunity. The genetic variants mostly have incomplete penetration and aHUS is frequently a two-hit disease. CFH mutation is the most frequent mutation identified with aHUS but 30–50% patients do not have an identifiable mutation. However, these results can take weeks to months and do not guide initial treatment (Fig. 28.2).

Diagnosis

1. Hemolysis and thrombocytopenia.
2. ADAMTS13 > 10% levels.

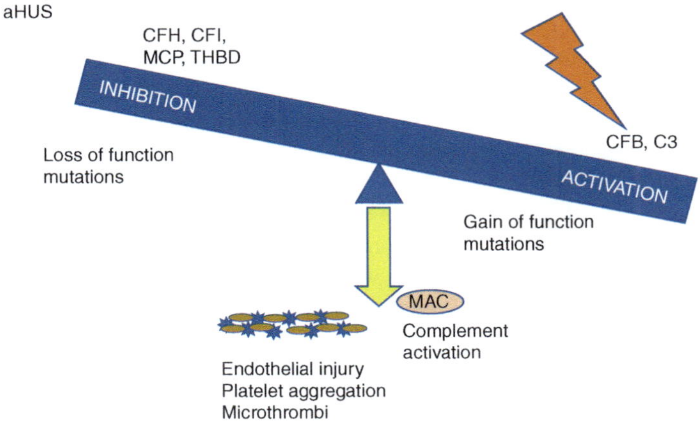

Fig. 28.2 Pathogenesis of TTP

3. Genetic mutation testing: While this does not guide initial treatment, patients with complement mutations have higher risk of relapse and hence warrant closer monitoring when considering cessation of treatment. Along-term therapy with eculizumab should be considered in aHUS with confirmed gene mutation. The panel of candidate genes used for diagnosis of aHUS should include CFH, CD46, CFI, C3, CFB, and diacylglycerol kinase ε (*DGKε*) genes.
4. Normal plasma levels of C3, C4, and complement factors do not exclude the diagnosis of complement mediated TMA.

Prognosis

aHUS genetic mutations CFH, CD46, CFI, C3, CFB, and diacylglycerol kinase ε (*DGKε*) genes predict higher probability of relapse.

Treatment

1. Eculizumab (anti-C5 monoclonal antibody): Induction: 900 mg weekly for four doses; maintenance: 1200 mg at week 5 and every 2 weeks thereafter [7].
2. Ravulizumab (long acting C5 inhibitor): administered every 8 weeks. Annual cost of maintenance is lower with ravulizumab compared to eculizumab, but cost is higher in first year. Efficacy and side effect profile are similar [8].

   - This leads to an improvement in platelet function and considerable time dependent improvement in renal function.
   - The risk of meningococcal infection is significantly increased and vaccination is important. However, vaccination is not fully protective in patients with anti-C5 antibodies. Therefore, prophylactic antibiotics (mostly phenoxymethylpenicillin) should be started and continued for 2 months after drug has been discontinued in these patients.

- Both these medications are safe in pregnancy and should be continued during pregnancy given that pregnancy is also identified as a potential trigger for aHUS.

Response Assessment

The median time for platelet count recovery occur 10 days after given C5 blockade. Response to C5 blockade is based on a platelet count normalization, LDH level decrease <2 folds over the upper limit of normal, and a decrease in serum creatinine of >20% or exchange from dialysis after 10 days of treatment initiation.

In the absence of response by day 10, aHUS diagnosis should be reconsidered and complement inhibition should be reevaluated and kidney biopsy should be considered. This would aid exclude other differentials such as lupus nephritis, C3 glomerulopathy, cryoglobulinemic glomerulonephritis, IgA nephropathy, and irreversible kidney fibrosis.

Maintenance therapy using anti-C5 treatment routinely lasts for at least 3–6 months after the acute phase of aHUS until the kidney function has plateaued. The goal trough level for eculizumab is >100–150 μg/L, to maintain optimal complement blockade in case of superimposed infections or other complement activation triggers. If trough level measurement is not available, CH50 (<20%) can be used as a marker for circulating eculizumab levels.

Discontinuation of Therapy

Discontinuation of therapy is considered if:

- The thrombotic microangiopathy has resolved and renal function has normalized, or new baseline has been achieved.
- No active triggers (complement amplifying condition identified).
- Closer monitoring of labs is possible.

The relapse rate is 20–30% prompting retreatment salvaged patients without further impairment in renal function. However, the relapse rate may be higher in patients with complement mutations:

- CFH variant: 72% (8/11)
- MCP variant: 50% (4/8)
- No variants: 0% (0/16)

Plasma exchange is recommended only if the modified French score (or PLASMIC score) is highly suggestive (≥2) of ADAMTS13 deficiency and/or if the patient has severe extrarenal manifestations, mainly neurological and cardiac. Plasma-based therapies theoretically could help not only via the replacement of normal levels of CFH, CFI, factor B, and C3, but also via the removal of mutated complement factors and CFH autoantibodies via plasma exchange.

In patients unable to achieve a hematologic response or renal improvement with plasma exchange over the first 3–5 days, the pretreatment ADAMTS13 activity provides valuable information for determining the next most appropriate course of therapy. Severely deficient pretreatment ADAMTS13 activity would confirm the diagnosis of acquired TTP and would be an indication for the addition or intensification of immune-suppressive therapy. However, the finding of pretreatment ADAMTS13 activity that was not severely deficient, in a patient not responding to plasma exchange, would be more consistent with a diagnosis of aHUS. In the absence of an alternative clinical explanation for their TMA (sepsis, malignancy, and autoimmune disorder), plasma exchange should be discontinued and therapy with eculizumab should be considered.

Caveats

- aHUS is caused by dysregulation of complement and 40–60% of patients harbor complement gene mutations.
- A trigger such as infection, surgery, or pregnancy is often identified.

- Terminal complement inhibition with a C5 inhibitor (eculizumab or ravulizumab) is the standard of care.
- C5 inhibition carries the risk of meningococcal infection (vaccination!)

Board Question

1. 27-year-old African American female who delivered a healthy infant at 37 weeks gestation was readmitted 5 days after discharge with fatigue, diarrhea, and generalized weakness. Her blood pressure was elevated at 170/90. Laboratory testing was significant for acute kidney injury with creatinine 3.6 mg/dl, thrombocytopenia with platelet counts 96, microangiopathic hemolytic anemia (hemoglobin 8.4 g/dL, LDH 3 times upper limit of normal, undetectable haptoglobin and schistocytes on the peripheral smear.

   What is the best next step in management?

A. Collect ADAMTS13 levels and await results before finalizing management plan.
B. Collect ADAMTS13 levels and initiate plasma exchange.
C. Collect ADAMTS13 levels and initiate eculizumab.
D. Collect ADAMTS13 levels, awaits results and start phenoxymethylpencillin

Answer: C

2. Which of the following must be administered prior to initiation of eculizumab?

   A. quadrivalent A, C, W, and Y conjugate
   B. quadrivalent A, C, W, and Y conjugate and B meningococcal vaccines
   C. prophylaxis with methylpenicillin
   D. B and C

Answer: D

References

1. Joly BS, Veyradier A. Thrombotic thrombocytopenic purpura. Blood. 2017;129(21):2836–46.
2. Coppo P, Schwarzinger M, Buffet M, French reference center for thrombotic microangiopathies, et al. Predictive features of severe acquired ADAMTS13 deficiency in idiopathic thrombotic microangiopathies: the French TMA reference center experience. PLoS One. 2010;5(4):e10208. PMID: 20436664.
3. Bendapudi PK, Hurwitz S, Fry A, et al. Derivation and external validation of the PLASMIC score for rapid assessment of adults with thrombotic microangiopathies: a cohort study. Lancet Haematol. 2017;4(4):e157–64. Epub 2017 Mar 2. PMID: 28259520.
4. Page EE, Kremer Hovinga JA, Terrell DR, et al. Rituximab reduces risk for relapse in patients with thrombotic thrombocytopenic purpura. Blood. 2016;127(24):3092–4. Epub 2016 Apr 8. PMID: 27060171.
5. Scully M, Cataland SR, Peyvandi F, et al. Caplacizumab treatment for acquired thrombotic thrombocytopenic purpura. N Engl J Med. 2019;380(4):335–46. PMID: 30625070.
6. Fakhouri F, Schwotzer N, Frémeaux-Bacchi V. How I diagnose and treat atypical hemolytic uremic syndrome. Blood. 2023;141(9):984–95. PMID: 36322940.
7. Legendre CM, Licht C, Muus P, et al. Terminal complement inhibitor eculizumab in atypical hemolytic-uremic syndrome. N Engl J Med. 2013;368(23):2169–81. PMID: 23738544.
8. Dixon DP, Madris-Aris AD, Adams B, et al. Two-year efficacy and safety of ravulizumab in adults and children with atypical hemolytic uremic syndrome (aHUS): analysis of two phase 3 studies. Blood. 2021;138(Supplement 1):769.

Part IV

Bleeding Disorders

29 Hemophilia A and B

Khine Swe Shan, Nyein Thaw Dar,
and Manuel Martinez-Rio

Introduction

Hemophilia A and B are X-linked recessive bleeding disorders caused by inherited genetic mutations of the factor VIII (FVIII) and factor IX (FIX) genes on the X chromosome. However, 30% of hemophilia A and B are from sporadic mutations. Hemophilia comprises about 95% of inherited bleeding disorders. More than 1.2 million people worldwide are affected, mostly males because of their hemizygous state, but moderate-to-severe deficiencies can also be observed among females, resulting from extreme lyonization, Turner's syndrome, or homozygosity from both parents.

Determined by the level of the factor activity, the intensity of hemophilia A and B is categorized into mild (5–10%), moderate (1–4%), and severe (<1%), and clinical features vary from traumatic bleeding to spontaneous joint bleeding. Based on data from the Centers for Disease Control and Prevention, the median age of diagnosis for mild, moderate, and severe disease is 36 months, 8 months, and 1 month, respectively.

K. S. Shan (✉) · N. T. Dar · M. Martinez-Rio
Memorial Health Care, Memorial Cancer Institute, Hollywood, FL, USA
e-mail: KShan@mhs.net

L. Sokol, L. Zhang (eds.), *Non-Neoplastic Hematologic Disorders*,
https://doi.org/10.1007/978-3-031-62373-8_29

Pathogenesis

Hemophilia A has been associated with over 2100 mutations of the FVIII gene, with the most common mutation being an intron 22 inversion. The severity of the disease is influenced by genetic mutation types such as deletions, inversion, and missense mutations, resulting in functional defects, protein misfolding, and the impaired assembly of the FIXa and FVIIIa complexes. The complete lack of the intracellular membrane lectin ERGIC-53 causes an impaired secretion of both factor V and VIII. Mutations in the FVIII binding domain of the von Willebrand Factor (vWF) result in impaired clot-formation complex assembly.

Hemophilia B (Christmas disease) has been associated with over 1100 mutations of the FIX gene with the most common being missense mutations; however, nonsense and splicing mutations, large deletions, and even duplication of the FIX gene have caused hemophilia B.

The deficiency of FVIII or FIX impairs thrombin production and affects clot stability by interfering with fibrin cross linkage and decreasing thrombin-induced fibrinolysis inhibitor production.

Diagnosis

Patients present with mucocutaneous, deep tissue, or joint bleeding depending on the severity of the deficiency of factor VIII/IX levels. In severe cases, infants may experience excessive bleeding from venipuncture sites, increased bruising, joint or muscle hemorrhage with activity, or occasionally intracranial hemorrhage. Mild disease usually presents with traumatic bleeding rather than spontaneous bleeding.

Prenatal screening and chorionic villous biopsy should be performed on all carriers or patients with a family history of hemophilia. Since the factor IX level may be low in the neonatal period, screening and biopsy should be repeated in 6–12 months after birth before making diagnosing hemophilia B.

Initial evaluation begins with a detailed personal and family history of increased bleeding, thorough physical examination, and initial laboratory testing with platelet count, prothrombin time (PT), and activated partial thromboplastin time (aPTT). In most cases, aPTT is elevated and a mixing study is required to differentiate between hemophilia (aPTT is corrected in mixing study) and acquired hemophilia caused by the presence of inhibitors (aPTT is not corrected). Specific factor assays are needed to identify the deficient clotting factor. If clinical presentation is highly suspicious for hemophilia, factor assays can be ordered as part of the initial laboratory testing. The diagnosis of hemophilia A or B requires <40% of normal activity. If the activity level is ≥40%, confirmation with gene mutation studies is required. Since factor VIII is an acute phase reactant, it may be falsely elevated in the setting of acute inflammation.

Differential Diagnosis

Diagnosis of hemophilia A or B needs to be distinguished from other bleeding disorders with prolonged aPTT such as acquired factor deficiencies secondary to autoantibodies to factor VIII and Von Willebrand Disease (vWD). Acquired factor inhibitors are common in adulthood, and the aPTT will not correct with mixing studies. In vWD, patients may present with a normal or prolonged aPTT and decreased FVIII levels. However, clinically, the bleeding pattern is more mucosal than joint bleeding as is frequently observed in hemophilia. In vWD, there will be normal FVIII with low vWF antigen (vWF:Ag) and low vWF activity. The exception is vWD 2N type, a rare disease, which has a low factor VIII with normal multimers and behaves similarly to hemophilia A. Type lll vWD is rare with an undetectable factor VIII/vWF and multimer levels.

Prognosis

Patients with mild-to-moderate disease can have a good quality of life with a normal life expectancy. According to the Centers for Disease Control and Prevention in 2013, "in severe hemophilia (<1%) with appropriate primary prophylaxis initiated during childhood, average lifetime is near normal." Using prophylactic factor replacement reduces the risk of recurrent hemarthrosis. The development of inhibitors occurs in about 30% of hemophilia A and is associated with a poor prognosis. The morbidity depends on the frequency and severity of bleeding events which can lead to permanent disabilities.

Treatment

Prophylactic factor replacement is given as primary prophylaxis in severe hemophilia (<1%). Secondary prophylaxis is given after more than one episode of bleeding to prevent the development of joint damage, especially in those with severe disease who were not started on primary prophylaxis. Intermittent prophylaxis can be used for patients with mild-to-moderate disease and no prior bleeding. This is individualized based on factor level and physical activity and can be used in specific circumstances such as procedures or high-impact activities. The SPINART trial compared routine prophylaxis vs on-demand treatment of adults with severe hemophilia A. The trial demonstrated better joint function and better health-related quality of life and reduced median annualized joint-bleeding events in the prophylaxis group compared to on-demand recombinant FVIII use [1].

For primary prophylaxis, the target goal is to keep the trough-factor level between 1% and 2%. In on-demand therapy, the target goal is 30–40% in mild bleeding episodes or minor surgery; 80–100% for severe bleeding or major surgery; 20–40% postoperatively and 50% for invasive dental procedures. Treatment is usually continued until the bleeding event stops and healing occurs. The levels should be maintained for at least 3–5 days.

The choice of the factor concentrate may be from plasma derived or genetically engineered recombinant products. This depends on availability, cost, manufacturing method, and duration of half-life. Half-lives of the factor products can be prolonged by a 1.5-fold in factor VIII and 4- to 5-fold in factor IX by Fc-fusion or albumin-fusion technologies, e.g., factor VIII (BDD)-FC (Eloctate), factor IX-FC (Alprolix), factor IX albumin–infused product (Idelvion) [2]. These extended half-life products have the advantage of decreasing the frequency of administration while maintaining therapeutic factor levels.

A major complication of factor replacement therapy is the formation of inhibitors, measured in Bethesda units, which interfere with factor replacement therapy and the ability to achieve adequate levels needed for hemostasis. Inhibitors develop in up to 35% of hemophilia A and 13% of hemophilia B, and this risk is higher among cases of major gene defects, with the use of recombinant replacement therapy, and in minority (Hispanic/Latino) population. Immune-tolerance induction therapy with frequent infusion of FVIII/IX daily overtime with the goal of inducing peripheral tolerance has shown promise in overcoming inhibitor resistance.

Other strategies for managing hemophilia include using bypassing agents such as FVIII inhibitor bypass activity, activated prothrombin complex concentrates, and recombinant factor VIIa (Novo Seven). Nonfactor replacement therapies include emicizumab, desmopressin (DDAVP), and antifibrinolytic agents such as aminocaproic acid (Amicar). Emicizumab is a recombinant humanized bispecific monoclonal antibody that binds to the factors IX and X, acting as a substitute for the role of FVIII in the tenase complex of hemostasis. It was FDA approved for treating hemophilia A patients with or without inhibitors [3, 4]. DDAVP is a synthetic analog of vasopressin that promotes the release of FVIII and vWF from platelet storage granules and endothelial cells. This can be used for patients with mild hemophilia for minor cuts, mucosal bleeding, or before minimally invasive procedures. A test dose of DDAVP needs to be performed to evaluate its efficacy, and it cannot be used in hemophilia B patients because FIX is not present in storage pools [5].

Patients with hemophilia are advised to avoid contact sports including the American football and basketball because of inherent intracranial bleed which has high mortality (60%) despite the treatment with factor replacement therapy

Specific situations	
Dental extraction	One dose of factor concentrate to bring the level to 50% before the procedure or antifibrinolytic therapy (first dose 4 h before the procedure followed by therapy for the next 5 days)
Biopsy	50% before the procedure
Epidural anesthesia	50% before the procedure
Postpartum phase	Infusion of factor concentrate on days 3, 4, and 5 following delivery (factor VIII is an acute-phase reactant which increases during pregnancy and precipitously drops in the immediate postpartum period)
Acute hemarthrosis	1–2 days of factor (to achieve 25%)
Intramuscular hematoma	Patients with intramuscular hematoma may need a longer duration (even up to 15 days) of therapy
Major surgical procedures	Factor level to 100% before the procedure and maintain this level for the next 5 days
Intracranial bleed	Factor level kept at 100% until a response in the neurological status

Promising Clinical Studies

Gene therapy—The basic principle of gene therapy is the transduction of selected genes into target cells by injecting artificially designed segments of DNA on an adeno-associated virus (AAV) vector to incorporate genetic material into target tissues or cells, primarily the liver (construct carrying vectors). The duration of effect, hepatic toxicity, genetic integration and development of oncogenes, toxicity, and immunity to vector and vector transmission are all current challenges to this type of gene therapy.

For hemophilia A, valoctocogene roxaparvovec (Roctavian) was conditionally approved by the European Medicines Agency to use in severe hemophilia A without inhibitors and without immunity to adeno-associated viral serotype in the European Union in 2022 [6]. SPK-8011 with AAV-LK3 vector carrying a liver-specific promoter and a codon-optimized B domain deleted F8 gene and Giroctocogene fitelparvovec (formerly SB-525) are still under investigation. For hemophilia B, Verbrinacogene setparvovec (formerly FLT 180a), Fidanacogene elaparvovec (formerly SPK-9001), and Etranacogene dezaparvovec (formerly AMT-061) have been under investigation. Etranacogene dezaparvovec (Hemgenix) was approved by the FDA in 2022 [7].

Efanesoctocog alfa is a new class of factor VIII replacement therapy designed to decouple the recombinant factor VIII from endogenous VWF and overcome the VWF-imposed half-life ceiling. In a trial of 133 patients with severe hemophilia A, the median annualized bleeding rate was 0 (interquartile range, 0–1.04) with Efanesoctocog alfa.

Other investigational approaches include cellular therapies such as the implantation of autologous dermal fibroblasts or bone marrow cells and transplantation of liver sinusoidal endothelial cells from donor or polymer-encapsulated human cells. In addition, anti-tissue factor pathway inhibitor therapies (anti-TFPI) such as concizumab and fitusiran (siRNA that targets antithrombin for degradation in liver cells to enhance thrombin generation and increase fibrin clot formation) are also promising approaches for hemophilia treatment [8].

Caveats

- About 5–10% of patients with severe hemophilia (<1%) do not bleed because of the associated coinheritance of hypercoagulable states (factor V Leiden/prothrombin gene mutation).
- If patients on prophylactic therapy fail to respond (with recurrent mucosal bleeding or hemarthrosis), allo-immunization with factor VIII inhibitor should be suspected and appropriate tests should be done to exclude this complication.
- Patients receiving bispecific antibody (emicizumab) should not receive factor VIII bypassing agent because of the associated prothrombotic effects.

- Antifibrinolytic agents including tranexamic acid and aminocaproic acid are not indicated for patients with frank hematuria because of *clot colic* in the urothelial tract.
- Osteoarthrosis is a late complication of hemophilic arthropathy which may need surgical intervention.

Questions

1. A 52-year-old female with a history of uterine fibroids presented to her primary care clinic to have a pre-operative assessment for an elective hysterectomy. She was healthy and denied a history of bleeding disorder, but she does not know her family history because she was adopted. The physical examination was unremarkable. Laboratory tests showed normal complete blood count, comprehensive metabolic panel, and prothrombin time test/international normalized ratio but prolonged aPTT at 58 s. A repeated aPTT in 1 week showed 52 s. What would be the next step in management?

   A. Recommend proceeding with the surgery as aPTT is slightly prolonged in adult age.
   B. Check a mixing study, factor 8, factor 9, factor 11, and factor 13 screening assays to know the activity level of coagulation factors.
   C. Check a mixing study and phospholipid syndrome panel.
   D. Recommend against hysterectomy procedure as she is post menopause and risks outweigh benefits.

   Answer: C. In the setting of prolonged aPTT, one should rule out the presence of factors inhibitors (acquired hemophilia) which is common among adult patients and is commonly associated with antiphospholipid syndrome that is more prone to clotting rather than bleeding.

2. A 23-year-old female with a history of systemic lupus erythematosus presented to the emergency department with generalized weakness, dyspnea on exertion, and heavy menstrual periods. Her maternal uncle had a bleeding problem, however,

she did not know which type. She never had any trauma or a major surgical procedure. On examination, she had bruises on her lower extremities and pallor on eyes and lips. Testing showed hemoglobin was 7 g/dL, MCV 77, platelets 149,000, WBC 9000, PT 12 s, international normalized ratio 1.0, aPTT 48 s, and a normal liver function test. aPTT improved to 28 s upon mixing with normal serum; factor VIII activity was 41%; factor IX activity was normal range; and vWD panel was normal. What would be the next step in management?

A. Transfuse whole blood
B. Transfuse factor 7 concentrate
C. Fresh frozen plasma
D. Tranexamic acid

Answer: D. Patient has mild deficiency of FVIII activity (41%) and anemia which is likely caused by heavy menstrual blood loss. The bleeding can be controlled with tranexamic acid. Skin bruises can be seen in mild disease. B and C can be used in severe bleeding and severe disease.

References

1. Manco-Johnson MJ, Lundin B, et al. Effect of late prophylaxis in hemophilia on joint status: a randomized trial. J Thromb Haemost. 2017;15(11):2115–24.
2. Mitragotri S, Burke PA, Langer R. Overcoming the challenges in administering biopharmaceuticals: formulation and delivery strategies. Nat Rev Drug Discov. 2014;13(9):655–72.
3. Oldenburg J, Mahlangu J, Kim B, et al. Emicizumab prophylaxis in hemophilia A with inhibitors. N Engl J Med. 2017;377:809–18.
4. Mahlangu J, Oldenburg J, Paz-Priel I, et al. Emicizumab prophylaxis in patients who have hemophilia A without inhibitors. N Engl J Med. 2018;379:811–22.
5. Nolan B, White B, Smith J, O'Reily C, Fitzpatrick B, Smith OP. Desmopressin: therapeutic limitations in children and adults with inherited coagulation disorders. Br J Haematol. 2000;109(4):865.
6. ROCTAVIAN, INN-valoctocogene roxaparvovec. European Medicines Agency. Available at: https://www.ema.europa.eu/en/documents/product-

information/roctavian-epar-product-information_en.pdf. Accessed 02 Nov 2022.
7. FDA approves first gene therapy to treat adults with hemophilia B. US Food and Drug Administration. Available at: https://content.govdelivery.com/accounts/USFDA/bulletins/3396c72. Accessed 22 November 2022.
8. Butterfield J, Hege KM, Herzog RW, Kaczmarek R. A molecular revolution in the treatment of hemophilia. Mol Ther. 2020;28(4):997–1015.

Von Willebrand Disease

30

Sanjay Bridgelall and Mandy O'Leary

Introduction

The von Willebrand disease (vWD) is the most common inherited bleeding disorder that comprises seven types of qualitative and/or quantitative inherited abnormalities of vWD. vWD has a prevalence of approximately 1:100. Normally, von Willebrand factor (vWF) plays a role in primary hemostasis by mediating platelet adhesion (via the GP1b receptor) to exposed collagen at the site of vascular injury and secondarily serves as a protective transporter of factor VIII (the von Willebrand multimer carries receptors for platelet glycoprotein and factor VIII antigen). Without vWF, factor VIII is rapidly cleared. vWF is stored in the Weibel-Palade bodies and produced by megakaryocytes. Quantitative abnormalities of vWD occur in types 1, 1C, and 3, whereas qualitative abnormalities occur in types 2A, 2B, 2M, and 2N. vWD can also be acquired and is seen as recent onset with no personal or family history of bleeding propensity. Some patients have an autosomal-dominant defect in platelet GP1b receptors that results in enhanced binding of vWF that can mimic vWD type 2B, termed platelet type vWD (Table 30.1). Type 1 vWD represents approximately 75% of all cases. Common symptoms of vWD include mucocutaneous

S. Bridgelall (✉) · M. O'Leary
USF/Moffitt Cancer Center, Tampa, FL, USA

L. Sokol, L. Zhang (eds.), *Non-Neoplastic Hematologic Disorders*,
https://doi.org/10.1007/978-3-031-62373-8_30

Table 30.1 Types, genetics, and characteristics

	Genetic inheritance	Description
vWD type 1 (quantitative)	Autosomal dominant	Quantitative decrease in vWF with preserved ratios between vWF antigen, activity, and factor VIII; normal multimer distribution
vWD type 3 (quantitative)	Autosomal recessive	Virtually complete deficiency of vWF
vWD type 2A (qualitative)	Autosomal dominant (or recessive)	Decreased platelet-dependent vWF activity with loss of high-molecular-weight multimers
vWD type 2B (qualitative)	Autosomal dominant	Increased vWF affinity for GP1b with increased platelet clearance
vWD type 2M (qualitative)	Autosomal dominant (or recessive)	Decreased vWF-dependent platelet function
vWD type 2N (qualitative)	Autosomal recessive	Markedly decreased vWF binding to factor VIII
Acquired vWD		Decreased vWF and particularly loss of high-molecular-weight multimers caused by shearing from mechanical forces, adsorption on tumors, or autoimmune inhibitor formation
Platelet type vWD	Autosomal dominant	Enhanced binding of normal vWF to platelets and in its clearance from plasma caused by a gain-of-function defect in platelet GP1b

Ag antigen, *vWD* von Willebrand disease, *vWF* von Willebrand factor

bleeding, bruising without recognizable trauma, prolonged and/recurrent nosebleeds, bleeding gums, or menorrhagia.

Pathogenesis

See Table 30.1.

Diagnosis

Screening tests for all types of vWD: complete blood count, activated partial thromboplastin time (aPTT), prothrombin time (PT), and PFA-100 (Table 30.3) [1].

Diagnostic assays for vWD (Table 30.2) [2]

vWF antigen (vWF: Ag): determines the quantity of vWF protein

- Measured by two types of assays
  - Enzyme-linked immunoabsorbance (ELISA)
  - Latex immunoassay (LIA)

FVIII activity (Table 30.3)

Table 30.2 vWF activity

Assay	Measurement	Characteristics
Ristocetin cofactor activity assay (vWF: RCo)	To measure ability of vWF to agglutinate platelets in response to ristocetin	Gold standard
vWF:GP1bR	To measure ability of patient's vWF to bind to recombinant platelet GP1b receptor; ristocetin added to enhance binding	More sensitive than vWF: RCo, automated
vWF:GP1bM	To measure ability of patient's vWF to bind to recombinant mutated GP1b receptor; ristocetin not needed because of gain-of-function mutation in recombinant GP1b	More sensitive than vWF: RCo, automated
vWF: Ab	To measure binding of specific monoclonal antibody to GP1b binding site on vWF	Automated
Collagen-binding activity assay (vWF: CB)	To measure ability of vWF to bind collagen-coated plates	

vWF von Willebrand factor

Table 30.3 Assay results [3]

	Platelet count	PT or PTT	vWF activity	vWF antigen	vWF: RCo/vWF: Ag	Factor VIII	Multimer distribution	RIPA
Type 1	Normal	Normal to prolonged	Decreased	Decreased	>0.7	Normal or decreased	Normal but decreased	Normal or decreased in severe disease
Type 2A	Normal	Normal or prolonged aPTT, normal PT	Decreased, out of proportion to decrease in VWF: Ag	Decreased	<0.7	Normal or decreased	Absent HMWM or IMWM	Decreased
Type 2B	Low to normal	Normal or prolonged aPTT, normal PT	Decreased, out of proportion to decrease in vWF: Ag	Decreased	<0.7	Normal or decreased	Absence of HMWM	Normal Increased with low-dose RIPA
Type 2M	Normal	Normal or prolonged aPTT, normal PT	Decreased vWF activity (vWFR: Co) out of proportion to decrease in vWF: Ag	Decreased	<0.7	Normal or decreased	Normal	Decrease

Type 2N	Normal	Prolonged aPTT, normal PT	Normal or decreased	Normal or decreased	>0.7	Decreased (5–15%)	Normal	Normal
Type 3	Normal	Prolonged aPTT, normal PT	Severely decreased	Severely decreased	>0.7	Severely decreased	Absence of all multimers	Absent
Acquired vWD Patterns similar to types 1, 2A, or 2B	Normal	Prolong aPTT at low FVIII activity levels	Decreased vWF activity by ristocetin cofactor activity assay (vWF: RCo) or collagen-binding activity assay (vWF: CB)	vWF antigen may be normal or decreased		Normal or decreased	Absence of HMWMs	
Platelet type vWD	Low		Decreased vWF activity by ristocetin cofactor activity assay (vWF: RCo)	Decreased	<0.7	Normal or decreased	Absence of HMWMs	Normal Increased with low-dose RIPA

aPTT activated partial thromboplastin time, *RIPA* ristocetin-induced platelet aggregation, *vWD* von Willebrand disease, *vWF* von Willebrand factor

- Measured using two types of assays
  - aPTT-based 1-stage clotting assay
  - Chromogenic factor activity assay

vWD subtyping assays (Table 30.3)

- Ristocetin-induced platelet aggregation (RIPA)
  - To measure ability of vWF to agglutinate platelets at various low concentrations of ristocetin
- Multimer analysis (Table 30.3)
  - Sodium dodecyl sulfate-agarose electrophoresis

    To assess multimers in plasma
  - Multimers are classified as high, intermediate, or low molecular weight.
- Genotyping can be used to identify mutations and can be useful for differentiating between various types of vWD

Reference intervals:

- Normal vWF antigen: 50–150%
- Normal vWF: RCo: 50–150%
- Normal vWF: CB: 50–150%
- Normal vWF multimeric analysis: normal multimeric distribution
- Normal FVIII activity: 50–150%

Major Differential Diagnosis of Each vWD Subtype

- Type 1: acquired vWD
- Type 2A:
  - Acquired vWD
  - Mild hemophilia A
  - Type 2N

- Type 2B: platelet type or pseudo-vWD–similar phenotype
- Type 2N: mild hemophilia A
- Type 3:
  - Acquired vWD
  - Hemophilia A
- Acquired vWD: vWD types 2A and 2B
- Platelet type vWD: vWD 2B

Prognosis

- vWD is an inherited bleeding disorder that varies in severity from mild to severe (type III) hemostatic disorder that can be managed acutely and prophylactically. Clinically, severe hemorrhage in vWD is largely seen with trauma or invasive procedures.

Treatment[4]

- Type 1
  - Bleeding

    Direct pressure
    Topical hemostatic agents

    - Gelatin/foam matrix
    - Topical thrombin
    - Fibrin sealants
- Antifibrinolytics
  - Tranexamic acid
  - ε-aminocaproic acid
  - Useful for minor surgical or dental procedures to prevent and/or treat bleeding

- Directly increasing VWF and FVIII
  - Desmopressin/DDVAP

    Promotes release of stored vWF with peak effects in 30–60 min
  - Estrogen

    May increase synthesis of vWF
    Decrease menorrhagia in women
  - VWF/FVIII concentrates

    For patients who do not respond to DDVAP or have adverse effects to DDVAP
    Patients undergoing major or multiple surgery
    Goal: maintain peak ratio VWF:RCo and FVIII activity levels at >100% and trough >50% until hemostasis is achieved

- Type 2
  - Increasing the level of vWF

    DDVAP challenge: Test the patients' response before therapeutic use
    Response to DDVAP: variable

    - Type 2A: often show adequate response
    - Type 2B: generally contraindicated
      - Leads to severe thrombocytopenia and bleeding
    - Type 2M: do not respond well
    - Type 2N: 2× to 9× increase in vWF and FVIII lasting approximately 3 h
- Type 3
  - VWF/FVIII concentrates

    Weight-based dosing

Infusions given every 12–24 h
Patients do not respond to desmopressin

- Acquired vWD
  - Treatment of acute bleeding

    Similar to treatment for types 1 and 2
    DDVAP and VWF/FVIII concentrates
    Antifibrinolytic

  - High-dose IVIG

    Decreases antibody response

    - Decreased clearance or decreased inhibition of vWF

    Plasmapheresis

    - Decreases antibody titer
      - Decreased clearance or decreased inhibition of vWF

    Recombinant activated factor VII (rFVIIa)

  - Treatment of underlying cause

    Antibodies

    - Treat with high-dose IVIG
    - Immunosuppressive therapy
    - Plasmapheresis

    Myeloproliferative disorders

    - Cytoreduction

    Cardiovascular abnormalities

    - Repair congenital defects
    - Valve replacement
    - Discontinue ventricular assist device (VAD) with transplant

- Platelet type vWD
  - Administration of:

    Platelet concentrates
    VWF-rich concentrates

Caveats [5]

- Patients with type O blood have approximately 30% decreased vWF levels compared to patients with blood types A and B.
- Hypothyroidism is shown to be associated with decreased vWF while inflammation increases vWF.
- In menorrhagia secondary to vWD, local measures (oral contraceptive medication intrauterine device are preferred over systemic therapy with vWF).
- Angiodysplasia of gastrointestinal tract is associated with lack of high-molecular-weight multimers in 2% of type 2B and 4.5% of type 3 vWD. vWF replacement has no significant role in controlling gastrointestinal bleeding. Vascular endothelial growth factor inhibitors have a beneficial effect with gastrointestinal bleeding caused by angiodysplasia.
- In acquired vWD—including states of hypervascularity (ventricular septal defect, severe mitral valve prolapse, or external membrane oxygenation), replacement of vWF has been shown to have minimal effect.
- vWF multimer assay is normal in type 2N/2M subtypes of VWD.

Board Question

1. Which of the follow shows a similar phenotype to von Willebrand Type 2B?

   A. von Willebrand type 1
   B. von Willebrand type 3

C. von Willebrand type 2A
D. Acquired vWD
E. Platelet type vWD

Answer: E) Platelet type vWD

Explanation: Both type 2B and platelet type vWD disease exhibit low platelets, decreased VWF activity, decreased VWF antigen, absence of HMWMS, normal or decreased FVIII activity, vWF:RCo/vWF:Ag <0.7, normal or increased response to low-dose RIPA. Modified RIPA and genetic studies can be used to distinguish between the 2 types.

2. Decreased binding to FVIII is found in which of the following?

A. von Willebrand type 1
B. von Willebrand type 2A
C. von Willebrand type 2N
D. Platelet type vWD

Answer: C) von Willebrand type 2N

Explanation: Of the above choices, vWD type 2N shows decreased FVIII binding activity. vWD type 1, vWD type 2A, and platelet type vWD can show normal FVIII activity.

3. An autosomal recessive inheritance pattern is found in which of the following?

A. von Willebrand type 1
B. von Willebrand type 3
C. Platelet type vWD
D. Acquired vWD
E. von Willebrand type 2A

Answer: B) von Willebrand type 3

Explanation: Of the above choices, only von Willebrand type 3 is the type that has autosomal recessive inheritance. vWD type 1, platelet type vWD, acquired vWD, and vWD type 2A all exhibit autosomal-dominant inheritance.

References

1. James PD, et al. ASH ISTH NHF WFH 2021 guidelines on the diagnosis of von Willebrand disease. Blood Adv. 2021;5(1):280–300.
2. Rick ME, et al. von Willebrand disease. In Kitchens C et al: Consultative thrombosis and hemostasis. 3rd ed. Elsevier. 90–102, 2013.
3. Miller JL, et al. Platelet Disorders and von Willebrand Disease. In: McPherson R, et al., editors. Henry's clinical diagnosis and management by laboratory methods. 23rd ed. Saunders; 2017. p. 829–32.
4. Connell NT, et al. ASH ISTH NHF WFH 2021 guidelines on the management of von Willebrand disease. Blood Adv. 2021;5(1):301–25.
5. Nichols WL, et al. von Willebrand disease (VWD): evidence-based diagnosis and management guidelines, the National Heart, Lung, and Blood Institute (NHLBI) Expert Panel report (USA). Haemophilia. 2008;14(2):171–232.

Rare Familial Deficiencies of Coagulation Factors II, V, VII, X, XI, and XIII

31

Abida Babu

Introduction

Hemophilia A (factor VIII [FVIII] deficiency), hemophilia B (factor IX [FIX] deficiency/Christmas disease), and von Willebrand disease (vWD) compose 95–97% of all coagulopathies. The remaining coagulation factor deficiencies, including fibrinogen, prothrombin (factor II [FII]), factor V (FV), factor VII (FVII), factor X (FX), factor XI (FXI), factor XIII (FXIII), and congenital deficiency of vitamin K-dependent factors (VKDCFDs), compose the rare coagulation disorders (RCDs). Here, we discuss the less prevalent RCDs, including FII, FV, FVII, FX, FXI, and FXIII deficiencies [1].

A. Babu (✉)
Department of Hematology Oncology, H Lee Moffitt Cancer Center, University of South Florida, Tampa, FL, USA
e-mail: Abida.Babu@moffitt.org

L. Sokol, L. Zhang (eds.), *Non-Neoplastic Hematologic Disorders*, https://doi.org/10.1007/978-3-031-62373-8_31

Epidemiology

RCDs are rare autosomal recessive forms of inherited bleeding disorders. Incidence rates include the following:

Factor II	1 in 2,000,000
Factor V	1 in 1,000,000
Factor VII	1 in 500,000
Factor XI	1 in 1,000,000
Factor XIII	1 in 2,000,000
Factor V + VIII	1 in 2,000,000

FXI deficiency (hemophilia C/Rosenthal syndrome) is unique to the Jewish population. The disease is highly prevalent among Ashkenazi and Iraqi Jewish populations, at a frequency of 6% for heterozygous disease and 0.1–0.3% for homozygous disease.

Pathogenesis

Rare coagulation disorders (RCDs) present a diagnostic and treatment challenge to physicians in areas where consanguineous marriages are prevalent. RCDs follow an autosomal recessive pattern of inheritance and thus require both parents to carry the gene and pass it to their children. In FII/prothrombin deficiency, there is either less normal prothrombin protein produced or dysprothrombinemia (production of dysfunctional prothrombin protein). The most frequent defect genotyped are missense mutations for FII deficiency. Factor V inherited deficiency is a result of several mutations in the *F5* gene, including missense, nonsense, null, and frameshift mutations. The *F5* gene is located on the long arm of chromosome 1q24.2, spanning 25 exomes. Another deficiency that is distinct from FV deficiency is a combination of FV and FVIII (FV + FVIII) deficiency. FV + FVIII deficiency is caused by genetic variants of the *LMAN1* or *MCFD2* genes, which encode the ER/Golgi intermediate compartment proteins involved in the intracellular transportation of FV and FVIII. Two-thirds of FVII deficiency is due to missense mutations, and the remaining cases are due to mutations which reduce or eliminate expression of factor VII (null mutations). The *F7* gene is located on chromosome 13, close to the gene encoding FX. Approximately, three-fourths of FX–deficient patients have missense mutations. A few factor X-deficient patients have stop codon deletions in *F10,* and there are no known nonsense mutations. FXI deficiency is attributed to more than 65 mutations of the *F11* gene. Interestingly, among the Jewish population, as low as two to three mutations are found. An exon 5 nonsense mutation (Glu117Stop) in Ashkenazi Jews leads to the trivial factor XI expression. FXIa is formed via two pathways. In an activated partial thromboplastin time- (aPTT-) based assay, protease results from activation by FXIIa in conjunction with high-molecular-weight (HMW) kininogen and kallikrein. In vivo, thrombin acts as the activator of FXI. The activation of thrombin by tissue factor/FVIIa activates FXI on the platelet surface, which contributes to further thrombin formation. Defects in *F13A* (mostly due to missense mutations in exons) and *F13B* genes lead to FXIII deficiency, the majority of them due to the former.

FV deficiencies can have a thrombotic effect like that seen in FV Leiden homozygotes. FV gene mutation leads to an activated protein C resistance phenotype. This mutation has a "trans" association to the FV Leiden deficiency. Figure 31.1 demonstrates the intrinsic and extrinsic coagulation cascade. The specific 20210a mutation of prothrombin can lead to venous thromboembolism or other type of thrombosis, with a prevalence of 2% in Caucasians.

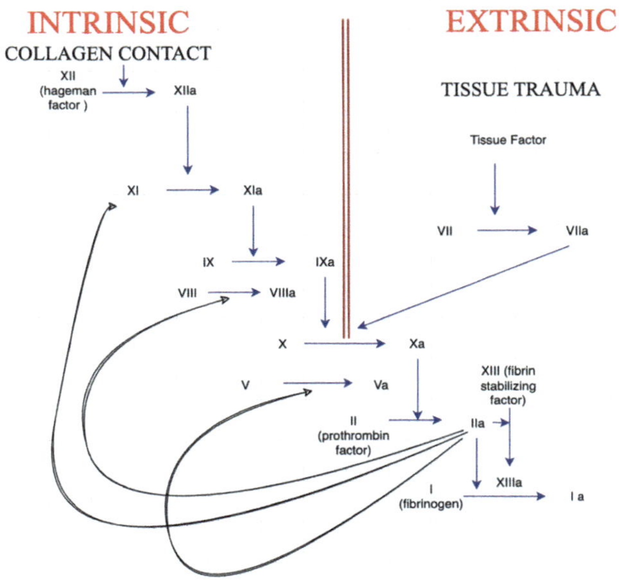

Fig. 31.1 Coagulation cascade

Diagnosis

Morphology/Histopathology/Cytology

Clinical symptoms of RCDs vary significantly, even between patients with the same disorder. The common clinical manifestations are bleeding of subcutaneous and mucosal tissues as well as excessive bleeding during invasive procedures, childbirth, and circumcision. Life-threatening manifestations, such as intracranial bleeding and hemarthroses, are mostly associated with afibrinogenemia, factor X deficiency, and factor XIII deficiency. Women with these coagulation factor deficiencies can have menorrhagia, bleeding complications during pregnancy, and childbirth.

Key Laboratory Findings

See Table 31.1.

Laboratory Diagnosis

After receiving abnormal screening coagulation results (Table 31.1), coagulation mixing studies (50:50 of patient's plasma to control) are performed for exclusion of an inhibitor. After mixing studies are corrected, the deficiency is identified through factor assays. Screening coagulation test results are normal for FXIII deficiency. A quantitative FXIII activity assay detects all types of FXIII deficiency. The assay is based on the measurement of ammonia released during the transglutaminase reaction and measurement of labeled amine incorporated into a protein substrate. If the FXIII activity is low, FXIIIA or FXIIIB levels are measured via a FXIII immunological antigen assay. This process helps to ensure classification and treatment are correct.

Table 31.1 Laboratory and molecular diagnosis

Deficiency factor	Gene diagnosis	Laboratory diagnosis			
		TT	APTT	PT	Specified assays
Factor II	*F2* (11p11-q12)	Normal	Increased	Increased	NA
Factor V	*F5* (1q24.2)	Normal	Increased	Increased	NA
Factor V and VIII combined deficiency	*LMAN1* (18q21.3-q22) *MCFD2* (2p21-p16.3)	Normal	Increased	Increased	NA
Factor VII	*F7* (13q34)	Normal	Normal	Increased	NA
Factor X	*F10* (13q34)	Normal	Increased	Increased	NA
Factor XI	*F11* (4q35.2)	Normal	Increased	Normal	NA
Factor XIII	*F13A1* (6p24-p25) *F13B* (1q31-q32.1)	Normal	Normal	Normal	Required

Molecular Diagnosis

Clinically relevant RCDs are mostly compound heterozygotes or homozygotes [2]. The affected genes in RCDs are listed in Table 31.1. The lack of repetitive mutations makes genotyping difficult, so the gene's entire coding region and the surrounding area must be sequenced.

Global Hemostasis Tests

Global hemostasis tests (i.e., thromboelastographic testing, thrombin generation testing), help assess the total thrombin generation, clot formation, and polymerization of fibrin in vivo. These tests are particularly useful in assessing hemostasis in patients with factor V or factor XI deficiency. They can also be used to monitor RCD treatment for FXI deficiency especially, for which standard assays fail to correlate bleeding risk.

Major Differential Diagnosis

Clinical assessment, pertinent family/personal history, and laboratory findings are effective ways to determine the cause of a patient's bleeding disorder. Some other diagnoses to consider when evaluating for RCDs are vWD, acquired coagulation disorders, and hemophilia.

Acquired Coagulation Disorders

Bleeding manifestations in acquired coagulation disorders can mimic inherited coagulation disorders. They are differentiated from inherited disorders by obtaining collateral information, such as clinical history, physical examination, and other laboratory tests. Some conditions with acquired coagulation disorders are as follows:

- Liver disease due to impaired production of coagulation factors, such as factor I, FII, FV, FVII, FIX, FX, and FXI

- Long-term use of medications, such as antibiotics containing N-methyl-thio-tetrazole (NMTT), vitamin E, alcohol, and anticoagulants
- Impaired vitamin K absorption from the intestines
- Acquired FX deficiency related to amyloidosis due to binding of the protein to amyloid fibrils
- Antibodies to prothrombin factor, seen in patients with antiphospholipid antibodies
- Poisoning by vitamin K antagonists, such as rat poison, or with the use of synthetic cannabinoids contaminated with an anticoagulant rodenticide or over dosage of Warfarin.

Von Willebrand Disease

vWD is suspected when patients have slightly prolonged aPTT and a moderate decrease in FVIII levels. When vWD is suspected, more specific tests, like assays of FVIII, von Willebrand factor antigen, and von Willebrand factor activity (measured by a ristocetin cofactor assay), are required to make a diagnosis.

Hemophilia A and B

Once hemophilia is suspected based on clinical and family history, laboratory values like prolonged aPTT, normal prothrombin time (PT), normal platelet count, reduced FVIII (hemophilia A) levels, and reduced FIX (hemophilia B) levels help differentiate hemophilia from other RCDs.

Prognosis

One of the most useful prognosticating values is the factor level itself. Absence of factor II is not compatible with life. Hypoprothrombinemia manifests as prolonged postinjury bleeding time, hematomas, and hemarthrosis, whereas patients with prothrombin levels >30–40% or with dysprothrombinemia may

Table 31.2 Clinical bleeding severity categorization

Bleeding severity	Definition
Asymptomatic	No prior bleeding episodes
Grade I	Bleeding due to trauma or drug ingestion
Grade II	Bruising, ecchymosis, small wounds, oral mucosal bleeding, epistaxis, menorrhagia, and minor spontaneous bleeds
Grade III	Major spontaneous bleeds, hematomas, hemarthrosis, intraparenchymal brain bleeds, gastrointestinal, and umbilical cord bleeds

remain asymptomatic. A study by the European Network of Rare Bleeding Disorders Group (EN-RBD) demonstrated a notable link between severity of bleeding and lower activity of coagulants, particularly regarding FXIII, fibrinogen, FX, and combined FV/VIII deficiencies. A weaker association existed for FVII and FV deficiencies. Notably, there was no correlation between FXI deficiency manifestations and residual factor levels. Another element that determines prognosis is the severity of bleeding (Table 31.2). The higher the grade of bleeding, the worse the prognosis.

Treatment

RCD treatment is "*on-demand*," meaning that treatment is given at the onset of bleeding. Prophylactic treatment is determined by the frequency of spontaneous bleeding and the associated risks, as well as by the disability from multiple bleeds which could accumulate over time with on-demand treatment only (Table 31.3) [3].

Antifibrinolytics

ε-Aminocaproic acid (EACA) and tranexamic acid (TA) can be used for menorrhagia and mild mucosal bleeding. They are also useful when replacement products are unavailable. These drugs

Table 31.3 Half-lives, therapeutic target levels, treatment options, on-demand, and prophylactic dosages for each RCD treatment

Factor deficiency	Factor half-life	Therapeutic target level (European Network of Rare Bleeding Disorders, EN-RBD)	Available treatment	On-demand dosages	Long-term prophylaxis dosages
FII	3–4 days	>10%	FFP (virus inactivated plasma preferable)	15–25 mL/kg	–
			PCC	20–40 U/kg	20–40 U/kg once/week
Factor V	36 h	10%	FFP (virus inactivated plasma preferable)	15–25 mL/kg	20 mL/kg 2 times/week
			Alloimmunization required for platelet transfusions		
Factor V and Factor VIII	Factor VIII 10–14 h	40%	FV deficiency as above, mild FVIII deficiency: DDAVP. Moderate and severe FVIII deficiency: plasma derived—or rFVIII concentrates		
FVII	6 h	>20%	FFP (virus inactivated plasma preferable)	–	10–15 ml/kg/2 times/week
			Platelet derived-FVII concentrate	30–40 U/kg	30–40 U/kg 3 times/week
			rFVIIa	15–30 ug/kg every 4–6 h	20–40 mg/kg 2–3 times/week

(continued)

Table 31.3 (continued)

Factor deficiency	Factor half-life	Therapeutic target level (European Network of Rare Bleeding Disorders, EN-RBD)	Available treatment	On-demand dosages	Long-term prophylaxis dosages
FX	40–60 h	>40%	FFP (virus inactivated plasma preferable)	10–20 mL/kg	–
			PCC	20–30 U/kg	20–40 U/kg 2 times/week
			Platelet derived-FX/FXI concentrate	10–20 U/kg	20 U/kg/weekly
			Platelet derived- FX	25 U/kg	25 U weekly
FXI	50 h		FFP (virus inactivated plasma preferable)	15–20 mL/kg	Not indicated
			Platelet derived-Factor XI concentrate	15–20 U/kg	
FVIII	9–12 days	30%	Cryoprecipitate	2–3 bags	–
			FFP (virus inactivated plasma preferable)	3–5 mL/kg	–
			Platelet derived-FXIII concentrate	20–40 U/kg	20–40 U/kg/4 weeks
			rFXIII-A	35 U/kg	35 U/kg/4 weeks (2–3 weeks in pregnant women)

block sites where lysine binds the plasminogen molecules, decreasing the affinity of fibrin to plasminogen. This process results in the antifibrinolytic activity. Tranexamic acid is more effective than EACA and has completely replaced EACA in clinical practice. TA can be administered topically or orally. When TA is used for hemorrhagic bleeding, it can be used to a maximum dose of 4–6 g.

Promising Clinical Studies

Most novel treatment options for RCDs are based on previous experiences with hemophilia patients. A novel RNA interference therapeutic targeting antithrombin (ALN-AT3) has shown to increase thrombin generation in patients with hemophilia. This investigational drug could be extrapolated for use with RCD patients. Also, a novel plasma-derived FV concentrate has been recently developed, which showed correction of PT, aPTT, and PT when used in vitro for FV-deficient patients. This product is in the clinical trial stages and its effect on factor V deficient patients is yet to be studied. Finally, a gene therapy approach using adeno-associated viral (AAV) serotype delivery of FVII transgene in a large-animal model with <1% FVII activity showed a clinically therapeutic expression of up to 15% for >1 year.

Caveats

- Be aware of the development of inhibitors after multiple treatments for patients with RCDs. For example, in FXI-deficient patients who develop inhibitors, fresh frozen plasma (FFP) and FXI concentrates should be avoided. These patients are treated with prothrombin complex concentrate (PCC)/activated PCC (aPCC) or recombinant activated FVII.
- Some rare bleeding disorders are associated with thrombotic events, such as venous and arterial thrombosis, and are most seen with afibrinogenemia, FVII deficiency, and FXI deficiency.

- Replacement therapy should be individualized based on prior and family history of bleeding/clotting.
- For most RCDs, factor level >10% is sufficient to attain hemostasis.

Board Questions

Surgery for a Patient with Normal PT/aPTT

1. A 43-year-old teacher has recurrent abdominal pain. The surgeon wants her to receive a laparotomy. Her previous medical history is significant for bleeding following dental extraction, tonsillectomy, and menorrhagia. Her complete blood count (CBC) shows that her white cell count is 4.5 x 10^9/L, hemoglobin is 15.2 g/dL, and platelet count is 295 x 10^9/L. Her PT is 12.4 seconds (s), aPTT is 26.8 s, and PTT is 11.5 s. Her fibrinogen is 220 mg/dL.

   What is the next step for the patient?

A. Patient has normal coagulation parameters and should proceed to surgery.
B. Patient needs further coagulation workup.
C. Patient should proceed to surgery with prothrombin complex concentrate.
D. Administer intravenous aminocaproic acid 4 g half or before surgery followed by 4 g every 6 h for the next 5 days.

Answer: B. Patient needs further coagulation workup.

This patient has had previous history of significant bleeding, warranting further workup despite normal PT, aPTT, fibrinogen, and platelet counts. The initial screening tests are normal for FXIII deficiency. For patients with a strong bleeding history, FXIII is assessed by the clot stability with 5 mol/L urea. If this suggests FXIII deficiency, then a FXIII assay must be done to assess the severity, and FXIII concentrate should be infused prior to surgery.

2. A 26-year-old White female with Jewish ancestry presents with no history of nosebleeds and no history of bleeding after tonsillectomy or appendectomy. She has been admitted for a cesarean section. The coagulation parameters requested show that her PT is 14.8 s, aPTT is 85 s, and fibrinogen is 185 mg. Her aPTT 50:50 mixing study is 28 s. The FXI level is 15%.

   What is next step for the peripartum management?

A. Proceed with surgery.
B. Order for cryoprecipitate.
C. Order for FVIII-specific inhibitors.
D. Patient needs fresh frozen plasma.

Answer: A. Proceed with surgery

Patients with FXI deficiency do not bleed, even with low FXI levels. This patient, who has had previous surgical interventions without bleeding, does not need blood product support prior to an interventional procedure, including surgery.

References

1. Menegatti M, Peyvandi F. Treatment of rare factor deficiencies other than hemophilia. Blood. 2019;133(5):415–24. PMID: 30559262.
2. Palla R, Peyvandi F, Shapiro AD. Rare bleeding disorders: diagnosis and treatment. Blood. 2015;125(13):2052–61.
3. Mannucci PM, Duga S, Peyvandi F. Recessively inherited coagulation disorders. Blood. 2004;104(5):1243–52. PMID: 15138162.

Congenital Afibrinogenemia, Hypofibrinogenemia, Dysfibrinogenemia

32

Robert Killeen

Introduction

Afibrinogenemia is a rare genetic disorder of hemostasis occurring with an estimated prevalence of approximately 1 in 1,000,000. This is an autosomal recessive disorder mostly seen in communities where consanguinity is prevalent (India, Pakistan, and the Middle East). Afibrinogenemia results in altered hemostasis, poor inflammatory response (fibrinogen is an acute-phase reactant), and delayed wound healing because of a distorted cellular and matrix interaction. Dysfibrinogenemia is an autosomal-dominant disorder causing bleeding and thrombosis. Thrombosis occurs among about 20% of patients with dysfibrinogenemia. There appears to be no direct correlation between functional fibrinogen and clinical features in dysfibrinogenemia. Until recently, fresh frozen plasma and cryoprecipitate were the mainstays of treatment, but the newer fibrinogen concentrates are favored because of the infective/allergic complications of the blood products. However, the fibrinogen concentrates (4 FDA-approved agents) are still not advised for dysfibrinogenemia with thrombotic symptoms. Furthermore, acquired causes of hypo-/dysfibrinogenemia

R. Killeen (✉)
Moffitt Cancer Center, Tampa, FL, USA

L. Sokol, L. Zhang (eds.), *Non-Neoplastic Hematologic Disorders*,
https://doi.org/10.1007/978-3-031-62373-8_32

are by far more common, and these should be excluded from evaluating patients with defective fibrinogen synthesis.

Pathogenesis

Fibrinogen is produced by hepatocytes with a molecular weight of 340 kD (Fig. 32.1). The serum concentration is 200 to 400 mg/mL. The production of fibrinogen is under control of three separate genes located on chromosome 4 [1]. Fibrinogen has a half-life of 80 hours. It is converted to fibrin by thrombin forming insoluble fibrin to attain hemostasis. Fibrinogen is needed for platelet aggregation by binding to platelet glycoprotein IIb/IIIa, attachment to a tissue-matrix protein such as fibronectin and serves as a carrier protein for factor XIII. Hence, defects of fibrinogen synthesis may lead to mucosal bleeding, defective wound healing, and hemostasis.

Afibrinogenemia occurs secondary to mutations in the gene encoding of the fibrinogen alpha chain. Defective synthesis of fibrinogen occurs from several mechanisms at the DNA level, at the RNA level by affecting mRNA splicing or stability, or at the protein level by affecting protein synthesis, assembly, or secretion [2].

Dysfibrinogenemia occurs as an autosomal-dominant trait. Molecular defects in dysfibrinogenemia:

Genetic defects in dysfibrinogenemia result in impaired release of fibrinopeptides, defects in fibrin polymerization, and defective crosslinking by factor XIIIa (Table 32.1). Approximately 25% of patients present with a history of bleeding and about 20% result in thrombotic states [3].

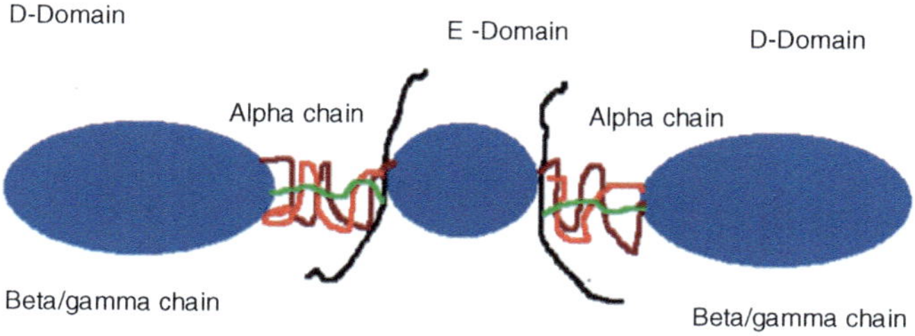

Fig. 32.1 Fibrinogen molecule

Table 32.1 Molecular variants of abnormal fibrinogen

Type	Molecular defect
Fibrinogen Detroit	Arg38Ser
Fibrinogen Mahdia	Frameshift Gly323GlufsX79
Fibrinogen Canterbury	Missing polymerization site AaV20D
Fibrinogen Baltimore	Defective D:D site function yG292V
Fibrinogen Kyoto	Substitution of Pro with Leu A18
Fibrinogen Tokyo	Substitution R275C

Clinical Features

Symptoms of bleeding in afibrinogenemia can range from minimal to life-threatening bleeding episodes. Fatal umbilical-cord bleeding (60%) and intracranial bleeding (24%) may occur in severe afibrinogenemia [4]. Other bleeding symptoms include muscle hematoma, postoperative bleeding, ecchymosis, and mucosal bleeding including gastrointestinal and genitourinary bleeding. In women, menorrhagia, spontaneous abortion, and pregnancy-associated hemorrhage (peripartum) may occur.

In dysfibrinogenemia, thrombotic episodes occur in about 20% and bleeding episodes in about 25% of patients. The bleeding symptoms are noted with functional fibrinogen levels below 50 mg/dL. Among about 50% of patients with dysfibrinogenemia, there is no evidence of bleeding or thrombosis [5]. Life-threatening bleeding in dysfibrinogenemia is rare. However, the bleeding symptoms include menorrhagia, subcutaneous bruises, postoperative bleeding, gastrointestinal bleeding, and rarely, intracranial retroperitoneal bleeding and muscle hematoma.

Diagnosis

As with other bleeding disorders, a family or personal history of mucocutaneous bleeding including unexplained menorrhagia, unexplained umbilical-cord/intracranial/postoperative bleeding from childhood or unexplained bleeding associated with thrombosis in the family should raise the suspicions of afibrinogenemia and dysfibrinogenemia. A detailed history to exclude acquired causes including chronic liver disorders, consumptive coagulopathy, and medication-induced (asparaginase) must be taken.

Basic tests of hemostasis including prothrombin time, activated partial-thromboplastin time, and thrombin time should be the initial screening tests. Prolongation of screening tests—especially prolonged thrombin time—suggests abnormal fibrinogen (reptilase time should be done to exclude heparin contamination). Antigenic and functional fibrinogen should be requested (functional fibrinogen less than 50% of antigenic fibrinogen suggests dysfibrinogenemia). If there is a family history, genotyping and sequencing fibrinogen should be requested. This will identify individuals who are asymptomatic in the family. This may help the individual with abnormal menstrual cycles, preconception planning, and in genetic counseling during pregnancy [6].

Differential Diagnosis

Acquired causes of afibrinogenemia/dysfibrinogenemia are by far much more common than the inherited variety. Chronic liver disease including cirrhosis of the liver, disseminated intravascular coagulation, therapy-induced (thrombolytic therapy, asparaginase), neoplastic (prostate, lung cancer), paraproteinemia from myeloma or lymphoma, and storage disorders should be excluded before the diagnosis of inherited hypo-/dysfibrinogenemia.

Management

Management of hypo-/dysfibrinogenemia is aimed to prevent and treat serious bleeding and thrombosis. For women, treatment is needed to control menorrhagia, intrauterine death, and prevent obstetric complications. Not all patients require intervention as mild hypofibrinogenemia and dysfibrinogenemia without symptoms do not need treatment. The sources of fibrinogen include fresh frozen plasma, cryoprecipitate, and fibrinogen concentrates. Fibrinogen concentrate is preferred over the plasma products because of the lower risk of transfusion reactions and volume overload. Currently, lyophilized pasteurized human-fibrinogen concentrates are available for patients with afibrinogenemia and patients with dysfibrinogenemia with a history of bleeding. A multinational, prospective, open-label, uncontrolled study of afibrinogenemia among patients 6 years or older to assess the pharmacokinetic profile, clot integrity, and safety profile indicated that fibrinogen concentrate was safe to restore hemostasis [7].

Principles of Treatment

- For major surgery, a target level of >100 mg/dL with a trough of >50 mg per dL is needed to achieve hemostasis. Patients with afibrinogenemia do not need prophylactic fibrinogen concentrate. However, prior to major surgical procedures and delivery the patient may need to have fibrinogen concentrate infused, aiming for 150 mg/dL prior to intervention (X one dose) - FIBRYGA: Dose (in mg) = weight (in kg) × desired increase (in mg/dL) ÷ 1.8. For FIBRYGA in children, divide by 1.4 instead of 1.8 or RiaSTAP and Haemocomplettan: Dose (in mg) = [weight (in kg) × desired increase (in mg/dL)] ÷ 1.7.
- Primary prophylaxis for afibrinogenemia is not needed unless the level is <10 mg/dL.
- Fibrinogen concentrates are not indicated for dysfibrinogenemia with history of thrombosis. Rather, patients with thrombotic episodes may need anticoagulation therapy with enoxaparin or with the newer oral anticoagulants.

Spontaneous or Posttraumatic Bleeding

For patients with afibrinogenemia who have spontaneous or posttraumatic bleeding, fibrinogen concentrate is infused to keep fibrinogen level > 100 mg/dL. However, for patients with intracranial or life-threatening bleed, the target level is >150 mg/dL.

Dental Extraction

For patients with afibrinogenemia who need dental extraction, one dose of fibrinogen concentrates to keep the level > 100 mg/dL before extraction or using oral antifibrinolytic therapy is advised to achieve hemostasis.

Elective Surgery

Patients with congenital afibrinogenemia with bleeding symptoms should receive fibrinogen concentrate or cryoprecipitate before surgery to keep the level > 100 mg/dL. Patients with no history of bleeding and a level > 50 mg/dL do not need prophylaxis before interventional procedures. Topical treatment with fibrin, cautery, or other local measures may be considered during surgery.

Menorrhagia

Patients with menorrhagia may benefit from oral contraceptive medication or oral aminocaproic acid or tranexamic acid. However, systemic antifibrinolytic therapy is not indicated for menorrhagia among patients with dysfibrinogenemia and history of thrombosis.

Pregnancy

Pregnancy-associated afibrinogenemia with a history of recurrent miscarriages, stillbirth, abruptio placentae, subchorionic hematomas, and postpartum hemorrhage need prophylaxis during pregnancy. A high-risk obstetrics and gynecology specialist should be involved in treatment planning. Once the pregnancy is confirmed, the patient should receive fibrinogen concentrate every 80 hours to keep the trough level of fibrinogen >50 mg per dL.

Prophylaxis

For patients with afibrinogenemia having bleeding symptoms with serum fibrinogen <10 mg/dL, primary prophylaxis with fibrinogen concentrate may be considered. Prophylactic therapy is advised after life-threatening bleed such as intracranial bleeding. However, in a retrospective study of prophylaxis vs on-demand therapy, there was no appreciable difference (0.5 vs 0.7 bleeding events) [8]. Repeated exposure to fibrinogen concentrates has complications including infections, allergy, development of inhibitors, and thromboembolism.

Managing Patients with Dysfibrinogenemia

Patients with dysfibrinogenemia with a history of bleeding symptoms can be managed with fibrinogen concentrate. However, if patients have thrombotic symptoms, fibrinogen concentrates are not indicated.

Managing Thrombosis in Hypofibrinogenemia/Dysfibrinogenemia

Antithrombotic therapy can be safely given if the fibrinogen level is >50 mg per dL. The antithrombotic therapy of choice is enoxaparin and for long-term use, warfarin. The role of the newer oral anticoagulant therapy is not known.

The systemic antifibrinolytic therapy (intravenous aminocaproic acid or tranexamic acid) is not advised in managing bleeding episodes. Oral antifibrinolytic therapy is only advised with dental procedures.

Prognosis

The prognosis of hypo-/dysfibrinogenemia depends on the severity of the disease. Catastrophic bleeding occurs with intrauterine death, umbilical-cord bleeding (85%), neonatal intracranial bleeding, splenic rupture, and major bleeding following surgical intervention (in undiagnosed patients with afibrinogenemia). However, the prognosis in the adult age group is good. For pregnant woman with afibrinogenemia, once lyophilized fibrinogen concentrate is initiated as soon as pregnancy is confirmed, the pregnancy runs an uneventful course. Complications of treatment include infective complications from cryoprecipitate, antifibrinogen antibodies following use of fibrinogen-factor concentrates, and thrombosis in dysfibrinogenemia (these patients present with both bleeding and thrombosis).

Prenatal Diagnosis

As these are genetic disorders (afibrinogenemia is autosomal recessive and dysfibrinogenemia autosomal dominant), pregnant women with a family history of consanguinity need appropriate genetic counseling. If the mother's genetic profile is known, chorionic villous biopsy and the genetic makeup of the fetus will help the obstetrician to decide on the mode of delivery. Fetal blood sampling must be avoided. Fetal cranial ultrasound should be done to detect early intracanal bleed and to assess the need for appropriate therapy.

Caveats

- It may be challenging to diagnose disorders of fibrinogen synthesis. Detailed personal and family history should help in diagnosing and managing.
- The diagnosis should be based on clinical findings and laboratory tests—there may not be direct correlation between laboratory findings and the clinical course.
- Gene sequencing of fibrinogen is done in the referral centers. This will help in the prenatal diagnosis of consanguineous parents.
- Pregnant women with a history of fetal loss should receive fibrinogen concentrate as soon as pregnancy is confirmed. High-risk obstetric team should be involved in the management.
- Thrombotic episodes in dysfibrinogenemia should be managed along with other thrombotic events following the appropriate guidelines (short term vs long term). The role of the newer oral anticoagulants in this setting is debatable.

Board Questions

1. A 35-year-old Caucasian male presents with lower-extremity deep vein thrombosis and pulmonary embolism. The patient's mother and maternal grandfather have had histories of pulmonary embolism. Coagulation screening shows a prothrombin time of 18 seconds (12–14 seconds), activated partial thromboplastin time of 42 seconds (28–35 seconds), and a thrombin time of 17 seconds (12–14 seconds). Mixing studies did not correct prolonged thrombin time. The fibrinogen was 215 mg per dL (200–400 mg).

   Which of the following tests would most likely make the diagnosis in this patient?

   A. Lupus anticoagulant assay
   B. Ristocetin cofactor assay
   C. Functional fibrinogen assay
   D. Factor X assay
   E. Factor V assay

Answer – C

Educational objective

To suspect dysfibrinogenemia with a strong family history and prolonged thrombin time

Critique

The patient presents with an episode of venous thromboembolism. The first thing in this patient is to establish the diagnosis. Patients with lupus anticoagulant syndrome have thrombotic events but no family history of thromboembolism. Patients with factor V and X deficiencies have prolonged thrombin time but they do not present with thrombosis.

1. A 35-year-old Asian American born to consanguineous parents presents with a history of epistaxis since childhood and a recent history of febrile illness associated with flu-like symptoms and ecchymosis and was admitted to the hospital. The complete blood cell count at the time of admission shows a white blood cell count of 5300/μL, hemoglobin of 9.3 g/dL, hematocrit of 28.2%, mean corpuscular volume of 99 fL, and platelet count of 164 300/μL. His D-dimer of 0.3 μ/mL (Normal <0.4). The prothrombin time is 21 seconds (12–14); partial-thromboplastin time is 45 seconds (28–35); and thrombin time is 22 seconds (12–14).

   Which of the following is the most likely diagnosis?

   A. Disseminated intravascular coagulation
   B. Primary fibrinogenolysis
   C. Acquired hemophilia A
   D. Afibrinogenemia
   E. von Willebrand disease

Answer – D

Educational objective

To suspect afibrinogenemia with history of consanguinity, history of mucocutaneous bleeding, and prolonged coagulation profile with normal D-dimer

Critique

Primary fibrinogenolysis is mostly an acquired disorder secondary to use of tissue plasminogen activator therapy for managing myocardial infarction or thrombotic stroke or underlying neoplasia including prostate or lung cancer. This is seldom an inherited disorder. von Willebrand disease and acquired hemophilia are defects of the intrinsic pathway. Disseminated intravascular coagulation is very unlikely because of normal D-dimer.

References

1. Olaisen B, Teisberg P, Gedde-Dahl T. Fibrinogen γ chain locus is on chromosome 4 in man. Hum Genet. 1982;61(1):24–6.
2. Vu D, Neerman-Arbez M. Molecular mechanisms accounting for fibrinogen deficiency: from large deletions to intracellular retention of misfolded proteins. J Thrombs Haemost. 2007;5:125–31.
3. Ebert RF. Index of variant human fibrinogens. CRC Press; 1994.
4. Casini A, von Mackensen S, Santoro C, et al. Clinical phenotype, fibrinogen supplementation, and health-related quality of life in patients with afibrinogenemia. Blood. 2021;137(22):3127–36.
5. Casini A, Blondon M, Lebreton A, et al. Natural history of patients with congenital dysfibrinogenemia. Blood J Am Soc Hematol. 2015;125(3):553–61.
6. Casini A, Blondon M, Tintillier V, et al. Mutational epidemiology of congenital fibrinogen disorders. Thromb Haemost. 2018;118(11):1867–74.
7. Manco-Johnson M, Dimichele D, Castaman G, et al. Pharmacokinetics and safety of fibrinogen concentrate. J Thromb Haemost. 2009;7(12):2064–9.
8. Peyvandi F, Haertel S, Knaub S, et al. Incidence of bleeding symptoms in 100 patients with inherited afibrinogenemia or hypofibrinogenemia. 2006.

Acquired Inhibitors of Coagulation Factors

33

Ashley M. Rose and Nathan Visweshwar

Introduction

Acquired inhibitors of coagulation factors are antibodies that inhibit the production or clearance of a coagulation factor. The most common autoantibodies occur against factor VIII. The incidence is 1.4 cases per million per year. This condition is termed acquired hemophilia A (AHA). Common etiologies for acquired inhibitors are postpartum, autoimmune disease, malignancy, and drug induced (Table 33.1). However, 50% are idiopathic [1]. Acquired inhibitors occur in a bimodal distribution because of some patients being associated with pregnancy and others in older age. The median age of onset is 77 years. Patients typically present with bleeding, such as postoperative bleeding, postpartum hemorrhage, melena, hematuria, and bleeding into skin or muscle. In contrast to congenital hemophilia, hemarthroses are uncommon [2]. Bleeding in AHA may be more severe than congenital

A. M. Rose (✉)
Department of Hematology and Oncology, H. Lee Moffitt Cancer Center and Research Institute, Tampa, FL, USA

Department of Hematology and Oncology, University of South Florida, Tampa, FL, USA

N. Visweshwar
Department of Hematology and Oncology, University of South Florida, Tampa, FL, USA

L. Sokol, L. Zhang (eds.), *Non-Neoplastic Hematologic Disorders*,
https://doi.org/10.1007/978-3-031-62373-8_33

Table 33.1 Etiology

Cause	Entities
Idiopathic—50%	
Immunological	Autoimmune hemolytic anemia, rheumatoid arthritis, myasthenia gravis, ulcerative colitis, psoriasis, and graves' disease
Pregnancy/post Partum related	
Malignancy	Prostate, stomach, cervical, breast, and lung
Hematologic	Chronic lymphatic leukemia, non-Hodgkin's lymphoma, Waldenstrom's macroglobulinemia
Drugs	Alpha methyldopa, fludarabine, penicillin, sulfa and alpha interferon

hemophilia despite similar factor levels. Autoantibodies to other clotting factors may be associated with a variety of disorders and present with variable clinical findings (Table 33.2).

Pathogenesis

Acquired factor inhibitors are immunoglobulin G (IgG) antibodies that inhibit the activity of a specific factor leading to symptoms of mucocutaneous bleeding. Acquired coagulation factor inhibitors may occur:

1. Spontaneously
2. From alloimmunization (secondary to factor replacement therapy)
3. Antiphospholipid antibodies (lupus anticoagulant)

In this section, we will focus on the spontaneous (de novo) autoantibody production against a specific factor. Among the specific inhibitors, AHA is by far the most common. This is a disease of older patients and occurs with equal sex incidence. An acquired factor VIII inhibitor is an IgG antibody (with no complement binding). Factor VIII contains three different types of domains, namely A1-A2-B-A3-C1-C2. The anti-A2 inhibitors are present

Table 33.2 Other factor inhibitors

Factor	Associated condition	Clinical presentation	Treatment	Special considerations
Prothrombin (factor II) inhibitors	aPL Antiprothrombin Ab (accelerated clearance, tests will be consistent with deficiency rather than inhibitor)	Bleeding diathesis rather than clotting in patient with aPL Mixing study consistent with deficiency rather than inhibitor	FFP 15–20 ml/kg with target prothrombin level > 30% Modalities used to treat factor VIII inhibitors	Antiphosphatidyl serine Ab (an aPL Ab) causes function interference with prothrombin assay
Thrombin (factor IIa) inhibitors	Rare Exposure to bovine thrombin found in topic thrombin or fibrin glue used in surgery Less commonly: SLE, RA, MGUS	May cause clinical bleeding if cross-react with human thrombin or factor V Prolonged TT	Corticosteroids, cyclophosphamide, other IS medications, PLEX	Patients with inhibitor related to autoimmune disease may have severe bleeding, while those with exposure to bovine thrombin/fibrin glue can have increased TT without clinical bleeding
Factor V inhibitors	Exposure to bovine thrombin found in topic thrombin or fibrin glue used in surgery (incidence 38% after cardiac or neurosurgery) Malignancy, post-partum, autoimmune	Variable bleeding, may be severe Prolonged aPTT and PT but normal TT and decreased FV activity. TT will be prolonged if there is concomitant inhibitor to thrombin	Most inhibitors disappear within months Platelet transfusion, PLEX, IVIG (for acute bleeding) Corticosteroids, cyclophosphamide, rituximab	Bind to C2 domain of protein similar to some FVIII inhibitors

(continued)

Table 33.2 (continued)

Factor	Associated condition	Clinical presentation	Treatment	Special considerations
Factor VII inhibitors	Rare	Prolonged PT, normal aPTT Variable bleeding diathesis	PLEX, corticosteroids, cyclophosphamide	
Factor IX inhibitors	Rare Two cases reported postpartum	Prolonged aPTT with normal PT	Managed similarly to FVIII. Use of IVIG and corticosteroids have been reported	
Factor X inhibitors	Rare Acute respiratory infections Amyloidosis can lead to deficiency of FX due to binding of protein to amyloid fibrils.	May result in sudden onset of severe, acute bleeding Prolonged aPTT and PT. May have transient and severe FX deficiency May have clinical signs of amyloidosis	Corticosteroids and other IS medications may be used	Tests may reveal a deficiency rather than inhibitor in cases due to amyloidosis
Factor XI inhibitors	SLE	Typically, mild or no bleeding despite long aPTT		Minor or no bleeding due to FXI tertiary role in activating FX

Factor	Associated condition	Clinical presentation	Treatment	Special considerations
Factor XIII inhibitors	Rare SLE or other autoimmune disease, lymphoid malignancy, drugs [4]	Delayed bleeding after surgery due to initial clot being weak and unstable Spontaneous hematoma or intracranial hemorrhage Normal aPTT/PT, abnormal clot stability	Corticosteroids, cyclophosphamide, IVIG, rituximab, PLEX Infusion of FXIII concentrates	May occur due to inhibition of activation, interference with enzymatic function, or prevention of binding to fibrin

Ab antibody, *aPCC* activated prothrombin complex concentrates, *aPL* antiphospholipid antibody, *aPTT* activated partial thromboplastin time, *CLL* chronic lymphocytic leukemia, *CR* complete remission, *DDAVP* desmopressin, *FEIBA* factor VIII inhibitor bypassing agent, *FFP* fresh frozen plasma, *IS* immunosuppressive, *IVIG* intravenous immunoglobulin, *MGUS* monoclonal gammopathy of undetermined significance, *PLEX* plasma exchange, *PT* prothrombin time, *RA* rheumatoid arthritis, *SLE* systemic lupus erythematosus, *TT* thrombin time or clotting time

in 71% of hemophilic plasmas but only in 33% of autoantibody plasmas [3]. The factor VIII inhibitor interferes with phospholipid binding. Factor VIII–phosphatidylserine binding is prevented by factor VIII inhibitor that has strong factor VIII light-chain reactivity. In another study, it was confirmed that the inhibitory activity of some human factor VIII inhibitors may be caused by inhibition of factor VIII functions within the C2 domain.

Clinical Features

Patients may present with symptoms of severe mucocutaneous bleeding. The bleeding manifestations are extensive ecchymosis, intracranial, retroperitoneal, gastrointestinal bleeding (hematemesis/melena), genitourinary bleeding (painful hematuria with clots), peripartum hemorrhage, and soft-tissue hematoma. The presentation of acquired hemophilia is different from the inherited type in which patients present with recurrent hemarthrosis and muscle hematomas. Severe bleeding occurs in up to 90% of acquired hemophilia cases. Preoperatively, if acquired factor VIII is not suspected, uncontrollable bleeding may occur during the procedure, resulting in increased morbidity and mortality.

Diagnostic Workup

Onset of sudden bleeding in older patients, such as a large hematoma, ecchymoses, postoperative, or sudden postpartum bleeding should prompt workup for an acquired factor VIII inhibitor. Workup includes baseline complete blood cell count, prothrombin time, activated partial thromboplastin time (aPTT), thrombin time, and fibrinogen assay. Patients with acquired factor VIII inhibitor have normal platelet count, prothrombin time, and serum fibrinogen but unduly prolonged aPTT. The next step is to do a mixing study (1:1 mix of normal plasma/patient's plasma). In an acquired factor VIII inhibitor, there is immediate correction of aPTT with normal plasma, but aPTT will be prolonged after incubation at 37 °C for 1 to 2 hours—confirming acquired inhibitor (delayed factor VIII inhibitor). For patients with factor VIII deficiency, aPTT will correct with the immediate and delayed phases. Patients with lupus anticoagulant syndrome will have prolonged aPTT with no correction with normal plasma anytime.

Antibody Titration

Once delayed factor VIII inhibitor is confirmed, then the intensity of the antibody is quantified with the Bethesda assay. The patient's plasma is mixed with normal plasma at serial dilutions and incubated at 37 °C for 2 hours, and the factor VIII activity is measured. The dilution of patient plasma that results in the 50 percent factor VIII activity is ascertained (Bethesda unit). Patients with acquired hemophilia have high elevated titers (>10 Bethesda units).

Differential Diagnosis

Factor deficiencies, von Willebrand disease, heparin, or other anticoagulant use, disseminated intravascular coagulation, vitamin K deficiency, liver disease, lupus anticoagulant, deficiency of prekallikrein, or high-molecular-weight kininogen (not associated with bleeding diathesis but will have prolonged aPTT).

Principles of Treatment

1. Control of bleeding
2. Removal of IgG antibody
3. Immunosuppression to eliminate the production of the factor VIII inhibitor

Agents to Arrest the Bleeding

Agents used in the immediate control of bleeding include desmopressin (DDAVP), factor VIII concentrates, factor VIII inhibitor bypassing activity (FEIBA), recombinant human factor VIIa (rFVIIa), and recombinant porcine factor VIII concentrate. Because acquired hemophilia has a high antibody titer (>10BU), DDAVP and factor VIII concentrates are of limited value. rFVIIa infusion with a starting dose of 90 mcg/kg IV every 2 hours will help control bleeding through the extrinsic pathway. The factor VIII bypassing agent (FEIBA—contains activated factors II, IV, IX, and X) at a dose of 75 units/kg IV every 12 hours may be used along with rFVIIa. In the study by Morrison et al., the mean initial dose of porcine factor VIII (*Obizur*) infused was 84 IU/kg, which increased the plasma factor VIII:C activity to 0.85 IU/mL [4]. The median duration of therapy was 8.5 days. A clinical response was seen among 78% of recipients [4].

Removal of the Factor VIII Inhibitor

Factor VIII inhibitor is an IgG antibody with a half-life of 21 days. The severity of the disease depends on the titer and avidity of the antibody. The high-titer antibody circulating in the system must be eliminated among patients with critical illness, including life-threatening intracranial bleeding. In this setting, high-volume plasmapheresis may be initiated before the specific therapy directed against the inhibitor.

Elimination of the Antibody with Immunosuppressive Agents

Spontaneous disappearance of the inhibitor can occur; however, treatment to eliminate the inhibitor is recommended to avoid further bleeding. Treatment is recommended even for patients without clinical signs of bleeding. Prednisone (1 mg/kg per day) or prednisone plus oral cyclophosphamide (1–2 mg/kg per day) for at least 5 weeks is typically given for first-line treatment. There is no difference in outcomes among patients treated with steroids alone vs steroids in combination with cytotoxic agents [5]. Patients with lower titers (BU <20) are more likely to respond to corticosteroids alone. Thus, corticosteroids plus cyclophosphamide may be used upfront among patients with high titers (BU >20). Cyclosporin A 200 to 300 mg/day alone or with prednisone may be used as second-line therapy. High-dose immunoglobulin of 1.0 g/kg per day for 2 days may be used in association with other treatments (steroids, immunoadsorption). IV rituximab of 375 mg/m^2 weekly for 4 weeks is useful in relapse associated with steroids. Emicizumab is a monoclonal antibody that functions to restore the missing activated factor VIII and shows promise among patients with AHA [6].

Monitor inhibitor titer levels every 2 to 4 weeks. Check factor activity level at 4 weeks after immunosuppression is stopped. Treatment of the underlying disorder (malignancy, autoimmune disease, stopping offending drug, and delivery of child) may result in disappearance of the inhibitor.

Prognosis

Bleeding in the setting of acquired inhibitors of coagulation may be more severe than in congenital hemophilia. Bleeding can be more severe earlier in the course of the disease and is often diagnosed at the time of bleeding rather than by routine labs. Fatal bleeding occurs among 22% of patients [7]. Most studies evaluated patients with FVIII inhibitors as it is the most common type of acquired inhibitor. Complete remission rates (as defined by undetectable inhibitor levels, factor VIII level > 70 IU/mL, and off immunosuppression) occurred among up to 70% of patients in a median time of 5 weeks. Complete remission with rituximab took twice as long as those cases with steroids and/or immunosuppressive agents. Second-line therapy was successful among 60% of cases that did not respond to first-line therapy. Postpartum disease was associated with 97% 2-year overall survival and 100% complete remission by 30 months. Patients with low antibody titers (BU <5) tend to have faster remissions than those with high titers. Treatment of the underlying condition may result in disappearance of the inhibitor. Some patients may even have spontaneous disappearance of the inhibitor. For all patients with AHA, the relapse rate after the first complete remission is estimated to be around 20%, with 70% of these patients achieving a second complete remission. The relapse rate in pregnancy is lower but rarely can affect fetal FVIII levels, resulting in life-threatening hemorrhage in a subsequent pregnancy.

Promising Clinical Studies

Emicizumab is a monoclonal antibody with a bispecific factor IXa and factor X antibody that functions to restore the missing activated factor VIII. A series of 12 patients with AHA treated with emicizumab showed effective control of bleeding among all patients, even those refractory to FEIBA [6].

Board Questions

1. A 73-year-old male presents to the emergency department with complaints of dark, tarry stools for the last 3 days. He is found to have diffuse ecchymoses. He has no history of bleeding. Vital signs are stable. Hemoglobin is 8.1 g/dL, and the remainder of the CBC is normal. PT/international normalized ratio is within normal limits; however, aPTT is 81 seconds (normal 21–35 seconds). Fibrinogen is normal.

   Which of the following tests should be performed next?

   A. Esophagogastroduodenoscopy
   B. ADAMTS13
   C. 1:1 mixing study
   D. BCR-ABL

   Answer: C. This patient has clinical signs of mucocutaneous bleeding in the setting of elevated aPTT. Given his age and lack of bleeding history, an acquired coagulation-factor inhibitor should be suspected. The next step in workup is a 1:1 mixing study. Esophagogastroduodenoscopy may be performed at a later time since the patient is stable, and a bleeding disorder should be ruled out before procedures. ADAMTS13 is not helpful, as thrombotic thrombocytopenic purpura is not suspected in this patient with normal platelet count. BCR-ABL is used to evaluate for chronic myelocytic leukemia which is not suspected in this patient.

2. A 79-year-old female presents to the emergency department with uncontrolled epistaxis resulting in respiratory failure. The patient is intubated on arrival. CBC is within normal limits. PT/international normalized ratio are within normal limits; however, aPTT is 92 seconds (normal 21-35 seconds). Fibrinogen, D dimer, and fibrin split products are normal. She has not received any anticoagulants. A 1:1 mixing study shows initial correction of aPTT; however, prolongation to 85 seconds after 2 hours of incubation. She is found to have a factor VIII inhibitor with titers of 20 BU.

   All the following may be included in this patient's treatment except:

   A. Factor 8 inhibitor bypassing agent (FEIBA)
   B. Prednisone and cyclophosphamide
   C. Intravenous immunoglobulin
   D. Brentuximab vedotin
   E. rFVIIa

   Answer: D. Brentuximab vedotin is not used in the setting of acquired FVIII inhibitor, as it is a monoclonal antibody directed at CD30. Rituximab can be used in relapsed/refractory cases of AHA. FEIBA and rFVIIa may be used in this patient to control bleeding. Prednisone with or without cyclophosphamide as well as intravenous immunoglobulin may be used to eliminate the inhibitor.

Caveats

- Acquired inhibitors of coagulation factors are antibodies that inhibit the production or clearance of a coagulation factor, most commonly occurring against factor VIII.
- The most common causes of acquired factor inhibitors are autoimmune diseases, malignancies, medications, and pregnancy; however, the majority of cases idiopathic.
- The goals of treatment are to control bleeding and remove and eliminate the inhibitor.
- FEIBA, rFVIIa, and porcine FVIII concentrates are often used to control bleeding, while steroids with or without cytotoxic medications are used to eliminate the inhibitor.

References

1. Franchini M, Mannucci PM. Acquired haemophilia A: a 2013 update. Thromb Haemost. 2013;110(12):1114–20.
2. Delgado J, Jimenez-Yuste V, Hernandez-Navarro F, et al. Acquired haemophilia: review and meta-analysis focused on therapy and prognostic factors. Br J Haematol. 2003;121(1):21–35.
3. Prescott R, Nakai H, Saenko EL, et al. The inhibitor antibody response is more complex in hemophilia A patients than in most nonhemophiliacs with factor VIII autoantibodies. Blood J Am Soc Hematol. 1997;89(10):3663–71.
4. Morrison A, Ludlam C, Kessler C. Use of porcine factor VIII in the treatment of patients with acquired hemophilia. 1993;81:1513.
5. Green D, Rademaker AW, Briët E. A prospective, randomized trial of prednisone and cyclophosphamide in the treatment of patients with factor VIII autoantibodies. Thromb Haemost. 1993;70(11):753–7.
6. Knoebl P, Thaler J, Jilma P, et al. Emicizumab for the treatment of acquired hemophilia A. Blood. 2021;137(3):410–9.
7. Green D, Lechner K. A survey of 215 non-hemophilic patients with inhibitors to factor VIII. Thromb Haemost. 1981;45(03):200–3.

34 Disseminated Intravascular Coagulation

Mohammad Ammad Ud Din
and Nathan Visweshwar

Introduction

Disseminated intravascular coagulation (DIC) is an uncommon but potentially fatal acquired syndrome resulting from the aberrant systemic activation of the clotting cascade that leads to the consumption of procoagulant factors and platelets causing both micro- and macrovascular thrombi and hemorrhage simultaneously. The phenomenon is seen among approximately 1% of admissions to tertiary hospitals and has been described in two distinct phases: acute DIC, which is usually catastrophic and characterized by widespread thrombi with subsequent multiorgan failure and/or major hemorrhage, or chronic DIC, which is a more subclinical syndrome stemming from advanced mucin-secreting adenocarcinoma. The DIC is almost always secondary to a triggering condition, most commonly sepsis. Up to half of all cases of DIC are seen among patients with severe sepsis, while approximately 10% of cases are seen among patients with trauma, malignancy,

M. A. U. Din (✉)
Department of Hematology/Oncology, H Lee Moffitt Cancer Center and Research Institute, Florida, USA
e-mail: Mohammad.ammad-ud-din@moffitt.org

N. Visweshwar
Hematology/Oncology, University of South Florida, Tampa, Florida, USA

L. Sokol, L. Zhang (eds.), *Non-Neoplastic Hematologic Disorders*,
https://doi.org/10.1007/978-3-031-62373-8_34

or obstetrical complications (Table 34.1). Acute DIC carries a grim prognosis, with some studies showing a 28-day mortality rate ranging from 25% to 50%, which is significantly higher compared to critically ill hospitalized patients that do not fulfill the criteria of DIC. Since DIC is driven by an underlying trigger, the treatment relies on management of the inciting condition, with supportive measures aimed at repleting the coagulation proteins.

Table 34.1 Summary of underlying triggers for disseminated intravascular coagulation

Clinical condition	Causes of DIC
Sepsis for severe infection	Gram-negative bacteria Viral infection (COVID-19, enteric viral hemorrhagic fever, dengue, ebola) Malaria, rickettsia
Trauma	Severe burns Head injury Fat embolism Heat stroke
Malignancy associated	Solid tumors (pancreas, stomach, colorectal cancer, or any mucin-secreting adenocarcinoma) Acute leukemia (classically acute promyelocytic leukemia)
Liver disease	Acute decompensated cirrhosis Fulminant liver failure
Obstetrical complications	Placental abruption Placenta previa Eclampsia Hemolysis, elevated liver enzymes, and low platelets (HELLP) syndrome Amniotic fluid embolism
Vascular abnormalities	Vasculitis Aortic aneurysm Giant hemangiomas (Kasabach–Merritt syndrome)
Severe toxic or immunological reactions	Snake bite (particularly snakes from the genus *Echis*) Acute graft vs host disease Acute graft rejection ABO-incompatible transfusion reaction

Pathogenesis

Several mechanisms that lead to an awry activation of the coagulation cascade in DIC have been identified. All pathways lead to the initiation and self-sustenance of a prothrombotic state that in turn causes consumption of the physiologic coagulation factors. The formation of thrombi consumes the natural anticoagulants as well as for the clot-dissolving processes, leading to widespread clotting, and bleeding. Key inflammatory agents involved in these processes include tumor necrosis factor (TNF)-α and interleukin (IL)-1 and IL-6. Recent research suggests that intravascular webs (neutrophil extracellular traps), composed of DNA released from apoptotic cells entangled with neutrophils, platelets, fibrin, and cationic proteins like histones, may also play a significant role in the formation of thrombi [1].

The production of thrombin in DIC is initiated through the activation of the tissue-factor/factor VII(a) pathway, leading to the generation of factors Xa and IXa. Tissue factor can be exposed by activated mononuclear cells, endothelial cells, or cancer cells. In DIC, all natural anticoagulation pathways are impaired. There is a significant imbalance between the reduced function of tissue-factor pathway inhibitor and increased tissue factor-dependent clotting activation. Moreover, a significant deficiency in the protein-C system further hinders the effective inhibition of thrombin production. This deficiency is caused by a decrease in the expression of thrombomodulin on endothelial cells and a reduction in the synthesis and increased degradation of protein C. Additionally, levels of antithrombin, the main inhibitor of thrombin, are significantly reduced in DIC because of concurrent use, decreased synthesis, and degradation by elastase from activated neutrophils. Furthermore, natural blood clot–dissolving processes are inactive because of an elevated level of plasminogen activator inhibitor-1 (PAI-1), which regulates the activation of plasminogen and plasmin generation [1, 2].

Clinical Manifestations

Depending on the underlying trigger, degree of coagulation activation, and consumption of anticoagulation pathways, DIC may present as either:

Compensated/chronic DIC resulting from continuous, low-grade hemostatic dysfunction, resulting in an increased risk of thrombosis without obvious concomitant hemorrhage. This phase is usually associated with chronic long-term triggers like pregnancy, autoimmune diseases, and, occasionally in, malignancy. In usual cases, emergent use of blood products for rapid restoration of the coagulation profile is not needed, and correction of the procoagulant state can be achieved by treatment directed toward reducing the systemic inflammatory state. Chronic DIC can progress to acute DIC in cases of an added insult to the existing compromised coagulation regulatory mechanisms.

Acute overt DIC is associated with both thrombotic and major bleeding manifestation resulting from a severe disturbance of the hemostasis mechanisms. The most commonly associated trigger is acute sepsis. Because of the rapid consumption, coagulopathy in overt-hemorrhage patients requires repeated transfusion support for repletion of procoagulant factors while the underlying trigger is being medically managed. Acute DIC carries a high mortality because of the subsequent multiorgan dysfunction. Patients are usually critically ill with concomitant shock, respiratory failure, and renal and/or hepatic dysfunction [2, 3, 4].

Laboratory Investigations

DIC is a clinical and laboratory diagnosis. All laboratory testing should be ordered in the appropriate clinical scenario as no single test can confirm or dismiss the diagnosis of DIC. In cases in which the clinical suspicion of DIC is high, supporting laboratory workup includes complete blood count, prothrombin time (PT) and activated partial thromboplastin time (aPTT), fibrinogen, fibrin split products, D-dimer, and review of the peripheral blood smear. The common abnormalities in these parameters are summarized in Table 34.2. As mentioned earlier, these tests are sensitive but not specific for DIC and can be deranged in a variety of other pathologic conditions as mentioned in Table 34.2.

Generally, acute DIC presents with laboratory evidence of consumption of coagulation factors and platelets (e.g., prolonged PT, aPTT, and low fibrinogen) and fibrinolysis (e.g., increased D-dimer and fibrin split products) in the absence of other competing diagnoses. Chronic DIC, by contrast, may only have evidence of fibrinolysis (e.g., increased D-dimer) in the absence of another etiology. Of note, though fibrinogen is mostly low in DIC, it is an acute phase state, and thus, its plasma level might be false within normal range because of massive overproduction in systemic inflammatory conditions such as sepsis and malignancy. The peripheral blood smear can be normal, but a classic feature associated with DIC is microangiopathic hemolytic anemia with schistocytes and helmet cells, although these changes are less pronounced compared to other thrombotic microangiopathies [3, 4, 5].

Table 34.2 Laboratory investigation and differential diagnosis of disseminated intravascular coagulation

Laboratory investigation	Result	Other pathologies besides DIC with similar results
Platelet count	Decreased	Acute venous thrombotic event, hypersplenism, sepsis-related bone marrow suppression, microthrombotic angiopathies
Prothrombin time	Prolonged	Liver failure, vitamin K deficiency, acute major hemorrhage
Activated partial thromboplastin time	Prolonged	Heparin use, liver failure, acute major hemorrhage
Fibrinogen	Decreased	Liver failure, acute major hemorrhage, use of direct thrombin inhibitors, autoantibody formation in myeloma, or drug induced
Fibrin split products	Increased	Hematoma, autoimmune flares

Treatment Strategies

The fundamentals of treating DIC revolve around successful mitigation of the precipitating condition. However, supportive measures are needed to ameliorate coagulopathy for severe cases. For DIC patients with thrombocytopenia or clotting factor deficiency, transfusion of platelets or cryoprecipitate is usually not warranted, based on deranged laboratory investigations alone, and is reserved for patients with active hemorrhage or those scheduled for surgery or interventions associated with bleeding. Though the beneficial of transfusing plasma, fibrinogen concentrate, cryoprecipitate, or platelets have not been established through randomized controlled trials, most expert guidelines recommend 1 or 2 units of platelet concentrate (5 donors/unit) to increase the platelet count to at least $20–30 \times 10^9$/L among such patients with hemorrhage and at least 50×10^9/L among patients scheduled for a major procedure [6]. Similarly, coagulation-factor replacement should also be considered for cases of significantly prolonged PT or aPTT or a fibrinogen level <50 mg/dL. Commonly used options include fresh frozen plasma, frozen within 24 hours after collection and cyoprecipitate. The goal of these supportive measures again is to control bleeding, not to correct the laboratory derangements [6, 7]. Using antifibrinolytic agents like tranexamic acid or epsilon-aminocaproic acid is discouraged in DIC as inhibition of the fibrinolytic system potentially increases risk of thrombosis, but their use can be considered exclusively for cases of hypofibrinolytic states. Similarly, using prothrombin complex, concentrates is contradicted because of the heightened risk of thrombosis [6, 8].

Usage of anticoagulation to tackle the risk of thrombosis in DIC has remained controversial. Though experimental studies have shown heparin to be beneficial in blocking the coagulation cascade, data from large trials supporting this intervention are still lacking. Recently, however, a randomized controlled study among patients with sepsis demonstrated a small benefit of heparin on mortality and did not show significant adverse effects. Generally, using heparin is accepted with DIC in the setting of high-volume tumor burden and in purpura fulminans where thrombotic complications outweigh bleeding events. Additionally, patients with DIC who are not actively bleeding should receive prophylactic anticoagulation with heparin or low molecular weight heparin, particularly in the intensive care unit [6, 7].

Questions

1. A 26-year-old female presents to the emergency department in labor at 38 weeks of gestation. This is her first pregnancy. She is admitted for delivery, but her labor fails to progress after 19 hours. She thereafter has a cesarean section and delivers a healthy male infant. Shortly after the procedure, she begins to have heavy vaginal bleeding and is diagnosed with placental abruption. She is fluid-resuscitated, and 3 units of packed red blood cells are administered. On physical examination, she is afebrile; blood pressure is 92/64 mmHg; and pulse rate is 102/minute. Moderate persistent vaginal bleeding is noted. Laboratory studies revealed elevated D-dimer, prolonged activated partial thromboplastic time and PT, hemoglobin: 7.1 g/dl, platelet count: 65 000/Ul, and fibrinogen: 75 mg/dl (normal range, >150–350 mg/dl).

   What is the most appropriate infusion for further management?

   A. Cross-matched whole blood
   B. Cryo-poor plasma
   C. Single-donor platelets
   D. Fresh frozen plasma and cryoprecipitate

   Answer: D. Fresh frozen plasma and cryoprecipitate

   Explanation: Bleeding from DIC usually requires transfusion support while the underlying cause is addressed. Fresh frozen plasma and cryoprecipitate is the treatment of choice for patients with ongoing bleeding and hypofibrinogenemia.

2. A 28-year-old male presents to the emergency department for worsening fatigue and dyspnea on exertion for the past 4 days.

This morning, he felt feverish and had low-grade epistaxis. He denies any substance abuse or prior medical history. On physical examination, temperature is 100.5 °F, blood pressure is 104/68, pulse rate is 112/minute, and respiration rate is 23/minute. Dried blood is noted in the nares. Petechiae is noted on bilateral lower extremities. Laboratory studies revealed pancytopenia, hemoglobin 9.8 g/dl, leukocyte count 2900/uL (20% neutrophils, 35% lymphocytes, 4% bands, and 20% large, atypical cells), platelet count 14 000/Ul. Coagulation studies demonstrated an elevated D-dimer, prolonged aPTT and PT, and fibrinogen: 81 mg/dl (normal range, >150–350 mg/dl).

What is the most likely diagnosis?

A. Aplastic anemia
B. Acute promyelocytic leukemia
C. Chronic granulocytic leukemia
D. Sezary syndrome

Answer: B. Acute promyelocytic leukemia

Explanation: This patient has new onset pancytopenia with peripheral blood count showing atypical large cells most consistent with acute leukemia. Acute promyelocytic leukemia is a subset of acute myeloid leukemia that typically presents with bleeding and coagulopathy resulting from DIC. Presence of DIC should prompt initiation of supportive transfusion measures with fresh frozen plasma, cryoprecipitate (for hypofibrinogenemia), and platelets (for thrombocytopenia) to reduce risk of early mortality. Coagulopathy, because of acute promyelocytic leukemia, also responds to all-trans retinoic acid, which targets the underlying differentiation of blast cells.

References

1. Papageorgiou C, Jourdi G, Adjambri E, et al. Disseminated intravascular coagulation: an update on pathogenesis, diagnosis, and therapeutic strategies. Clin Appl Thromb Hemost. 2018;24(9_suppl):8s–28s.
2. Levi M, Toh CH, Thachil J, Watson HG. Guidelines for the diagnosis and management of disseminated intravascular coagulation. Br J Haematol. 2009;145(1):24–33.

3. Wada H, Matsumoto T, Yamashita Y. Diagnosis and treatment of disseminated intravascular coagulation (DIC) according to four DIC guidelines. J Intensive Care. 2014;2(1):15.
4. Toh CH, Dennis M. Disseminated intravascular coagulation: old disease, new hope. BMJ. 2003;327(7421):974–7.
5. Gando S, Levi M, Toh CH. Disseminated intravascular coagulation. Nat Rev Dis Primers. 2016;2:16037.
6. Levi M, Scully M. How I treat disseminated intravascular coagulation. Blood. 2018;131(8):845–54.
7. Saba HI, Morelli GA. The pathogenesis and management of disseminated intravascular coagulation. Clin Adv Hematol Oncol. 2006;4(12):919–26.
8. Levi M. Pathogenesis and diagnosis of disseminated intravascular coagulation. Int J Lab Hematol. 2018;40(S1):15–20.

Liver Disease and Coagulopathy

35

Jerrin Joy Pullukkara

Introduction

The liver is associated with all three phases of hemostasis—primary hemostasis, coagulation, and fibrinolysis. In the Unites States, 4.5 million people are diagnosed with liver disease. Alcohol-associated cirrhosis accounts for 48% of deaths caused by cirrhosis. Therefore, coagulopathy caused by liver disease is a common occurrence. There is growing evidence that liver dysfunction results in deficiencies in procoagulant and anticoagulant factors, leading to a rebalanced homeostasis [1]. However, any tipping of this balance can result in a risk of bleeding or clotting. Thus, patients with coagulopathy caused by liver dysfunction require close monitoring and clinically oriented management—rather than correcting abnormal prothrombin time (PT), activated partial thromboplastin time (aPTT), or platelet count.

J. J. Pullukkara (✉)
Department of Internal Medicine, University of South Florida, Tampa, FL, USA
e-mail: jjoypullukkara@usf.edu

L. Sokol, L. Zhang (eds.), *Non-Neoplastic Hematologic Disorders*,
https://doi.org/10.1007/978-3-031-62373-8_35

Pathogenesis

Primary Hemostasis

Liver dysfunction is associated with mild-to-moderate thrombocytopenia caused by:

- Congestive splenomegaly causing platelet sequestration.
- Bone marrow suppression secondary to alcohol, antiviral therapy like interferon and folate deficiency, and medications like azathioprine (treatment of autoimmune hepatitis) and fluroquinolones (treatment of peritonitis).
- Impaired hepatic synthesis of thrombopoietin (TPO).
- Accelerated TPO clearance by binding to platelets in spleen.
- Hypersplenism caused by exaggerated function of splenic macrophages.
- Immune-mediated platelet dysfunction in hepatitis C and primary biliary cholangitis [2].

Coagulation System

The liver has a major role in synthesizing all clotting factors except factor VIII (along with von Willebrand factor), which is produced by vascular endothelial cells. It is also associated with the synthesis of clotting factors, natural anticoagulants, as well as several fibrinolytic proteins (see Table 35.1).

Chronic liver disease results in reduced synthesis of procoagulant proteins factors II, V, VII, IX, X, and XI. The factor levels correlate with progression of the disease. Patients develop acquired dysfibrinogenemia in 50% to 78% of cases as regenerating hepatocytes synthesize an abnormal fibrinogen with increased sialic acid residues, which impair the polymerization of fibrin monomers. The half-life of clotting factors varies from 6 hours for factor VII to 5 days for fibrinogen. Factor VIII levels are also

Table 35.1 Clotting-factor production site and half-life

Clotting factor	Site of synthesis		Vitamin K dependency	Half-life
	Hepatocyte	Endothelial cells		
I	+	+		2 d–4 d
II	+		+	3 d–4 d
III		+		
IV				
V	+			36 h
VI				
VII	+		+	4 h–6 h
VIII		+		8 h–12 h
IX	+		+	18 h–24 h
X	+		+	40 h–60 h
XI	+			40 h–70 h
XII	+			60 h
XIII	+			11 d–14 d

increased several-fold secondary to increased synthesis caused by cytokine release and inflammatory response, triggering production of factor VIII from the endothelium. This is taken advantage of while differentiating coagulopathy from liver disorder and disseminated intravascular coagulation.

The following inhibitors are synthesized in the liver independently of vitamin K: AT-III, protein-C inhibitor, C1-esterase inhibitor, alpha-2 macroglobulin, and histidine-rich glycoprotein. The levels of antithrombin, protein-C, and protein-S levels range from 10% to 65% of normal among patients with liver disease. Tissue-factor pathway inhibitor is synthesized by endothelial cells, and their levels are normal or elevated among patients with chronic liver disease. However, this is functionally impaired by low levels of protein S, which functions as a cofactor for tissue-factor pathway inhibitor-mediated downregulation of thrombin generation.

Fibrinolysis

All profibrinolytic and antifibrinolytic proteins are synthesized by the liver except tissue plasminogen activator (tPA) and PAI-1, which are synthesized by endothelial cells. PAI-1 is produced by a variety of sources, including adipose tissue. Plasma levels of tPA are usually elevated because of the release by activated endothelial cells and reduced hepatic clearance while there is a reduction in the levels of plasminogen, α2-antiplasmin, thrombin-activatable fibrinolysis inhibitor, and FXIII. Peritoneal fluid contains the fibrinolytic activity shown by high levels of plasminogen and plasmin-antiplasmin complexes, and reabsorption of ascitic fluid into systemic circulation may cause accelerated fibrinolysis, disrupting the balance [3].

Due to the rebalancing of the hemostasis system as seen in Table 35.2 (lack of production of coagulation and anticoagulation factors), ruptured esophageal varices causing mechanical bleeding are clinically the most relevant bleeding problem in cirrhosis (this is relevant because when a patient has massive hematemesis, usage of a Sengstaken–Blakemore tube is more useful than plasma products).

Table 35.2 Coagulation steps and functions affected by liver dysfunction

Promote bleeding	Rebalance	Promote thrombosis
Thrombocytopenia and platelet function defects Enhanced production of nitric oxide and prostacyclin	Primary hemostasis	Elevated levels of VWF Decreased levels of ADAMTS-13
Low levels of coagulation factors II, V, VII, IX, X, and XI Vitamin K deficiency Dysfibrinogenemia	Secondary hemostasis	Elevated levels of FVIII Decreased levels of protein C, protein S, antithrombin, alpha 2 macroglobulin, and heparin cofactor II
Low levels of alpha 2 antitrypsin, factor XIII, and TAFI Elevated tPA levels	Fibrinolysis	Low level of plasminogen

TAFI thrombin-activatable fibrinolysis inhibitor, *tPA* tissue plasminogen activator, *VWF* van Willebrand factor

Diagnosis

1. PT/international normalized ratio (INR)
   PT is performed by recalcifying citrated plasma in the presence of tissue factor and phospholipid and determining the time to form a fibrin clot. This assesses the extrinsic and common pathways of coagulation and is developed for patients on standard anticoagulation with vitamin K antagonists like warfarin. The INR is calculated from patient PT standardized by control PT adjusted for the international standardized index (ISI). The reduction of procoagulant factors can result in PT and aPTT prolongation; however, these results do not correlate with bleeding risk because they do not reflect the parallel reduction in anticoagulant factors. So, they are not considered as a good marker of coagulation function in liver disease and are not validated in chronic liver disease. Since the INR has been adopted in the model for the end-stage liver disease score, there have been proposals to use ISI liver for standardization among liver patients. But ISI liver has been found to have interlaboratory variant and logistical challenges and is not widely used.
2. Platelet count and function
   This has been found to be more predictive of bleeding than INR. A platelet count of <65–70 × 10^9/L was associated with increased risk of bleeding. There is no threshold that has been proposed, as the utility of platelet count to predict bleeding among patients with cirrhosis is still uncertain. Low platelet counts may reflect progression and severity of the underlying liver disease, accompanying portal hypertension and hypersplenism to a greater extent than bleeding risk at baseline. Platelet function is measured using platelet aggregometry, but it is not widely available and is unreliable among individuals with thrombocytopenia and may show false results with medications such as NSAIDs, SSRIs, and antiplatelet agents.
3. Viscoelastic testing
   Viscoelastic testing has received growing attention as an alternative marker for bleeding risk. It is also known as a global

hemostasis assay as it evaluates the entire hemostatic process from platelet activation and the coagulation cascade to clot formation and lysis. It is usually performed during major surgery like cardiac and liver transplantation as well as in trauma and postpartum hemorrhage. Thromboelastography (TEG) was able to accurately reflect the balance of hemostasis among patients with chronic liver disease outside of surgery in limited studies, but it has not been validated for predicting procedural bleeding risk using prospective studies.

(a) TEG
TEG is the more commonly used viscoelastic test and is measured using a cylindrical cup that holds a whole-blood sample at 37 °C and is oscillated to and from with a rotation cycle of 10 seconds. As the clot forms, the torque of the rotating cup is transmitted to an immersed pin which is converted to an electrical signal and monitored on a chart. The strength increases during clot development and decreases during clot lysis (Fig. 35.1 and Table 35.3).

(b) Rotational thromboelastography
Rotational TEG is an adaptation of TEG in which the cup remains stationary and the pin rotates

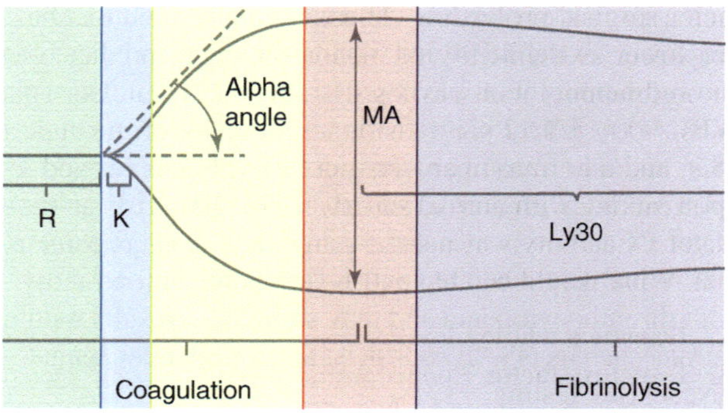

Fig. 35.1 Normal thromboelastography

Table 35.3 TEG interpretation and treatment recommendations

Component	Definition	Normal	Problem with	Treatment
ACT	Rapid time to first fibrin formation	80 s–140 s	Clotting factors	>140 s: FFP
R time	Actual time to first significant clot formation	5 min–10 min	Clotting factors	>10 min: FFP
K time	Time until achievement of fixed clot strength	1 min–3 min	Fibrinogen	>3 min: Cryoprecipitate
α angle	Speed of fibrin accumulation	53°–72°	Fibrinogen	<53: Cryoprecipitate
Maximum amplitude	Maximum strength of clot	50 mm–70 mm	Platelets	<50 mm: Platelets and/or DDAVP
Lysis at 30 min	% of amplitude reduction 30 min after maximum amplitude	0%–3%	Excess fibrinolysis	>3%: Tranexamic acid and/or aminocaproic acid

ACT activated clotting time, *DDAVP, FFP* fresh frozen plasma, *TEG* thromboelastography

4. Thrombin generation test (TGT)

   The TGT measures the total amount of thrombin generated during in vitro coagulation. In the presence of thrombomodulin, TGT measures the balance between procoagulant and anticoagulant factors in liver disease. Despite prolonged PT/INR and PTT levels among stable cirrhosis patients, TGT was found to be normal, demonstrating the rebalance of the coagulation system. This is currently a research tool and is not validated for bleeding risk among patients with liver disease.

   These are few tests that were used before the development of the new standardized testing [4].

- Quick's value: test for thrombin and fibrin formation in percentage, combination of PT, and PTT.
- Koller's test: differentiating test between lack of coagulation factors caused by hepatocellular damage vs vitamin K deficiency. Tested by intravenous administration of 10 mg vitamin K as well. See correction of Quick's value from <70% to >75% in 24 hours favoring vitamin K deficiency.
- Colombi index: percentage sum of factors II, V, and VII.

Major Differential Diagnosis

Differential diagnoses for coagulopathy caused by liver disease may include other etiologies of thrombocytopenia or bleeding disorders. An important differential diagnosis to rule out is disseminated intravascular coagulopathy (DIC), as clinical features and laboratory findings are similar to those in liver disease (low platelets, elevated PT/PTT/INR, low fibrinogen). Factor VIII levels are typically normal or high in liver-associated coagulopathy, as FVIII is made by vascular endothelial cells rather than the liver. FVIII is typically low in DIC caused by consumption. DIC and liver-associated coagulopathy may also coexist. Other differential diagnoses include microangiopathic hemolytic anemias (MAHAs), such as TTP, ITP, or thrombocytopenia caused by infections or marrow suppression, coagulation-factor deficiency or inhibitors, and iatrogenic disease.

Treatment

Bleeding can occur because of portal hypertension, thrombocytopenia, or intercurrent problems that disturb the balance between procoagulant and anticoagulant factors. The risk of bleeding among patients with cirrhosis is variable, and characteristics unique to cirrhosis, such as the presence of advanced Child–Turcotte–Pugh cirrhosis, presence of acute or chronic liver failure, acute kidney injury, or infections play a role in altering the balance of coagulation. Asymptomatic patients do not require any treatment for correction of abnormal laboratory values. It is important to recognize that these patients are also at risk for thrombosis, and inappropriate treatment to correct laboratory values could result in a further increased risk of thrombosis.

Prevention of Bleeding

The American Gastroenterology Association recommends against the use of TPO-receptor agonists (TPO-RA) or fresh frozen plasma (FFP)/platelets for bleeding prophylaxis for low-risk procedures. They also suggest standard anticoagulation prophylaxis over no anticoagulation for venous thromboembolism (VTE) prophylaxis for cirrhosis patients, given the thrombotic risk [5].

Vitamin K

Vitamin K supplementation should be considered if a deficiency is suspected, especially among patients with biliary disease or gut sterilization from broad-spectrum antibiotics who are at increased risk of deficiency. Cirrhotic patients have reduced synthetic function, and routine vitamin K has no proven benefit.

FFP

Prophylactic transfusion of FFP has not been shown to have any benefit before invasive procedures. Thrombin generation was normal among patients with cirrhosis, despite prolonged routine coagulation tests, suggesting that prophylactic infusion of FFP before invasive procedures is unlikely to have any clinical benefit and might be detrimental because of volume overload and worsening portal hypertension, thus increasing the risk of bleeding.

Platelet Transfusion

Correction of modest thrombocytopenia is unnecessary among patients with liver disease and might be unnecessary in low-risk procedures even if platelets are less than 50×10^9/L. Transfusion may be considered in high-risk procedures if platelets are less than 50×10^9/L, but there is no consensus on transfusion threshold.

Thrombopoietin-Receptor Agonists

TPO production is disrupted in chronic liver disease; thus, thrombopoietin agonists can be used to raise the platelet count to reduce the risk of procedure-related bleeding. The use of romiplostim and eltrombopag was associated with a reduction in platelet transfusion intraprocedure but at the cost of increased incidence of portal vein thrombosis. Second-generation oral agents avatrombopag (ADAPT-1 and ADAPT-2) and lusutrombopag (L-PLUS-1 and L-PLUS-2) are now approved for use among patients with thrombocytopenia related to liver disease who are undergoing an elective procedure. They are administered in patients with platelets $<50 \times 10^9$/L and had no prior history of thrombosis starting 7 to 10 days before the procedure.

Spleen-Directed Therapies

Partial-spleen embolization or laparoscopic splenectomy might have a role if TPO-RA fails, and a patient is not a candidate for transfusions. This procedure carries a risk of abscess, rupture, and sepsis and will only lead to a transient rise in platelets.

Management of Bleeding in Chronic Liver Disease

Patients experiencing active bleeding can be treated with:

- Cryoprecipitate to increase fibrinogen levels to greater than 100 mg/dL.
- Platelet transfusions to maintain platelet count greater than 50×10^9/L.
- Red blood cell transfusions should aim for target hemoglobin of 7 to 8 g/dL.
- Recombinant factor VIIa has not been shown to be beneficial in active bleeding even though it normalizes PT/INR and is not recommended.
- Prothrombin complex concentrates are costly and associated with thrombotic complications and should not be routinely used in managing coagulopathy of liver disease.
- Desmopressin did not improve clinical outcome among these patients.
- Antifibrinolytic agents were shown to reduce blood loss during liver transplantation but did not show any benefit in gastroin-

testinal bleeding as seen by HALT IT trial (hemorrhagic alleviation with tranexamic acid—intestinal system).

There is tremendous progress around the area of coagulopathy in liver disease with a move toward restrictive transfusions and testing as patients with liver disease appear to be in hemostatic balance. **Conventional laboratory testing has not been designed to reflect this, and optimal diagnostic and treatment strategies are needed for preventing bleeding and thrombosis among patients with liver disease**.

Board Question

1. A 49-year old woman comes to the emergency department with abdominal pain. Medical history is significant for alcohol associated cirrhosis with grade 1 esophageal varices. She takes spironolactone and furosemide. Temperature is 37.2 °C (99°F); blood pressure is 90/50 mm Hg; pulse is 104/min; and respirations are 18/min. Ecchymoses are noted on the upper and lower extremities. Ascites is present, and the abdomen is diffusely tender on palpation. aPTT at 35 s, D-dimer at 0.7 μg/mL, hemoglobin at 9.4 g/dL, WBC at 12 000/μL, platelets at 68 000/μL, PT at 17 s, and fibrinogen at 75 mg/dL.

   Which of the following tests will be most helpful in evaluation of the patient's coagulopathy?

   A. Factor II level
   B. Factor VIII level
   C. Factor X level
   D. Thrombin time

   Answer: B. Factor VIII is often normal or elevated among patients with liver disease because factor VIII is produced in hepatic and nonhepatic endothelial cells; however, factor VIII is consumed in DIC. A normal or elevated factor VIII level will support liver disease as the cause of this patient's coagulopathy.

References

1. Andriulli A, Angelo A, Angeli P, et al. Hemostatic balance in patients with liver cirrhosis: report of a consensus conference. Dig Liver Dis. 2016;48(5):455–67.
2. Lim HI, Cuker A. Thrombocytopenia and liver disease: pathophysiology and periprocedural management. Hematology Am Soc Hematol Educ Program. 2022;1:296–302.
3. Kujovich JL. Coagulopathy in liver disease: a balancing act. Hematology Am Soc Hematol Educ Program. 2015;1:243–9.
4. Kuntz E, Kuntz HD. Hepatology, principles and practice: history, morphology, biochemistry, diagnostics, clinic, therapy. 2nd ed. Springer-Verlag; 2006.
5. O'Shea RS, Davitkov P, Ko CW, et al. AGA clinical practice guideline on the Management of Coagulation Disorders in patients with cirrhosis. Gastroenterology. 2021;161(5):1615–1627.e1.

Therapeutic Principles of Bleeding Disorders

36

Ajay B. Iyer and Ashley M. Rose

Introduction

The approach to a patient with excessive bleeding should start with a history and physical exam. The onset of bleeding at birth or childhood may suggest a congenital bleeding disorder, while onset later in life suggests an acquired disorder. Bleeding may be spontaneous or after a procedure or surgery. The pattern of bleeding, whether it is mucocutaneous or soft-tissue bleeding, may also aid in coming to a diagnosis. Patients with disorders of primary hemostasis (platelets and von Willebrand disease [vWD]) often experience mucocutaneous bleeding, while those with disorders of secondary hemostasis (coagulation pathway disorders) will experience deep-tissue or central nervous system bleeding. It is critical to discuss medications, surgical history including dental procedures, past medical history, and family history to further understand the possible etiology of bleeding. It is of utmost importance to discern normal bleeding from abnormal bleeding. Treatment of recurrent bleeding with normal coagulation-factor assays depends on the cause and severity of bleeding. In this

A. B. Iyer
Department of Internal Medicine, HCA Healthcare, Sarasota, FL, USA

A. M. Rose (✉)
Department of Hematology and Oncology, H. Lee Moffitt Cancer Institute and Research Center, FL, USA

L. Sokol, L. Zhang (eds.), *Non-Neoplastic Hematologic Disorders*,
https://doi.org/10.1007/978-3-031-62373-8_36

chapter, we will discuss the general treatment of bleeding including bleeding caused by trauma and disorders or hemostasis.

Pathogenesis

Bleeding may be caused by a wide range of disorders affecting platelets, von Willebrand factor (vWF), or coagulation factors. The condition may be caused by quantitative or qualitative defects. The details about the pathogenesis of various disorders can be seen in the specific chapters dedicated to those disorders.

Diagnosis

Initial screening tests for abnormal bleeding include platelet count, prothrombin time (PT), and activated partial thromboplastin time (aPTT). Low platelet count should prompt workup for thrombocytopenia. Elevated PT or aPTT should prompt workup for coagulation-factor disorders, in which the next step would be a 1:1 mixing study. Test correction indicated a factor deficiency, while no correction indicated a factor inhibitor. Platelet function analyzer (PFA-100) can be used to screen for platelet dysfunction including vWD. Screening tests are sensitive to specimen handling and may need to be repeated. Clinical suspicion should prompt further workup if initial screening tests are negative.

Major Differential Diagnosis

Disseminated intravascular coagulopathy (DIC), immune thrombocytopenic purpura, vWD, heparin-induced thrombocytopenia, hemophilia A or B, rare coagulation-factor deficiency or inhibitor, platelet dysfunction caused by medications (including aspirin, anticoagulants, antibiotics, selective serotonin reuptake inhibitors, alcohol, clopidogrel NSAIDs, vitamin E, garlic, and gingko biloba), liver disease, renal disease, acute leukemia, or trauma.

Prognosis

Patients living with congenital bleeding disorders can expect to live full, productive lives with appropriate medical treatment, education, and a management plan in case of trauma or surgery. Life expectancy in congenital bleeding disorders, especially in hemophilia, varies, depending on whether patients receive appropriate treatment. Prognosis for patients with or without bleeding disorders depends on the cause and severity of bleeding.

Treatment

Treatment of bleeding varies depending on the cause and severity of bleeding. Initial management should include evaluation of hemodynamic status, recognizing life-threatening injuries, such as cardiac tamponade or intracerebral hemorrhage, preventing further blood loss, and restoring intravascular volume if necessary for the patient's specific condition.

Blood Products

Transfusion of blood products should be given if needed. Red blood cells (RBC) are typically given in the setting of hemoglobin level less than 7 g/dL. RBC transfusion might also be needed in the case of rapid, severe bleeding, or trauma (even with Hb. >9 g., especially with acute gastrointestinal bleed). Fluid resuscitation with lactated ringers may be used with caution until blood products are available. In moderate-to-severe bleeding in the adult trauma patient, blood products (i.e., RBC, fresh frozen plasma [FFP], and platelets) should be given in equivalent amounts in a 1:1:1 ratio. Whole blood can be used if available [1]. Recent studies have shown that aggressive intravenous fluid administration can at times be significantly harmful. Limited volume replacement intended to maintain minimally adequate organ perfusion with a goal of systolic blood pressure greater than

70 mmHg may improve outcomes [2]. This strategy has been referred to as delayed fluid resuscitation, controlled hypotension, or permissive hypotension [3]. The rationale behind this strategy is that aggressive fluid administration may dilute clotting factors and produce hypothermia which could disrupt thrombus formation and thus paradoxically enhance bleeding, leading to worsened outcomes.

For patients with nonsevere but ongoing significant bleeding (e.g., more than 4 units of packed RBC are transfused in the first few hours or significant continued drainage from drain), using the same transfusion ratios (1:1:1 ratio of PRBCs, FFP, and platelets) as mentioned above would be a reasonable and cautious approach. Where available, thromboelastography (TEG) and rotational thromboelastometry provide faster and more accurate assessment of coagulopathy. Using this in an appropriate manner can help guide treatment with clotting factors and reduce unnecessary transfusions.

Antifibrinolytics and Vitamin K

For patients with signs of significant, active hemorrhage who present within 3 h of injury, antifibrinolytics such as tranexamic acid (TXA) should be administered. The rationale behind this is that significant trauma can result in a marked inhibition of fibrinolysis. Antifibrinolytic agents can reduce all-cause and bleeding-related mortality if given within 3 h of injury in patients with significant hemorrhage [4]. Where available, TEG can be used to guide treatment, but if TEG is unavailable, empiric treatment with TXA should be given except for patients with isolated, severe traumatic brain injury. The initial dose is 1 g given over 10 min. The possibility of vitamin-K deficiency can be evaluated by measuring PT/international normalized ratio, both of which would be prolonged in vitamin-K deficiency. When the deficiency is mild, only the PT may be prolonged because of a predominant effect on factor VII. Vitamin K can be administered intravenously or orally to patients with bleeding while receiving warfarin and who are found to have a supratherapeutic INR. Individuals with major bleeding are given 10 mg of vitamin K by slow intravenous infusion. Further details about warfarin reversal are mentioned in Table 36.2.

FFP contains factor VIII and vWF, but large volumes are needed to obtain adequate factor levels (20–25 mL/kg). Because of the need for large volumes, fluid overload is a concern with FFP. Cryoprecipitate is a human plasma-derived product containing high levels of concentrated factor VIII, vWF, and fibrinogen (factor I). Cryoprecipitate is less likely to cause volume overload and associated complications, such as transfusion-associated circulatory overload when compared to FFP. The absence of factor IX in cryoprecipitate negates its use in hemophilia B. The details of specific indications for different blood products in bleeding scenarios are stated in Table 36.1.

Stopping Anticoagulation

When a major bleeding occurs, temporarily stopping the anticoagulant and initiating measures to control the bleeding source are required. Specific coagulation studies can be used to evaluate the significance of anticoagulant-induced bleeding. Normal INR would exclude warfarin-induced bleeding in patients taking the medication. A normal thrombin time or aPTT usually excludes clinically relevant levels of dabigatran. Anti-factor Xa levels (either general or drug-specific) can be used to exclude clinically relevant levels for factor Xa inhibitors. Reversal agents should be strongly considered for life-threatening bleeding or major bleeding that does not resolve with initial conservative management. Further details about bleeding-reversal strategies are mentioned in Table 36.2.

Table 36.1 Blood products: indications in bleeding and specific considerations

Blood Product	Indications	Special Considerations
Platelet	• Actively bleeding patients for platelet count <50,000/μL. • Platelets <100,000/μL if there is CNS bleeding. • Moderate-to-severe bleeding in trauma patients in a 1:1:1 ratio with pRBC and FFP.	• PTP is a rare transfusion reaction in which thrombocytopenia develops 5–10 days following transfusion because of lack of platelet antigen PIA1. Treatment is with IVIG.
DDAVP	• Minor bleeding/minor surgical procedures in individuals >2 years of age with vWD: mild-to-moderate type 1 and type 2. • Mild hemophilia A.	• Contraindicated in type 3 vWD. • No use in life-threatening bleeding because of slow onset of action. • Avoid use in >65 years of age because of increased risk of thrombosis. • Use with caution in epilepsy because of risk of hyponatremia.
Factor VIII	• Hemophilia A (severe bleeding)—50 IU/kg to raise the factor VIII level to 100%. • Hemarthrosis: 25 IU/kg of factor VIII to raise the factor VIII level by 50%. • Severe, refractory bleeding with factor VIII Inhibitors—for patients with low titer (<5 BU) or a low-responding inhibitor. Full replacement dose as above, plus an additional 50% correction for every BU of inhibitor.	• Patients on emicizumab for prophylaxis, factor replacement is needed for acute bleeding. Standard aPTT-based assay for factor VIII activity is falsely normalized/elevated with emicizumab.

(continued)

Blood Product	Indications	Special Considerations
FFP	• Warfarin reversal if PCC is not available. • Active bleeding, planned surgery or invasive procedure in patients with history of coagulation disorders. • TTP or factor deficiency with no alternate therapy available. • Moderate-to-severe bleeding in trauma patients in a 1:1:1 ratio with pRBC and platelets.	• Cirrhotic and heart failure patients poorly tolerate as high infusion volumes are necessary to achieve adequate hemostatic levels of coagulation factors. • CMV and graft-versus-host disease cannot be transmitted as there are no viable leukocytes.
Cryoprecipitate	• Postpartum hemorrhage. • Massive transfusion protocol for certain trauma. • DIC. • Uremia for which desmopressin is ineffective. • Acquired hypofibrinogenemia.	• Only contains factors VIII, XIII, fibrinogen, and von Willebrand factor.
APCC	• First line treatment for acquired hemophilia when factor VIII inhibitor >5 BU. • Reversal for non-VKA inhibitors if specific reversal agents unavailable.	• Avoid in hemophilia A with inhibitors receiving emicizumab because of risk of thrombotic microangiopathy. • Contraindicated in DIC.
Antifibrinolytics	• Active hemorrhage within 3 h of injury. • Routine administration in cardiac bypass. • Alternative agent for abnormal uterine bleeding. • Adjunctive treatment for tooth extraction in vWD, hemophilia A.	• Do not exceed maximum tranexamic-acid dose (50–100 mg/kg) because of potential neurotoxicity.

APCC activated prothrombin complex concentrate, *aPTT* activated partial thromboplastin time, *CMV* cytomegalovirus, *CNS* central nervous system, *DIC* disseminated intravascular coagulation, *FFP* fresh frozen plasma, *IVIG* intravenous immunoglobulin, *pRBC* packed red blood cells, *PTP* post-transfusion purpura, *TTP* thrombotic thrombocytopenic purpura, *TXA* tranexamic acid, *VKA* vitamin-K antagonist, *vWD* von Willebrand disease, *vWF* von Willebrand factor

Table 36.2 Bleeding-reversal strategies. PCC: prothrombin complex concentrate; FEIBA: factor 8 inhibitor bypassing activity.* Use activated PCC only if idarucizumab is unavailable and/or if continued bleeding is likely to be fatal within hours

Type of bleeding	Agent	Possible interventions
Life-threatening or imminently fatal bleeding (e.g., intracranial, retroperitoneal, compartment syndrome, massive gastrointestinal)	Dabigatran	• Idarucizumab. • Activated PCC* (e.g., FEIBA). • Antifibrinolytic agent (e.g., TXA). • Anticoagulant discontinuation. • Oral-activated charcoal (if last dose within prior 2 h). • Hemodialysis.
	Rivaroxaban, apixaban, edoxaban	• Andexanet alfa **or** 4F unactivated PCC (e.g., Kcentra). • Antifibrinolytic agent (e.g., TXA). • Anticoagulant discontinuation. • Oral-activated charcoal (if last dose recent enough).
	Warfarin	• **Preferred approach:** Give 4F PCC 1500–2000 units IV over 10 min. Check INR 15 min after completion of infusion. If INR is not ≤1.5, give additional 4F PCC. • Vitamin K 10 mg IV over 10–20 min. • **If 4F PCC is not available:** Give 3F PCC 1500 to 2000 units IV over 10 min. Check INR 15 min after administration. If INR is not ≤1.5, give additional 3F PCC. • Give factor VIIa 20 mcg/kg IV **OR** give FFP 2 units IV by rapid infusion. Factor VIIa preferred if volume overload is a concern. • Give vitamin K 10 mg IV over 10–20 min. • **If neither 4F PCC nor 3F PCC are available**: Give FFP 2 units IV by rapid infusion. Check INR 15 min after administration. If INR ≥1.5, administer 2 additional units of FFP IV. Repeat process until INR ≤1.5. Consider loop diuretic between FFP infusions if volume overload is a concern. • Give vitamin K 10 mg IV over 10 to 20 min.

4F-PCC 4-factor prothrombin complex concentrate, *FFP* fresh frozen plasma, *INR* international normalized ratio, *IV* intravenously, *PCC* prothrombin complex concentrate

Promising Clinical Studies

Recombinant FVIIa is reserved as salvage therapy to control microvascular bleeding when conventional therapy with transfusions and antifibrinolytic therapies has failed to control the bleeding. Another potential indication for rFVIIa is trauma or surgery in an individual who declines blood transfusions, such as a Jehovah's Witness, or an individual for whom compatible blood is not available. A 2005 randomized trial involving 301 patients with blunt or penetrating trauma found that compared to transfusions, rFVIIa (administered after the eighth unit of RBCs at a dose of 200 μg/kg, followed by a dose of 100 μg/kg 1 and 3 h later) was associated with a reduction in transfusions [5].

Caveats

- If the patient has history of significant postoperative and post-dental bleeding (needing blood products), then normal PT, partial thromboplastin time, and thrombin time do not exclude significant bleeding disorder (coagulation screening tests are normal among patients with a factor level > 25%).
- Platelet disorders (qualitative/quantitative) rarely produce life-threatening bleeding (intracranial bleed in patients with immune thrombocytopenic purpura is <1%).
- For patients with significant postoperative bleeding with negative factor assay, testing FFP (about 3–4 units) will be sufficient to attain hemostasis. In rare bleeding disorders (factor II, V, or VII deficiencies), a level of 10% is sufficient to attain hemostasis.
- For severe thrombocytopenia with refractoriness to platelets secondary to alloimmunization, empiric treatment with antifibrinolytics may be needed to avoid intracranial bleeding.
- DDAVP is contraindicated in type 3 vWD. It should be used with caution among patients with epilepsy because of the risk of hyponatremia and among elderly individuals (>65 years) because of the risk of thrombosis.

- Post-transfusion purpura is a rare transfusion reaction to any platelet-containing product, in which thrombocytopenia develops 5–10 days following transfusion because of the lack of platelet antigen PIA1. Treatment is with IVIG.
- The cryoprecipitate contents fibrinogen, factor VIII, vWD, factor XIII, and fibronectin. Hence, cryoprecipitate has no role in other bleeding disorders including factor IX deficiency.
- For patients with nonsevere but ongoing severe bleeding, such as requiring multiple units of blood in the first few hours, an approach to transfuse pRBC, platelets, and FFP in a 1:1:1 approach would be reasonable.
- For patients with no history of interventional/postoperative/postdental bleeding, significant bleeding following the procedure intervention/surgery is *silk-suture syndrome*, i.e., failure to achieve hemostasis during the interventional procedure causing local bleeding.

Board Questions

Question 1

A 48-year-old man with chronic liver disease is hospitalized after massive hematemesis. Medical history is notable for alcohol dependence. He takes no medications. On physical examination, temperature is normal, blood pressure is 102/68 mm Hg, pulse rate is 118/min, and respiratory rate is 22/min. He has hepatomegaly, jaundice, and spider angiomata. Hemoglobin is 9.5 gm/dl; platelets are 45,000/μL; PT is 17.8 s; PTT is 45 s; D-dimer is 5800 mg/L; and fibrinogen is 66 mg/dl. He receives volume resuscitation with fluids, erythrocyte and platelet transfusions, and vitamin K. Which of the following should also be provided to manage this patient's coagulopathy?

A. Activated factor VII concentrate.
B. Four-factor prothrombin complex concentrate.
C. Tranexamic acid.
D. Cryoprecipitate.

- This patient should receive a transfusion with cryoprecipitate. He has the coagulopathy of liver disease, characterized by thrombocytopenia, prolonged aPTT, PT, elevated D-dimer level, and hypofibrinogenemia. Vitamin K will help correct the PT, and thrombocytopenia is addressed with platelet transfusion. Fibrinogen levels less than 100 mg/dL (1 g/L) associated with active bleeding should be corrected. Cryoprecipitate contains more fibrinogen than FFP and is the blood component of choice for treating this patient. It is often difficult to distinguish between DIC and the coagulopathy of liver disease, but a normal or increased factor VIII-level points to liver disease instead of DIC. The management of these coagulopathies is often the same.
- Recombinant activated factor VII is recommended to treat patients with acquired hemophilia associated with high titers of antibody directed against factor VIII. It may also be used to treat uncontrolled bleeding in patients with liver disease unresponsive to replacement of platelets, FFP, vitamin K, and cryoprecipitate.
- Accelerated fibrinolysis plays some role in the coagulopathy of bleeding in liver disease, and TXA may reduce bleeding in some of these patients. No laboratory test correlates fibrinolysis with bleeding risk, and TXA should not be used before treating more objective measures of coagulopathy, such as low fibrinogen levels.
- Four-factor prothrombin complex concentrate is used to treat patients with warfarin toxicity and life-threatening bleeding. It should not be used more routinely to treat patients with the coagulopathy of liver disease and bleeding until conventional component support proves ineffective.

Question 2

A 75-year-old man is evaluated for new onset left-sided weakness that started 3 h ago. He had sudden onset symptoms without any precipitating events. He has a pertinent history of atrial fibrillation on warfarin. On evaluation, he had an elevated INR of 10.5. CT scan showed a right-sided intracranial hemorrhage. Complete blood count is normal with a hemoglobin of 13, platelet count of 200,000/μL. Which of the following is the next best step?

A. FFP.
B. Intravenous (IV) vitamin K.
C. FFP + vitamin K.
D. Four-factor PCC + vitamin K.

Answer: D. Four-factor PCC + vitamin K

- This patient is having a life-threatening bleed with right-sided intracranial hemorrhage and is on warfarin with an elevated INR. He meets the criteria for administration of urgent reversal agents. The reversal agent of choice would be to give 4F-PCC, 1500 to 2000 units IV over 10 min. The next step would be to check INR 15 min after completion of the infusion. If INR is not $\leq$1.5, give additional 4F- (4-factor) PCC. This should be accompanied by vitamin K, 10 mg IV over 10–20 min.
- FFP is the third agent of choice for warfarin reversal if 4F-PCC or 3F PCC are not available.
- Administering IV vitamin K by itself would not be the agent of choice in this patient who is having a life-threatening bleed caused by warfarin use as its onset of action is slower compared to PCC.

Question 3

A 27-year-old male patient with a history of hemophilia A is diagnosed with a right-sided subdural hematoma. He is scheduled to have a craniotomy for decompression in the operating room. In addition to ordering factor VIII concentrate, what pharmacologic adjunct should be given intravenously to help minimize surgical bleeding?

A. FFP.
B. Factor IX.
C. TXA.
D. Antithrombin III.

- TXA is an antifibrinolytic that will competitively inhibit the inactivation of plasminogen, which thereby reduces the conversion of plasminogen to plasmin.
- In this case, factor VIII would be the initial treatment of choice, but TXA would serve as an excellent adjunct to help stabilize clot formation and minimize further bleeding.
- Antithrombin III is a protease that inhibits coagulation by neutralizing the enzymatic activity of thrombin. Antithrombin III is indicated in the following scenarios: heparin resistance, DIC, and hereditary antithrombin III deficiency. It would, therefore, be of no clinical value in this scenario.
- Factor IX infusions have no clinical benefit for a patient with hemophilia A. Since this patient is already planning to receive factor VIII infusions, administering FFP would provide no additional benefit.

References

1. Spahn DR, Bouillon B, Cerny V, et al. The European guideline on management of major bleeding and coagulopathy following trauma. Crit Care. 2019;23(1):98. . 5th edition. Published 27 Mar 2019. https://doi.org/10.1186/s13054-019-2347-3.
2. Stern SA, Dronen SC, Birrer P, Wang X. Effect of blood pressure on hemorrhage volume and survival in a near-fatal hemorrhage model incorporating a vascular injury. Ann Emerg Med. 1993;22(2):155–63. https://doi.org/10.1016/s0196-0644(05)80195-7.
3. Tran A, Yates J, Lau A, Lampron J, Matar M. Permissive hypotension versus conventional resuscitation strategies in adult trauma patients with hemorrhagic shock: A systematic review and meta-analysis of randomized controlled trials. J Trauma Acute Care Surg. 2018;84(5):802–8. https://doi.org/10.1097/TA.0000000000001816.
4. Roberts I, Shakur H, Coats T, et al. The CRASH-2 trial: a randomized controlled trial and economic evaluation of the effects of tranexamic acid on death, vascular occlusive events and transfusion requirement in bleeding trauma patients. Health Technology Assessment, No. 17.10.
5. Boffard KD, Riou B, Warren B, et al. Recombinant factor VIIa as adjunctive therapy for bleeding control in severely injured trauma patients: two parallel randomized, placebo-controlled, double-blind clinical trials. J Trauma. 2005;59(1):8–18. https://doi.org/10.1097/01.ta.0000171453.37949.b7.

Part V

Clotting Disorders

Familial Thrombophilia

37

Jerel David, Wissam Hanayneh, and Michael Jaglal

Introduction

Familial thrombophilia is an encompassing term used to describe multiple inherited disorders that increase the risk of developing venous thromboembolism (VTE). There are several types of familial thrombophilia, each caused by unique genetic mutations. The most common types are factor V Leiden and prothrombin gene mutation which together account for 50–60% of cases [1]. The relative thrombosis risk for patients who harbor heterogeneous or homozygous Factor V Leiden mutations is 3–7 times or 50–100 times than those without, respectively. Other types of familial thrombophilia include protein C deficiency, protein S deficiency, and antithrombin (AT) deficiency. The probability of developing thrombosis compared with those with no defect was 8.5 times higher for carriers of protein S deficiency, 8.1 for AT

J. David
Hematology Oncology Fellow, Moffitt Cancer Center/University of South Florida, Tampa, FL, USA

W. Hanayneh
Our Lady of Lourdes- JD Moncus Cancer Center, Lafayette, LA, USA

M. Jaglal (✉)
Moffitt Cancer Center, University of South Florida, Tampa, FL, USA
e-mail: michael.jaglal@moffitt.org

L. Sokol, L. Zhang (eds.), *Non-Neoplastic Hematologic Disorders*,
https://doi.org/10.1007/978-3-031-62373-8_37

deficiency, 7.3 for protein C deficiency, and 2.2 for factor V Leiden [2]. Despite some case reports indicating a possible link with an increased risk of arterial thrombosis, this has not been validated nor substantiated in larger studies [3–5]. The book chapter will focus on the common familial thrombophilia and summarize the standard clinicopathologic features, underlying mechanisms, and prophylactic and treatment strategy. Rarely thrombophilia syndromes, such as hereditary hyperhomocysteinemia, elevated FVIII level, hereditary dysfibrinogenemia, Factor XII deficiency, and plasminogen activator inhibitor, can lead to thrombosis [6].

Pathogenesis

The pathogenesis of familial thrombophilia is under investigation. Mutations involving the genes in control of hemostasis and coagulation pathway are attributable to the following common familial thrombophilia (Table 37.1).

Factor V Leiden Deficiency

This condition is caused by a mutation in the gene that codes for the procoagulant protein factor V (F5). A single point mutation results in the replacement of Arg506 in one of the activated protein C (APC) cleavage sites with a Gln, which impairs the degradation of FVa by APC [7]. It carries 4–5 times increased risk of VTE. The mutation is heterozygous in 99% of people with FVL. The other 1% are homozygous for FVL or, in extremely rare situations, have pseudo-homozygosity for FVL, because they have heterozygous FVL plus a variation on the other F5 allele that causes factor V deficiency, leaving FVL as the only type of factor V in their circulation [8–10].

Table 37.1 Genetics of the most common inherited thrombophilia

Disorder	Mode of inheritance	Genotypic mutation	Altered coagulation pathway
Activated protein C resistance/ factor V Leiden mutation	AD	Commonly a heterozygous point mutation at 1691 G → A	Mutated gene is resistant to cleavage at position 506 by activated protein C.
Prothrombin gene mutation	AD	Point mutation at 20210 G → A in prothrombin gene	Multiple imbalances in hemostasis
Protein C deficiency	AD	Mutations in the *PROC1* gene on chromosome 2	Uninhibited procoagulant factors Va and VIIIa.
Protein S deficiency	AD	Mutations in the *PROS1* gene on chromosome 3	Uninhibited procoagulant factors Va and VIIIa.
Antithrombin deficiency	AD with variable penetrance	Mutations and other genetic alteration in the *AT3* gene on chromosome 1	Uninhibited thrombin (factor IIa), factor Xa, and other serine proteases in the coagulation cascade.

AD autosomal dominant

Prothrombin Gene Mutation

This condition is caused by the single point G to A mutation at position 20,210 affects the 3′ untranslated region of the prothrombin gene (F2). This results in an increased level of prothrombin in the blood in addition to gain of function of the protein which in turn increases the risk of VTE by 2–4 times [1].

Protein C Deficiency

This condition can be inherited or acquired. Protein C is one of the vitamin K-dependent anticoagulants. Protein C gene mutations can lead to quantitative (type I deficiency) or qualitative (type II deficiency) defects, and circulating levels of protein C may be reduced in a number of conditions that affect protein C synthesis (right heart failure with hepatic congestion, severe liver disease, malnutrition, or disseminated intravascular coagulation [DIC]) [11]. Protein C deficiency increases the risk of thrombosis by 7–10 times.

Protein S Deficiency

Like protein C deficiency, this condition can be inherited or acquired. The inherited form can lead to quantitative (type I), qualitative (type II), or selective free protein S deficiency (type III). Protein S serves as a cofactor for APC, which inactivates procoagulant factors Va and VIIIa, reducing thrombin generation. A deficiency can also be acquired due to conditions, such as pregnancy, acute thrombosis, liver disease, nephrotic syndrome, or DIC [12]. It carries a 5–8-time increased risk of thrombosis.

Antithrombin Deficiency

AT deficiency can also be inherited or acquired. Inherited deficiencies are due to AT3 gene mutations which lead to quantitative (type I) or qualitative (type II) deficiencies. Acquired AT deficiencies occur from protein losses, impaired production of functional AT, and accelerated consumption [13]. AT deficiency is associated with the highest increased relative risk of thrombosis of all thrombophilias reaching 16 times the risk in the general population (Fig. 37.1).

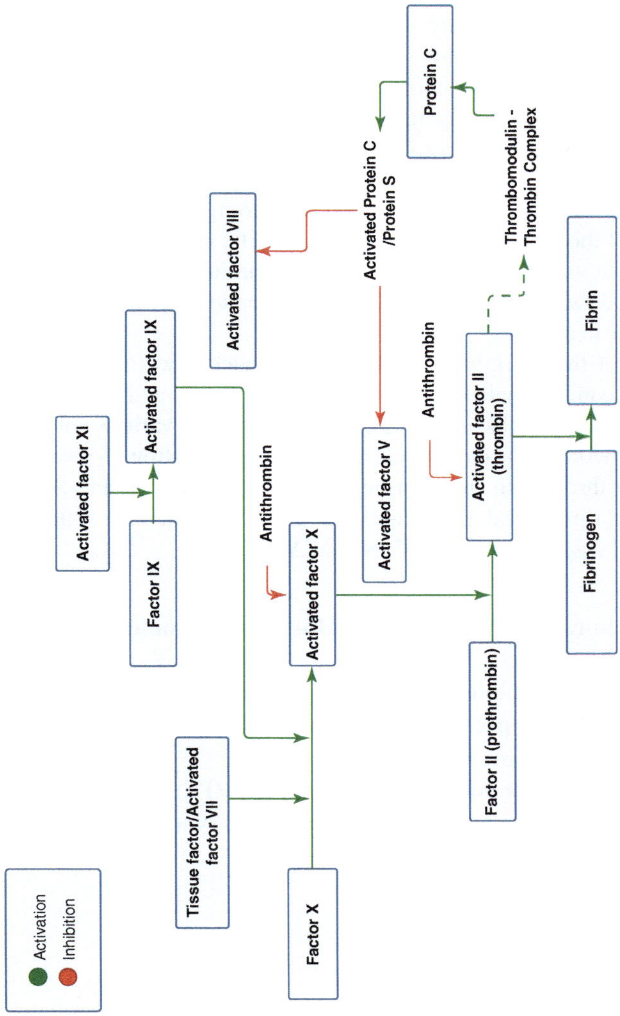

Fig. 37.1 Coagulation system highlighting the effects of natural anticoagulants

Diagnosis

Evaluation for inherited thrombophilia is generally not indicated for patients presenting with their first VTE. Consideration for a thrombophilia workup should be made for patients presenting with a first-degree family history of VTE, recurrent thrombosis, thrombosis at a young age (<45), and thrombosis at multiple sites or in unusual locations (mesenteric/splanchnic vessels and cerebral veins).

Physical examination can reveal findings associated with the site of thrombosis, but there are no specific findings to indicate the specific underlying disorder. Warfarin-induced skin necrosis can be seen with protein C deficiency in patient recently started on warfarin alone.

If a thrombophilia workup is indicated, the timing of these tests can be challenging as acute thrombosis, and other comorbidities (liver disease and kidney disease) and various anticoagulant medications can affect the reliability of testing. For example, acute thrombosis and warfarin can lower protein C and S levels, while direct oral anticoagulants (DOACs) interfere with functional assays for protein C, S, and AT.

A Laboratory Workup, When Indicated, Should Include

- **Complete blood count, kidney, and liver function testing: to rule out pre-existing comorbidities which can affect the anticoagulant chosen.**
- **Routine coagulation studies** (PT, aPTT, INR): which can reveal and underlying antiphospholipid syndrome with an artificially prolonged aPTT.

- **Factor V Leiden (FVL)/Activated Protein C (APC) resistance:** FVL can be detected by functional coagulation test for APC resistance using a "second-generation" assay or by genetic testing (DNA testing). DNA testing is not affected by acute thrombosis or anticoagulation.
- **Prothrombin gene mutation:** The prothrombin 20210A gene mutation is detected by molecular analysis. This is also not affected by acute thrombosis or anticoagulation.
- **Proteins C and S:** The best screening test for protein C deficiency is a functional assay that detects both quantitative and qualitative defects. The best screening test for protein S deficiency is the free protein S antigen assay. As noted above, the timing for testing should taken into account the chronicity of the VTE and anticoagulant used. Interruption of anticoagulation and transitioning to a heparin-based treatment might be required for accurate testing.
- **Antithrombin:** The AT–heparin cofactor assay using factor Xa, or thrombin detects all currently recognized subtypes of familial AT deficiency. Heparin use can lower AT levels and the timing of testing should be considered.

Differential diagnoses include all following listed, but not limited to, acquired hyperthrombotic state (Table 37.2). It is crucial to distinguish familial from acquired thrombophilia, as the diagnosis and treatment for the acquired forms should also target to the underlying diseases.

Table 37.2 Differential diagnosis for acute or recurrent thrombosis

Major differential diagnosis	What happen to coagulation
Malignancy	Hypercoagulable state due to the production of procoagulant substances.
Pregnancy	Increased risk of thrombosis due to obstruction of venous return by the uterus, as well as the hypercoagulable state.
Oral contraceptives or hormone replacement therapy	Increases the levels of coagulation proteins and decreases the levels of anticoagulant proteins leading to increased thrombosis risk.
Liver dysfunction	The liver produces endogenous inhibitors of coagulation. Liver disease may contribute to a prothrombotic state because these natural inhibitors may be reduced.
Heart failure	Increased risk of thrombosis due to poor blood flow.
Antiphospholipid syndrome	The presence of antibodies directed against plasma proteins bound to phospholipids. Patients may present with venous or arterial thrombosis
Paroxysmal nocturnal hemoglobinuria	A multidimensional prothrombotic state due to the pathological effects of platelet activation, intravascular hemolysis, and neutrophil/monocyte activation. Platelet and endothelial microparticles as well as oxidative stress may play a role.
Myeloproliferative neoplasms, especially *JAK2* mutated	Thrombosis is a manifestation of disease associated with hyperviscosity secondary to increased plasma viscosity, an increased number of red or white blood cells, or decreased deformability of cells
Nephrotic syndrome	Among the natural anticoagulant proteins, plasma antithrombin levels are often reduced due, at least in part, to increased urinary excretion.
Obesity	Promotes chronic inflammation and impaired fibrinolysis, both of which lead to an increased risk of thrombosis.
Surgery, trauma, or immobilization	Activation of the coagulation system following surgery or trauma are incompletely understood but may include decreased venous blood flow in the lower extremities, diminished fibrinolysis, the release or exposure of tissue factor, and depletion of endogenous anticoagulants.

Prognosis

The overall outcome for frequent thrombotic episodes and non-compliance to anticoagulation therapy is suboptimal. Survival data for hereditary thrombophilia are sparse; however, retrospective studies have not shown an increased risk of mortality for patients with hereditary thrombophilia on therapeutic anticoagulation compared to the general population.

Treatment

Treatment for familial thrombophilia typically involves lifelong anticoagulation. The most used anticoagulants include **DOACs** (e.g., apixaban and rivaroxaban) in addition to older generation anticoagulants (e.g., warfarin) and low molecular weight heparin (enoxaparin and dalteparin). It is important to note that bridging with parenteral anticoagulation is necessary for patients with protein C deficiency if warfarin is selected to decrease the risk of skin necrosis (Table 37.3).

Table 37.3 Anticoagulation options

Generic name	Brand name	Mechanism of action	Indication
Warfarin	Coumadin, Jantoven	Inhibits vitamin K-dependent coagulation factors	Anti-phospholipid syndrome, renal disease, cost.
Heparin	Various	Enhances the activity of antithrombin III, which neutralizes coagulation factors	Anti-phospholipid syndrome, liver disease, pregnancy, short-half life.
Dabigatran	Pradaxa	Directly inhibiting thrombin, a key enzyme in the coagulation cascade	Oral therapy and no monitoring preferred.
Rivaroxaban	Xarelto	Inhibiting factor Xa, a key enzyme in the coagulation cascade	Once daily oral therapy and no monitoring preferred.
Apixaban	Eliquis	Inhibiting factor Xa, a key enzyme in the coagulation cascade	Oral therapy and no monitoring preferred.
Edoxaban	Savaysa	Inhibiting factor Xa, a key enzyme in the coagulation cascade	Once daily oral therapy and no monitoring preferred.
Fondaparinux	Arixtra	Enhances the activity of antithrombin III, which neutralizes coagulation factors	For those with a history of heparin intolerance.

Promising Clinical Studies

There have been ongoing developments in other anticoagulation targets. Furthermore, two currently active clinical trials are investigating prophylactic protein C and AT concentrates:

1. A Study of TAK-662 for Japanese Patients with Congenital Protein C Deficiency. ClinicalTrials.gov Identifier: NCT04984889.

2. Efficacy of Atenativ in Patients with Congenital AT Deficiency Undergoing Surgery or Delivery. ClinicalTrials.gov Identifier: NCT04918173.

Caveats

- Testing for thrombophilia is not indicated for most patients affected by their first VTE episode. It should be considered for patients with a strong family history of VTE, recurrent VTE, VTE at a young age, and VTEs in unusual locations.
- The timing of testing regarding the time of most recent DVT and anticoagulant used is of paramount importance for correct interpretation of laboratory test results.
- The management of familial thrombophilia is highly individualized and involves correct anticoagulant therapy, lifestyle modifications, and clinical and laboratory close monitoring for the potential development of blood clots.
- Patients frequently require lifelong therapy.

Board Question

1. A 35-year-old Caucasian woman comes for follow-up evaluation a week after being diagnosed with deep venous thrombosis in the emergency department. Apixaban was initiated at the time of diagnosis, and she reports that her symptoms are improving. This is her first episode of VTE. Hypercoagulability testing is drawn before initiating anticoagulation therapy.

   Which of the following findings is most likely to show up on hypercoagulable workup?

   A. Heterozygosity for mutation in factor V Leiden
   B. Antithrombin 3 deficiency
   C. Positive lupus anticoagulant on two occasions 12 weeks apart

D. Protein C deficiency
E. Protein S deficiency

Answer A. Heterozygosity for mutation in factor V Leiden.

2. A 25-year-old female with the history of cholecystectomy 3 weeks ago was found to have right ankle swelling. She was later found to have a right femoral DVT, right popliteal vein and right femoral vein. Apixaban therapy was initiated, and her symptoms decreased within 2 weeks.

   Which of the following is the most appropriate duration of anticoagulant therapy?

   A. 6 weeks
   B. 9 weeks
   C. 3 months
   D. 6 months
   E. indefinitely

Answer C. 3 months

References

1. Mateo J, Oliver A, Borrell M, Sala N, Fontcuberta J. Laboratory evaluation and clinical characteristics of 2,132 consecutive unselected patients with venous thromboembolism--results of the Spanish Multicentric Study on Thrombophilia (EMET-Study). Thromb Haemost. 1997;77(3):444–51.
2. Martinelli I, Mannucci PM, De Stefano V, Taioli E, Rossi V, Crosti F, et al. Different risks of thrombosis in four coagulation defects associated with inherited thrombophilia: a study of 150 families. Blood. 1998;92(7):2353–8.
3. Rosendaal FR, Siscovick DS, Schwartz SM, Beverly RK, Psaty BM, Longstreth WT Jr, et al. Factor V Leiden (resistance to activated protein C) increases the risk of myocardial infarction in young women. Blood. 1997;89(8):2817–21.
4. Juul K, Tybjaerg-Hansen A, Steffensen R, Kofoed S, Jensen G, Nordestgaard BG. Factor V Leiden: the Copenhagen City heart study and 2 meta-analyses. Blood. 2002;100(1):3–10.

5. Lalouschek W, Schillinger M, Hsieh K, Endler G, Tentschert S, Lang W, et al. Matched case-control study on factor V Leiden and the prothrombin G20210A mutation in patients with ischemic stroke/transient ischemic attack up to the age of 60 years. Stroke. 2005;36(7):1405–9.
6. Khan S, Dickerman JD. Hereditary thrombophilia. Thromb J. 2006;4:15.
7. Bertina RM, Koeleman BP, Koster T, Rosendaal FR, Dirven RJ, de Ronde H, et al. Mutation in blood coagulation factor V associated with resistance to activated protein C. Nature. 1994;369(6475):64–7.
8. Simioni P, Scudeller A, Radossi P, Gavasso S, Girolami B, Tormene D, et al. "Pseudo homozygous" activated protein C resistance due to double heterozygous factor V defects (factor V Leiden mutation and type I quantitative factor V defect) associated with thrombosis: report of two cases belonging to two unrelated kindreds. Thromb Haemost. 1996;75(3):422–6.
9. Zehnder JL, Jain M. Recurrent thrombosis due to compound heterozygosity for factor V Leiden and factor V deficiency. Blood Coagul Fibrinolysis. 1996;7(3):361–2.
10. Reitsma PH, Bernardi F, Doig RG, Gandrille S, Greengard JS, Ireland H, et al. Protein C deficiency: a database of mutations, 1995 update. On behalf of the subcommittee on plasma coagulation inhibitors of the scientific and standardization committee of the ISTH. Thromb Haemost. 1995;73(5):876–89.
11. Mannucci PM, Vigano S. Deficiencies of protein C, an inhibitor of blood coagulation. Lancet. 1982;2(8296):463–7.
12. Esmon CT. Protein S and protein C biochemistry, physiology, and clinical manifestation of deficiencies. Trends Cardiovasc Med. 1992;2(6):214–9.
13. Dahlback B. Advances in understanding pathogenic mechanisms of thrombophilic disorders. Blood. 2008;112(1):19–27.

Antiphospholipid Syndrome 38

Dimitrios Drekolias, Wissam Hanayneh,
and Michael Jaglal

Introduction

Antiphospholipid syndrome (APS) is an autoimmune systemic disorder characterized by venous or arterial thrombosis and/or pregnancy complications among patients with laboratory evidence of autoantibodies against phospholipid-bound proteins (aPL) [1]. The most common autoantibodies against these proteins include the anticardiolipin antibody (aCL), and the anti-beta-2 glycoprotein I (anti-beta2 GPI) antibody, which are part of the diagnostic criteria.

Based on the predominant clinical manifestation, APS is further classified into three categories:

1. *Thrombotic—presenting with vascular thrombosis with persistent aPL positivity*
2. *Obstetric—presenting with pregnancy morbidity linked to APS*
3. *Catastrophic—catastrophic APS (CAPS) presents with acute multi-organ failure in the setting of widespread vascular thrombosis*

D. Drekolias · M. Jaglal (✉)
Moffitt Cancer Center, University of South Florida, Tampa, FL, USA
e-mail: Michael.Jaglal@moffitt.org

W. Hanayneh
Our Lady of Lourdes- JD Moncus Cancer Center, Lafayette, LA, USA

L. Sokol, L. Zhang (eds.), *Non-Neoplastic Hematologic Disorders*,
https://doi.org/10.1007/978-3-031-62373-8_38

Among patients without any history of autoimmunity, aPL have been identified in approximately 14% presenting with stroke, 11% presenting with myocardial infarction, 10% presenting with deep vein thrombosis, and 9% with pregnancy loss [2].

About half of APS cases are designated as primary APS. Secondary APS transpires within underlying autoimmune disease, with systemic lupus erythematous (SLE) being the most common (35% of cases) [3].

Etiology and Pathogenesis

The underlying etiology of APS is not yet definitively established. Accumulating evidence has pointed to the possibility that the phenomenon of molecular mimicry may underlie and trigger the formation of aPL in certain individuals. Autoreactive T and B cells have been found to cross-react with epitopes expressed by commensal bacteria and, subsequently, to trigger the formation of aPL [4].

The pathogenesis of APS is primarily driven by the prothrombotic effects of the aPL as they interact with the physiologic mechanisms of anticoagulation, including antifibrinolytic and direct procoagulant properties [5]. In addition, several studies have indicated significant interaction of the aPL with components of inflammation [6]. Anti-beta2 GPI antibodies have been found to interact with complement in various ways, inducing deposition of C5b-9. In APS-induced nephropathy, aPL appear to stimulate the mTOR/PI3K/AKT pathway . In obstetric APS, anti-beta2 GPI antibodies disrupt trophoblast proliferation, secretion of human chorionic gonadotropin, and syncytialization.

Diagnosis

Suspicion for APS arises in certain clinical scenarios, such as: unexplained vascular thrombotic event (especially among younger patients or at unusual body sites, e.g., retinal, portal, renal vein, and cerebral venous sinus); age < 50 years with ischemia attack;

and adverse pregnancy-related outcome (e.g., multiple pregnancy losses, fetal death after the tenth week of gestation; or premature birth in the setting of preeclampsia or placental insufficiency). The suspicion should be further augmented in the presence of SLE, livedo reticularis (irregular, branched vascular pattern), heart disease, or cerebrovascular event without an apparent explanation.

Laboratory Workup

- **Complete blood count (CBC):** thrombocytopenia is variable.
- **Routine coagulation studies** (prothrombin time [PT], activated partial thromboplastin time [aPTT])**:** which detects a prolonged aPTT/PT for lupus anticoagulant (LA) testing. Most LA affects the aPTT pathway.
- **Renal function testing:** may reveal kidney injury, indicating potential APS-induced vascular events.
- **Antiphospholipid titers:** immunoglobulin G (IgG)/immunoglobulin M (IgM), anticardiolipin antibodies (aCL) by enzyme-linked immunosorbent assay, and IgG/IgM anti-beta-2 glycoprotein I (anti-beta-2 GPI) by enzyme-linked immunosorbent assay.
- **Lupus anticoagulant (LA):** coagulation assay.

The hallmark of the LA coagulation assay is the correction of the prolonged PT or aPTT with the addition of a phospholipid, but not with the addition of control plasma, indicating that the inhibitor of coagulation is phospholipid dependent in vitro.

The IgG isotype of the immunoassays carries stronger clinical significance than the IgM counterpart [7]. Although immunoglobulin-A (IgA) isotypes of the abovementioned immunoassays are frequently performed by most laboratories along with the IgG and IgM, their clinical significance remains controversial. Triple aPL positivity supports the strongest clinical significance and is the one most strongly associated with vascular events.

Time of testing is critical. The immunoassays (aCL and beta2GPI) are not affected by the acuity of the thrombotic event. However, the LA coagulation assay may be confounded by the acute thrombosis, since the latter may falsely normalize the aPTT in the acute setting. The initial aPL positivity after acute thrombosis should always be followed by confirmatory re-testing at least 12 weeks later, because transient aPL positivity can occur in a variety of settings (e.g., certain infections and drug exposures). Two positive tests, 12 weeks apart, are required for laboratory diagnosis of aPL. Furthermore, anticoagulant use may cause false positive LA testing. If possible, repeat testing should occur, while the patient is off anticoagulation.

Based on the revised Sapporo APS Classification Criteria (Table 38.1), APS requires the presence of at least 1 of the following clinical criteria and at least 1 of the following laboratory criteria.

Table 38.1 Revised Sapporo criteria

Clinical criteria	Laboratory criteria tested on 2 or more occasions at least 12 weeks apart
Thrombosis: At least 1 episode of venous or arterial thrombosis with unequivocal imaging or histologic evidence of thrombosis. Superficial venous thrombosis does not satisfy this criterion.	IgG and/or IgM aCL by ELISA *with titer > 40 units.*
	IgG and/or IgM anti-beta-2 GPI by ELISA *with titer > 40 units.*
Pregnancy complication: At least 1 unexplained death of a normal fetus at $\geq$10 weeks gestation or 1 or more premature births of a normal neonate before the 34th week of gestation caused by eclampsia, preeclampsia, or placental insufficiency or at least 3 or more consecutive spontaneous losses at $<$10 weeks gestate; one or no chromosomal/maternal/hormonal causes.	LA coagulation assay.

aCL anticardiolipin antibodies, *anti-beta-2 GPI* anti-beta-2 glycoprotein, *ELISA* enzyme-linked immunosorbent assay, *IgG* immunoglobulin G, *LA* lupus anticoagulant

Table 38.2 Differential diagnosis

Diseases
Hereditary or acquired thrombophilia
SLE
Heparin-induced thrombocytopenia
Paroxysmal nocturnal hemoglobinuria
Myeloproliferative neoplasms, especially *JAK2*-mutation positive
Vaccine-induced thrombocytopenia
Pregnancy-related causes of miscarriages: Chromosomal abnormalities, anatomic variations, or abnormalities of the uterus, as well as endocrine disorders (e.g., hypothyroidism)
Surgery, trauma, or immobilization

SLE systemic lupus erythematous

Major Differential Diagnosis (Table 38.2)

Other Conditions with Positive Antiphospholipid Antibodies

- Infections: leptospirosis, syphilis, Lyme disease, tuberculosis, hepatitis A, hepatitis B, HIV, cytomegalovirus, and Epstein–Barr virus can lead to transient aPL positivity, most commonly low-level IgM aCL, and, rarely, result in thrombotic events.
- Medications: phenytoin, hydralazine, amoxicillin, chlorothiazide, oral contraceptives, and propranolol have been linked to a transient (most commonly IgM) titer.

Prognosis

APS has been linked to increased overall mortality and morbidity. Approximately 90% of APS patients experience decreased life expectancy during a 10-year follow-up period [8]. During that period, the main causes of death included vascular thrombosis (31%), sepsis (27%), malignancy (14%), hemorrhage (11%), SLE (8%), and CAPS (5%).

Treatment (Fig. 38.1)

Foot note: aPTT: activated partial thromboplastin; DOCAs: direct oral anticoagulants, INR: international normalized ratio, LMWH: low molecular weight heparin; PT: prothrombin time; UFH: unfractionated heparin.

Acute Thrombosis

In the setting of acute thrombosis, anticoagulation with unfractionated heparin or low molecular weight heparin (LMWH) should be initiated until the diagnostic workup for the etiology of the thrombosis is determined.

Long-Term Thrombosis Prevention

For most cases, warfarin remains the mainstay of long-term anticoagulation in APS. There have been several studies assessing the role of direct oral anticoagulants (DOACs) in APS vs warfarin; however, DOACs s remain less efficacious [9]. In cases of venous thrombotic event (VTE), evidence supports anticoagulation with warfarin with a target of an international normalized ratio (INR) of 2.5 (2–3), rather than a higher INR of 3–4 [10]. LMWH should be used in the event of pregnancy and in patients for whom INR monitoring is problematic. Low-molecular-weight heparin prevents aPL-inhibited human endometrial endothelial cells angiogenesis, both in vitro and in vivo, and is able to restore the aPL-inhibited NF-κB and/or STAT-3 activity, the VEGF secretion, and the matrix metalloproteinase activity. In the event of arterial thrombosis, such as ischemic cerebrovascular event or myocardial infarction, the evidence is less conclusive, with most approaches recommending warfarin (INR 2–3) with the addition of low-dose aspirin. For most cases, the duration of anticoagulation should be indefinite because of the high likelihood of recurrence in the absence of anticoagulation.

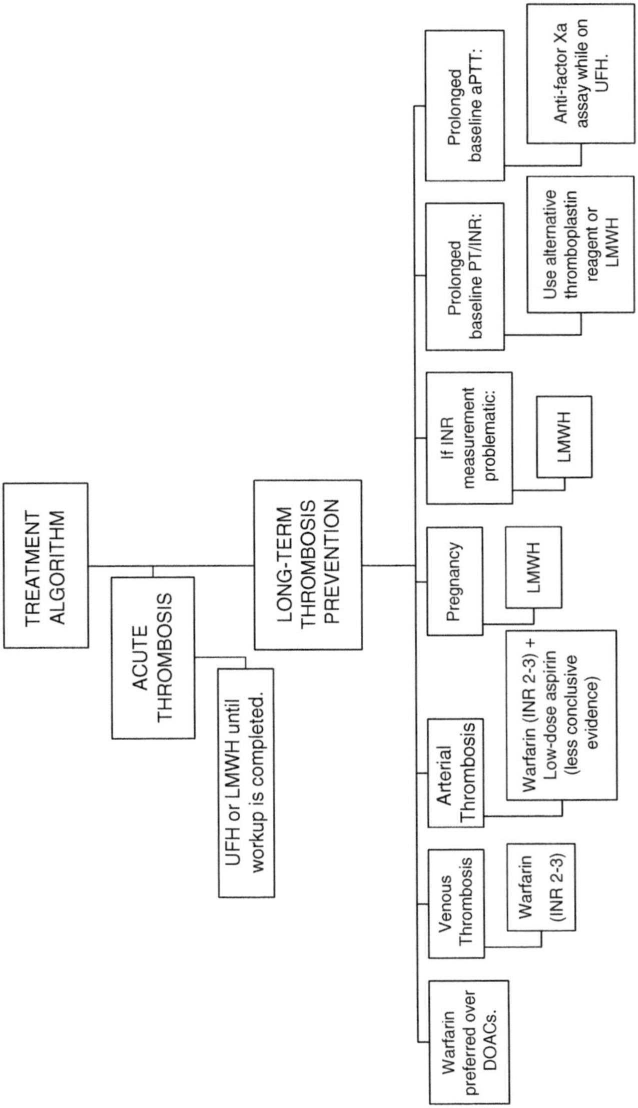

Fig. 38.1 Treatment algorithm

In the event of prolonged baseline PT/INR, an alternative thromboplastin reagent (either a combination of thromboplastins or a reagent that is not affected by aPL) should be utilized after discussion with the lab to determine availability.

In the event of prolonged baseline aPTT (more commonly encountered due to the LA phenomenon), anti-Xa factor assay can be used to monitor therapeutic effect of unfractionated heparin. LMWH can be used without routine monitoring.

Promising Clinical Studies

- An open-label phase 2 trial targeting the noncriteria manifestations of APS (thrombocytopenia, skin ulcers, and cognitive decline) with the use of rituximab recruited 19 patients with the results showing symptomatic effect in certain cases .
- Eculizumab, a monoclonal antibody that targets complement protein C5, has been used in cases of refractory APS as well as in cases of CAPS.

Caveats

Confirmatory aPL antibody at least 12 weeks after the initial testing is essential for diagnosing APS:

- Baseline coagulation panel (PT, aPTT) should be obtained for all patients both for LA testing and for future treatment monitoring purposes.
- Warfarin remains the mainstay of treatment in the event of vascular thrombosis with high suspicion for APS or confirmed APS diagnosis.

Board Questions (Multiple Choice)

1. A 34-year-old woman referred for consultation regarding anticoagulation choice. She has no history of deep vein thrombosis and no recent risk factors for thrombosis. She was diagnosed with left femoral occlusive venous thrombosis. She was examined in the emergency room and initiated therapy with apixaban 10 mg orally twice a day for 7 days followed by 5 mg PO BID. Thrombophilia workup revealed positive IgG anti-cardiolipin antibodies (65 GPL units) and positive LA. Results of lupus anticoagulant test performed 5 days after discontinuing apixaban were also positive 3 months later. Her baseline INR is 1.03.

   Which of the following is the most appropriate next step in management of this patient?

   A. Do not restart anticoagulation.
   B. Continue apixaban indefinitely.
   C. Switch to warfarin with target INR of 2–3.
   D. Switch to dabigatran 150 mg orally twice a day.
   E. Switch to warfarin and target INR 2.5–3.5.

   Answer C Switch to warfarin with target INR of 2–3.

2. A 26-year-old was diagnosed with SLE 3 months ago. She has malar rash, diffuse arthralgias, and pleurisy, no history of thrombosis. Her rheumatologist ordered an LA panel that was positive. Her lupus confirmatory laboratory test was positive 3 months later.

   Which of the following is the next best step?

   A. Do not start anticoagulation and repeat LA test 12 weeks later.
   B. Start apixaban for an indefinite time period.
   C. Start warfarin with target INR of 2–3.
   D. Start dabigatran 150 mg orally twice a day.
   E. Start warfarin with target INR of 2.5–3.5.

   Answer A. Do not start anticoagulation and repeat LA test 12 weeks later.

References

1. Miyakis S, et al. International consensus statement on an update of the classification criteria for definite antiphospholipid syndrome (APS). J Thromb Haemost. 2006;4(2):295–306.
2. Andreoli L, et al. Estimated frequency of antiphospholipid antibodies in patients with pregnancy morbidity, stroke, myocardial infarction, and deep vein thrombosis: a critical review of the literature. Arthritis Care Res (Hoboken). 2013;65(11):1869–73.
3. Roubey RA. Autoantibodies to phospholipid-binding plasma proteins: a new view of lupus anticoagulants and other "antiphospholipid" autoantibodies. Blood. 1994;84(9):2854–67.
4. Ruff WE, et al. Pathogenic autoreactive T and B cells cross-react with Mimotopes expressed by a common human gut commensal to trigger autoimmunity. Cell Host Microbe. 2019;26(1):100–113.e8.
5. Garcia D, Erkan D. Diagnosis and Management of the Antiphospholipid Syndrome. N Engl J Med. 2018;378(21):2010–21.
6. Zhou H, Wolberg AS, Roubey RA. Characterization of monocyte tissue factor activity induced by IgG antiphospholipid antibodies and inhibition by dilazep. Blood. 2004;104(8):2353–8.
7. Kelchtermans H, et al. IgG/IgM antiphospholipid antibodies present in the classification criteria for the antiphospholipid syndrome: a critical review of their association with thrombosis. J Thromb Haemost. 2016;14(8):1530–48.
8. Cervera R, et al. Morbidity and mortality in the antiphospholipid syndrome during a 10-year period: a multicentre prospective study of 1000 patients. Ann Rheum Dis. 2015;74(6):1011–8.
9. Cohen H, et al. Rivaroxaban versus warfarin to treat patients with thrombotic antiphospholipid syndrome, with or without systemic lupus erythematosus (RAPS): a randomised, controlled, open-label, phase 2/3, non-inferiority trial. Lancet Haematol. 2016;3(9):e426–36.
10. Holbrook A, et al. Evidence-based management of anticoagulant therapy: antithrombotic therapy and prevention of thrombosis, 9th ed: American College of Chest Physicians Evidence-Based Clinical Practice Guidelines. Chest. 2012;141(2 Suppl):e152S–84S.

Principles of Antithrombotic and Fibrinolytic Therapy

39

Ruoyu Miao, Wissam Hanayneh, and Michael Jaglal

Introduction

Venous thromboembolism (VTE), including deep vein thrombosis (DVT) and pulmonary embolism (PE), occurs in approximately 2–3 per 1000 person-years among adults in the United States, with an estimated 60,000–100,000 deaths per year. DVT refers to thrombosis involving deep veins, including popliteal, femoral, and iliac veins of lower extremity and brachial, axillary, subclavian, and brachiocephalic veins of upper extremity. Proximal DVT involves the popliteal or more proximal veins, whereas distal (below the knee) DVT involves vessels distal to the trifurcation of the popliteal vein. Massive PE is defined as any PE that causes hemodynamic instability with systemic arterial hypotension. Submassive PE is associated with evidence of right ventricular dysfunction without systemic hypotension.

R. Miao · M. Jaglal (✉)
Moffitt Cancer Center, University of South Florida, Tampa, FL, USA
e-mail: michael.jaglal@moffitt.org

W. Hanayneh
Our Lady of Lourdes- JD Moncus Cancer Center, Lafayette, LA, USA

L. Sokol, L. Zhang (eds.), *Non-Neoplastic Hematologic Disorders*,
https://doi.org/10.1007/978-3-031-62373-8_39

Pathophysiology

Virchow's triad proposed that VTE occurs because of three contributing factors: vascular stasis, hypercoagulable state, and vascular trauma. The causes of VTE can be divided into two risk groups: hereditary and acquired. However, VTE is typically a complex multifactorial disorder involving one or more genetic and/or environmental risk factors.

Diagnosis

The diagnosis of VTE typically depends on the location. Upper and lower extremity DVT are diagnosed via Doppler ultrasound, while thrombi in inaccessible vessels by ultrasound (splanchnic, iliac, and pulmonary) require computed tomography (CT) with contrast.

Treatment

Acute Therapy of VTE

Direct oral anticoagulants (DOACs) (including the oral anti-Xa inhibitors rivaroxaban, apixaban, edoxaban, and betrixaban and the oral direct thrombin inhibitor dabigatran) are favored over vitamin K antagonists (VKAs) because of lower risk of intracranial and fatal bleeding and more rapid and predictive onset of action. Subcutaneous low-molecular-weight heparin (LMWH) or fondaparinux with weight-based dosing and intravenous unfractionated heparin (UFH) with activated partial thromboplastin time (aPTT) monitoring and dosing are also effective options. Parenteral anticoagulants require at least 5 days overlapping with warfarin until the INR is ≥2.0 for 24 h or before starting dabigatran or edoxaban.

For selected patients with massive acute iliofemoral DVT with symptom duration of fewer than 14 days and low risk of bleeding, catheter-directed thrombolysis with or without mechanical thrombus fragmentation and aspiration can be considered to decrease acute symptoms, but it does not improve post thrombotic syndrome.

Systemic thrombolytic therapy is indicated for massive life-threatening PE. It is not warranted for most hemodynamically stable patients with acute PE because of major bleeding increased risk. Patients with submassive PE require close monitoring after rapid initiation of anticoagulation, as rescue thrombolytic therapy may benefit patients who develop cardiovascular deterioration.

An inferior vena cava (IVC) filter is indicated for patients with acute proximal DVT or PE who have an absolute contraindication to anticoagulation (e.g., active bleeding, hemorrhagic stroke immediately after neurosurgical, severe thrombocytopenia, or ophthalmologic procedures). The presence of an IVC filter is a risk factor for recurrent VTE. Retrievable filters should be removed as soon as the patients are no longer at high risk of developing PE and can tolerate anticoagulation. Anticoagulant therapy should be administered as soon as the risk of bleeding allows among patients with IVC filters, since filters increase the risk for recurrent VTE.

Angioplasty and stenting are sometimes used in treating venous occlusive disease, such as May–Thurner syndrome, although there is no high-quality evidence that these interventions reduce the risk of recurrent VTE or post-thrombotic syndrome. The presence of a venous stent may be considered as a potential risk factor for recurrent VTE.

Therapeutic anticoagulants reduce the risk of VTE extension or recurrence by 80–90%. Causes of anticoagulation failure may include cancer, antiphospholipid syndrome (APS), an anatomic cause, or noncompliance. Apart from addressing the identifiable causes, treatment options are either to increase the target INR if on VKA, increase LMWH dose by 25%, add another anticoagulant or antiplatelet agent, or switch to another anticoagulant.

Duration of Anticoagulant Therapy

Time-limited anticoagulation for 3 months is recommended for a VTE secondary to a major transient risk factor since the risk of recurrence is low. For patients with unprovoked proximal DVT or PE, extended anticoagulant therapy should be strongly considered. Clinical factors that favor extended anticoagulation include male sex, history of recurrent VTE, PE rather than DVT, persistent D-dimer elevation, obesity, older age, persistent underlying risk factor, strong thrombophilia, and well-tolerated anticoagulant therapy. Other factors to consider are bleeding risks and personal preferences. The risks and benefits should be re-evaluated periodically if extended anticoagulation is chosen. Low-dose apixaban or rivaroxaban after therapeutic dose for 6 months decreases the incidence of recurrent VTE with a low overall risk of bleeding. Daily low-dose aspirin appears to reduce the VTE risk by 30% and may be considered for patients who discontinue anticoagulation or have no access to DOACs but are at increased risk for recurrent VTE.

Special Site of VTE

Superficial Thrombophlebitis

Patients with extensive or intractable superficial thrombophlebitis benefit from a short course of anticoagulant therapy—6 weeks of subcutaneous prophylactic-dose fondaparinux, low-dose DOAC, or LMWH. Non-extensive thrombophlebitis (<5 cm in length and not close to the deep venous system) requires symptomatic therapy only. Follow-up ultrasound should be considered for patients with extensive thrombophlebitis if anticoagulation is not given.

Upper-Extremity DVT

About 80% upper-extremity DVT is associated with central venous catheters or cancer. LMWH, UFH, DOACs, or fondaparinux may be used in the acute setting. Anticoagulation should be continued for at least 3 months. Catheter removal is not necessary if the catheter is functional and needed.

Visceral Thrombosis

Hepatic vein thrombosis (Budd–Chiari syndrome) is most associated with myeloproliferative neoplasms (MPNs), JAK2 mutation without overt MPN, and paroxysmal nocturnal hemoglobinuria. Thrombolytic therapy should be considered for acute fulminant thrombosis. Angioplasty and stenting, shunt procedures, and/or liver transplantation may be necessary. Most patients require chronic anticoagulation.

Portal vein thrombosis (PVT) is associated with cirrhosis, MPNs, JAK2-positive status, paroxysmal nocturnal hemoglobinuria, and intra-abdominal problems, including neoplasia, inflammation, infection, trauma, and surgery. Patients with acute PVT are usually anticoagulated for at least 3–6 months to prevent progression of thrombosis.

Mesenteric vein thrombosis may be secondary to progression of PVT, pancreatic disease, and other causes similar to those in PVT. Patients are managed with anticoagulation alone or in combination with surgical intervention. Duration of anticoagulation depends on the presence of transient or permanent risk factors.

Splenic vein thrombosis is associated with pancreatitis, pancreatic malignancies, or other intra-abdominal problems. The role and length of anticoagulation is not well defined. Splenic vein thrombosis after splenectomy is likely a physiological adaptation to the presence of a blind venous stump, and anticoagulation is generally not indicated.

For renal vein thrombosis, thrombolytic therapy should be considered in the acute setting, particularly if there is bilateral thrombosis or impending renal failure. Therapeutic anticoagulation is indicated, and the length depends on the presence of transient or permanent risk factors.

Cerebral Sinovenous Thrombosis (CSVT)

LMWH or UFH (if neurosurgical decompression is anticipated) is recommended in acute CSVT, even with some parenchymal hemorrhage. Decompressive surgery may be lifesaving for patients with brain displacement and herniation. There is limited evidence for DOACs, although small case series have reported effective results. The length of anticoagulation is recommended for 3 months with a transient risk factor, and long term with a high-risk thrombophilia or recurrent event.

Retinal Vein Thrombosis

Retinal vein occlusion has been associated with classic arterial cardiovascular risk factors rather than inherited or acquired thrombophilia. There is little high-quality evidence on the usefulness of antiplatelet or anticoagulant therapy.

Perioperative Management of Antithrombotic Therapy

The perioperative management of antiplatelet or anticoagulant agents is based on the risk of perioperative bleeding and risk of thromboembolism.

Warfarin should be discontinued approximately 5 days before major surgery until normalization of the INR. Bridging anticoagulation with therapeutic-dose LMWH or UFH is indicated for high risk of perioperative thromboembolism, e.g., atrial fibrillation with CHA_2DS_2–VASc [1] scores of ≥7; recent (≤3 months) cerebrovascular accident or VTE; mechanical mitral valves; rheumatic valvular heart disease; or severe thrombophilia (e.g., APS; deficiencies of antithrombin, protein C, or protein S). Bridging may be considered for patients at moderate risk, e.g., atrial fibrillation with CHA_2DS_2–VASc 5–6; VTE or cerebrovascular accident within the last 3–12 months; or heterozygous factor V Leiden mutation or factor II mutation. Warfarin may be continued for minor dental (use oral antifibrinolytic agent, if needed) or dermatologic procedures and cataract surgery.

DOACs should be discontinued 48 h before major surgery without the routine needs for bridging, given their predictable, short half-life. Longer intervals may be necessary with renal or hepatic impairment, older age, or concurrent antiplatelet agents. Hemostasis must be achieved before restarting DOAC postoperatively.

Aspirin may be continued for minor dental or dermatologic procedures and cataract surgery but needs to be withheld for at least 7 days before major noncardiac surgery. Antiplatelet agents are typically suspended for intracranial, ocular, or high-bleeding-risk surgery. Elective surgery should be deferred 6 weeks after placement of bare-metal coronary stents or 6 months after placement of drug-eluting coronary stents. If surgery cannot be delayed, dual antiplatelet therapy should be continued. After above period, the $P2Y_{12}$ inhibitor may be suspended temporarily for surgery. Patients undergoing coronary artery bypass grafting may need to remain on antiplatelet medications perioperatively.

Prevention of VTE in Hospitalized or Surgical Patients

VTE prophylaxis should be considered for every hospitalized patient based on the individual's risk stratification. The American College of Chest Physicians guidelines use two validated risk-stratification models (Rogers score and Caprini score) for patients undergoing nonorthopedic surgery. Prophylactic measures include early ambulation, mechanical prophylaxis (e.g., intermittent compression devices and graduated compression stockings), and pharmacological prophylaxis with an anticoagulant or antiplatelet agent. Extended prophylaxis may be given if the VTE risk extends after discharge. Pharmacological prophylaxis for a minimum of 10–14 days postoperatively is recommended for most adult patients undergoing major orthopedic surgery. Patients undergoing hip fracture repair, total hip arthroplasty, or total knee arthroplasty benefit from post-discharge prophylaxis for up to 5 weeks. Pharmacological prophylaxis for patients undergoing major surgery for cancer should be continued for at least 7–10 days.

Extended prophylaxis for up to 4 weeks postoperatively is recommended for high-risk abdominal or pelvic cancer surgery patients.

Pregnancy and Estrogen Exposure

The risk of VTE is increased during pregnancy. It is highest in the first 6-week postpartum and gradually returns to normal at 12-week postpartum. Table 39.1 summarizes the 2018 American Society of Hematology guidelines to prevent VTE in pregnancy.

The anticoagulant of choice in pregnancy is LMWH, which has a better safety profile than UFH. Warfarin carries the highest fetal risk but may be used in selected patients with mechanical heart valves as it appears more effective than heparin in preventing valvular thrombosis. LMWH and VKAs are both acceptable options postpartum and safe with breastfeeding. DOACs should not be used in pregnancy or while breastfeeding.

Therapeutic-dose LMWH (1 mg/kg q12 h or 1.5 mg/kg daily) is recommended for treating VTE in pregnancy. The duration should be at least 3 months and include the 6-week postpartum period. Anti-Xa level monitoring may be considered in select high-risk VTE cases (e.g., patients with renal dysfunction or obesity).

LMWH is suggested for treating superficial vein thrombosis in pregnancy to minimize the risk of recurrence and progression to DVT, with a common duration of at least 6 weeks.

Anticoagulation is indicated for patients with symptomatic or extensive postpartum ovarian vein thrombosis. Antibiotics should be given if infection is suspected. Treatment is usually not required for asymptomatic ovarian vein thrombosis in the postpartum period and in the general population. The duration of anticoagulation is most commonly 3 months.

Testing for antiphospholipid antibodies is recommended for patients with recurrent pregnancy loss. For patients with APS and prior pregnancy loss who fulfill the revised Sapporo criteria, LMWH and aspirin are recommended to prevent recurrent pregnancy loss. For women with prior thrombotic events, therapeutic-dose LMWH is recommended, often in combination with low-dose aspirin. Screening for inherited thrombophilia and LMWH are otherwise not recommended for women with a history of pregnancy loss or complications.

Table 39.1 2018 American society of hematology guidelines to prevent VTE in pregnancy

Condition	Recommendation
Homozygous factor V Leiden	Antepartum and postpartum: suggests antithrombotic prophylaxis
Homozygous prothrombin gene mutation	Antepartum: without family history of VTE: suggests against antithrombotic prophylaxis; with family history of VTE: panelists favored prophylaxis Postpartum: suggests antithrombotic prophylaxis
Compound heterozygosity	Antepartum and postpartum: suggests antithrombotic prophylaxis
Heterozygous for factor V Leiden or prothrombin gene mutation	Antepartum and postpartum: suggests against antithrombotic prophylaxis
Protein C deficiency or protein S deficiency	Antepartum: suggests against antithrombotic prophylaxis Postpartum: without family history of VTE: suggests against antithrombotic prophylaxis; with family history of VTE: suggests antithrombotic prophylaxis
Antithrombin deficiency	Antepartum: without family history of VTE: suggests against antithrombotic prophylaxis; with family history of VTE: suggests antithrombotic prophylaxis Postpartum: without family history of VTE: suggests against antithrombotic prophylaxis; with family history of VTE: recommends antithrombotic prophylaxis
Prior VTE that was unprovoked or associated with a hormonal risk factor	Antepartum and postpartum: recommends anticoagulant prophylaxis
Prior VTE associated with a nonhormonal temporary provoking risk factor and no other risk factors	Antepartum: suggests against anticoagulant prophylaxis Postpartum: recommends anticoagulant prophylaxis
No or 1 clinical risk factor (excluding a known thrombophilia or history of VTE)	Antepartum and postpartum: suggests against prophylaxis

VTE venous thromboembolism

Prophylactic LMWH for 3 months is suggested for severe ovarian hyperstimulation syndrome induced by assisted reproductive therapy.

Exogenous hormones (e.g., combined hormonal contraceptives [CHCs], depot medroxyprogesterone, menopausal hormone therapy [HT], and male-to-female HT) may increase the risk of thrombosis. Women with a history of thrombosis who are on long-term anticoagulation and use CHCs or menopausal HT are no more likely to develop recurrent VTE and, therefore, may continue the exogenous hormones. Women with a history of thrombosis or at high risk of thrombosis who are not on long-term anticoagulation should be counseled to avoid CHCs, depot medroxyprogesterone, and oral menopausal HT. Transgender women with a history of thrombosis will need to continue the male-to-female HT and, therefore, will need anticoagulation.

Antiphospholipid Syndrome

Please refer to Chap. 38 for a detailed discussion on APS and previous discussion in *Pregnancy* for anticoagulation management during pregnancy.

Patients with APS and history of unprovoked VTE should be maintained on anticoagulation indefinitely. The anticoagulant of choice is warfarin with a target INR range of 2.0–3.0. If the prothrombin time is prolonged at baseline, INR should be compared to a chromogenic factor X assay to confirm the validity of INR while on warfarin. Point-of-care INR should be corelated with that from a phlebotomy sample periodically since aPL titers can fluctuate over time. If the aPTT is prolonged at baseline, UFH therapy should be monitored with an antifactor Xa assay. DOACs should be avoided in high-risk patients (e.g., triple positive, history of arterial events) because of an increased risk of recurrent thrombosis relative to warfarin. DOACs may be considered for patients with lower risk (e.g., single venous thrombosis, low-risk aPL profile with isolated anticardiolipin or anti-beta-2 glycoprotein I at low-to-medium titer); however, patients should be informed about the available evidence and possible reduced benefit of a DOAC.

Cancer-Associated Thrombosis (CAT)

LMWH has been the recommended treatment for the first 6 months after acute CAT, given the superior efficacy compared to warfarin. Edoxaban or rivaroxaban have been demonstrated to be noninferior to LMWH for the composite endpoint of recurrent VTE and major bleeding in randomized trials but are associated with an increased risk of major gastrointestinal (GI) bleeding, predominantly in patients with GI cancers. Apixaban has been shown to be noninferior to LMWH in preventing recurrent VTE, and there was no difference in the risk of major bleeding, including GI bleeding. Overall, DOACs represent a reasonable alternative to LMWH in treating CAT.

Heparin-Induced Thrombocytopenia

Please refer to Chap. 27 for a detailed discussion.

Acute Coronary Syndrome and Ischemic Stroke

Please refer to the latest guidelines from the American Heart Association, American College of Cardiology, American College of Chest Physicians, and American Stroke Association for using antithrombotic and fibrinolytic therapy in preventing and treating acute coronary syndrome or ischemic stroke. For most patients with nonvalvular atrial fibrillation who do not have a specific indication for VKAs, a DOAC is preferred over a VKA for stroke prevention. DOACs should not be used in patients with moderately or severe mitral stenosis or a mechanical heart valve.

Anticoagulants

Tables 39.2 and 39.3 summarize the oral and parental anticoagulants, respectively.

Table 39.2 Oral anticoagulants

Name	Dabigatran	Apixaban	Betrixaban	Edoxaban	Rivaroxaban	Warfarin
Mechanism	Direct anti-FIIa	Direct anti-FXa	Direct anti-FXa	Direct anti-FXa	Direct anti-FXa	VKA
Half-life (h)	12–17	8–15	19–27	10–14	5–9 (11–13 in elderly)	20–60
Dosing	VTE treatment after 5–10 days of parenteral anticoagulation, CrCl >30 mL/min: 150 mg po bid. Recurrent VTE prophylaxis, CrCl >30 mL/min: 150 mg po bid. Prophylaxis of VTE following hip replacement, CrCl >30 mL/min: 110 mg po first day then 220 mg qDay. NVAF: CrCl >30 mL/min: 150 mg po bid. CrCl 15–30 mL/min: 75 mg po bid.	VTE treatment: 10 mg po bid × 7 days then 5 mg po bid. No dose adjustment for renal impairment. VTE prophylaxis: 2.5 mg po bid. NVAF: 5 mg po bid. 2.5 mg po bid if at least 2 of the following: age ≥ 80 years, weight ≤ 60 kg, or serum creatinine ≥1.5 mg/dL.	VTE prophylaxis: CrCl >30 mL/min: 160 mg po first day then 80 mg once daily. CrCl 15–30 mL/min: 80 mg po first day then 40 mg once daily.	VTE treatment after 5–10 days of parenteral anticoagulation: CrCl >50 mL/min: 60 mg po qDay. CrCl 15–50 mL/min or weight ≤ 60 kg: 30 mg po qDay. NVAF: CrCl >95 L/min: avoid use. CrCl 50–95 mL/min: 60 mg po qDay. CrCl 15–50 mL/min: 30 mg po qDay.	VTE treatment: 15 mg po bid with food × 21 days then 20 mg po qDay with food. Avoid use if CrCl <15 mL/min. VTE prophylaxis: 10 mg po qDay. Avoid use if CrCl <15 mL/min. NVAF: 20 mg (CrCl >50 mL/min) or 15 mg (CrCl ≤50 mL/min) po qDay with food. CAD or PAD: 2.5 mg po bid, in combination with aspirin 75–100 mg po qDay.	Individualize dosing regimen and adjust based on INR response.

Hepatic impairment	A large intersubject variability among patients with moderate hepatic impairment (Child–Pugh B) but no evidence of a consistent change in exposure or pharmacodynamics.	Severe hepatic impairment: not recommended.	Avoid in patients with moderate and severe hepatic impairment or with any hepatic disease associated with coagulopathy.	Moderate or severe hepatic impairment: not recommended.	Avoid use in Child–Pugh B and C hepatic impairment or hepatic disease associated with coagulopathy.	Use caution.
Drug interactions	P-gp	P-gp and CYP3A4	P-gp	P-gp	P-gp and CYP3A	CYP2C9 (primary), 1A2, 3A4, etc.
Reversal agent	Idarucizumab	Andexanet alfa	NA	NA	Andexanet alfa	Vitamin K, prothrombin complex concentrate.

CAD, *INR* international normalized ratio, *PAD*, *NA* not available, *NVAF* nonvalvular atrial fibrillation, *VTE* venous thromboembolism

Table 39.3 Parental anticoagulants

Name	Heparin (UFH)	Enoxaparin (LMWH)	Dalteparin (LMWH)	Fondaparinux	Bivalirudin	Argatroban
Mechanism	Indirect FIIa and FXa inhibitor	Indirect FXa inhibitor	Indirect FXa inhibitor	Indirect FXa inhibitor	Direct FIIa inhibitor	Direct FIIa inhibitor
Half-life	0.5–2 h	3.5–7 h	3–5 h	17–21 h	25 min	40–50 min
Dosing	VTE treatment: 80 units/kg IV bolus followed by 18 units/kg/h IV. VTE prophylaxis: 5000 units SQ q8-12h.	VTE treatment: CrCl ≥30 mL/min: 1 mg/kg SQ q12h or 1.5 mg/kg SQ qDay. CrCl <30 mL/min: 1 mg/kg SQ qDay or use UFH. VTE prophylaxis: CrCl ≥30 mL/min: 30 SQ q12h or 40 mg SQ qDay depending on specific indication. CrCl <30 mL/min: 30 mg SQ qDay or use UFH.	Extended treatment of VTE in adult patients with cancer: 200 IU/kg SQ qDay for Month 1, then 150 IU/kg SQ qDay for Months 2–6. VTE prophylaxis: 2500 IU or 5000 IU SQ qDay depending on specific indication.	VTE treatment: 5 mg (body weight < 50 kg), 7.5 mg (50–100 kg), or 10 mg (>100 kg) SQ qDay. VTE prophylaxis: 2.5 mg SQ qDay. CrCl 30–50 mL/min: use with caution. CrCl <30 mL/min: avoid use.	PCI with or at risk of HIT: 0.75 mg/kg IV bolus dose followed by 1.75 mg/kg/h (CrCl ≥30 mL/min) IV infusion for the duration of the procedure. Infusion rate should be reduced to 1 mg/kg/h if CrCl <30 mL/min and 0.25 mg/kg/h if on hemodialysis.	For HIT without hepatic impairment: 2 mcg/kg/min continuous infusion, adjust with aPTT target range of 1.5–3 × baseline value (not to exceed 100 s).

Name	Heparin (UFH)	Enoxaparin (LMWH)	Dalteparin (LMWH)	Fondaparinux	Bivalirudin	Argatroban
Hepatic impairment	Use with caution.	Use with caution.	Metabolism is not affected by hepatic failure. Use with caution.	Mild-to-moderate hepatic impairment: no adjustment recommended. Severe hepatic impairment: not defined, observe closely.	No dosage adjustment	Adjust starting dose and titrate carefully in patients with HIT who have moderate or severe hepatic impairment.
Reversal agent	Protamine sulfate	Only partially reversed by protamine sulfate	Only partially reversed by protamine sulfate	NA	NA	NA

aPTT activated partial thromboplastin time, *HIT* heparin-induced thrombocytopenia, *IV* intravenous, *LMWH* low-molecular-weight heparin, *NA* not available, *PCI*, *UFH* unfractionated heparin, *VTE* venous thromboembolism

Board Review Questions

1. A 24-year-old woman with no past medical history was found to have a 6-h history of severe frontal headache. She has no family history of DVT. Her physical exam depicts no neurologic deficits. CT venogram depicts a thrombus in the left cerebral sinus with a moderate amount of hemorrhage but no evidence of cerebral shift.

   Which of the following is the next best therapy to administer?

   A. Aspirin
   B. Fresh frozen plasma
   C. LMWH
   D. Fibrinolytic therapy and activated factor 7
   E. Activated factor 7

   Answer C. LMWH

2. A 35-year-old female was admitted to the hospital for right-leg pain after a motorcycle accident. She was later found to have a femur fracture and underwent surgery. Five days later, she had chest pain, and a CT angiogram showed a segmental right lower-lobe PE. Dopplers of the legs revealed an acute occlusive thrombosis of the left femoral vein.

   Which of the following is the next best step?

   A. IVC filter
   B. IVC filter and apixaban
   C. Thrombolytics administered via interventional radiology
   D. Thrombolytics given peripherally
   E. Heparin drip

   Answer: E. Heparin drip

Reference

1. Lip GY, Nieuwlaat R, Pisters R, et al. Refining clinical risk stratification for predicting stroke and thromboembolism in atrial fibrillation using a novel risk factor-based approach: the euro heart survey on atrial fibrillation. Chest. 2010;137(2):263–72.

Part VI

Transfusion Medicine

Principles and Clinical Applications of Human Blood Groups and Human Leukocyte Antigen System

40

Caroline Stanek and Nirupama Singh

Human Blood Groups

ABO blood group is the most important blood group system in transfusion medicine. In blood, ABO antigens are present on red cells and platelets. ABO antigens are also expressed on many other tissues, including those of the endothelium, kidney, heart, pancreas, etc. and, therefore, important for organ transplant. ABO typing is mostly performed by serology in identifying antigens on red cells (forward typing) and antibodies in the serum (reverse typing). A molecular assay is also available for ABO typing in special situations as the assay is expensive, tedious, and not widely available.

C. Stanek
Department of Pathology, University of Alabama at Birmingham, Birmingham, AL, USA

N. Singh (✉)
Division of Laboratory Medicine, Department of Pathology, University of Alabama at Birmingham, Birmingham, AL, USA
e-mail: nirupamasingh@uabmc.edu

L. Sokol, L. Zhang (eds.), *Non-Neoplastic Hematologic Disorders*,
https://doi.org/10.1007/978-3-031-62373-8_40

Clinical Applications

Selection of red cells for transfusion

	Packed red cells		Whole blood
Patient	1st	2nd	Low titer*
A	A	O	O
B	B	O	O
AB	AB	O, A, B	O
O	O	O	O

*Low titer anti-A and anti-B

Selection of platelets and plasma for transfusion

	Platelets and plasma			
Patient	1st	2nd	3rd	4th
A	A	AB	B	O
B	B	AB	A	O
AB	AB	A	B	O
O	O	AB	A	B

Use low titer (below 50)/PAS platelets for 2nd–4th choices for platelets

Transfusion options with history of mismatched bone-marrow transplant

Recipient	Donor	Red cells	Plasma and platelets			
			1st	2nd	3rd	4th
O	A	O	A	AB	B	O
O	B	O	B	AB	A	O
O	AB	O	AB	A	B	O
A	O	O	A	AB	B	O
B	O	O	B	AB	A	O
AB	O	O	AB	A	B	O
A	B	O	AB	A	B	O
B	A	O	AB	B	A	O
A	AB	A	AB	A	B	O
B	AB	B	AB	B	A	O
AB	A	A	AB	A	B	O
AB	B	B	AB	B	A	O

*3rd and 4th choices should be used only after consult with the bone-marrow transplant

Human Leukocyte Antigen System Introduction

The human leukocyte antigen (HLA) system is the major histocompatibility complex in humans. Located on chromosome 6 and grouped into three regions (class I, class II, and class III); these highly polymorphic genes produce surface antigens that present peptides to T-cell receptors. Critical for the regulation of immune response, these antigens also dictate tissue compatibility.

	Class I	Class II
Genes	HLA-A, HLA-B, HLA-C	HLA-DP, HLA-DQ, HLA-DR
Expression on	Cytotoxic CD8+ T cells	Helper CD4+ T cells
Location	Nucleated cells	Antigen presenting cells

Methods for HLA Typing (Antigen or Allele)

Serology

HLA typing was originally done with serologic assay known as complement-dependent cytotoxicity (CDC). In CDC assay, lymphocytes are added to plates with known antibody specificities, and incubated with complement. When embedded antibody in the plate binds to lymphocyte antigen, it triggers activation of complement that injures the cell and allows the entrance of dye into the cell, creating a pattern of reactivity to be visually scored [1]. This method thus detects the epitopes of HLA molecules, where an antibody binds. Currently to evaluate HLA, molecular methods are required by regulatory agencies in the United States for solid-organ transplant and hematopoietic stem cell transplant (HSCT) instead of serology where molecular methods identify the HLA alleles compared to serology which identifies HLA epitope/antigen.

Molecular

In contrast to serology, molecular typing has the potential to identify all known alleles where DNA-based assays use polymerase chain reaction to identify genes (alleles) of interest. The routinely used DNA-based procedures include sequence-specific primer (SSP), sequence-specific oligonucleotide probes (SSOP), sequence-based typing (SBT), and next generation sequencing (NGS). The advantages of DNA-based methods are: (1) higher sensitivity and specificity; (2) small sample volume; (3) no need for cell viability; and (4) comparable to serology for cost, time, and labor [2]. Currently, most small laboratories use SSP/SSOP where high resolution can provide allele typing. SSP/SSOP are used for STAT typing of deceased donor and solid-organ transplant, whereas SBT and NGS are the gold standard for HSCT for accuracy of allele match with obvious disadvantages of complexity of the assay, long turnaround time, and increase costs. Of note, different typing methods are reflected in different nomenclature, as they reflect varying degrees of specificity. Different institutions and dates of typing can result in different entries, which should be viewed with care [3].

Methods to Identify HLA Antibodies

Cell-Based Assays

CDC assay was used in the past to identify HLA antibodies.

Solid-Phase Assays

More sensitive and reproducible solid-phase assays are currently used to identify HLA antibodies. The newer methods use beads or microparticles coated with HLA class I or class II antigens derived from cultured lymphocyte or recombinant HLA antigens (single-antigen beads). Fluorescent labeled anti-human globulin is used to identify antibody binding. The presence of antibody is detected by enzyme-linked immunosorbent assay, flowcytometry, and flow microarrays.

Clinical Applications

Role of HLA in Transfusion

Most nucleated cells participate in the modulation of immune response via presentation of their HLA antigens on the cell surface, to communicate with T-cell receptors. Mature red cells do not have nucleus and only express low levels of few HLA antigens [4]. Different from RBCs, even though anucleate, platelets still retain a high concentration HLA Class I antigens (predominately HLA A and B). In addition, platelets express human platelet antigen (HPA) glycoproteins as well as ABO antigens. Similar to the red blood cell antigens (non-ABO) eliciting antibodies only on exposure, HLA antibodies can be produced after exposure to foreign HLA antigens, such as pregnancy, transplantation, and blood transfusion. In the US, almost all cellular products are leukoreduced that has up to 50% reduction in HLA alloimmunization (16% to 7–8%) [5]. Recipients with HLA antibodies against class I HLA antigen can cause platelet refractoriness, flagging donor platelets for early destruction. Platelet refractoriness is defined as suboptimal response to platelet transfusion, which can be due to immune or non-immune factors.

Non-immune factors such as splenomegaly, sepsis, bleeding, and DIC are responsible for up to 80% of the refractoriness. Immune-mediated platelet refractoriness is caused by the recipient's antibodies against HLA class I antigens, and infrequently to HPA or ABO antigen. To differentiate immune versus non-immune platelet refractoriness, two sequential Corrected Count Increment (CCI) is calculated at 10–60 min after platelet transfusion where CCI < 5000 μL suggests immune cause of platelet refractoriness: [6]

$$\text{CCI} = \frac{\text{platelet count increment} \times \text{body surface area}}{\#\text{of platelets transfused} \times 10^{11}}$$

In addition, a good history and physical examination is must to rule out non-immune platelet refractoriness. To resolve non-immune refractoriness, correcting and removing the cause are the solution. Once immune-mediated refractoriness is suspected, cross-matched platelets are the first degree of additional testing and solution for platelet refractoriness. In platelet cross match, patient serum is combined with the aliquots of platelets from 12 to 14 different donors. In a solid-phase red cell adherence assay, the binding of a patient's alloantibody (HLA or HPA) to donor platelet can be visualized by the addition of indicator cells coated with anti-IgG. Donor platelet bound with alloantibody and indictor cells will coat the microplate well with a monolayer (Fig. 40.1). Patient alloantibody not bound to donor platelet will be removed in a washing step. Without alloantibody–platelet interaction, the subsequent indicator cells will remain unbound, and form a pellet upon centrifugation (Fig. 40.1). Crossmatched platelets are the solution for patients with short-term need for transfusion. For patients who are sustained transfusion dependent or attempting to avoid additional HLA alloimmunization prior to organ transplant, HLA-matched platelets would be the appropriate choice. To provide HLA match platelets, the patient is evaluated for HLA antigen type and HLA antibodies to determine HLA Calculated Panel Reactive Antibodies (cPRA). This also serves as a measure to quantify patient sensitization, where a low cPRA indicates less sensitization. As cPRA is calculated with population data, it represents the probability of finding a good match, where cPRA >20% suggests presence of some component of alloimmunization.

HLA matching (HLA class I antigen and HLA antibodies) can be the solution for immune-mediated refractoriness, but it may prevent the recipient immune system from recognizing donor T cells as foreign, allowing their proliferation, and causing transfusion-associated graft versus host disease (TA-GVHD), and therefore, HLA-matched platelets must be irradiated to prevent GVHD .

The role of HLA system is also important in other complications of transfusion, for example, febrile non-hemolytic

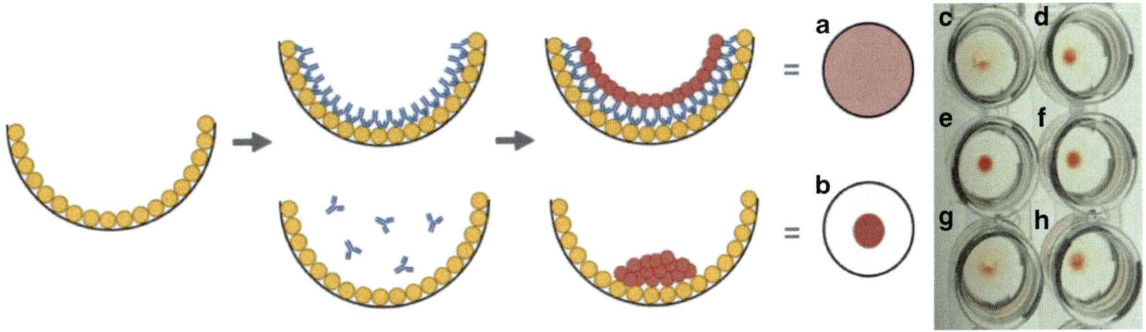

Fig. 40.1 Red cell adherence assay. Schematic demonstrating side and top-down view of microwells with (**a**) and without patient antibody (**b**)—donor platelet interaction and photograph (created with Biorender.com). (**c**, **g**): incompatible; (**e**, **f**) microwells represent cross match compatible; (**d**, **h**): are partial compatible

transfusion reactions (FNHTR), transfusion-related acute lung injury (TRALI) and TA-GVHD [2].

FNHTR

The pathogenesis of FNHTR is associated with HLA-mediated antigen–antibody reactions and cytokines released from leukocytes in blood products during storage. HLA antibodies in recipient or donor can interact with HLA antigen of donor or recipient, respectively, leading to decomposition and release of pyrogens from leukocytes or platelets. Incidence of FNHTR has decreased after universal leukoreduction leading to decreased cytokines in blood products. Currently, antipyretics is not recommended to prevent FNHTR but only used as treatment modality.

TRALI

Donor HLA and neutrophil antibodies when react with recipient's antigen lead to TRALI. In the US, to prevent TRALI, all plasma donors are usually male with no history of transfusion or tested for HLA antibodies. Occasionally, patients with HLA antibodies can react to donor HLA antigen leading TRALI.

Role of HLA Typing in Transplant

HLA testing is a part of solid-organ transplant, and HSCT to identify matched donor. HLA match is important for engraftment and reduce risk of GVHD, because donor immune cells recognize the recipient as "non-self" via these foreign HLA. Extensive HLA testing for HLA match is crucial for HSCT, whereas ABO compatibility is the most important for graft survival in solid-organ transplant with limited HLA testing for better outcomes. For HSCT, testing is performed for HLA alleles for class I and class II for donor and recipient along with HLA antibodies for the recipient. To identify compatible kidney, donors are tested for preformed HLA antibodies along with HLA allele typing for class I and class II in recipients. A crossmatch between recipient serum and donor lymphocytes is required before kidney transplantation to avoid acute graft rejection which is caused by donor HLA antibodies.

Recipient's HLA antibodies (cPRA) because of previous transplant, transfusion and pregnancy can delay organ transplantation.

Note: Currently, in the US, all cellular products (red cells and platelets) are leukocyte reduced and it decreases the risk of HLA immunization.

Caveats

1. HLA class I antigens are expressed on all nucleated cells, including T cells but also on platelets. HLA class II antigens are expressed on antigen presenting cells, including B lymphocytes. Activated T cells can express HLA II antigens.
2. Platelets have high concentration of HLA class I antigens in contrast to red blood cells which express only very low concentration. Platelet transfusion recipients with HLA antibodies against class I HLA antigen can cause platelet refractoriness.
3. Comprehensive HLA testing is very important for outcome of patients undergoing HLA matched HSCT in contrast to ABO compatibility that is the most important factor for solid-organ graft survival.

Board Questions

1. Suspecting immune-mediated platelet refractoriness secondary to multiple pregnancies, platelet cross match is ordered on a patient. The resulting plate contains 5 microwells with a monolayer of indicator cells and 9 microwells with pellets. Which of the following is the correct interpretation?

   A. 5/14 platelet compatibility,
   B. 9/14 platelet compatibility,
   C. 64 cPRA
   D. 36 cPRA

Answer: B. Patient serum alloantibody bound to platelet aliquots from five donors, and did not react with aliquots from 9 donors, indicating no antibody–platelet interaction with 9/14 donors. This solid-phase red cell adherence assay thus indicates 9/14 compatibility. cPRA is an index of HLA matching.

2. HLA system is associated with which of the following transfusion complications?

   A. Acute hemolytic transfusion reaction (AHTR)
   B. Hypotensive transfusion reaction
   C. Transfusion related acute lung injury (TRALI)
   D. Anaphylactic transfusion reaction

Answer: C. HLA plays a role in febrile non-hemolytic, TRALI, TA-GVHD, immune platelet refractoriness and solid and HPC transplant rejection.

3. Given the following patient histories, which of the following patients is least likely to have HLA antibodies?

   A. A nulliparous female with transfusion dependent thalassemia
   B. A male with previous history of prolonged ICU stays after multiple gunshot injury
   C. A multiparous female
   D. A male currently in DIC

Answer: D. Pregnancy and previous transfusion are the most common immunizing events that can lead to the formation of HLA alloantibodies (A, C). Assuming patient B likely received multiple transfusions during a prolonged ICU stay. Option D, male with no history of prior transfusion is least likely to have HLA antibodies.

4. To provide HLA matched units for immune refractoriness which class of HLA antigen is evaluated?

   A. HLA class I antigen
   B. HLA class II antigen
   C. HLA class I and II antigen
   D. HLA class III

Answer: A. Platelets express ABO and HLA class I antigen

References

1. Bontadini A. HLA techniques: typing and antibody detection in the laboratory of immunogenetics. Methods. 2012;56(4):471–6.
2. Fung MK. The HLA system, AABB technical manual. 19th ed.
3. Fang, D. AM23-MN-09-L. Platelet refractoriness management – how to treat refractory patients when nothing else works. AABB, 2023.
4. Daniels. Chapter 32 HLA (Human Leucocyte-Associated) Class I antigens on red cells, Human Blood Groups. Wiley; 2013.
5. Trial to Reduce Alloimmunization to Platelets Study Group (TRAP). Leukocyte reduction and ultraviolet B irradiation of platelets to prevent alloimmunization and refractoriness to platelet transfusions. N Engl J Med. 1997;337(26):1861–9.
6. Davis KB, Slichter SJ, Corash L. Corrected count increment and percent platelet recovery as measures of posttransfusion platelet response: problems and a solution. Transfusion. 1999;39(6):586–92.

Red Cell Transfusion

41

Mishi Bhushan, Pankit Vachhani, and Nirupama Singh

Introduction

Blood transfusion is a key therapeutic procedure for patients with hematological and oncological malignancies. In the last two decades with the advancement of newer testing methods for infectious disease screening and optimization of transfusion guidelines, blood transfusion is a much safer procedure. Blood collection and dispensation is a complex process, and for simplicity, we will cover history, pre-transfusion testing of blood components, blood product modifications, guidelines to transfuse, and adverse events of transfusion (Fig. 41.1).

The discovery of the ABO blood groups and other red blood cell antigens led to the discovery of transfusion. The advancements in technology for blood testing, for example, the early

M. Bhushan
Department of Pathology, University of Alabama Birmingham, Birmingham, AL, USA

P. Vachhani
Division of Hematology/Oncology, Department of Medicine, University of Alabama at Birmingham, Birmingham, AL, USA

N. Singh (✉)
Division of Laboratory Medicine, Department of Pathology, University of Alabama at Birmingham, Birmingham, AL, USA
e-mail: nirupamasingh@uabmc.edu

L. Sokol, L. Zhang (eds.), *Non-Neoplastic Hematologic Disorders*,
https://doi.org/10.1007/978-3-031-62373-8_41

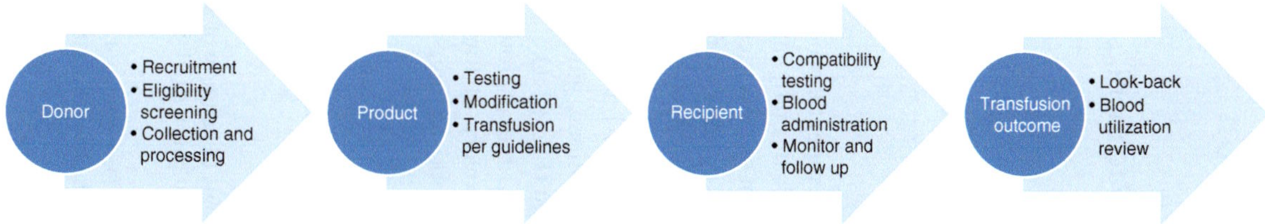

Fig. 41.1 The complex process of blood transfusion: details the different processes involved in blood transfusion from donor recruitment to post-transfusion quality control measures. (Reference: Association for the advancement of Blood and Biotherapies, aabb)

2000s, were marked by the introduction of nucleic acid amplification testing to detect viruses (HIV, HCV, HBV, and West Nile virus) and recent addition of pathogen-reduced technology has significantly reduced infectious complications of transfusion, which is capable of inactivating viruses, parasites, and bacteria and further reduces the risk of transfusion-transmitted infections and currently available for platelets only in the US.

Pre-transfusion Testing

The process of blood donation is complex: a potential blood donor must meet eligibility requirements with respect to age, weight, hemoglobin, blood pressure, and medical history. A full list of eligibility criteria can be found at redcrossblood.org/faq.html#eligibility. Each donor is evaluated for ABO and Rh type and screened for a host of infectious diseases, such as HBV, HCV, and HIV. Testing of recipient blood for ABO and Rh type, RBC antibody screen, and the crossmatch ensures ABO compatibility and decreases post-transfusion adverse events. Transfusion services perform hemovigilance to minimize adverse events and promote safe and effective use of blood [1].

- ABO grouping
  - ABO grouping (Fig. 41.2a)
    Forward Type: Testing of red cells with anti-A and anti-B reagents
    Reverse Typing: Testing of plasma/serum with A1 and B reagent red cells
  - Rh typing
    Anti-D reagent

In Fig. 41.2b, a gel card showing blood group A, Rh positive.

a

Forward Typing		Reverse Typing		
Patient's Red Cells		Patient's Serum		
Anti-A	Anti-B	Anti-A1	Anti-B	ABO group
4+	0	0	4+	A
0	4+	4+	0	B
4+	4+	0	0	AB
0	0	4+	4+	O

b

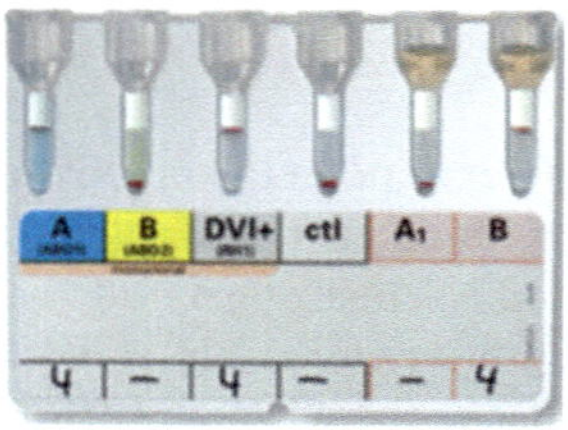

Fig. 41.2 ABO grouping with forward and reverse typing for each blood group (**a**), and sample test (**b**)

- RBC antibody screen: Identifies red cell alloantibodies in recipient acquired through transfusion or pregnancy
  - 2–4 reagent group O test cells are used (Fig. 41.3) showing three group O test cells). This is an example of a negative antibody screen
  - Usually, approximately 15–20 clinically significant antibody specificities to the following antigens are assessed: Rh (D, C, c, E, e), Duffy (Fy^a, Fy^b), Kidd (Jk^a, Jk^b), Kell (K, k), and SsU (S, s, U)
  - If the screen is positive, an antibody panel (Fig. 41.4) is performed to identify red cell alloantibodies. Figure 41.4 shows an example of anti-D in patient's plasma (agglutination is seen in presence of D antigen only, lanes 1–10, 20)
- Crossmatch:
  - Computer crossmatch: Permissible in patients with a negative antibody screen
  - Serologic crossmatch for patients with RBC alloantibodies (Fig. 41.5)

			Rh-hr								KELL						DUFFY		KIDD		Sex-linked	LEWIS		MNS				P	Lutheran		Special Antigen typing	Cell #	Test Results
Cell #	Rh-hr	Donor Number	D	C	E	c	e	f	Cw	V	K	k	Kp^a	Kp^b	Js^a	Js^b	FY^a	FY^b	JK^a	JK^b	Xga	Le^a	Le^b	S	s	M	N	P1	Lu^a	Lu^b			
1	R1R1	316782	+	+	0	0	+	0	0	0	0	+	0	+	/	+	+	0	+	0	+	0	+	+	0	+	0	+S	0	+		1	**0**
2	R2R2	318390	+	0	+	+	0	0	0	0	+	+	0	+	/	+	0	+	+	+	+	0	+	0	+	0	+	0	0	+		2	**0**
3	rr	323954	0	0	0	+	+	+	0	0	0	+	0	+	/	+	0	+	0	+	+	+	0	+	+	+	+	+S	0	+		3	**0**
	Patient Cells																																

Fig. 41.3 Antibody screen (**a**) with workup summary (**b**)

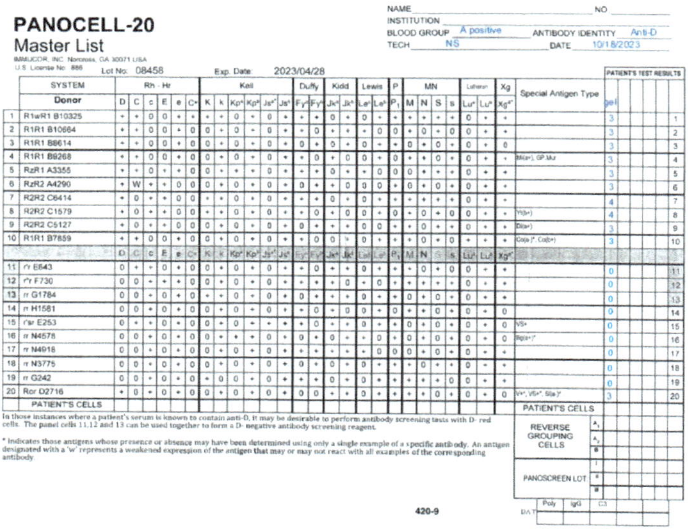

PANOCELL-20
Master List
IMMUCOR, INC. Norcross, GA 30071 USA
U.S. License No. 886 Lot No: 08458 Exp. Date: 2023/04/28

NAME ______ NO ______
INSTITUTION ______
BLOOD GROUP A positive ANTIBODY IDENTITY Anti-D
TECH NS DATE 10/18/2023

	SYSTEM	Rh - Hr						Kell						Duffy		Kidd		Lewis		P	MN				Lutheran		Xg	Special Antigen Type	PATIENT'S TEST RESULTS	
	Donor	D	C	c	E	e	Cw	K	k	Kpa	Kpb	Jsa	Jsb	Fya	Fyb	Jka	Jkb	Lea	Leb	P1	M	N	S	s	Lua	Lub	Xga		gel	
1	R1wR1 B10325	+	+	0	0	+	+	+	+	0	+	0	+	+	+	0	+	0	+	+	+	+	+	+	0	+	+		3	1
2	R1R1 B10664	+	+	0	0	+	0	0	+	0	+	0	+	+	0	+	+	+	0	0	+	0	+	0	0	+	+		3	2
3	R1R1 B8614	+	+	0	0	+	0	0	+	0	+	0	+	0	+	0	+	0	+	+	0	+	0	+	0	+	0		3	3
4	R1R1 B9268	+	+	0	0	+	0	0	+	0	+	0	+	+	0	+	0	0	+	0	+	+	0	+	0	+	+	Mi(a+), GP.Mur	3	4
5	RzR1 A3355	+	+	0	+	+	0	0	+	+	+	0	+	+	+	0	+	+	0	0	0	+	+	+	0	+	+		3	5
6	RzR2 A4290	+	W	+	+	0	0	0	+	0	+	0	+	0	+	+	0	0	0	+	0	+	0	+	0	+	+		3	6
7	R2R2 C6414	+	0	+	+	0	0	+	+	0	+	0	+	+	+	0	+	0	+	+	+	+	+	+	0	+	+		4	7
8	R2R2 C1579	+	0	+	+	0	0	+	+	0	+	0	+	+	0	+	0	0	+	0	+	0	+	0	0	+	+	Yt(b+)	4	8
9	R2R2 C5127	+	0	+	+	0	0	0	+	0	+	0	+	0	+	+	+	0	0	+	+	0	+	+	0	+	+	Di(a+)	3	9
10	R1R1 B7859	+	+	0	0	+	0	0	+	0	+	0	+	+	0	0	+	0	+	+	+	0	+	0	+	+	+	Co(a-)*, Co(b+)	3	10
		D	C	c	E	e	Cw	K	k	Kpa	Kpb	Jsa	Jsb	Fya	Fyb	Jka	Jkb	Lea	Leb	P1	M	N	S	s	Lua	Lub	Xga			
11	r'r E643	0	+	+	0	+	0	0	+	0	+	0	+	+	0	+	+	0	+	+	+	0	+	0	0	+	+		0	11
12	r''r F730	0	0	+	+	+	0	0	+	0	+	0	+	+	+	+	0	+	0	+	+	+	+	+	0	+	+		0	12
13	rr G1784	0	0	+	0	+	0	+	+	0	+	0	+	0	+	+	+	0	+	+	0	+	0	+	0	+	+		0	13
14	rr H1581	0	0	+	0	+	0	0	+	0	+	0	+	+	0	+	0	0	+	0	+	+	0	+	0	+	0		0	14
15	r'sr E253	0	+	+	0	+	0	0	+	0	+	+	+	+	0	+	+	0	+	+	0	+	0	+	0	+	0	VS+	0	15
16	rr N4578	0	0	+	0	+	0	0	+	+	+	0	+	0	+	0	+	+	0	+	0	+	0	+	0	+	0	Bg(a+)*	0	16
17	rr N4918	0	0	+	0	+	0	0	+	0	+	0	+	+	+	+	+	+	0	0	0	+	0	+	0	+	+		0	17
18	rr N3775	0	0	+	0	+	0	0	+	0	+	0	+	0	+	0	+	0	+	+	+	0	+	+	0	+	+		0	18
19	rr G242	0	0	+	0	+	0	+	0	0	+	0	+	+	+	0	+	0	+	+	+	+	+	0	0	+	+		0	19
20	Ror D2716	+	0	+	0	+	0	0	+	0	+	0	+	0	0	+	+	0	+	+	+	+	0	+	0	+	0	V+*, VS+*, Sl(a-)*	3	20
	PATIENT'S CELLS																											PATIENT'S CELLS		

In those instances where a patient's serum is known to contain anti-D, it may be desirable to perform antibody screening tests with D- red cells. The panel cells 11,12 and 13 can be used together to form a D- negative antibody screening reagent.

* Indicates those antigens whose presence or absence may have been determined using only a single example of a specific antibody. An antigen designated with a 'w' represents a weakened expression of the antigen that may or may not react with all examples of the corresponding antibody.

REVERSE GROUPING CELLS A1 A2 B
PANOSCREEN LOT I II III
DAT Poly IgG C3

420-9

Fig. 41.4 Antibody Panel performed showing anti-D where plasma is reacting with reagent cells which are D antigen positive and negative in absence of D antigen

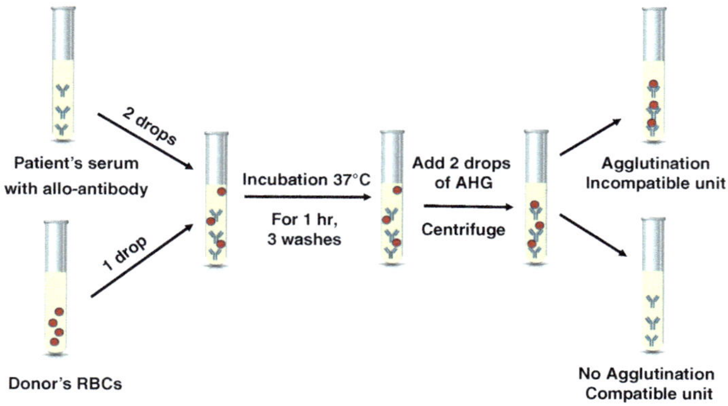

Fig. 41.5 Illustration of the serologic cross-match

- The following infectious diseases are screened in each allogeneic blood donation.
  - Hepatitis B virus
  - Hepatitis C virus
  - Human Immunodeficiency viruses, Types 1 and 2 (HIV-1,2)
  - Human T-Lymphotropic virus (HTLV-1/2)
  - West Nile virus
  - *Treponema pallidum* (Syphilis)
  - *Trypanosoma Cruzi*
  - Babesiosis

Component Manufacturing

In the US and other developed nations, whole blood was replaced with component therapy where blood is separated into red blood cell, platelets, and plasma [2]. Currently, apheresis is also used to obtain components, such as double RBCs, apheresis platelets, and plasma.

Blood Product Modification

Blood product modifications increase the cost and may delay the availability of the component; however, the benefits of these modifications usually outweigh the risk.

- **Leukoreduction:** Leukocyte reduction significantly decreases the number of leukocytes in red blood cell and platelet units. The regulatory standards in the US require that 95% of tested units must contain fewer than 5×10^6 residual leukocytes after beginning with billions of white cells. Most blood components in the United States are now leukoreduced. Leukoreduction is not an alternative to irradiating blood products.

- **Advantages:**
  - Decreases human leukocyte antigen (HLA) alloimmunization and, therefore, reduces immune platelet refractoriness
  - Decreases febrile non-hemolytic transfusion reactions
  - Decreases risk of cytomegalovirus (CMV) transmission (a leukoreduced component is considered equivalent to a CMV-seronegative blood component and is known as "CMV safe." CMV safe blood is acceptable for hematopoietic stem cell transplant (HSCT) recipients at high risk for severe CMV disease [3])
- **Irradiation:** Irradiation is indicated for prevention of transfusion-associated graft vs host disease (TA-GVHD) by preventing proliferation of donor T-lymphocytes. In the US, 25Gy is required for irradiation of cellular products, such as RBCs and platelets. Components such as plasma and cryoprecipitate do not need irradiation. Either gamma rays or X-rays can be used for irradiation. The newer pathogen reduction technology for platelets uses UVA light irradiation in the process and does not need further irradiation.
- **Indications:**
  - HSCT recipients
  - Intrauterine transfusion or premature infants
  - HLA-matched or directed blood product (transfusions from blood relatives)
  - Lymphoma
  - Congenital immunodeficiency
  - Chemotherapy with purine analogs or purine antagonists (fludarabine and bendamustine)
- **Washed products:** Washing of cellular products significantly reduces plasma proteins, and the component is resuspended in normal saline.
- **Indications:**
  - Recurrent or severe allergic reactions
  - Intrauterine transfusions, and red cell units for neonates with hyperkalemia

Drawbacks:

- Shortens product life (transfuse within 24 h of washing)
- Not available for plasma and cryoprecipitate

Note: Platelets can also be washed but usually not recommended/required. There is loss of up to 30% of platelet yield and platelet units expire within 4 h of washing.

- **CMV-negative**: This product is equivalent to leukocyte-reduced red cells (CMV safe). Currently, CMV seronegative units are in use for intrauterine transfusion and premature neonates only.

Transfusion Guidelines for RBCs

Millions of RBC units are transfused in the US annually and professional associations, such as AABB, and are actively updating transfusion guidelines [4].

These recommendations include*:

- A restrictive RBC transfusion threshold: of 7.0–8.0 g/dl for hospitalized adult patients who are hemodynamically stable.
- A restrictive RBC transfusion threshold of 8.0 g/dL for patients with a pre-existing cardiovascular disease and requiring major surgery, such as orthopedic or cardiac surgery.
- Single unit transfusion should be standard for non-bleeding hospitalized patients.

*Exceptions include patients with severe thrombocytopenia and chronic transfusion-dependent anemia.

Post-transfusion Complications

A transfusion should be suspended whenever a transfusion reaction is suspected. After pausing or cessation of the transfusion, and providing supportive care, a transfusion reaction study is initiated. Fresh blood samples should be sent to the blood bank. The transfusion reaction study includes a clerical check, inspection for hemolysis, a repeat ABO grouping, and a direct antiglobulin test with comparison of results to a pre-transfusion sample. A transfusion service physician reviews the workup to classify the reaction and determine whether additional testing is required. Types of transfusion reactions are detailed in Table 41.1 [5, 6].

Caveats

1. Irradiation of blood products prevents transfusion-associated graft vs host disease by eliminating T-lymphocytes. Radiation doses of 25 Gy are required for irradiation of cellular products in the USA.
2. RBC transfusion threshold is 7.0–8.0 g/dl for adult patients who are hemodynamically stable and 8.0 g/dL for patients with a pre-existing cardiovascular disease.
3. Washed blood products are recommended in severe recurrent allergic transfusion reaction, intrauterine transfusions, and for neonates with hyperkalemia.

Board Questions

1. What is the most common antibody associated with acute hemolytic transfusion reactions?

   A. Anti-D
   B. Anti-Kidd
   C. Anti-A/B
   D. Anti-Kell

Answer C. All other antibodies are usually associated with delayed hemolytic transfusion reactions.

Table 41.1 Types of Transfusion reaction: diagnosis and treatment

Type of reaction	Criteria	Incidence	Pathophysiology	Treatment & follow-up
Febrile, nonhemolytic transfusion reaction (FNHTR)	Occurs during or within 4 h of cessation of transfusion Fever (greater than or equal to 38C/100.4F oral and at least a change of 1C/1.8F from pre-transfusion value) Or: chills/rigor	Most common 1 in 200 transfusions	Mediated by cytokines released by white blood cells in the stored unit of blood	Antipyretics Transfusion with leukocyte reduced products
Allergic/ ANAPHYLACTIC transfusion reaction (ATR)	Following signs/symptoms during or within 4 h of cessation of transfusion: Mild: Pruritis (itching), Urticaria (hives) Severe: Hypotension, Bronchospasm, Angioedema	1 in 300 transfusions	An allergen in the donor blood product initiates IgE-mediated, type 1 hypersensitivity reactions	Symptomatic treatment for mild reaction, it is ok to pause the transfusion and restart once symptoms subside with treatment

(continued)

Table 41.1 (continued)

Type of reaction	Criteria	Incidence	Pathophysiology	Treatment & follow-up
Acute hemolytic transfusion reaction (AHTR)	Occurs during, or within 24 h of cessation of transfusion with new onset of the following signs/symptoms: Fever, Back/flank pain, Hematuria, Hypotension Elevated bilirubin & LDH Hemoglobinemia & Hemoglobinuria	Between 1 in 6000 and 1 in 30,000	Usually, Intravascular Related to ABO incompatibility	Stop transfusion Provide hemodynamic support Severity related to amount of red cells transfused
Delayed hemolytic transfusion reactions (DHTR)	Inadequate rise of post-transfusion hemoglobin level or rapid fall in hemoglobin back to pre-transfusion levels usually within 24 h & 28 days Newly identified RBC alloantibody in recipient plasma Positive DAT with elution of new alloantibodies	1 in 1500 transfusions	Delayed immunological reaction of host to alloantibodies	Identify the responsible antibody and avoid further exposure to it

Transfusion-transmitted infection (TTI)	Laboratory evidence of a pathogen in the transfusion recipient *Clinical presentation*: Transfusion recipient experiences high fever and shock	Incidence of transfusion-transmitted sepsis: 1/250,000 in platelet transfusions	Bacteria originate from donor skin or less commonly from donor blood Most common with platelet transfusion (since stored at room temperature)	Broad spectrum antibiotics and hemodynamic support following cessation of the transfusion Culture recipient blood
Transfusion associated graft versus Host disease (TA-GVHd)	A rare complication occurring from 2 days to 6 weeks after cessation of transfusion characterized by: Characteristic rash, Diarrhea, Fever Hepatomegaly, Liver dysfunction Marrow aplasia, Pancytopenia	Fatal (>90%) complication	Due to the introduction of immunocompetent lymphocytes into susceptible hosts: the allogeneic lymphocytes engraft, proliferate, and destroy host cells	None Prevention: irradiation of cellular blood products (red cells, platelets and granulocytes) for recipients at risk

(continued)

Table 41.1 (continued)

Type of reaction	Criteria	Incidence	Pathophysiology	Treatment & follow-up
Transfusion associated Acute lung injury (TRALI)	NO evidence of acute lung injury (ALI) prior to transfusion AND ALI onset during or within 6 h of cessation of transfusion AND hypoxemia defined by any of the following methods: PaO_2/FiO_2 less than or equal to 300 mmHg Oxygen saturation less than 90% on room air AND Radiographic evidence of bilateral infiltrates AND No evidence of left atrial hypertension	1/5000 transfusions	Noncardiac pulmonary edema following transfusion of plasma containing blood products Donor antigranulocyte and/or anti-HLA/HNA antibodies target recipient granulocytes, producing microaggregates in the pulmonary circulation	Stop the transfusion Supportive Prevention: exclusion of implicated donors from future transfusion

Transfusion-Associated Circulatory Overload (TACO)	New onset or exacerbation following within 12 h of cessation of transfusion: Evidence of acute or worsening respiratory distress (dyspnea, tachypnea, decreased oxygen saturation) and/or Radiographic or clinical evidence of acute or worsening pulmonary edema (crackles on lung auscultation, orthopnea, cough AND Elevated brain natriuretic peptide (BNP) or NT-pro --BNP relevant biomarker Evidence of fluid overload	Most common cause of transfusion fatality	Infusion volume cannot be effectively processed by the recipient either due to high rate and/or volume of infusion or an underlying cardiac or pulmonary pathology	Diuretics for symptomatic relief Prevention: slow rate of transfusion

(continued)

Table 41.1 (continued)

Type of reaction	Criteria	Incidence	Pathophysiology	Treatment & follow-up
Post transfusion purpura (PTP)	Alloantibodies in the patient directed against Human Platelet Antigen (HPA) system or platelet specific detected at or after development of thrombocytopenia and thrombocytopenia to less than 20% of pre-transfusion count Profound thrombocytopenia 2–14 days following RBC or platelet transfusions	2% of the population is HPA1a negative and capable of producing antibodies	Platelet alloantibodies, most commonly anti-HPA1a cause destruction of both donor and recipient platelets	Intravenous immunoglobulin (IVIG) results in rapid platelet recovery within 3–5 days
Hypotensive transfusion reaction	All other adverse reactions presenting with hypotension are excluded and hypotension occurs during or within 1 h after cessation of transfusion: Adults (≥18 years): Drop in systolic blood pressure (SBP) ≥ 30 mmHg and SBP ≤80mmHG Infants, children, and adolescents (1 year to <18 years): ≥25% drop in SBP from baselines			Supportive

Ref.: NHSN hemovigilance, https://www.aabb.org/docs/default-source/default-document-library/resources/aabb-quick-reference-guide-nhsn-hemovigilance-module.pdf?sfvrsn=30f1600b_6

2. Which of the following is true for leukoreduced blood products?

   A. Decreases the risk of febrile non-hemolytic transfusion reactions
   B. Decreases the risk of TA-GVHD
   C. Decreases the risk of TA-HIV
   D. Decreases the risk of TA-syphilis

Answer A. Leukocyte reduction decreases FNHTR and makes red cell CMV safe. All other transfusion reactions cannot be avoided by leukoreduction.

3. Which patient requires irradiated blood products?

   A. Patient with CLL on fludarabine
   B. HIV-infected patient
   C. Newly diagnosed breast cancer patient
   D. Child admitted with influenza

Answer A. GVHD is not seen in other patients.

4. A 65-year-old man with coronary artery disease and duodenal ulcer presented with systolic BP of 100 mm Hg, pulse 80/min and RR 20/min He was urgently transfused 2 red cell and 2 plasma units. His pretransfusion hemoglobin was 5.0 g/dL. After the transfusions he had chest tightness and dyspnea with systolic BP 130 mmHg, pulse 118/min, RR 30/min and was afebrile. Chest X-ray showed bilateral opacities and Blood Bank reported no acute hemolysis. What is the most likely diagnosis?

   A. Transfusion-associated circulatory overload (TACO)
   B. Transfusion-related acute lung injury (TRALI)
   C. Transfusion-associated dyspnea (TAD)
   D. Transfusion-associated hypertension

Answer A. Decompensated heart with increase in Blood pressure and no fever favors TACO.

References

1. Technical Manual, 21st Edition. AABB, 2022, chapter 4 ISBN 978-1-56395-370-5.
2. Acker JP, Marks DC, Sheffield WP. Quality assessment of established and emerging blood components for transfusion. J Blood Transfus. 2016:2016.
3. Bowden RA, Slichter SJ, Sayers M, et al. A comparison of filtered leukocyte-reduced and cytomegalovirus (CMV) seronegative blood products for the prevention of transfusion-associated CMV infection after marrow transplant. Blood. 1995;86:3598–603.
4. Carson JL, Guyatt G, Heddle NM, et al. Clinical practice guidelines from the AABB: red blood cell transfusion thresholds and storage. JAMA. 2016;316(19):2025–35. https://doi.org/10.1001/jama.2016.9185.
5. Carson JL, Triulzi DJ, Ness PM. Indications for and adverse effects of red-cell transfusion. N Engl J Med. 2017;377(13):1261–72. https://doi.org/10.1056/NEJMra1612789. PMID: 28953438.
6. AABB Quick Reference Guide NHSN Hemovigilance Module: Adverse Reaction Definitions. https://www.aabb.org/docs/default-source/default-document-library/resources/aabb-quick-reference-guide-nhsn-hemovigilance-. Accessed 27 Jan 2023.

Platelet Transfusions

42

Avani M. Singh and Kaaron Benson

Introduction

Platelet transfusions are an essential component of medical care, with around two million units transfused annually in the United States [1]. Platelets may be needed in diverse settings such as trauma, surgery, procedures, hematologic malignancies, pregnancy, and more. Once obtained by donors, they are stored at room temperature (20–24°C) for 5–7 days. Because they are not refrigerated, such as RBC and whole blood units, platelets pose a higher bacterial contamination risk. Extra precautions to screen for such contamination may include bacterial cultures or use of pathogen-reduction technology (PRT). Additional platelet modifications are available for special patient populations to prevent reactions.

A. M. Singh (✉)
Department of Hematology & Oncology, University of South Florida/Moffitt Cancer Center, Tampa, FL, USA
e-mail: Avani.Singh@Moffitt.org

K. Benson
Department of Pathology, H. Lee Moffitt Cancer Center, Tampa, FL, USA

L. Sokol, L. Zhang (eds.), *Non-Neoplastic Hematologic Disorders*, https://doi.org/10.1007/978-3-031-62373-8_42

Platelet Component Types

Platelets are obtained either by apheresis from a single donor or pooled from several whole blood units. The vast majority, approximately 92%, of platelets are obtained by apheresis donations [1]. A standardized dose of one unit of platelets contains either one unit of apheresis platelets or 4–6 pooled units from whole blood. Whole blood-derived (WBD) platelets can be prepared by the buffy-coat method, typical in Europe and Canada, or by the platelet-rich plasma method, typical in the United States. These two preparation methods differ primarily in centrifugation speed and steps. WBD and apheresis platelets are generally considered equally effective and safe [2].

Platelet Specifics

A platelet unit must contain a minimum of 300 billion (3×10^{11}) platelets per Food and Drug Administration (FDA) regulation. Most platelets are stored at room temperature (20–24 °C) with a 5–7-day shelf-life. Cold-stored platelets (1–6 °C) have been researched to lengthen the life span of platelet units and reduce the bacterial contamination risk. These cold-stored platelets may be effective for trauma patients in providing temporary hemostasis.

Unlike RBCs, platelets only weakly express ABO group A and B antigens and do not express Rh antigens. Platelet units contain some donor RBCs, which, if Rh-positive will express the Rh antigen. Therefore, platelet units should be selected by ABO and Rh type whenever possible but mismatched units are commonly transfused. Platelets are suspended in about 200 mLs plasma, so plasma compatible units should be considered whenever it is possible. ABO-incompatible platelets (e.g., group A platelets to O patient) may result in a lower but satisfactory platelet increment as compared to ABO-compatible platelets (O platelets to A patient) due to the weak A antigen expression on the donor platelets. Plasma-incompatible platelets (group O platelets to A patient) may rarely cause acute hemolysis, especially when transfusing a small-size patient. Efforts to minimize such hemolysis include avoiding plasma-incompatible transfusions in at-risk recipients.

Platelet Transfusion Guidelines

Indications

Platelet transfusions can be given prophylactically, or therapeutically for bleeding. Platelets are often given prophylactically to thrombocytopenic patients to prevent spontaneous bleeding. Thrombocytopenia is especially prevalent and significant in the critically ill patient population, with 9–30% of intensive care unit patients requiring platelet transfusion, primarily for bleeding prophylaxis [3]. In general, the transfusion threshold for bleeding prophylaxis is set at 10,000/uL based on randomized controlled trials demonstrating the prior 20,000/uL threshold could be safely lowered [4]. With any active bleeding, the platelet threshold is generally 50,000/uL, and with any intracranial or central nervous system bleeding, the threshold is 100,000/uL. Other factors that may increase a patient's risk of bleeding include fever and sepsis.

In the preoperative or pre-procedure setting, platelet thresholds are guided by the level of invasiveness and can be categorized into minimally invasive (e.g., endoscopy, central lines, angiography, lumbar puncture, bronchoscopy, and paracentesis), invasive procedures (e.g., laparotomy, transbronchial biopsy, liver biopsy, and cardiac surgery), and neurosurgical interventions. Factors that may affect the platelet threshold include antiplatelet/anticoagulant medications, underlying disease process, and anticipated bleeding. Though there are no randomized controlled studies to understand platelet threshold in the perioperative setting, standardized thresholds most often guide practice. In the minimally invasive setting, platelet count of 20,000–30,000/uL is considered acceptable to minimize bleeding risk. With most invasive procedures and cardiac surgery, a threshold of 50,000/uL is used. Finally with neurosurgery or CNS invasive procedures, the threshold is generally raised to 100,000/uL [1, 3, 5]. If bleeding can be controlled with pressure, such as with skin or bone marrow biopsy, platelet transfusion is generally not needed.

In the obstetric setting, studies have demonstrated improved outcomes with platelet goals of 50,000–80,000/uL. Obstetric patients often require epidural anesthesia, and this platelet goal minimizes bleeding risk with this procedure as well as vaginal and cesarean deliveries [3]. The indications of transfusion of platelets in neonates are slightly different from the adult ones. However, transfusion is always necessary if platelet count $<20 \times 10^9$/L. The indications for transfusion of platelets in adults are summarized in Table 42.1.

Disseminated intravascular coagulation (DIC) can be a common process in critically ill patients and is associated with a high risk of bleeding. Consumption of coagulation factors and platelets leads to the risk of both thrombosis and bleeding, and platelet transfusions are thus used with caution. Platelet transfusions in DIC are used for those actively bleeding, undergoing procedures, or otherwise severely ill, such as in the setting of sepsis. Patients presenting with new acute promyelocytic leukemia are at increased risk of DIC and fibrinolysis; early in their clinic course a revised platelet transfusion threshold is often necessary. This may vary slightly per institution; however, a goal of >30,000–50,000/uL is typical. With platelet dysfunction due to hereditary conditions, such as Glanzmann thrombasthenia, platelet function must be measured to guide transfusions.

Table 42.1 Platelet transfusion threshold values for adults

Indications	Platelet count ($\times 10^9$/L)
Surgery with active bleeding	<50 (often), >100 (rarely)
Invasive procedure or major surgery without active bleedings	<=50
Neurosurgery or eye surgery	<=100
Stable situation without bleeding	<10
Stable situation without bleeding, but with fever >100.4°F or undergoing invasive procedure	<20

Contraindications

Some disease processes in which platelet transfusions should be avoided include disorders, such as heparin-induced thrombocytopenia (HIT), thrombotic thrombocytopenic purpura (TTP), and immune thrombocytopenia (ITP). In these diseases, platelets are being consumed or destroyed; transfusing additional platelets can be deleterious in the setting of both HIT and TTP, increasing the risk of thrombosis.

Response to Platelet Transfusion and Platelet Refractoriness

After a platelet transfusion, the measured platelet count can be expected to fully equilibrate intravascularly after 1 h [6]. Typical survival of transfused platelets should be at least 3 days with an initial increase of at least 10,000/uL. To standardize the platelet response across patients and institutions, the corrected count increment (CCI) may be used. The CCI utilizes platelet increment, body surface area, and number of platelets to standardize patient response. Below is the formula:

$$\text{CCI} = \frac{\begin{array}{c}\text{post-transfusion platelet count} -\\ \text{pre-transfusion platelet count}\left(/\text{uL}\right)\times \text{BSA}\left(\text{m}^2\right)\end{array}}{\text{number of platelets transfused}}$$

An example: platelet increment 25,000/uL × 2.0 m^2/4 [× 10e11] platelets = 12,500;

CCI >7500 at 1-h rules out immune platelet refractoriness

When platelet values do not fully respond as expected after a transfusion, platelet refractoriness must be considered. Platelets may be refractory for immune reasons, but the majority are due to non-immune reasons, such as infection, sepsis, medications (amphotericin B, vancomycin), splenic sequestration, active bleeding, or a consumptive process, such as DIC or microangiopathic hemolytic anemia [5–7]. To determine if a patient may have immune platelet refractoriness, timed post-transfusion measurements must be taken.. Measurement of the platelet response soon after transfusion, e.g., 10 min or 1-h post-transfusion helps diagnose immune versus nonimmune platelet refractoriness (Fig. 42.1). A poor response soon after transfusion is consistent with immune-mediated platelet refractoriness. When non-immune refractoriness is diagnosed, more frequent platelet transfusions may be needed to prevent or control bleeding. Addressing an underlying consumptive process or changing medication may also be helpful.

Human leukocyte antigens (HLA)-A and -B are expressed on platelets, along with human platelet antigens (HPA). HLA antibodies may exist in the patient, leading to a poor response to transfusion (platelet refractoriness). While platelet refractoriness is often due to nonimmune factors, e.g., infection, splenomegaly, immune platelet refractoriness is especially problematic and most often due to HLA alloimmunization. HLA matching of the platelet donor with the patient may result in greater transfusion efficacy. Platelet crossmatching has been shown to be equivalent to HLA-matching in HLA/HPA-alloimmunized platelet transfusion recipients.

Alloimmunization is the term indicating recipient anti-platelet antibodies, commonly to donor HLA and rarely to HPA antigens.

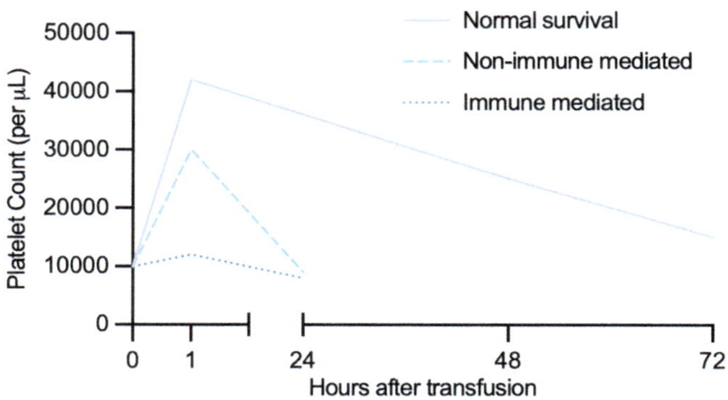

Fig. 42.1 Post-transfusion platelet level to determine etiology of refractoriness

HLA alloimmunization is often the cause of immune-related refractoriness to platelet transfusions. Platelets carry HLA class I antigens (HLA-A and HLA-B) but not class II antigens. In most immune-mediated refractory cases, class I antigens on donor platelets become the target of a patient's HLA alloantibodies. Women who have been pregnant one or more times are at higher risk of developing HLA class I antibodies. Chronically transfused patients, such as those with hematologic malignancies or stem cell transplants, are another population that develop alloimmunization. Alloantibodies to HLA class I antigens are much more common than those to HPA. Alloimmunization to HPAs is found in 2–8% of those who have received multiple transfusions [6].

Prevention of HLA alloimmunization is important and can be achieved by providing only leukocyte-reduced RBCs and platelets. Alloimmunization, once developed, can be managed by HLA-matching platelet units to recipients or by crossmatching platelets. Screening of a patient is initially performed to determine the presence of HLA or HPA antibodies. When present, either HLA-matched or crossmatch-compatible platelets should be transfused. Both HLA-matched and crossmatched platelet units are similarly effective [7].

A more detailed description of the HLA system is in Chap. 40, Principles of clinical applications of human blood groups and HLA system.

Transfusion Infectious Risks and Platelet Modifications

All transfusions carry a small risk of transmission of bloodborne pathogens, such as human immunodeficiency virus (HIV) and hepatitis B and C viruses (HBV, HCV). The rate of HIV transmission per unit of blood is one in 1.6–2.3 million, the rate of HBV is one in 1.0–1.5 million, and the rate of HCV is one in 2.0–2.6 million [8]. Other bloodborne pathogens include bacteria (anaplasmosis, brucellosis, and ehrlichiosis), parasites (malaria, babesiosis, and chagas), and viruses (dengue, west Nile, Zika, and yellow fever). Pathogens within platelet units may be residual donor skin flora, despite skin cleansing, or gut microbiota in bacteremic donors. An estimated 1 in 3000 units of platelets are found to have bacterial contamination, and sepsis is about 1 in 100,000 recipients [9].

PRT is a method of platelet modification approved by the US FDA in 2014. This technology is aimed to further reduce the risk of bloodborne transmissible diseases, rates of bacterial contamination leading to sepsis, and transfusion-associated graft-versus-host disease (GVHD) [3]. PRT is performed by treating the platelets with amotosalen/UV, riboflavin/UV, or UV alone [5, 10]. The advantages and disadvantages of PRT are listed in Table 42.2.

Cytomegalovirus (CMV) is an important intracellular pathogen; much of the population has been exposed to during their lifetime and generally results in mild or asymptomatic disease, however, unexposed (CMV-seronegative), immunosuppressed patients (e.g., stem cell transplant, hematologic malignancy, and premature newborns) are at risk of transfusion-transmitted CMV and severe disease. Preventing this viral disease is best accomplished with "CMV-safe" blood which is either leukocyte-reduced or CMV-seronegative. These methods have been deemed equivalent in mitigating transfusion-transmitted CMV. Vulnerable populations should receive leukocyte-reduced RBCs and platelets.

Leukoreduction of platelets before storage is the standard at most centers. This technique decreases white blood cells in donor products which decreases risks of CMV transmission, febrile

Table 42.2 Pathogen-reduction technology for platelet modification (pros and cons)

Pros	Cons
Inactivation of bacteria, viruses, parasites, fungi	Expensive and is about twice the cost of best culture methods for bacterial mitigation
T-cell inactivation prevents TA-GVHD so no irradiation is needed	Lower platelet yield with each unit
Eliminates need for CMV serology and potentially other current donor assays	Unable to inactivate prions

nonhemolytic reactions, HLA alloimmunization, and its associated platelet refractoriness.

Irradiation of platelets prior to transfusion is another modification, used to reduce the risk of transfusion-associated GVHD. Irradiation of 2500 cGy to the product stops donor T-lymphocyte replication, without changing the storage interval [1, 5]. Irradiated RBC and platelets are typically used for leukemia and lymphoma patients, stem cell transplant patients, transfusions from blood relatives, and intrauterine transfusions [1].

Platelets are suspended in about 200 mLs of donor plasma. Saline washing of platelets will clear donor plasma proteins, antibodies, and electrolytes. This protects IgA-deficient recipients with anti-IgA alloantibodies from potential anaphylactic transfusion reactions. Saline-washed platelets will have a lower yield resulting in fewer platelets transfused [5].

Finally, volume reduction of platelets removes excess plasma and may be useful for patients sensitive to volume-overload and helps reduce exposure to plasma proteins [1]. Both saline washing and volume reduction will result in lower platelet yields, and recipients may require more transfusions.

Adverse Effects of Platelet Transfusion

Platelets are the most implicated component associated with transfusion reactions. Fortunately, most common reactions include mild allergic reactions (e.g., urticaria) and febrile nonhemolytic transfusion reactions. These reactions may cause patient anxiety and mild discomfort but are generally transient and may respond to antihistamines (mild allergic), antipyretics (for fever), or narcotic analgesic (for chills/rigors). The key with these common reactions is to rule out the rare, but more harmful severe allergic reactions, such as anaphylaxis or acute hemolytic transfusion reaction, due to donor plasma ABO-incompatibility.

Respiratory reactions such as transfusion-associated circulatory overload (TACO) and transfusion-related acute lung injury (TRALI) can have high morbidity, and death can occur. Early recognition is crucial in managing these disorders. Stopping an implicated unit of blood product quickly and providing aggressive supportive measures may reduce the morbidity. Mitigation strategies such as slowing the infusion rate and diuresing patients with a history of congestive heart failure may prove helpful to prevent TACO. TRALI risks have decreased with male-only plasma donors and HLA serologic screening of parous female platelet and plasma donors as TRALI is often due to donor HLA alloantibodies.

Caveats

1. CMV safe blood products are either leukocyte reduced or from CMV seronegative donors.
2. Platelet transfusions should not be administered in diseases such as HIT, TTP, and ITP.
3. Platelet transfusion threshold for bleeding prophylaxis is 10×10^9/L. Generally, in actively bleeding patients, Plt count of 50×10^9/L is recommended. In patients with CNS bleeding, Plt cout of 100×10^9/L should be achieved to stop bleeding.

Board Questions

1. Which of the following procedures and preprocedural platelet counts is an indication for a platelet transfusion?

    a. Bone marrow biopsy with platelet count of 7000/uL
    b. Epidural placement with platelet count of 14,000/uL
    c. Bronchoscopy with a platelet count of 28,000/uL
    d. Cardiac by-pass graft (CABG) with platelet count of 52,000/uL
    e. Resection of intracranial mass with platelet count of 110,000/uL

Answer: b. Epidural placement with platelet count of 14,000/uL

2. A patient with AML has been hospitalized for induction chemotherapy for 25 days. She has required multiple RBC and

platelet transfusions to maintain her counts. Her course has been complicated by pneumonia, oral mucositis, and a bacteremia, but she is currently doing well and is hemodynamically stable. Her platelet count is 8000/uL and receives 1 unit of platelets to prevent bleeding. The next day, her platelet count is 7000/uL. She receives an additional unit of platelets, and 1-h post-transfusion her platelet count is 7000/uL.

What is the most likely reason for her failure to respond to the platelet transfusion?

a. IV antibiotic use
b. HPA antibodies
c. HLA-I antibodies
d. HLA-II antibodies
e. Ongoing bacteremia

Answer: c. HLA-I antibodies

References

1. Storch EK, et al. Review of current transfusion therapy and blood banking practices. Blood Rev. 2019;38:100593.
2. Heddle NM, et al. Comparing the efficacy and safety of apheresis and whole blood-derived platelet transfusions: a systematic review. Transfusion. 2008;48(7):1447–58.
3. Etchill EW, et al. Platelet transfusion in critical care and surgery: evidence-based review of contemporary practice and future directions. Shock. 2017;47(5):537–49.
4. Rebulla P, et al. The threshold for prophylactic platelet transfusions in adults with acute myeloid leukemia. Gruppo Italiano Malattie Ematologiche Maligne dell'Adulto. N Engl J Med. 1997;337(26):1870–5.
5. Savage WAC, ST. Transfusion medicine. ASH; 2021. p. 350–85.
6. Cohn CS. Platelet transfusion refractoriness: how do I diagnose and manage? Hematology Am Soc Hematol Educ Program. 2020;2020(1):527–32.
7. Stroncek DF, Rebulla P. Platelet transfusions. Lancet. 2007;370(9585):427–38.
8. Kleinman S. Blood donation and transfusion (Beyond the Basics). January 26, 2022.

9. Bacterial Contamination of Platelets, Centers for Disease Control and Prevention. 2022 September 29, 2022 [cited 2023 February 16, 2023]. Available from: https://www.cdc.gov/bloodsafety/bbp/bacterial-contamination-of-platelets.html#:~:text=Bacterial%20contamination%20of%20platelet%20components%20occurs%20because%20the%20storage%20temperature,bacteria%20(Levy%2C%202018)
10. Mowla SJ, et al. A comparison of transfusion-related adverse reactions among apheresis platelets, whole blood-derived platelets, and platelets subjected to pathogen reduction technology as reported to the national healthcare safety network hemovigilance module. Transfus Med Rev. 2021;35(2):78–84.

Plasma Product Transfusion: Fresh Frozen Plasma, Cryoprecipitate, Intravenous Immunoglobulin, and Albumin

43

Jesse J. Hubbard and Savan S. Shah

Introduction

The indications for use of plasma products in transfusion medicine are diverse. Fresh frozen plasma (FFP) and cryoprecipitate are among the most overused transfusion products in medicine with many of their real-world clinical uses not supported by evidence. Here, we will review FFP, cryoprecipitate, intravenous immunoglobulin (IVIG), and albumin infusions with particular emphasis on preparation and components, administration, indications for use, and potential adverse events (AEs) (summarized in Table 43.1).

J. J. Hubbard (✉) · S. S. Shah
Moffitt Cancer Center, Tampa, FL, USA
e-mail: jjhubbard@usf.edu; Jesse.Hubbard@Moffitt.org

L. Sokol, L. Zhang (eds.), *Non-Neoplastic Hematologic Disorders*, https://doi.org/10.1007/978-3-031-62373-8_43

Table 43.1 Comparison of FFP, cryoprecipitate, IVIG, and albumin

Product	Preparation	Approx. volume	Contents	Indications for use	Potential AEs
FFP	Apheresis	200–250 cc	All coagulation factors, all blood proteins	Massive transfusion, multiple coagulation factor deficiencies, single coagulation factor deficiencies in absence of single factor concentrates, reversal of warfarin with severe bleeding, TTP (plasma exchange)	Allergic and febrile non-hemolytic reactions, TRALI, TACO, anaphylactic reactions, infection
Cryoprecipitate	Coagulation factors precipitated from FFP	15 cc	Fibrinogen, factor VIII, factor XIII, von Willebrand factor, fibronectin	Hypofibrinogenemia due to massive blood loss or congenital defect, DIC, uremic bleeding	Infection
IVIG	Isolated from pooled plasma	Variable, dosed in mg/kg	Highly purified polyvalent IgG, variable IgA, variable ABO antibodies	Primary and secondary immunodeficiency, neuroimmunologic conditions, autoimmune/inflammatory conditions, infection, and infection-related conditions, alloimmune processes	Anaphylaxis in selective IgA deficiency (rare), hemolytic anemia (in patients with non-O blood types), acute kidney injury, thrombosis, infection

Product	Preparation	Approx. volume	Contents	Indications for use	Potential AEs
Albumin	Isolated from pooled plasma	5% (100 cc–500 cc), 25% (50 cc–100 cc)	Albumin, 5% or 25% in	Intravascular volume expansion in ARDS, cirrhotic ascites, hepatorenal syndrome type 1, and hypovolemia; prevention of renal failure in spontaneous bacterial peritonitis; prevention of hypoproteinemia in plasma exchange	Severe allergic and anaphylactic reactions, TACO, dilution coagulopathy

DIC Disseminated intravascular coagulation, *FFP* Fresh frozen plasma, *TACO* Transfusion-associated cardiovascular overload, *TRAIL* Transfusion-related acute lung injury, *TTP* Thrombotic Thrombocytopenic Purpura

Fresh Frozen Plasma (FFP)

- Preparation and contents: apheresis. Contains all blood proteins including all coagulation factors.
- Indications for use [1]:
  - Massive transfusion with packed red blood cells (PRBC): platelet: FFP ratio of 1:1:1
  - Multiple coagulation factor deficiencies with bleeding
  - Single coagulation factor deficiency with bleeding if no single factor concentrate is available
  - Reversal of warfarin overdose with severe bleeding
  - Plasma exchange therapy for TTP
- Administration: intravenous (IV) route.
- AEs [2]:
  - Febrile and allergic reactions: urticaria is common at 1–3%, febrile non-hemolytic reaction 01.–1.0%. No evidence to support reduced incidence with premedication (e.g., acetaminophen and diphenhydramine).
  - Transfusion-associated cardiovascular overload (TACO): incidence >1%.
  - Transfusion-related acute lung injury (TRALI): incidence <0.01%.
  - Anaphylactic reactions: in patients with IgA deficiency and anti-IgA antibodies, incidence 1 in 20,000 to 1 in 50,000.
  - Infection: similar incidence as other blood products (<1 in 1 million).

Cryoprecipitate

- Preparation and components: insoluble proteins (coagulation factors) precipitated from whole plasma products. Contains coagulation fibrinogen, factor VIII, factor XIII, von Willebrand factor, and fibronectin.

- Indications for use [1]:
  - Hypofibrinogenemia due to massive blood loss (e.g., trauma and surgery) or congenital defects. Usually given during rounds 1 and 2 only of massive transfusion protocols
  - Disseminated intravascular coagulation with fibrinogen <100
  - Uremic bleeding
- Administration: IV.
- AEs:
  - Infection: similar incidence as other blood products (<1 in 1 million).

Intravenous Immune Globulin (IVIG)

- Preparation and components: Isolated from pooled human plasma from >1000 donors. Pathogens removed via various inactivation methods and nanofiltration. Contains concentrated polyvalent IgG, variable IgA, variable anti-ABO.
- Indications for Use [3]:
  - Primary and secondary immunodeficiencies including inborn errors affecting immunity, hematologic malignancies, post-hematopoietic stem cell transplant (HSCT), and severe protein loss. Neuroimmunologic disorders including chronic inflammatory demyelinating polyneuropathy, Guillain–Barré syndrome (GBS) and GBS, and myasthenia gravis. May provide benefit in relapsing–remitting MS.
  - Autoimmune/inflammatory disorders including Graves ophthalmopathy, immune thrombocytopenic purpura, *Henoch*–Schönlein purpura, and dermatomyositis, among many others. The use of IVIG in the treatment of autoimmune/inflammatory disorders has decreased in recent years due to the introduction of various biologic and immunomodulating agents.
  - Infection and infection-related disorders: Kawasaki disease, neonatal sepsis, secondary infection prophylaxis in pediat-

  ric HIV, rotaviral enterocolitis, CMV pneumonitis in solid-organ transplant recipients, bacterial infections in patients with lymphoproliferative disorders, and toxic shock syndrome.
  - Alloimmune processes: infection prophylaxis and prevention of aGVHD after allo-HSCT, prevention of acute humoral rejection in allogeneic renal transplant recipients.
- Administration: Dosed in mg/kg based on ideal body weight or adjusted body weight, no evidence for dose adjustments in patients with elevated BMI. Available in low and high titer formulations. May be given IV, subcutaneous (SC), or intramuscular.
- AEs: Start at lowest infusion rate to minimize AEs. If AEs occur, future administrations may be given SC, which is associated with lower incidences of all AEs.
  - Anaphylaxis in patients with selective IgA deficiency is rare, but very-low IgA products are available to reduce risk.
  - IVIG-induced hemolysis due to presence of ABO antibodies (particularly anti-A) may occur; highest incidence among patients with blood types A and AB, lowest in type O; monitor hemoglobin after infusion [4].
  - Low titer products are hyperosmolar and may precipitate acute kidney injury.
  - Thrombosis may occur secondary to activated Factor XI present in the product, give IV hydration to reduce risk.
  - Infection incidence similar to other blood products (<1 in 1 million), higher for non-enveloped viruses (e.g. hepatitis A, Parvovirus B19) in products treated with detergents for infectious prevention.

Albumin Infusion

- Preparation: isolated from pooled plasma.
- Administration: IV. Available in 5% and 25% concentrations. Some products require use of a filter. Maximum administration rate 1–2 mL/min in patients without shock.

- Indications for use:
  - Intravascular volume expansion increases oncotic pressure, moving fluid intravascularly from interstitial spaces; specific clinical situations include acute respiratory distress syndrome (decreases pulmonary edema), cirrhotic ascites, hypovolemia, and hepatorenal syndrome type 1.
  - Spontaneous bacterial peritonitis: administration on days 1 and 3 post-diagnosis decreases incidence of acute renal failure.
  - Prevention of severe hypoproteinemia during plasma exchange therapy.
- AEs [5]:
  - Severe hypersensitivity and anaphylactic reactions
  - TACO
  - Dilution coagulopathy

Caveats

1. Massive transfusions with packed red blood cells require infusions of platelets and FFP in equal ratios to prevent coagulopathy.
2. FFP contains coagulation factors including fibrinogen, factor VIII, factor XIII, von Willebrand factor, and fibronectin.
3. AEs associated with IVIG administration include anaphylaxis in patients with IgA deficiency, hemolysis in subjects with anti-ABO antibodies especially anti-A, kidney injury secondary to hyperosmolar products and thrombosis due to activated factor XI included in the product.

Board Questions

1. A patient presenting after motor vehicle accident is transfused with 10 units of pRBCs and 3 units of platelets. He was stabilized with appropriate hemostasis. He received prophylaxis for hyperkalemia and was also given intravenous calcium supple-

mentation. Six hours later, his nurse reports difficulty controlling oozing at venipuncture sites. He is hemodynamically stable, reports no headache or worsening abdominal pain. Stat labs were obtained and revealed the following: hemoglobin 9.4 g/dL, platelets 126,000/μL, INR 4.4, aPTT 93 seconds, and fibrinogen 159 mg/dL.

What is the most appropriate therapy for this patient?

A. RBC transfusion
B. Platelet Transfusion
C. DDAVP
D. Cryoprecipitate
E. FFP

Answer: E. Following massive blood transfusions, dilutional coagulopathy develops and is best treated with fresh frozen plasma (FFP) containing all coagulation factors.

2. A 38-year-old man presents with fatigue, night sweats and bruising. Extensive ecchymoses are noted on exam. Laboratory testing shows a markedly elevated INR and aPTT, platelet count of 18,000/μL, and a fibrinogen level of 33 mg/dL. Hemoglobin is 7.3 g/dL and hematocrit is 22%. Total WBC is 2000 cells/μL with rare blasts noted on peripheral blood smear. What is the best next step to correct her coagulopathy?

A. RBC transfusion
B. Heparin infusion
C. DDAVP
D. Cryoprecipitate
E. FFP

Answer: D. Cryoprecipitate. APL is characterized by frequent and severe hemorrhage that can result from DIC and primary fibrinolysis. Treatment of the DIC is of high importance until definitive treatment can be initiated. Transfusions of platelets and cryoprecipitate should be initiated to maintain the platelet count above ≥30,000 to 50,000/μL and plasma fibrinogen >150 mg/dL. Heparin infusion in this setting does not have a proven benefit.

References

1. O'Shaughnessy DF, Atterbury C, Maggs PB, et al. Guidelines for the use of fresh–frozen plasma, cryoprecipitate and cryosupernatant. Br J Haematol. 2004;126(1):11–28. https://doi.org/10.1111/j.1365-2141.2004.04972.x.
2. Uhl L. 2022. Clinical use of plasma components. *UpToDate*. Retrieved April 21, 2023, from https://www.uptodate.com/contents/clinical-use-of-plasma-components?search=plasma%20products&source=search_result&selectedTitle=1~150&usage_type=default&display_rank=1#H5
3. Perez EE, Orange JS, Bonilla F, Chinen J, Chinn IK, Dorsey M, El-Gamal Y, Harville TO, Hossny E, Mazer B, Nelson R, Secord E, Jordan SC, Stiehm ER, Vo AA, Ballow M. Update on the use of immunoglobulin in human disease: a review of evidence. J Allergy Clin Immunol. 2017;139(3S):S1–S46. https://doi.org/10.1016/j.jaci.2016.09.023. Epub 2016 Dec 29.
4. Desborough MJ, Miller J, Thorpe SJ, Murphy MF, Misbah SA. Intravenous immunoglobulin-induced hemolysis: a case report and review of the literature. Transfus Med. 2014;24(4):219–26. https://doi.org/10.1111/tme.12083. Epub 2013 Oct 25.
5. China L, Freemantle N, Forest E, Kallis Y, Ryder SD, Wright G, Portal AJ, Salles NB, Gilroy DW, O'Brien A, Trial ATTIRE, Investigators. A randomized trial of albumin infusions in hospitalized patients with cirrhosis. N Engl J Med. 2021;384(9):808–17. https://doi.org/10.1056/NEJMoa2022166.

Recombinant Human Plasma Proteins in Clinical Practice

44

Zaker Schwabkey, Hassan Abushukair, Syeda Saba Kareem, and Kaaron Benson

Introduction

Recombinant proteins (RP) are crucial in medical conditions where a protein is either lacking or not properly produced. The development and utilization of such RPs have been optimized for therapeutic use and created more consistency in protein production. One of the most prominent examples of RP utilization is coagulation factors and their wide use in hematological conditions,

Z. Schwabkey (✉)
Division of Hematology and Hematologic Malignancies, Huntsman Cancer Institute at University of Utah, Salt Lake City, UT, USA
e-mail: Zaker.Schwabkey@hci.utah.edu

H. Abushukair
Department of Medicine, Jordan University of Science and Technology, Irbid, Jordan

S. S. Kareem
Department of Malignant Hematology, Moffitt Cancer Center, Tampa, FL, USA

K. Benson
Department of Pathology, H. Lee Moffitt Cancer Center, Tampa, FL, USA

L. Sokol, L. Zhang (eds.), *Non-Neoplastic Hematologic Disorders*,
https://doi.org/10.1007/978-3-031-62373-8_44

such as hemophilia. In this chapter, we aim to discuss the current use of coagulation-related RPs in hematological conditions.

Clinical Indications and Applications of Available Recombinant Proteins

Factor VIII and Factor IX

Hemophilia A and B are X-linked inherited coagulation deficiency disorders affecting factor VIII (fVIII) and factor IX (fIX), respectively. Other less common causes of fVIII and fIX deficiencies are acquired fVIII and fIX inhibitors. Multiple available recombinant fVIII (rfVIII) and recombinant fIX (rfIX) proteins have become available to treat these generally lifelong bleeding disorders, followed by some modifications to prolong the half-life, such as fusions with Fc portion of IgG1 (e.g., Eloctate) or addition of polyethylene glycol (PEGylation) (e.g., Adynovate, Esperoct, and Jivi). These modifications were more successful for rfIX. The available rfVIII and rfIX are listed in Table 44.1. Additional factors are listed in Table 44.2. Emicizumab (Hemlibra®), a non-factor replacement, is a recombinant humanized bispecific monoclonal antibody that works by substituting the role of factor VIIIa by binding to factors IXa and Xa as a cofactor. Treatment starts with a loading dose of 3 mg/kg subcutaneously 1/per 1 week for 4 weeks, followed by a maintenance dose with either 1.5 mg/kg, 1/per 1 week, or 3 mg/kg, 1/per 2 weeks, or 6 mg/kg subcutaneously, 1/per 4 weeks. It is not effective for acute bleeding, and thrombotic events were major complications observed in patients with inhibitors.

Prophylactic treatment in hemophilia is divided into primary, secondary, or tertiary; primary prophylaxis is a continuous treatment from time of diagnosis and before the second episode of large joint bleed. Secondary prophylaxis starts after the second episode of large joint bleed but before developing complications of chronic arthropathy. Tertiary prophylaxis aims to prevent further damage beyond chronic arthropathy.

Table 44.1 Currently commercially available recombinant factor VIII (rfVIII) and recombinant factor IX (rfIX)

Recombinant factor (alphabetical)	Half-life (h)	ADULTS: Recommended starting prophylactic dose #	PEDIATRIC: Recommended starting prophylactic dose #	Most common adverse reaction	Other
Recombinant factor VIII					
Advate	12	20–40 IU/kg every other day (3–4 times a week)	Same as adult	Pyrexia, headache, cough, nasopharyngitis, vomiting, arthralgia,	
Kogenate FS	11 to 15	25 IU/kg every other day	25 IU/kg every other day	Inhibitor formation, hypersensitivity	To be discontinued in 2023
Kovaltry	14	20–40 IU/kg 2–3 times a week	20–50 IU/kg 2–3 times a week	Inhibitor formation, pyrexia, headache, rash	
Novoeight	12	20–50 IU/kg 3 times weekly OR 20–40 IU/kg every other day	Age < 12: 25–60 IU/kg 3 times weekly	Inhibitor formation, pyrexia	
Nuwiq	17	30–40 IU/kg every other day (adult),	Age < 12: 30–50 IU/kg every other day	Headache, pyrexia, upper respiratory infection, cough, arthralgias	
Recombinate	11	Varies		Inhibitor formation	Adult only
Xyntha	11	30 IU/kg 3 times weekly	25 IU/kg every other day	Headache, arthralgia, pyrexia, and cough	

(continued)

Table 44.1 (continued)

Recombinant factor (alphabetical)	Half-life (h)	ADULTS: Recommended starting prophylactic dose #	PEDIATRIC: Recommended starting prophylactic dose #	Most common adverse reaction	Other
Recombinant factor VIII (Extended Half-life products)					
Adynovate*	15	40–50 IU/kg twice weekly	Age < 12: 55 IU/kg twice weekly (max 70 IU/kg)	Headache, diarrhea, rash, nausea dizziness and urticaria	PEGylated
Afstyla*	14	20–50 IU/kg 2–3 times a week	Age < 12: 30–50 IU/kg 2–3 times a week	Dizziness and hypersensitivity	Single chain
Altuviio	48	50 IU/kg weekly	Same as adult	Headache, arthralgia, back pain	Approved February 2023
Recombinant factor (alphabetical)	Half-life (h)	ADULTS: Recommended starting prophylactic dose #	PEDIATRIC: Recommended starting prophylactic dose #	Most common adverse reaction	Other
Eloctate*	16	50 IU/kg every 4 days	Age < 6: 50 IU/kg, 2/per 1 week	Arthralgia, malaise, myalgia, headache, and rash	Fc fusion
Esperoct*	22	50 IU/kg every 4 days	Age < 12: 65 IU/kg 2/per 1 week	Inhibitor formation and hypersensitivity	glycoPEGylated
Jivi*	19	30–40 IU/kg twice a week	Same as adult	Headache, cough, nausea and fever	PEGylated

Obizur	About 10	Not recommended for prophylaxis. Used only for acquired hemophilia A (not congenital)		Hypersensitivity reaction, inhibitor formation	Porcine factor VIII (not human derived)
Recombinant factor IX					
BeneFIX	22	100 IU once weekly	Same as adult for age > 16	Pyrexia, cough, nausea, headache, and dizziness	
Ixinity	24	40–70 IU/kg twice weekly	Same as adult	headache	12 years and older
Rixubis	26	40–60 IU/kg twice weekly	Age < 12: 60–80 IU/kg twice weekly	Dysgeusia, arthralgia and positive test for Furin antibody	
Recombinant factor IX (Extended Half-life)					
Alprolix*	86	50 IU/kg, 1/pper 1 week or 100 IU/kg, 1/per 10 days	Age < 12: 60 IU/kg once weekly	Headache, oral paraesthesia, obstructive uropathy and inhibitor formation	FC fusion

(continued)

Table 44.1 (continued)

Recombinant factor (alphabetical)	Half-life (h)	ADULTS: Recommended starting prophylactic dose #	PEDIATRIC: Recommended starting prophylactic dose #	Most common adverse reaction	Other
Idelvion*	104	25–40 IU/kg once weekly, if controlled then can be switched to 50–75 IU/kg every 2 weeks	Age < 12: 40–55 IU/kg once weekly	Headache and dizziness	Albumin fusion, adult only
Rebinyn*	115	40 IU/kg weekly	Same as adult	Itching, rash	glycoPEGylated
Other					
Emicizumab (Hemlibra®)	29 days	Loading:3 mg/kg weekly × 4 weeks Maintenance: 1.5 mg/kg weekly OR 3 mg/kg Q 2 weeks OR 6 mg/kg Q 4 week	Same as adult	Injection site reaction, headache, diarrhea, fever	Bispecific mAB

*long-lasting, #doses listed are the prophylactic, but most can be used for on demand and emergently as well
FC Fragment, crystallizable, *IU* international units, *kg* kilograms, *mAB* monoclonal antibody, *rf* recombinant factor

Table 44.2 Other FDA approved recombinant proteins

Recombinant factor (alphabetical)	Half-life	ADULTS	PEDIATRIC	Most common adverse reaction	Other
Von Willebrand Factor (VWF)					
Vonvendi	19–23	Routine ppx: 40–60 IU/kg twice weekly Control bleeding episode/on-demand: Minor (epistaxis, oral bleeding, menorrhagia): LD 40–50 IU/kg; MD 20–30 IU/kg every 12–48 h Major: LD 50–80 IU/kg MD 40–60 IU/kg every 8–24 h for 2–3 days	Only approved in adults	Headache, nausea, vomiting, dizziness arthralgia. Antibody formation, hypersensitivity, thrombotic events	

(continued)

Table 44.2 (continued)

Recombinant factor (alphabetical)	Half-life	ADULTS	PEDIATRIC	Most common adverse reaction	Other
Factor VIIa					
Novoseven	3	90 mcg/kg every 2–6 h until hemostasis is achieved for most indications; Congenital Factor VII deficiency is 15–30 mcg/kg every 4–6 h	35–90 mcg/kg have been used; For Congenital Factor VII deficiency doses as low as 10mcg/kg have been used	Fever, hypertension, thrombosis, antibody development, headache, dizziness, nausea	
SevenFact	1.4	Mild–moderate bleeding: 75mcg/kg every 3 h until hemostasis is achieved OR : initial 225mcg/kg, then 9 h later (if needed) 75mcg/kg every 3 h Severe bleeding: initial 225mcg/kg, then 6 h later (if needed) 75mcg/kg every 2 h	Same as adults	Fever, hypertension, thrombosis, antibody development, headache, dizziness, nausea	Cummataive daily doses >900mcg/kg have not been studied and may be associated with greater risk of thromboembolic events

Recombinant factor (alphabetical)	Half-life	ADULTS:	PEDIATRIC:	Most common adverse reaction	Other
Factor XIII					
Tretten	5 days	35 IU/kg once monthly	Same as adult	Headache, pain in extremities, injection site pain, D dimer increase	Thrombosis risk can increase if administered concomitantly with factor VIIa
Antithrombin (AT)					
ATryn	11–17	Dosage based on formulas utilizing baseline AT activity level. AT level drawn 2 hafter initiation is used to make further adjustments	Only approved in adults	Hemorrhage, infusion site reactions	
C1-esterase inhibitor (C1INH)					
Ruconest	2.5	Treatment: <84 kg: 50 units/kg ≥84 kg: 4200 units May be repeated after 2–4 h if symptoms worsen (rarely needed) Long-term ppx: Duration twice weekly	Same as adults	Headache, nausea, diarrhea	Max daily dose = 8400 units

(continued)

Table 44.2 (continued)

Recombinant factor (alphabetical)	Half-life	ADULTS	PEDIATRIC	Most common adverse reaction	Other
Factor X					
Andexanet alfa (Andexxa®)	2.7–4	Low dose: 400 mg bolus followed by 4 mg/min up to 120 min High dose: 800 mg bolus followed by 8 mg/min up to 120 min	Only approved in adults	Infusion related reaction, antibody development, thrombotic events	Anti-FXa level maybe falsely elevated if drawn after administration of andexanet alpha

VWF von Willebrand factor, *RCo* Ristocetin cofactor, *LD* Loading dose, *MD* Maintenance dose, *AT* Antithrombin

Von Willebrand Factor (VWF)

Recombinant Von Willebrand Factor (rVWF) contains a higher amount of high-molecular weight multimers and has a longer half-life than the plasma-derived form VWF (pdVWF), and, unlike pdVWF, it does not contain factor VIII. Therefore, an rFVIII must be given if the factor VIII level is less than 40%. The first rVWF was FDA approved in 2015 (Vonvendi™ by Baxalta US Inc.). Vonvendi is available in the intravenous route only which primarily has three indications with varying dosages [1]: (1) routine prophylaxis for adults with severe type 3 VWD, (2) on demand to control active bleeding: Minor bleeding is considered readily managed epistaxis, oral bleeding, and menorrhagia. Major bleeding would be severe or refractory epistaxis, menorrhagia, gastrointestinal bleeding, central nervous system trauma, traumatic hemorrhage, hemarthrosis (bleeding into join cavity), or if red blood cell transfusion is either required or potentially indicated. For each bleeding episode, an rFVIII needs to be given if the baseline levels of factor VIII are below 40% or are unknown, and (3) perioperative to prevent or control bleeding during or after surgery for the patients: For elective surgical procedure, a dose of Vonvendi may be given 12–24 h before surgery to allow the endogenous factor VIII levels to increase to at least 30% for minor surgery or 60% for major surgery with the recommendation to assess FVIII:C levels within 3 h before surgery. If the FVIII:C levels are at or above the recommended minimum target levels, a dose of Vonvendi alone is given within 1 h prior to the procedure. If the FVIII:C levels are below the recommended minimum target levels, rFVIII in addition to Vonvendi are given to raise VWF:RCo and FVIII:C.

Factor VIIa

In the US, there are two recombinant factors VIIa that are commercially available and FDA-approved, NovoSeven and Sevenfact. NovoSeven is approved for hemophilia A and B with inhibitors

(FVIII or FIX antibodies, respectively), acquired hemophilia, Glanzmann thrombasthenia, and congenital factor VII deficiency [2]. NovoSeven has a relatively longer half-life (2.6–6 h) compared to Sevenfact (1.4–1.7 h). In bleeding episodes, it is administered as 90 mcg/kg intravenous bolus every 2 h and every 3–6 h after hemostasis has been achieved. Notably, in clinical settings, doses higher than 90 mcg/kg have been found to increase efficacy in some hemophilia patients possibly due to their mechanism of action which does not saturate platelet binding. Sevenfact is approved for patients with hemophilia A and B with inhibitors who are at age of 12 years or older. Recombinant factor VIIa is unique in the sense that it includes the activated form rather than the precursor factors [2]. This translates to having a higher risk of thromboembolism in both hemophilia and non-hemophilia patients. Risk factors for such events include older age, vascular disease, recent cardiac surgery, and when combined with other prothrombotic drugs.

Factor XIII

The plasma-derived factor XIII (pFXIII) contains both A and B subunits, whereas the recombinant factor XIII (rXIII) contains only the A subunit which is solely needed in 95% of the factor XIII deficiency patients [3]. The first and only rFXIII (Tretten, Novo Nordisk Inc.) was FDA approved in 2013 for routine prophylaxis for Infants, children, and adolescent patients with autosomal recessive FXIII A-subunit deficiency [4]. Tretten is available in the intravenous route only and the recommended dose is 35 IU/kg once monthly to achieve a target level of FXIII activity at or above 10%. Adverse reactions are rare but mostly include headache and arthralgias [3]. Tretten has a drug interaction with rFVIIa.

Antithrombin (AT)

Recombinant AT (rAT) has a faster preparation time and a shorter half-life (~10 h) compared to plasma-derived AT [5]. In 2009,

ATryn, a rAT, was approved by the FDA for peri-operative and peri-partum thromboembolic events prevention in patients with hereditary antithrombin deficiency [5]. ATryn administration includes an initial intravenous dose followed by a continuous maintenance infusion. Notably, to avoid excess anticoagulation, monitoring ATryn's activity clinically and through laboratory testing {activated partial thromboplastin time and anti-factor Xa] is crucial for maintenance dosing. The most common adverse effects reported in clinical trials include hemorrhage (hemarthrosis, hematoma, and hematuria) as well as reactions at the site of infusions. Other uses for rAT include patients with heparin resistance and severe sepsis. Considering that rATs are produced in the milk of transgenic goats, they are contraindicated in patients with known hypersensitivity to goat milk proteins.

C1-Esterase Inhibitor (C1INH)

Hereditary angioedema (HAE) is caused by C1INH deficiency. Recombinant C1INH (Ruconest) is used for the treatment of acute HAE attacks at 50 units/kg up to 4200 units maximum as a lyophilized powder reconstituted in sterile water. In comparison with the plasma-derived product, the recombinant form has a shorter half-life which explains the required higher dose to reach proper plasma levels. Reported adverse effects include headache, nausea, and diarrhea. In addition, extra caution should be given to patients after administration to identify any possible signs and symptoms of an anaphylactic reaction although being rarely reported in previous cases. A small proportion of HAE patients may not respond or relapse (~2–3%); in such case, a second identical dose may be administered. Contraindications include a history of hypersensitivity reactions to C1INH or rabbit-derived products. Regarding acquired angioedema, which occurs with C1INH inhibitors, there are limited data supporting the use of recombinant C1INH considering its relatively shorter half-life which translates to requiring higher amounts to compensate for C1INH increased consumption.

Factor X

Currently, the only recombinant factor X approved by the FDA is andexanet alfa, which is a reversal agent for factor Xa inhibitors. It was approved in 2018 to counter anticoagulants, such as rivaroxaban and apixaban in patients with life-threatening or uncontrolled bleeding [6]. Andexanet alfa is given either as a low dose or high dose and that is based on the direct oral anticoagulant (DOAC) used and the time of last dose. Low dose is used for apixaban ≤5 mg or rivaroxaban ≤10 mg. High dose is used for apixaban >5 mg or rivaroxaban >10 mg or unknown doses for either agent. If last administration of DOAC was ≥8 h then low dose would be used. High dose has also been used if edoxaban or betrixaban was the DOAC of choice. The most common adverse events reported by patients and healthcare professionals include antibody development (6–17%) followed by cardiovascular events, such as deep vein thrombosis (6%), ischemic stroke (5%), and acute myocardial infarctions (3%). Infections such as urinary tract infection (~5%) and pneumonia (~5%) have been reported.

Alpha-1 Antitrypsin (AAT)

Recombinant AAT agents are yet to receive FDA approval and are being studied in patients with AAT deficiency. In a phase 2 trial of a recombinant adeno-associated viral vector expressing AAT, nine AAT-deficient patients received intramuscular injections of vector genomes and had tolerable adverse events with peak normal AAT levels (~ >20 microgram/ml) on day 30 with no evidence of antibodies to AAT [7]. Owing to differences in glycosylation of the AAT protein across different expression systems, there has been pushback on current forms of AAT as it is rapidly cleared from circulation if administered by IV route.

Promising Clinical Studies

Recent clinical trials investigating novel recombinant agents include the XTEND-1 pivotal trial which assessed Efanesoctocog Alfa (rFVIII Fc–VWF–XTEN Fusion Protein) in previously treated patients with severe hemophilia A, which consequently led to FDA priority review (on February 28th, 2023) [8].

In addition, recombinant ADAMTS13 (TAK-755) was recently granted FDA orphan drug designation for the treatment and prevention of congenital Thrombotic Thrombocytopenic Purpura (TTP) as well as fast track designation based on the phase 3 trial (NCT04683003) which compared prophylactic administration of TAK-755 and on-demand treatment with TAK-755 in patients with acute TTP events [9].

Caveats

1. rVWF has a longer half-life than the pdVWF due to increased content of high molecular weight vWF multimers. rVWF does not contain factor VIII; thus, a rFVIII must be administered if the factor VIII level is lower than 40%.
2. Emicizumab is a recombinant humanized bispecific monoclonal antibody that works by substituting the role of factor VIIIa by binding to factors IXa and Xa as a cofactor. This agent is not effective for acute bleeding.
3. Andexanet alfa is a reversal agent for factor Xa inhibitors, such as rivaroxaban and apixaban in patients with life-threatening or uncontrolled bleeding.

Board Questions

Q1: The parents of a 13-year-old boy with recently diagnosed severe VWD and a recent major bleed come to your office for counselling on treatment recommendations for their son. His factor VIII level is 28%. They agree with prophylactic treatment. Which one of the following would you recommend for this child?

A. pdVWF should be reserved for severe bleeds only
B. rVWF should be used with pdVWF for prophylaxis
C. rVWF can be used alone for prophylaxis
D. rVWF should be used with rFVIII for prophylaxis
E. Tranexamic acid is the only prophylaxis needed

Answer: D. rVWF should be used with rFVIII for prophylaxis

Q2: Which of the following situations warrants a close monitoring or avoidance with the use of recombinant factor VIIa:

A. Coronary artery disease
B. Pulmonary embolism.
C. Chronic deep vein thrombosis
D. Asthma
E. Chronic obstructive pulmonary disease

Answer: A. rfVIIa should be avoided or closely monitored in patients with coronary artery disease.

References

1. FDA. Vonvendi (von Willebrand factor [recombinant]) [prescribing information]. Lexington: Baxalta US Inc.; 2022.
2. Hedner U. Recombinant activated factor VII: 30 years of research and innovation. Blood Rev [Internet]. 2015 Jun 1 [cited 2023 Nov 6];29 Suppl 1(S1):S4–8. Available from: https://pubmed.ncbi.nlm.nih.gov/26073368/

3. Inbal A, Oldenburg J, Carcao M, Rosholm A, Tehranchi R, Nugent D. Recombinant factor XIII: a safe and novel treatment for congenital factor XIII deficiency. Blood [Internet]. 2012 Jun 5 [cited 2023 Nov 6];119(22):5111–7. Available from: https://pubmed.ncbi.nlm.nih.gov/22451421/
4. FDA. US Food and Drug Administration TRETTEN Product Information. 2018.
5. Pal N, Kertai MD, Lakshminarasimhachar A, Avidan MS. Pharmacology and clinical applications of human recombinant antithrombin. Expert Opin Biol Ther [Internet]. 2010 Jul [cited 2023 Nov 6];10(7):1155–68. Available from: https://pubmed.ncbi.nlm.nih.gov/20528611/
6. Heo YA. Andexanet Alfa: First Global Approval. Drugs [Internet]. 2018 Jul 1 [cited 2023 Nov 6];78(10):1049–55. Available from: https://link.springer.com/article/10.1007/s40265-018-0940-4
7. Flotte TR, Trapnell BC, Humphries M, Carey B, Calcedo R, Rouhani F, et al. Phase 2 clinical trial of a recombinant adeno-associated viral vector expressing α1-antitrypsin: interim results. Hum Gene Ther [Internet]. 2011 Oct 1 [cited 2023 Nov 6];22(10):1239–1247. Available from: https://pubmed.ncbi.nlm.nih.gov/21609134/
8. Sanofi. Press Release: FDA approves once-weekly ALTUVIIIO™, a new class of factor VIII therapy for hemophilia A that offers significant bleed protection. 2023.
9. Takeda. Pivotal Phase 3 Data Presented at ISTH 2023 Congress Spotlight TAK-755 Prophylaxis for Patients with Congenital Thrombotic Thrombocytopenic Purpura (cTTP). 2023.

Basics of Therapeutic Apheresis

45

Mariola Vazquez Martinez,
Joseph Schwartz, and Hien D. Liu

Introduction (Definition, Epidemiology, Etiology, Novel Findings)

Apheresis is the separation and removal of components of blood. Whole blood from a patient flows into an automated instrument that separates it into various components either by centrifugation (based on their specific gravity, Table 45.1) or by membrane filtration (size) [1]. For therapeutic apheresis (TA), the goal is generally to remove a specific pathologic component of blood to treat an underlying disease and return the remaining components back to the patient with or without replacement fluid. The replacement fluid is most often a crystalloid/colloid (albumin) or donor plasma. Common TA procedures include therapeutic plasma exchange (TPE), red blood cell exchange (RCE), and cellular reductions, including removal of platelets or white blood cells. Leukapheresis, the removal of white blood cells, can be for therapeutic purposes

M. V. Martinez · H. D. Liu (✉)
Department of Blood and Marrow Transplant and Cellular Immunotherapy, H. Lee Moffitt Cancer Center and Research Institute, Tampa, FL, USA
e-mail: hien.liu@moffitt.org

J. Schwartz
Department of Pathology/Hematopathology and Laboratory Medicine, H. Lee Moffitt Cancer Center and Research Institute, Tampa, FL, USA

L. Sokol, L. Zhang (eds.), *Non-Neoplastic Hematologic Disorders*,
https://doi.org/10.1007/978-3-031-62373-8_45

Table 45.1 Components of blood with specific gravity

Component of blood	Specific gravity
Plasma	1.025–1.029
Platelets	1.040
White blood cells	1.067–1.092 (Neutrophils) 1.065–1.066 (Monocytes) 1.050–1.061 (Lymphocytes)
Red blood cells	1.078–1.114

(such as leukoreduction for symptomatic hyperleukocytosis) or to obtain cells for preparation for immune effector cell therapies (such as hematopoietic progenitor cell transplantation or immune effector cell therapies). There are also special apheresis procedures for lipoprotein apheresis and for extracorporeal phototherapy (extracorporeal photopheresis). The purpose of this chapter is to discuss the basics of these apheresis procedures and the common indications for which they are performed.

Therapeutic Plasma Exchange

TPE aims to remove pathologic substances in a patient's plasma to treat an underlying disease condition. The plasma that is removed is then replaced with either albumin (most commonly) or donor plasma. Pathologic substances that are removed include autoantibodies, paraneoplastic antibodies, immune complexes, and cryoglobulins [2]. TPE is used to treat neurologic disorders, hematologic conditions, and renal and metabolic diseases. The process of TPE and indications for TPE will be discussed in detail in Chap. 46.

Red Blood Cell Exchange

In RCE, a patient's own diseased red blood cells are removed and replaced with allogeneic donor red blood cells. The most common indication for RCE is sickle cell disease (SCD), but it is also used to treat malaria or babesiosis (removal of parasite-infected red blood cells). For SCD, RCE is used to remove sickled red blood cells that contribute to vaso-occlusive complications in patients with SCD. This can be for acute or chronic indications. Acute indications include immediate treatment of acute chest syndrome (ACS), acute stroke, intrahepatic cholestasis, priapism, or acute symptomatic anemia. Chronic indications include prevention of ACS, silent infarcts, stroke prophylaxis, pregnancy, and preoperative risk management. While simple transfusion can be used for SCD, RCE has advantages including a more rapid and effective lowering of the hemoglobin S (HbS), less risk for circulatory volume overload, and minimizing iron overload. Disadvantages of RCE are that patients are exposed to more RBC units and, therefore, exposed to more red cell antigens, potentially increasing risk for alloimmunization [3].

Cellular Reductions

In cellular reductions, a particular cell type is removed to relieve or improve a patient's symptoms related to an underlying condition. Cell types most commonly removed are platelets (plateletpheresis), white blood cells (leukocytapheresis/leukapheresis), or red blood cells (erythrocytapheresis). The most common indications are myeloproliferative hematologic malignancies, including essential thrombocythemia, polycythemia vera, and leukemia. The excess diseased cells can contribute to increased viscosity, thrombosis, or bleeding for which rapid lowering of the cells is needed to prevent further damage or devastation.

Leukapheresis

Leukapheresis can be used to remove white blood cells for therapeutic purposes, such as symptomatic hyperleukocytosis (leukostasis) or for cell collection in preparation for cellular therapies. Leukocytes (e.g., monocytes, lymphocytes, and dendritic cells) have different specific gravities. Adjusting settings in the apheresis instrument during leukapheresis can allow for enriched fractions of specific white blood cells for different therapies: hematopoietic progenitor cells for peripheral blood cell transplantation, lymphocytes for donor lymphocyte infusion or chimeric antigen receptor T cell therapy, and monocytes for dendritic vaccine therapy.

Low-Density Lipoprotein Apheresis

In low-density lipoprotein apheresis (LDL-A), the goal is to remove low-density lipoprotein cholesterol (LDL-C) or lipoprotein A [Lp(a)]. LDL-A is more selective and effective than TPE in removing LDL-C and Lp(a). LDL-A is used in patients with homozygous and heterozygous familial hypercholesterolemia (FH), Lp(a) hyperlipoproteinemia, and focal segmental glomerulosclerosis (FSGS). In FSGS, the impaired lipid metabolism results in hypercholesterolemia which is nephrotoxic to podocyte function [4]. LDL-A is indicated in patients who are refractory to standard immunosuppressive therapy.

Extracorporeal Photopheresis

Extracorporeal photopheresis is a leukapheresis based treatment that involves collection of leukocytes, adding a photoactivating agent, 8-methoxypsoralen (8-MOP) to the leukocyte product, and then exposing the product to ultraviolet A light. This results in crosslinking of pyrimidine bases in DNA, causing these cells to under apoptosis. The treated cells are infused back to the patient, resulting in immune modulation in the patient. ECP is FDA approved for treatment of cutaneous T-cell lymphoma but is also used in treatment acute and chronic graft versus host disease and solid-organ transplant rejection. The exact mechanism of action is unclear, but evidence supports that ECP leads to activation and differentiation of monocytes into dendritic cells, changes in the activation of several types of T cells, and improved immune profile in the patient [5].

Apheresis Considerations

"One Compartment Model"

The amount of substance removed from a single TA procedure is estimated using a "one compartment model" which assumes that the rate of catabolism of substance is the same as the rate of production and that there is no significant movement between the intravascular and extravascular spaces. This is true for substances that are primarily in the intravascular space (such as fibrinogen or other clotting factors) and large immunoglobulins (classically IgM). There is a logarithmic relationship between the number of plasma volumes (PV), or blood volumes (BV) processed, and the amount of targeted component removed. The greatest efficiency of TPE is obtained with processing 1–1.5 PV, which generally removes 65–75% of the targeted plasma protein [2]. Note that for substances with high rates of production or large extravascular distribution, TPE will not be as effective. For patients undergoing cellular reductions, processing 1.5–2 total BV will reduce absolute counts about 30–50% [1].

Replacement Fluid and Fluid Balance

During TA procedures, particularly TPE, plasma is removed and exchanged with a replacement fluid. The replacement fluid is necessary for maintaining oncotic pressure in the intravascular space and preventing any deleterious hemodynamic changes. Depending on the patient age, size, hematologic parameters, and underlying medical conditions (including cardiac and renal function), each patient has a unique capacity for tolerating fluid shifts and ending fluid balance.

The type and amount of fluid replacement must be considered carefully. Normal saline alone does not provide adequate oncotic support and diffuses in the extravascular space quickly. Therefore, other types of replacement fluid are necessary. Depending on the disease indication, either albumin (alone or in combination with normal saline) or donor plasma is typically used for replacement fluid.

Clinical Decision Making

A comprehensive review of indications for TA and guidelines for disease management using TA is published by the American Society for Apheresis every 3 years. Peer-reviewed literature is used to categorize the evidence of clinical efficacy of TA and to provide a framework for clinical decision making for utilization of TA [6].

Medications

It is important to note what concurrent medications a patient is receiving with TA. TA can result in lower serum concentration of specific medications and potentially decrease the efficacy of these medications, particularly those that are bound to proteins. Medications with a low volume of distribution (Vd) and high plasma protein binding capacity will be significantly removed by TPE. A medication's half-life (how long it takes for it to move out of the intravascular fluid) is also an important factor in determining how much will be removed by TPE.

Angiotensin-converting enzyme inhibitors (ACE I) should be avoided prior to TA. Use of ACE I prior to TA leads to decreased ability to inactivate bradykinin that accumulates during a TA procedure, resulting in serious and immediate adverse events, including flushing, brisk hypotension, bradycardia, and dyspnea [7].

Vascular Access

Adequate vascular access (VA) is needed to perform TA. Several types of VA can be used for TA, including peripheral veins, central venous catheters, ports, and arteriovenous fistulas or grafts. If a patient has adequate veins, peripheral access should always be considered as first option for safety. However, the type of VA that is most appropriate for the patient depends on multiple variables, including frequent/duration of TA, setting of TA treatment (inpatient or outpatient facility), urgency of procedure, and age of the patient.

Citrate Toxicity, Hypocalcemia, and Electrolyte Abnormalities

Anticoagulation is necessary to prevent clotting in the extracorporeal circuit during TA. Citrate anticoagulation is most frequently used, though heparin is used for certain TA. Citrate anticoagulation is preferred based on safety profile and rapid systemic clearance. The mechanism of action of citrate anticoagulation is reversible chelation of divalent cations such as calcium and magnesium which can result in temporary hypocalcemia and hypomagnesemia. Patients are not at risk of systemic anticoagulation effect but may be at risk for developing symptomatic hypocalcemia. Symptoms of hypocalcemia can range from minor (metallic taste and acral or peri-oral paresthesias), moderate (nausea, vomiting, tremors, and hypotension), to major (carpal–pedal spasm and tetany, seizure). Depending on the type of TA procedure, risk of symptomatic hypocalcemia is reported in up to 50% of patients [8]. Patients who have severe hepatic or renal dysfunction or those receiving blood products as replacement fluid may be at increased risk of symptomatic hypocalcemia. Adjustments in the citrate infusion rate or administering supplemental calcium to the patient can ameliorate this risk.

Differences Between Apheresis and Hemodialysis

Apheresis and hemodialysis (HD) are both extracorporeal therapies; however, there are fundamental differences that are important, and they are not interchangeable procedures. TA is applicable to disease in which the expected pathogen has a higher molecular mass (since this is based largely on centrifugation) and a low volume of distribution. HD is filtration-based, targets smaller molecules, and largely does not affect cells. HD can remove extra fluid, in a fluid-overloaded patient (which TA cannot do this). HD flow rates are also much faster than TA (100–500 mL/min versus 15–165 mL/min).

Caveats

1. The most common indications for RBC exchange transfusion are SCD in clinical situations, such as acute cerebrovascular events, ACS with hypoxemia and priapism.
2. Low-density lipoproprotein apheresis is used for removal of LDL-C or lipoprotein A [Lp(a)] in patients with homozygous and heterozygous FH.
3. Extracorporeal photopheresis is FDA approved for treatment of Sezary syndrome and for therapy of acute and chronic graft versus host disease post-allogeneic hematopoietic stem cell transplantation and solid-organ transplant rejection.

Questions

1. **What is a common indication for Red Blood Cell Exchange?**

   a. Thrombotic thrombocytopenic purpura
   b. Polycythemia vera
   c. Sickle cell disease
   d. Essential thrombocythemia

   Correct answer: Sickle cell disease. The goal is to decrease HbS concentration to <30%.

2. **A 65-year-old woman with hepatic dysfunction undergoing leukapheresis develops a metallic taste and peri-oral numbness/tingling. What is the most likely cause?**

   a. ACE-inhibitors
   b. Zinc deficiency
   c. Hypocalcemia
   d. Renal failure

   Correct answer: c. Hypocalcemia has been observed in up to 50% of patients treated with leukapheresis due to acid citrate dextrose solution A administration.

References

1. Balogun RA, Aqui NA, Garcia A, et al. Principles of apheresis technology. 7th ed; 2020.
2. Weinstein R. Basic principles of therapeutic plasma exchange. Transfus Apher Sci. 2023; 62, online prior to print https://doi.org/10.1016/jtransci.2023.103675
3. Tanhehco YC, Shi PA, Schwartz J. Transfusion therapy in sickle cell disease. Ann Blood. 2022;7:9. https://doi.org/10.21037/aob-21-67.
4. Shah L, Hooper DK, Okamura D, et al. LDL-apheresis-induced remission focal segmental glomerulosclerosis recurrence in pediatric renal transplant recipients. Pediatr Nephrol. 2019;34(11):2343–50. https://doi.org/10.1007/s00467-019-04296-6.
5. Cho A, Jantschitsch C, Knobler R. Extracorporeal photopheresis – an overview. Front Med. 2018;5:236. https://doi.org/10.3389/fmed.2018.00236.
6. Connelly-Smith L, Alquist CR, Aqui NA, et al. Guidelines on the use of therapeutic apheresis in clinical practice – evidence-based approach from the Writing Committee of the American Society for Apheresis: the ninth special issue. J Clin Apher. 2023;38(2):77–278. https://doi.org/10.1002/jca.22043.
7. Owen HG, Brecher ME. Atypical reactions associated with use of angiotensin-converting enzyme inhibitors and apheresis. Transfusion. 1994;34(10):891–4. https://doi.org/10.1046/j.1537-2995.1994.341095026976.x.
8. Bray K, Lynde C, Vu T, et al. Prevalence of baseline hypocalcemia and symptomatic hypocalcemia during leukapheresis. J Clin Aph. 2023, online ahead of print https://doi.org/10.1002/jca.22076.

Therapeutic Plasma Exchange

46

Jaime Roman Diaz, Joseph Schwartz, and Hien D. Liu

Introduction

Therapeutic plasma exchange (TPE) is a type of apheresis procedure during which a patient's plasma is removed and replaced with either albumin or donor plasma. The goal of TPE is to remove pathologic substances present in a patient's plasma to improve the underlying condition. For some diseases, both the removal of the pathologic substance and the replacement fluid (with normal proteins/substances) likely contribute to the benefit from TPE. Pathologic substances that are removed include autoantibodies, paraneoplastic antibodies, immune complexes, lipoproteins, and cryoglobulins. Substances that are primarily in the intravascular system (i.e., proteins that are bound to plasma and have low volume of distribution) are most effectively removed [1]. TPE can be performed either by centrifugation or by membrane filtration. In membrane filtration, plasma can only be separated, and compo-

J. R. Diaz · H. D. Liu (✉)
Department of Blood and Marrow Transplant and Cellular Immunotherapy, H. Lee Moffitt Cancer Center and Research Institute, Tampa, FL, USA
e-mail: hien.liu@moffitt.org

J. Schwartz
Department of Pathology/Hematopathology and Laboratory Medicine, H. Lee Moffitt Cancer Center and Research Institute, Tampa, FL, USA

L. Sokol, L. Zhang (eds.), *Non-Neoplastic Hematologic Disorders*,
https://doi.org/10.1007/978-3-031-62373-8_46

nents removed by size, while with centrifugation, plasma can be separated, and blood components further fractionated by density (specific gravity). TPE is most commonly performed by centrifugation. The purpose of this chapter is to discuss the basics of TPE and review considerations for the patient undergoing TPE.

Indications

TPE is used to treat various conditions, including neurologic disorders, hematologic conditions, and renal and metabolic diseases. When considering initiation of TPE, it is important to understand the rationale for treatment, goals of treatment, and have a clear plan for the course of therapy (including length, duration, and frequency of TPE). A comprehensive review of indications for TPE and guidelines for disease management using TPE are published by the American Society for Apheresis (ASFA) every 3 years [2].

One-Compartment Model

The ideal target for removal by TPE is a substance that has high molecular weight, a slow rate of formation, long half-life, and low volume of distribution (Vd). The distribution of the substance within the intravascular space is also affected by how rapidly the substance moves between the intravascular and extravascular spaces. The amount of a substance removed by TPE depends on how much of the substance is in the intravascular compartment at the time of TPE. This is the "one-compartment model." Substances are generally in a steady state with removal of a substance occurring faster than replacement of it during TPE [3].

Exchange Volume and Prediction of Substance Removal

Based on the one-compartment model, a substance that is not rapidly synthesized and has low Vd, processing 1 PV results in the most efficient removal of protein (approximately 65–70% of the substance removed). Due to exponential nature of substance removal, additional PV processing results in much lower substance removal (2 PV = 20–25% substance removal and 3 PV 5–10% substance removal). For this reason, ASFA generally recommends 1–1.5 PV per session [2–4]. It is important to note that TPE is not a selective procedure. Not only are negative pathogens removed, but TPE also removes normal circulating proteins, such as glycoproteins, lipoproteins, and coagulation factors [5–7].

Care of the Patient Undergoing Therapeutic Plasma Exchange

Fluid Replacement

Fluid removed by TPE must be replaced to prevent detrimental volume depletion. The choice of fluid replacement, either donor plasma or albumin (alone or in combination with crystalloid) primarily depends on the indication for TPE; however, other considerations include risk of bleeding, infection, and anticipated need for concurrent procedure/surgery. Donor plasma is used when there is a need for replacement of plasma, in the case of thrombotic thrombocytopenic purpura (TTP). It is also used when patients are at risk of acute bleeding or anticipated need for surgery. For other indications and settings, albumin is preferred to reduce exposure to blood products and prevent complications, such as transfusion reactions and infections associated with blood product exposure. A combination of albumin and crystalloid solution can be used; however, the amount of crystalloid solution cannot exceed 50% of the total volume replaced as this would provide insufficient oncotic pressure to maintain adequate intravascular fluid volume [1].

Anticoagulation

Anticoagulation for TPE is required to prevent clotting in the extracorporeal circuit. Systemic heparin and citrate, in the form of Anticoagulant Citrate Dextrose Formula A (ACD-A), are the most common anticoagulant agents used. ACD-A is preferred because of its safety profile and short half-life. There is essentially no systemic anticoagulation, and therefore, no increased bleeding risk. ACD-A is primarily metabolized by the liver (65–90% by first pass metabolism) [7]. The main mechanism of action of ACD-A is temporary binding of calcium which can contribute to citrate-induced hypocalcemia and other electrolyte abnormalities. Heparin is primarily preferred for membrane-based TPE, LDL apheresis, or photopheresis but can be associated with bleeding complications and heparin-induced thrombocytopenia [8].

Vascular Access

Adequate vascular access is required for successful TPE, with flow rates ranging from 50 to 120 ml/min. ASFA recommends that peripheral venous access be used whenever possible. If, however, large-bore peripheral access is not possible, then central venous catheters (either non-tunneled or tunneled) can be used. There is also an FDA-approved port, the Bard PowerFlow®, which can be used for therapeutic apheresis procedures. Arteriovenous fistulas or grafts can also be used for TPE and are preferred in patients who will require long-term, frequent TPE.

Medications and Drug Removal by Therapeutic Plasma Exchange

ACE-Inhibitors

Angiotensin-converting enzyme (ACE) inhibitors are contraindicated prior to TPE. Use of ACE-I prior to TPE can result in flushing and hypotension, with published reports of severe hypotension and even hemodynamic collapse. These reactions are thought to be due to excessive bradykinin release, triggered by apheresis tubing kit exposure, albumin replacement fluid (which may have kallikrein activating substances), and inhibited bradykinin catabolism [9].

Therapeutic Drug Removal

TPE is commonly combined with other medications for treatment of the underlying condition. Timing of plasma exchange and medication administration is important, since TPE can remove and/or lower the efficacy of some medications. For highly protein bound drugs with low Vd, there can be a large amount of drug removal [10]. Therapeutic monoclonal antibodies (such as rituximab or eculizumab) are also significantly removed. If intravenous immune globulin is being administered, it should be planned for after TPE sessions.

Hypocalcemia and Therapeutic Plasma Exchange

Use of ACD-A and rapid infusion of substantial amounts of albumin can contribute to hypocalcemia reactions. Mild reactions can present as perioral and extremity paresthesia. Severe reactions can include tetany and arrythmias (associated with QT prolongation). Hypocalcemia reactions are more likely to occur in longer procedures and in patients with abnormal hepatic or renal function. Prophylactic calcium supplementation can used to decrease risk of symptomatic hypocalcemia [7].

Risks Associated with Therapeutic Plasma Exchange

Aside from the previously discussed considerations, there are other notable risks to consider during TPE. If donor plasma is replacement fluid, then patients can be at increased risk of transfusion reaction or infection. TPE using albumin alone or in combination with saline can result in a transient depletion of blood-clotting factors, especially if TPE is repeated on consecutive days [6]. Clinically significant bleeding is rare, but this should be considered if patients are scheduled for any procedure/surgery. Bleeding or hematoma can occur at venipuncture/line insertion sites can occur. Patients with non-tunneled or tunneled central venous catheters can also be at risk of developing central line associated infections or thrombosis. Metabolic acidosis can occur with albumin replacement due to the acidic nature of albumin. Metabolic alkalosis because of citrate metabolism can occur when plasma is used as replacement fluid, because stored plasma contains citrate; this is especially compounded when ACD-A is used as anticoagulant for TPE.

Caveats

1. ACE inhibitors are contraindicated concurrently with plasma exchange due to possible development of flushing and hypotension.
2. ACD-A that is used for prevention of clotting during TPE can result in hypocalcemia
3. Repeat TPE with only albumin and saline volume replacement can lead to transient depletion of coagulation factors, abnormal coagulation tests and increased propensity for bleeding.

Questions

1. **What is the preferred fluid replacement for patients with thrombotic thrombocytopenic purpura?**

   a. Albumin
   b. Albumin combined with normal saline
   c. Donor plasma
   Correct answer: c

Donor plasma is preferentially used in case of thrombotic thrombocytopenic purpura since it contains ADAMTS13 enzyme in contrast to albumin. Doner plasma is also preferred in patients with increased risk of bleeding or prior to surgery since TPE removes also coagulation factors.

2. **During therapeutic plasma exchange, a patient develops perioral and acral paresthesia symptoms. What is the most likely cause?**

   a. Volume depletion
   b. Hypocalcemia
   c. Hypokalemia
   d. Allergic reaction to albumin
   Correct answer: b

ACD-A transiently binds calcium. Along with rapid infusion of large amount of albumin, it can result in development of clinical manifestations of hypocalcemia.

3. **What characteristics make a target ideal for removal by TPE?**

   a. Large molecular weight
   b. Long half-life
   c. Low volume of distribution
   d. All of the above
   Correct answer: d

The ideal target for removal by TPE is a substance that has high molecular weight, a slow rate of formation, long half-life, and low volume of distribution (Vd).

References

1. Balogun RA, Aqui NA, Garcia A, et al. Principles of apheresis technology. 7th ed; 2020.
2. Connelly-Smith L, Alquist CR, Aqui NA, et al. Guidelines on the use of therapeutic apheresis in clinical practice – evidence-based approach from the Writing Committee of the American Society for Apheresis: the ninth special issue. J Clin Apher. 2023;38(2):77–278. https://doi.org/10.1002/jca.22043.

3. Weinstein R. Basic principles of therapeutic plasma exchange. Transfus Apher Sci. 2023;62, online prior to print https://doi.org/10.1016/jtransci.2023.103675.
4. Reverberi R, Reverberi L. Removal kinetics of therapeutic apheresis. Blood Transfus. 2007;5:164–74.
5. Pearlman ES, Litty CA, Edger N, et al. Effect of therapeutic plasmapheresis on coagulation parameters. J Clin Apher. 1994;9:202–3.
6. Zantek ND, Boral LI, Li Y, Yamada C, et al. Hemostasis management and therapeutic plasma exchange: results of a practice survey. J Clin Apher. 2018;33:604–10.
7. Bray K, Lynde C, Vu T, et al. Prevalence of baseline hypocalcemia and symptomatic hypocalcemia during leukapheresis. J Clin Apher. 2023;38:654–63.
8. Lee G, Arepally GM. Anticoagulation techniques in apheresis: from heparin to citrate and beyond. J Clin Apher. 2012;27(3):117–25.
9. Owen HG, Brecher ME. Atypical reactions associated with use of angiotensin-converting enzyme inhibitors and apheresis. Transfusion. 1994;34:891–4.
10. Cheng CW, Hendrickson JE, Tormey CA, et al. Therapeutic plasma exchange and its impact on drug levels: an ACLPS critical review. Am J Clin Pahol. 2017;148:190–8.

Part VII

Miscellaneous Disorders

Lipid Storage Diseases

47

Olga Sazanova, Brian D. Schlick,
Lugen Chen, and Prerna Rastogi

Lipid storage diseases are a diverse group of more than 70 rare, distinct disease conditions with the common characteristic of the buildup of metabolic precursors in lysosomes [1]. Intracellular lysosomes are responsible for the degradation of a variety of biomolecules, with several pathways involved. Deficiencies of one of these pathways will lead to accumulation of a substrate and subsequent cellular dysfunction. Various hematologic abnormalities across this spectrum of diseases have been described [2].

Lipid storage diseases have a cumulative frequency of 1 in 7000–8000 live births. They have an autosomal recessive mode of inheritance, with some exceptions (Table 47.1). Prevalence is higher than previously thought, with a significant proportion of cases diagnosed in adulthood and found across all population

O. Sazanova · P. Rastogi (✉)
Department of Pathology, University of Iowa, Carver College of Medicine, Iowa City, IA, USA
e-mail: prerna-rastogi@uiowa.edu

B. D. Schlick
Department of Internal Medicine, USF Health, Moffitt Cancer Center, Tampa, FL, USA

Tennessee Oncology, Nashville, TN, USA
e-mail: bschlick@tnonc.com; brian.schlick@moffitt.org

L. Chen
Department of Pathology, Tampa General Hospital, Tampa, FL, USA

L. Sokol, L. Zhang (eds.), *Non-Neoplastic Hematologic Disorders*,
https://doi.org/10.1007/978-3-031-62373-8_47

Table 47.1 Etiology and pathogenesis of selected lipid storage diseases involving the reticuloendothelial system

Disease	Mode of inheritance	Affected gene	Enzyme deficiency	Major accumulating metabolite	Incidence
Sphingolipidoses					
Gaucher disease	AR	GBA	Glucocerebrosidase	Glucosylceramide	1:60,000
Niemann–Pick disease, types A, B	AR	*SMPD1*	Acid-sphingomyelinase	Sphingomyelin	1:250,000
Niemann–Pick, types C1, C2	AR	*NPC1*, *NPC2*	Primary defect in non-enzymatic lipid transport	Unesterified cholesterol and glycolipids	1:120,000
Tay–Sachs disease	AR	*HEXA*, *HEXB*, *GM2A*	Hexosaminidase A	GM2 ganglioside	1:320,000
Sandhoff disease *O variant of Tay–Sachs disease	AR	*HEXB*	β-Hexosaminidase	GM2 ganglioside	1:384,000
Farber disease	AR	*ASAH1*	Lysosomal acid ceramidase	Ceramide	<1:1,000,000
Fabry disease	X-linked	*GLA*	Alpha-galactosidase A	Globotriaosylceramide (Gb3)	1:40,000
GM1 gangliosidosis Infantile, juvenile, adult types	AR	*GLB1*	Beta galactosidase	GM1 ganglioside	1:100,000–1:200,000

Mucolipidoses					
I-cell disease and pseudo-Hurler disease	AR	*GNPTAB*	Deficiency in phosphorylating enzymes in the mannose-6-phosphate pathway: N-acetyl glucosamyl-phosphotransferase	Mucopolysaccharide Glycolipid	1:1,000,000
Others					
Wolman disease (Acid lipase deficiency)	AR	*LIPA*	Lysosomal acid lipase	Triglycerol esters Triglycerides Phosphate esters	Rare
Metachromatic leukodystrophy late infantile, early juvenile, late juvenile, adult types	AR	*ARSA*	arylsulfatase A	Galactosyl-3-sulfate ceramides	1:40,000

AR autosomal recessive

groups. However, some diseases, including Gaucher disease and Niemann–Pick disease type A, are found at higher frequencies among people of Ashkenazi Jewish descent caused by the founder effect.

Etiology and Pathogenesis

Lipid storage diseases can result from genetic mutations causing:

- Enzyme deficiency
- Cofactor deficiency
- Alterations in cellular-sorting mechanisms

Defects in lipid transport protein hydrolytic enzymes with cofactors are responsible for the breakdown of lipid complex molecules within the acidic lysosomal compartment, so that breakdown components can be recycled. Enzyme or cofactor deficiency leads to substrate accumulation and interference with normal lysosomal function. Gaucher disease is caused by inactivating glucocerebrosidase mutations, leading to accumulation of glucocerebroside. Niemann–Picks disease types A and B are caused by inactivating sphingomyelinase mutations, leading to accumulation of sphingomyelin.

In addition, intact cellular transport machinery is required to transport the enzymes from their site of secretion in the endoplasmic reticulum and assembly in the Golgi apparatus to the lysosomal compartment. This requires post-translational modification by adding a mannose-6-phosphate that serves as a label to channel the proteins toward the lysosomes. Thus, defects in cellular-sorting mechanisms can also lead to an enzyme deficiency within the lysosomes and lipid storage diseases. The latter mechanism is encountered in mucolipidoses, such as I-cell disease (mucolipidosis type II) and pseudo-Hurler poliodystrophy. Those conditions are usually associated with the deficiency of multiple enzymes, since they share common transport mechanisms.

Finally, deficiency in lipid transport proteins can also be a causative mechanism as in the case of Niemann–Pick disease type C.

The nature of accumulating metabolites depends on the deficient enzyme, degree of enzyme deficiency, and organ involvement. For example, gangliosides are abundant in the nervous system; therefore, ganglioside–beta-galactosidase deficiency leads to neuronal dysfunction [3, 4]. Organs containing large numbers of phagocytic cells, such as the spleen, liver, and bone marrow, are affected frequently, since phagocytic cells are rich in lysosomes. In addition, patients with mutations eliminating enzymatic activity will have substantially more significant clinical manifestations than patients with mutations that leave some residual enzymatic activity. This forms the basis of the different disease categories (e.g., type 1 vs type 2 Gaucher disease). Substrate accumulation in lysosomes can lead to cellular damage in several ways:

- Storage material can spread to the other cellular compartments, impairing their function
- Defective transport across the lysosomal membrane which results in cell starvation
- Impaired autophagy
- Mitochondrial stress and apoptosis
- Dysregulation of redox processes

Diagnosis: General Approach

Positive family history is one of the important diagnostic clues, as many of these diseases are inherited in autosomal recessive or X-linked inheritance fashion. In many subtypes of lipid storage diseases, the onset is age-dependent; for example, Niemann–Pick disease type A has an early onset at age 3 months, and types B and C manifest mostly in childhood [5]. The majority of patients with lipid storage diseases who present to hematologists do so with hepatosplenomegaly, cytopenia, and, in some instances, bone pain and erosions. Based on presenting symptoms or family history, a common diagnostic approach is included in Fig. 47.1.

Bone-marrow biopsy is usually not necessary, and morphological findings are very nonspecific. However, if performed, three major morphologic patterns can be seen in the bone marrow:

1. **Gaucher cells:** These are distended histiocytes with fibrillary cytoplasm, which have often been compared to crinkled tissue paper (Fig. 47.2). They are found in the spleen, liver, and lymph nodes. Secretion of cytokines by macrophages erodes bone and produces bone pain in Gaucher disease. Pseudo-Gaucher cells, morphologically similar to Gaucher cells, are encountered in the following conditions: chronic myelogenous leukemia, acute leukemias, myelodysplastic syndrome, Hodgkin lymphoma, congenital dyserythropoietic anemias, hemoglobinopathies/thalassemia, bacterial infections, etc., as bystanders.
2. **Foamy histiocytes:** These are histiocytes with highly vacuolated appearance, often noted with Niemann–Pick types A and B, hereditary hypercholesterolemia, Farber disease (disseminated lipogranulomatosis), Tangier disease, and polyvinylpyrrolidone storage disease (Fig. 47.3).
3. **Sea-blue histiocytes:** Histiocytes filled with variably sized blue–green to sea-blue granules are found in Niemann–Pick type C, Fabry disease, Sandhoff disease, Wolman disease, hyperlipoproteinemia, total parenteral nutrition, myelodysplastic syndromes, myeloproliferative neoplasms, idiopathic thrombocytopenic purpura, etc.

The initial screening test includes an enzyme activity measurement in leukocytes or cultured fibroblasts. The test may not establish a specific phenotype (Niemann–Pick A subtype vs B subtype) or differentiate between a carrier and disease state. Enzyme activity assays by fluorometry and tandem mass spectrometry can test for metabolic disorders, and some are now included in newborn screening for lysosomal storage diseases, depending on the state and country of birth.

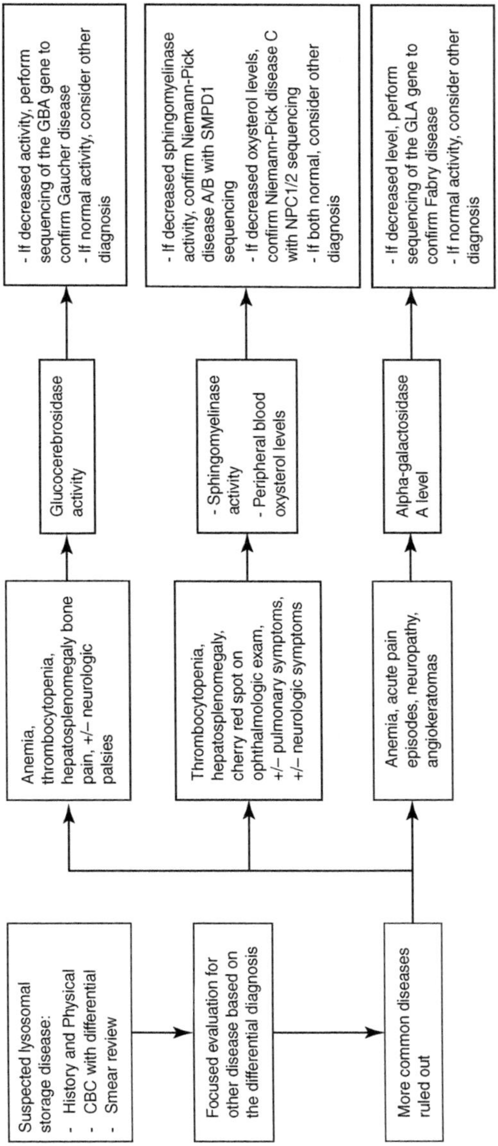

Fig. 47.1 Diagnostic algorithm of lysosomal storage diseases that may present to a hematologist

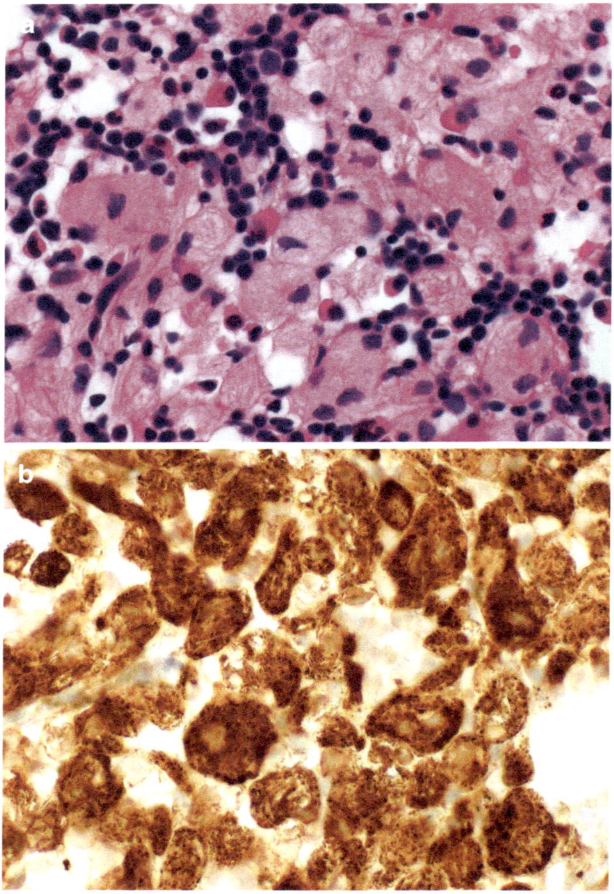

Fig. 47.2 Gaucher cells stained with PAS (**a**) and TRAP (**b**), magnification ×60

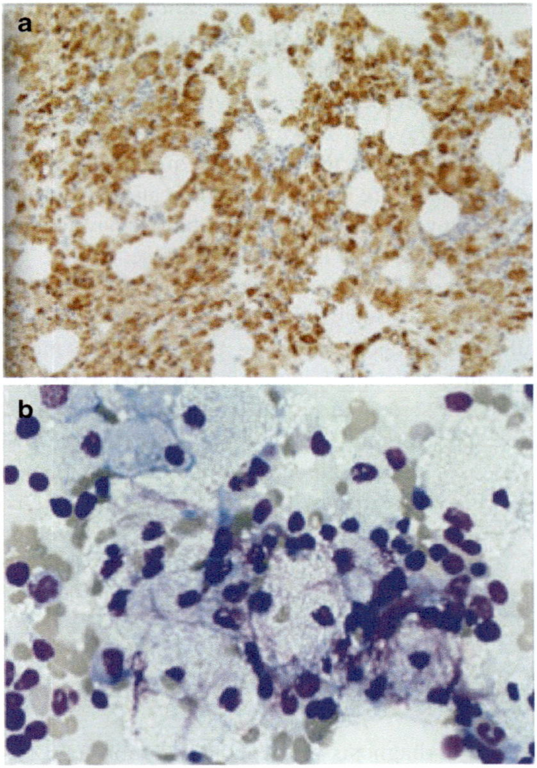

Fig. 47.3 Foamy histiocytes stained with CD68, magnification ×200 (**a**) and Wright Giemsa, magnification ×1000 (**b**) in a patient with familial hypertriglyceridemia

Molecular analysis with next-generation sequencing (NGS) is used to confirm diagnosis, to differentiate between heterozygous and homozygous state and, based on the identified pathogenic variant, to establish the disease subtype and prognosis. A negative molecular test may not, however, rule out diagnosis unless the entire coding region of the gene is sequenced, because diverse pathogenic variants are found to be implicated in the same phenotypes. For example, more than 100 mutations have been identified in the gene *GBA1* altered in Gaucher disease.

However, certain pathogenic variants are more frequent among people of Ashkenazi Jewish descent caused by founder effects and reach allelic frequencies of more than 1%. The most frequent variants identified among people of Ashkenazi Jewish descent are incorporated in screening panels available for families from the susceptible population. The screenings for the following lipid storage diseases are recommended for people of Ashkenazi Jewish descent: Tay–Sachs disease, mucolipidosis IV, Niemann–Pick disease type A, and Gaucher disease [6]. Of note, screening panels used for the Ashkenazi Jewish population may show a very low positive predictive value outside of the targeted population.

Differential Diagnosis

The differential diagnosis of the most common lipid storage disorders involving hematopoietic organs (spleen, liver, and bone marrow) is shown in Table 47.2.

Table 47.2 Differential diagnosis of lipid storage disorders involving hematopoietic organs (spleen, liver, and bone marrow)

		Lysosomal storage disorders	Indolent leukemias and lymphomas	PMF, fibrotic	ITP	Primary cirrhosis	Amyloidosis	Langerhans cell histiocytosis	Sarcoidosis	SLE	Infections
Age of onset		Childhood most frequent, but adults possible	Any	Adults	Bimodal distribution (childhood and adults)	Adults	Adults	Children most frequent, but adults possible	Young and middle-aged adults	Any	Any
Symptoms	Splenomegaly	Splenomegaly >> hepatomegaly	Variable	Prominent	None to minimal	Hepatomegaly >> splenomegaly	Yes	Possible	Possible	Possible	Variable
	Bone marrow involvement	Yes	Yes	Yes	No	No	Possible	Most frequent	Possible	No	Variable
	Nervous system involvement	Variable	Variable	No	No	Late-stage encephalopathy	Rare	No	Rare	Possible	Variable
	Peripheral blood	Anemia/ Thrombocytopenia	Variable: lympho-cytosis, atypical circulating cells, pancytopenia, or normal	Variable cytopenias, leukoerythro-blastosis	Isolated thrombo-cytopenia	Acanthocytes	Pancytopenia	Pancytopenia	Pancytopenia in the case of hyper-splenism	Pancytopenia	Variable

(continued)

Table 47.2 (continued)

		Lysosomal storage disorders	Indolent leukemias and lymphomas	PMF, fibrotic	ITP	Primary cirrhosis	Amyloidosis	Langerhans cell histiocytosis	Sarcoidosis	SLE	Infections
Morphology/ biopsy	Bone marrow	Gaucher cells/ foamy macrophages/ sea-blue histiocytes	Presence of malignant cells, "pseudo-Gaucher" cells	Increased reticulin fibrosis, atypical megakaryocytes	Megakaryocyte hyperplasia	Normal	Amyloid deposition, confirmed by Congo Red histochemical stain	Langerhans cells: CD1a+, S-100+, langerin+ by IHC	Compact non-caseating granulomas	Variable: sea-blue histiocytes, lipogranulomas, nonspecific findings	Granulomatous inflammation, possible caseating granulomas
	Spleen			Extramedullary hematopoiesis	Follicular hyperplasia and presence of foamy macrophages	Normal				Follicular hyperplasia, vasculitis, focal histiocytic collections with apoptotic debris	
	Liver				Normal	Cirrhosis				Nonspecific findings	
	Ancillary tests	Enzyme activity assay, genetic testing	Flow cytometry: aberrant phenotypes. Cytogenetics and molecular studies	Molecular studies: JAK, CALR, MPL mutations	None/ diagnosis of exclusion	Liver biopsy	Mass spectrometry for amyloid type determination	Molecular studies: BRAF V600E mutation	None/ diagnosis of exclusion	ANA, anti-dsDNA Coombs test, complement C3 and C4, immune complex assays	Cultures, microscopy

ANA antinuclear antibodies, *IHC* immunohistochemistry, *ITP* idiopathic thrombocytopenic purpura, *PMF* primary myelofibrosis, *SLE* systemic lupus erythematosus

Treatment and Prognosis

While the role of supportive treatments such as physical and occupational therapy, chest physiotherapy, and statin treatment for hyperlipidemia is invaluable, several new game-changing therapies have emerged. These include enzyme replacement therapy (ERT), chaperone therapy, substrate reduction therapy (SRT), bone-marrow transplantation, and gene therapy. An overview of treatments is included in Table 47.3.

ERT is based on the recombinant enzyme delivery to the affected cells by intravenous route. The recombinant enzyme secretion is usually induced in a cell line; then, the enzyme is bound to the mannose group to target it to the lysosomes and delivered intravenously. Olipudase alpha is now approved for the treatment of non-neurologic manifestations of Niemann–Pick types A and B disease. Patients treated with this medicine saw a 39% reduction in spleen volume, 28% decrease in liver volume, and 22% increase in DLCO [7]. Olipudase alpha is administered intravenously every 2 weeks, with dose escalation to 3 mg/kg. It does carry a black-box warning for anaphylaxis that may require a desensitization protocol. The major drawback of ERT is the inability for the enzyme to penetrate the blood–brain barrier. Therefore, its efficacy for patients with neural system involvement is limited.

When the enzyme deficiency results from secretion of a defective protein, it is often misfolded and not active or easily destroyed. In such instances, chaperone therapy, or enzyme stabilization therapy, can be beneficial. A chaperone is a small-molecule protein which binds the enzyme to enhance folding or prevent degradation. Since only a small amount of active enzyme is required for substrate degradation, chaperone therapy can be a viable option.

SRT works by inhibiting the enzyme responsible for the substrate production. Although the treatment is less effective than ERT, in some instances, it can reduce neurological progression of disease. For patients with Niemann–Pick type C disease, SRT with miglustat is generally associated with stabilization but not prevention of neurologic decline [8].

Table 47.3 Clinical features and treatment of selected lipid storage diseases involving the reticuloendothelial system

Disease	Age of onset	Peripheral blood	Bone marrow	Other hematopoietic organs	Other affected organs	Treatment
Gaucher						Type 1 and non-neuronopathic manifestations of Type 3: Imiglucerase (ERT) Taliglucerase alfa (ERT) Velaglucerase (ERT) Eliglustat (SRT) Type 3 (before symptom onset): Hematopoietic cell transplantation
Type 1	Adult	Anemia and/or thrombocytopenia	Gaucher cells	Hepatomegaly, splenomegaly with Gaucher cells	Interstitial lung disease Pulmonary hypertension Bony lytic lesions *No CNS involvement*	
Type 2 (acute)	Infantile	Anemia and thrombocytopenia	Gaucher cells	Hepatosplenomegaly with Gaucher cells	As in type 1 +: Hydrops fetalis Arthrogryposis *CNS involvement*	
Type 3 (chronic)	Juvenile	Anemia and thrombocytopenia	Gaucher cells	Hepatosplenomegaly with Gaucher cells	As in type 1 +: *CNS involvement*	

Niemann–Pick disease, type A and B	Newborn to mid-childhood	Anemia or pancytopenia	Foamy histiocytes	Hepatosplenomegaly	*Macula with cherry-red spot* Pulmonary infiltrates/ interstitial lung disease Failure to thrive/ developmental delay (type A) CNS involvement (type B)	Olipudase alfa (ERT)
Niemann–Pick disease, type C	Childhood		Sea-blue histiocytes/ foamy histiocytes	Hepatosplenomegaly	Interstitial lung disease, hyperlipidemia, possible CNS involvement	Miglustat (SRT)
Fabry	Young adult (30–40 years)	Anemia	Sea-blue histiocytes (not a significant involvement)	NA	Angiokeratomas Renal failure Cardiomyopathy Vascular disease Corneal deposits Neuropathy	Agalsidase alfa (ERT) Agalsidase beta (ERT) Pegunigalsidases alfa (ERT) Migalastat (chaperone)

CNS central nervous system, *ERT* enzyme replacement therapy, *NA* not applicable, *SRT* substrate reduction therapy

Hematopoietic stem cell transplant can be curative for many lipid storage diseases, since the cells with the ineffective enzyme are replaced by *healthy* donor cells. However, stem cell transplant is a very high-risk procedure and is of limited clinical utility unless performed before the onset of symptoms. Given the availability of ERT and SRT and the potential of gene therapy, hematopoietic stem cell transplant is reserved for severe cases before symptom onset.

Finally, gene therapy is the newest approach. It involves harvesting patient's stem cells and their ex vivo transfection with a virus vector carrying the normal gene encoding the fully functioning enzyme. After bone-marrow ablation with chemotherapy, host hematopoietic cells with genes coding for the defective enzyme are eliminated, and transfected cells are introduced to the bone marrow. Currently, gene therapy shows promising results in investigational studies.

Promising Clinical studies

Type 1 Gaucher

- AVR-RD-02: lentiviral vector gene therapy (NCT 04145037)

Niemann–Pick type C: trials aimed at removing excess lipids or preventing their accumulation.

- N-acetyl-L-leucine (NCT 05163288)
- Hydroxypropyl-β-cyclodextrin (NCT 04860960)
- AZ-3102 (NCT 05758922)

Board Questions

1. A 43-year-old female is referred to a hematologist for an incidentally discovered platelet count of 97×10^9/L and hemoglobin of 12.1 g/dL. Her white blood cell count and differential are within normal limits. On exam, she is noted to have hepatosplenomegaly, and on further discussion she endorses nondescript bone pains. Imaging study revealed multifocal lytic

lesions involving her spine and long bones. She is most likely to have which of the following mutations?

a. Nonsense mutation in glucocerebrosidase
b. A missense mutation in *MPL*
c. A missense mutation in glucocerebrosidase
d. A frame shift mutation in *DKC-1*
e. A silent mutation in *SMPD1*

Answer: c

The clinical presentation is consistent with Gaucher disease. Mutations in gene *GBA1* (glucocerebrosidase 1) are responsible for this condition. Numerous variants in this gene have been described. Missense mutations are frequent variants and often result in residual enzyme activity causing milder symptoms.

2. A 6-year-old boy of Ashkenazi Jewish heritage presents to his pediatrician with neurologic decline, hepatosplenomegaly, thrombocytopenia, and interstitial lung disease. Fundoscopic exam shows a cherry-red macula. Which is the most suitable test to order as a next step in the diagnosis?

a. Glucocerebrosidase enzyme activity
b. Acid-sphingomyelinase enzyme activity
c. NGS screening panel for Ashkenazi Jewish population
d. NGS for *SMPD1* gene
e. NGS for *NPC1* and *NPC2* genes

Answer: b

The clinical presentation is consistent with Niemann–Pick disease. Besides cytopenia and hepatosplenomegaly, approximately 100% and 33% of affected babies or children manifest with the cherry-red spot eye abnormality, in types A and B, respectively. Neurological impairment and lung damage are common. Enzyme assay for acid sphingomyelinase should always be performed first, with gene sequencing to follow once the biochemical diagnosis has been confirmed. NGS as a first step is not suitable since turnaround times are longer, and most variants are nonpathogenic or of unknown clinical significance. Therefore, NGS can be difficult to interpret without proper clinical context of decreased enzyme activity. Screening panels may not have sufficient coverage of the gene of interest and are not recommended for the confirmation of the diagnosis.

References

1. Schulze, H. and K. Sandhoff, Lysosomal lipid storage diseases. Cold Spring Harb Perspect Biol, 2011. 3(6) a004804.
2. Leal AF, et al. Hematological findings in lysosomal storage disorders: a perspective from the medical laboratory. Ejifcc. 2022;33(1):28–42.
3. Proytcheva MA. Diagnostic pediatric hematopathology. Cambridge: Cambridge University Press; 2011. p. xi. 577 p.
4. Wang RY, et al. Lysosomal storage diseases: diagnostic confirmation and management of presymptomatic individuals. Genet Med. 2011;13(5):457–84.
5. Abed Rabbo M, et al. Sphingolipid lysosomal storage diseases: from bench to bedside. Lipids Health Dis. 2021;20(1):44.
6. D'Amore S, et al. In-depth phenotyping for clinical stratification of Gaucher disease. Orphanet J Rare Dis. 2021;16(1):431.
7. Hoffman JD, et al. The Ashkenazi Jewish carrier screening panel: evolution, status quo, and disparities. Prenat Diagn. 2014;34(12):1161–7.
8. Wasserstein M, et al. A randomized, placebo-controlled clinical trial evaluating olipudase alfa enzyme replacement therapy for chronic acid sphingomyelinase deficiency (ASMD) in adults: one-year results. Genet Med. 2022;24(7):1425–36.

Benign Lymphadenopathy 48

Ahmed Arfa, Yu Yang,
and José D. Sandoval-Sus

Introduction

Benign lymphadenopathy is encompassed by all non-neoplastic processes occurring in a lymph node showing varying degrees of reactive changes, e.g., follicular, parafollicular/interfollicular, or mixed follicular and paracortical hyperplasia; progressive transformation of germinal centers (PTGCs); granulomatous or necrotic changes; vascular transformation; drug inducted (iatrogenic); foreign-substance deposition (lipid, silicone, metal, gold, and proteinaceous materials); and lymphadenopathies associated with clinical syndromes (e.g., Kimura, Rosai–Dorfman, rheumatoid, dermatopathic, Castleman, Kikuchi–Fujimoto, systemic lupus, and IgG4 lymphadenopathy). Following the emergence of advanced molecular diagnostic techniques, especially implication

A. Arfa
Department of Hematopathology, University of South Florida, Moffitt Cancer Center & Research Institute, Tampa, FL, USA

Y. Yang
Department of Pathology, Immunology and Laboratory Medicine, University of Florida College of Medicine, Gainesville, FL, USA

J. D. Sandoval-Sus (✉)
Department of Malignant Hematology and Cellular Therapy, Moffitt Cancer Center at Memorial Healthcare System, Pembroke Pines, FL, USA
e-mail: Jose.Sandoval@moffitt.org

L. Sokol, L. Zhang (eds.), *Non-Neoplastic Hematologic Disorders*,
https://doi.org/10.1007/978-3-031-62373-8_48

of next-generation sequencing (NGS) in clinical laboratories and research, people have better insights into non-neoplastic lymphadenopathies. Among them, several previously benign lymphadenopathy disorders (LPD) are now included in the fifth the edition of the *WHO Classification of Tumors* under "tumour-like lesions with B-cell or T-cell predominance." [1] These have been included in this section for completion, but the changes should be noted for the following:

Reactive Follicular Hyperplasia

Introduction

Benign proliferation of hyperplastic lymphoid follicles with prominent GCs. The most common pattern of reactive lymphoid proliferation, occurring in all age groups, origin unknown in many cases. Represents B-cell stimulation within the lymph node, leading to increases in the number and size of follicles. Localized or generalized.

Pathogenesis

Stimulation by different antigens, e.g., infections, vaccination, drugs, chemicals, etc.

Diagnosis

- **Morphology:** Hyperplastic follicles with variable size and shape with prominent polarized GCs (light-blue enterocyte zone and dark-blue centroblast zone), background tangible-body macrophages, and follicular dendritic cells (FDCs) with well-demarcated mantel zone. In some cases, the GCs may increase in size and coalesce with geographic appearance (florid follicular hyperplasia).
- Immunohistochemical (IHC) stain: usually clusters of differentiation (CD) 10+, BCL6+, and BCL2- in GCs with high Ki67 index with polarization.
- Ancillary studies: no monoclonal immunoglobulin heavy (IgH) rearrangement.

Major Differential Diagnosis

- Follicular lymphoma (Table 48.1)
- Pediatric-type follicular lymphoma
- PTGC
- Nodular lymphocyte-predominant Hodgkin's lymphoma (NLPHL)
- Hyaline-vascular Castleman disease

Prognosis

Usually a benign, reversible process (it depends on the underlying cause).

Treatment

Follow-up of localized lymphadenopathy up to 4 weeks, if not resolved, then additional examination is needed.

Caveats

Always consider other diseases that can be associated with reactive follicular hyperplasia: rheumatoid arthritis, Sjögren's syndrome, immunoglobulin G (IgG) 4-related lymphoproliferative disease, toxoplasmosis, syphilis, early phase HIV-associated lymphadenopathy, Kimura disease, and sometimes a neoplasm, etc.

Table 48.1 Follicular hyperplasia vs. follicular lymphoma: diagnostic differences

	Follicular hyperplasia	Follicular lymphoma
Follicles	Low density, variable size, and shape	Back-to-back, comparable size and shape
Tangible-body macrophages	Present	Absent
Mantle zone	Intact	Absent
Polarization	Present	Absent
Bcl-2	Negative	Positive
Ki-67	High, with polarization	Low, no polarization

Progressive Transformation of Germinal Center (PTGC)

Introduction

Typically, large nodules with a background of follicular hyperplasia. The nodules are disrupted by infiltrating mantel-zone B cells. Usually presents as asymptomatic cervical lymphadenopathy; however, it could present as generalized lymphadenopathy. In addition, it could be an incidental finding in lymphoma cases (e.g., NLPHL).

Pathogenesis

Unknown pathogenesis but could be related to an autoimmune or viral etiology, especially in the pediatric population.

Diagnosis

Morphology: The involved asynchronous follicles may be seen at any of the following various stages: (1) hyperplastic GCs with fusion of 2–3 examined centers; (2) destruction of the GCs by infiltrating mantle-zone B cells; (3) disappearance of the GCs with scattered remaining centroblasts and FDCs among the mantle-zone B cells; and (4) importantly, absence of malignant lymphocyte predominant (LP) cells.

- IHC stain: CD10+, BCL6+, and BCL2-GCs with disrupted FDCs and the follicular dendritic meshwork are CD21+ and CD23+. The mantle-zone B cells are IgM+, IgD+, BCL2+, CD10−, and BCL6 − .
- Ancillary studies: no monocytic population by flow cytometry study.

Major Differential Diagnosis

- NLPHL: the presence of LP cells with rosetting of CD3-positive and PD1-positive follicular helper T cells around the neoplastic CD20-positive LP cell
- Follicular lymphoma, floral variant (see Table 48.1)
- Lymphocytic-rich classic Hodgkin lymphoma (HL) (nodular variant)

Prognosis

It usually resolves spontaneously but may recur. Not considered a premalignant condition but can precede or coexist with HL.

Treatment

Active surveillance is recommended. Single-agent rituximab could be considered for symptomatic PTGC after successful treatment of HL (PMID: **21663508**).

Caveats

Positive transformation of germinal center is frequently associated with malignancy (NLPHL, HL), autoimmune, infection, or other reactive LPD (PMID: **35293684**). Recurrence of lymphadenopathies among patients with PTGC is common. Positron emission tomography–computed tomography (PET–CT) is not recommended as surveillance and should be done to assess for other diagnoses. Both PTGC and HL are avid on PET–CT and a fine-needle aspiration is suboptimal for diagnosis. Diagnosis should be made via an excisional biopsy or a core needle biopsy.

Histiocytic Necrotizing Lymphadenitis (Kikuchi–Fujimoto Disease)

Now classified under "tumour-like lesions with T-cell predominance" in the *WHO Classification* [1].

Introduction

It is a subacute necrotizing lymphadenopathy associated with mild fever, upper-respiratory infection-like symptoms, and tender cervical lymphadenopathy. It commonly affects young Asian women but can affect both sexes at any age and from any ethnicity. It is a self-limited process.

Pathogenesis

Unknown, however, there are hypotheses linking Kikuchi to autoimmune etiologies, medications (e.g., anti-IL23-antibody Risankizumab or phenytoin), and cytokine-mediated mechanisms (↑ INF-α, IL-6).

Diagnosis

- Morphology: paracortical proliferation of C-shaped histiocytes and plasmacytoid dendritic cells, with apoptosis and abundant karyorrhectic debris, and rare plasma cells in patchy, well-circumscribed areas of necrosis. Neutrophils and eosinophils should be absent. There are three histologic phases: proliferative, necrotic, and phagocytic.
- IHC stain: Histiocytes positive for CD4, CD68, and CD163, and plasmacytoid dendritic cells positive for CD123, CD303/BDCA2, TCF4, and TCL1. Flow cytometry shows CD8(+) T cells usually without aberrancies.
- Ancillary studies: No evidence of monoclonal T-cell receptor or rearrangement of IgH.

Major Differential Diagnosis

- Systemic lupus erythematosus (SLE) lymphadenitis: Morphologically identical, but the presence of hematoxylin bodies is only seen in SLE lymphadenitis.
- Cat-scratch disease: Show abundant acute inflammatory cells including numerous neutrophils and eosinophils.

Prognosis

Spontaneous resolution within 1–4 months, with 3–7% of recurrence rate.

Treatment

Symptomatic treatment with short-term course of nonsteroidal anti-inflammatory drugs or corticosteroids. Hydroxychloroquine has been used for recurrent or complicated cases (PMID: 2902144).

Caveats

Excellent prognosis without specific treatments. Important differential diagnoses are T-cell/histiocyte-rich large B-cell lymphoma (THRLBCL) and CD8-positive peripheral T-cell lymphoma.

Dermatopathic Lymphadenitis

Introduction

Paracortical hyperplasia (caused by underlying skin disease) consists of interdigitating dendritic cells (IDCs), Langerhans cells, and macrophages with melanin pigments. It usually presents as inguinal or axillary lymphadenopathy.

Pathogenesis

T-cell response to skin antigen presented and processed on dendritic cells and Langerhans cells.

Diagnosis

- Morphology: preserved lymph node architecture with follicular hyperplasia and paracortical expansion by IDCs. Langerhans cells and macrophages contain melanin pigmentation. The paracortical area may coalesce and compress the follicles.
- IHC stain: Langerhans cells and IDCs are positive for S100. CD1a often shows a variable intensity. Only Langerhans cells are positive Langerin/CD207.

Major Differential Diagnosis

- Langerhans cell histiocytosis: CD1a+/Langerin+ Langerhans cells and a subset of cases with *BRAF V600E* mutation
- Mycosis fungoides: atypical lymphoid cell infiltrate, commonly CD4+, cerebriform-appearing T cells that are CD26-negative. CD8+ MF occurs occasionally.
- Classic HL: CD45−, PAX-5 dim+, CD30+, and CD15+ Reed–Sternberg B cells.
- Anaplastic large-cell lymphoma: sinusoidal infiltration, filled with sheets of CD30+ large T cells, anaplastic lymphoma kinase (ALK) + or ALK−.
- Metastatic melanoma: positive for HMB-45, SOX10, and melanin-A and S100 (variable).

Prognosis
Depends on the underlying skin disease, if associated with underlying mycosis fungoides, it could have poor prognosis.

Treatment
Self-limited condition that often requires no specific treatment. Treatment should focus on the underlying condition.

Caveats
Looking for underlying reactive or neoplastic process of skin is warranted for patients who present with dermatopathic lymphadenopathy. It is commonly associated with MF, with or without disease involvement.

SLE Lymphadenitis

Introduction
An autoimmune disease that commonly affects middle-aged females. Can be systemic (affects multiple organs and skin, with lymph adenopathy among 60% of the patients) or cutaneous-only involvement [2, 3].

Pathogenesis
Type III hypersensitivity reaction mediated via autoantibodies include (anti-double-stranded DNA, antihistones, and antinucleosomes).

Diagnosis
- Morphology: The lymph node shows large areas of coagulative necrosis in background follicular hyperplasia with numerous plasma cells. Fibrinoid necrosis, increased apoptosis, and presence of "hematoxylin bodies (5–12 μm in size, amorphous extracellular necrotic clumps)" are characteristic. (Fig. 48.1a, b)

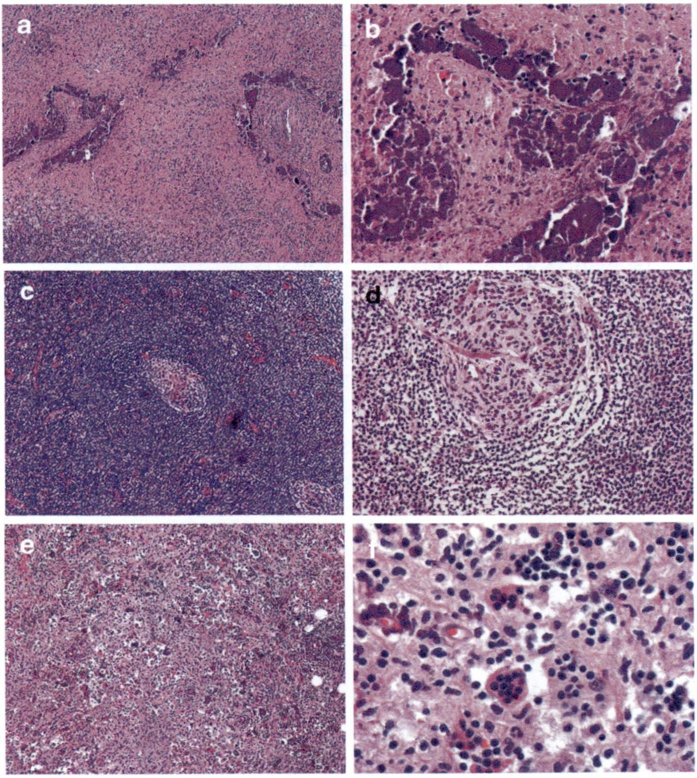

Fig. 48.1 (**a**, **b**) **SLE**: large areas of coagulative necrosis in background follicular hyperplasia with numerous plasma cells, with or without lymphocytic/immunoblastic expansion of the interfollicular zone. (**c**, **d**) **Castleman disease**: follicular hyperplasia with germinal center atrophy and concentric layering of the mantle-zone lymphocytes (onion-skin appearance). The follicles may contain ≥2 germinal (twinning) with hyalinized small vessels penetrating through the germinal centers (lollipop sign). RDD Rosai–Dorfman disease, SLE systemic lupus erythematosus. (**e**, **f**) **RDD**: histiocytic sinus dilatation and emperipolesis (RDD cells, histocytes engulf other cells including lymphocytes, neutrophils, and plasma cells)

- Presence of symptoms of SLE, such as fever, fatigue, malar rash, joint pain and swelling, renal malfunction-related symptoms, etc.
- Ancillary studies: Laboratory testing includes increased rheumatoid factor, C-reactive protein, antinuclear antibody, double-stranded DNA, and anti-Smith antibodies.

Major Differential Diagnosis

- Kikuchi–Fujimoto disease: See above.

Prognosis

It depends on the prognosis of the associated SLE.

Treatment

SLE-directed treatments are given and managed by rheumatology.

Caveats

Prognosis and treatment depend on the control of underlying SLE. Rheumatology always needs to be consulted.

Kimura Disease

Introduction

Chronic inflammatory disease mostly seen among young Asian males. It presents with subcutaneous slow-growing nontender masses in the head and neck; it also involves the major salivary glands (parotid and submandibular) with lymphadenopathy.

Pathogenesis

Unknown, it may be related to overexpression of cytokines such as IL4, IL5, and IL13 and proliferation of CD4 T-helper2 (Th2) in the lesions. (PMID: **35138349**).

Diagnosis

Morphology: Disruption of the lymph-node architecture with hyperplastic follicles and well-formed GCs (that may show proteinaceous material caused by immunoglobulin E [IgE] deposition). Interfollicular hyperplasia with abundant eosinophils with eosinophilic micro-abscesses, eosinophilic follicle lysis, and vascular proliferation and varying degrees of sclerosis. Ancillary studies: eosinophilia with elevated serum IgE level and erythrocyte sedimentation rate (ESR), nephrotic syndrome may occur among 20% of patients.

Major Differential Diagnoses

- Angio-lymphoid hyperplasia with eosinophilia, a benign vascular neoplasm, no SLE-associated clinical findings (PMID: 24580875).
- Langerhans cell histiocytosis (CD1a+/Langerin+ Langerhans cell with or without harboring *BRAF* V600E mutation).
- Dermatopathic lymphadenopathy: see above.
- Neoplasm: Myeloid sarcoma, T-cell lymphoma, or classic HL, mixed cellularity type.
- Parasitic infection.

Prognosis

Chronic disease with episodes of remission and relapses, but there are also case of spontaneous resolution.

Treatment

Surgical excision, but relapses are frequent. Systemic corticosteroids are effective for a brief time. Localized radiation therapy is also effective.

Promising Clinical Studies

There are several case reports of successful treatment of relapse Kimura disease with dupilumab (IL-4–receptor antagonists that inhibit IL-4 and IL-13 signaling).

Caveats
The basis of therapy is surgery and radiation of localized lesions and systemic corticosteroids of generalized disease.

Castleman Disease (CD)

Now classified under "tumour-like with B-cell predominance" in the *WHO Classification of Tumours* [1, 4, 5].

Introduction
CD is a group of heterogeneous disorders of lymphadenopathy with similar histological features but diverse clinical manifestations. Affects both genders between the fourth and seventh decades. Based on its clinical manifestations and disease course, it is classified into:

- Unicentric CD (UCD), a localized disease (i.e. mediastinal mass) involving a single lymph-node group.
- Oligocentric CD, which affects few regional lymph nodes without any other clinical manifestations and behaves like UCD.
- Multicentric CD (MCD) that is subdivided into three categories: (1) human herpesvirus-8-(HHV8-) associated MCD; (2) polyneuropathy, organomegaly, endocrinopathy, monoclonal plasma-cell disorder, skin changes-(POEMS-) associated MCD; and (3) idiopathic MCD.

Currently, the disease can be subcategorized according to HHV8 status. A subset of MCD is driven by HHV8 among HIV-infected or otherwise immunosuppressed patients, while HHV8-negative MCD is called idiopathic MCD (iMCD). iMCD shows an overlap with infectious, autoimmune, and malignant disease and is further subclassified as iMCD–NOS [not otherwise specified] or iMCD–TAFRO [thrombocytopenia, anasarca, fever, reticulin fibrosis, renal insufficiency, and organomegaly].

Pathogenesis

The pathogenesis of UCD is unclear, but recent data suggest that some cases could be related to neoplastic transformation of FDCs (PMID: 28087540). The pathogenesis of iMCD is not well understood, but IL-6 overexpression, elevated VEGF, and activation of mTOR pathway have been implicated. Monoclonal plasma cells are responsible for POEMS-associated MCD.

Diagnosis

Clinical diagnosis of HHV8-positive CD is based upon clinical history and morphology. Clinical diagnosis of HHV8-negative idiopathic CD is based on international evidence-based consensus diagnostic criteria (PMID: 28087540).

- Morphology diagnosis: It is pathologically classified into:
  - Hyaline-vascular type (HV): It is more prevalent in UCD, see Fig. 48.1c, d.
  - Plasma-cell type: It is more prevalent in MCD.
  - Mixed type: Lymph nodes have a combination of both hyaline-vascular type and plasma-cell type. It can be seen in UCD and MCD.
- IHC stain: CD21 or CD23 show concentric expansion of the FDCs meshwork with CD20+ and CD5+ expanded mantle-zone B cells. HHV8 stain is positive or negative.
- Ancillary studies: To differentiate between UCD and MCD, the following tests are recommended: PET–CT (or CT scan with contrast), complete blood count (CBC), ESR, complete metabolic panel (CMP), serum–protein electrophoresis with immunofixation, serum immunoglobulins, urinalysis, and HIV serology.

Major Differential Diagnosis

- HIV-associated lymphadenopathy.
- Angioimmunoblastic T-cell lymphoma: atypical proliferation of CD10+/PD1+/ICOS+/BCL6+ follicular T-helper cells outside of GCs and adjunct to high endothelial venules.
- Follicular lymphoma: See Table 48.1.

- Mantle-cell lymphoma (atypical, monotypic, and CD5+ and cyclin D1+).
- Epstein–Barr virus (EBV) infection.
- Autoimmune disorders (e.g., SLE, rheumatoid arthritis, etc.).
- FDC sarcoma (needs to be ruled-out in UCD).
- Plasmacytoma.
- Kaposi sarcoma: HHV8+, can be concurrent with HHV8+ CD.
- KSHV/HHV8 diffuse large B-cell lymphoma (DLBCL) and KSVH/HHV8+ germinotrophic LPD: HHV8+ DLBCL develops among MCD patients with HIV infections. CD is usually polyclonal, while its monoclonal Ig rearrangement is usually identified in DLBCL. CD is typically EBV negative, while germinotrophic LPD frequently EBV and HHV8 co-infected. Coexpression of LANA and vIL-6 favors GLP.

Prognosis

Depends on the CD type. UCD usually has a good prognosis with a 10-year survival of greater than 90% after complete resection (PMID: **22367441**), but it also has the highest risk of developing FDC sarcoma and both classic HL and non-Hodgkin's lymphoma (NHL). HHV8-associated MCD is at risk of developing NHL and Kaposi sarcoma.

Treatment

- UCD and oligocentric CD: complete resection is preferred, but asymptomatic unresectable disease can be monitored with active surveillance. Radiation therapy and local embolization can be used in localized symptomatic cases. Systemic treatment with rituximab or anti-IL-6 monoclonal antibodies (siltuximab/tocilizumab) can also be used, especially in cases that have associated inflammatory symptoms.
- HHV8-associated CD: weekly rituximab for 4 weeks. Antiretroviral therapy is started or continued for patients with HIV. Antiviral therapy directed at HHV8 (ganciclovir) is considered.

- POEMS-associated CD: If there are lytic bone lesions, multiple myeloma therapy should be used. In the absence of skeletal lesions, iMCD therapy can be used.
- iMCD: Siltuximab (an IL-6 directed antibody) is the preferred frontline therapy, but if it is not available, tocilizumab can be used. Corticosteroids are used for temporary symptom control. Second-line treatment options: rituximab, immunomodulatory therapies (e.g., sirolimus, etc.), chemo-immunotherapy (e.g., R-CVP, R-CHOP, etc.).

Promising Clinical Studies

All patients should be offered enrollment on the Castleman Disease Collaborative Network's ACCELERATE natural history registry (NCT02817997 at clinicaltrials.gov). A phase II study of sirolimus for previously treated patients with iMCD (NCT 03933904 at clinicaltrials.gov) is currently enrolling.

Caveats

- The histopathological subtypes of CD can be seen across the spectrum of CD and are not pathognomonic of any single clinical subtype. These subtypesare not directly associated with prognosis and used for a treatment decision regarding TAFRO syndrome [thrombocytopenia, anasarca, fever, reticulin fibrosis, and organomegaly] can be seen in conjunction with iMCD.

Rosai–Dorfman Disease (RDD)

Now classified under "tumour-like with T-cell predominance" in the *WHO Classification of Tumors* [1, 6].

Introduction

It is a benign histiocytic proliferation that usually presents with large bilateral painless cervical lymphadenopathy and is associated with B symptoms. RDD can be subclassified in the *sporadic* or familial category. The former includes classic nodal, extranodal (e.g., skin, central nervous system, and soft tissue), autoimmune-disease associated, or neoplasia associated.

Pathogenesis

Uncertain, recent studies identified certain recurrent mutations involving the RAS/MEK pathway (e.g., *ARAF*, *KRAS*, *NRAS*, *MAP2K1*, etc.), but further research is needed on the clonality of this entity.

Diagnosis

- Morphology: Preserved lymph-node architecture with histiocytic sinus dilatation and emperipolesis with follicular hyperplasia and background sclerosis (Fig. 48.1e, f)
- IHC stain: RDD cells are positive for S100, CD163, cyclin D1, and OCT2 and negative for CD1a and Langerin.
- Molecular studies: 30% of the cases show mutations in the MAPK pathway (KRAS and MAP2K1).
- Ancillary studies: PET–CT (or CT scans), CBC, CMP, ESR, neuroimaging (if symptoms of central nervous system), bone-marrow biopsy (for cytopenias), and serum immunoglobulins with IgG subclasses. NGS study of involved tissue is ordered for potential targeted therapy if refractory to conventional treatment.

Major Differential Diagnosis

- IgG4-related disease: IgG4-positive plasma cells can be increased in RDD, accounting for 40% of IgG-positive plasma cells. Composite RDD and IgG4 disease are common.
- Langerhans cell histiocytosis: CD1a+/Langerin+/BRAF V600E(VE1) + Langerhans cell per IHC study and *BRAF* V600E mutation detected by polymerase chain reaction (PCR) or NGS study.

Prognosis

Usually has good prognosis in nodal and cutaneous RDD. Patients with multifocal and extranodal RDD, and especially involving lungs, liver, and/or kidney, have a more aggressive course and poor prognosis.

Treatment

Asymptomatic nodal or cutaneous RDD can be observed or surgically resected, especially if there are related local symptoms. There is a role for radiation for localized symptomatic unresectable RDD. Relapsed disease can be treated with corticosteroids, immunosuppressants (e.g., sirolimus), chemotherapy (e.g., cladribine, methotrexate), or targeted therapies such as MEK inhibitors (e.g., cobimetinib).

Promising Clinical Studies

There is one study of lenalidomide and dexamethasone for RDD outside the United States (NCT04924647). There are no other upcoming clinical studies.

Caveats

RDD has a heterogenous clinical picture and is usually associated with a good clinical outcome. RDD-like lesions can be seen in classic HL, NHL, or myelodysplastic syndromes or after bone-marrow transplant for acute leukemia. RDD can be associated with autoimmune diseases, such as SLE, idiopathic juvenile arthritis, and commonly in IgG4-related diseases.

Rheumatoid Arthritis-Related Lymphadenopathy

Introduction

Lymphadenopathy related to underlying autoimmune rheumatoid arthritis, commonly seen among middle-aged HLA-DR1/HLA-DR4 females who smoke cigarettes.

Pathogenesis

Autoimmune disease that may be triggered by infections among genetically susceptible patients (HLA-DR1 and HLA-DR4).

Diagnosis

- Morphology: 2 major histologic changes, including marked follicular hyperplasia with interfollicular plasmacytosis. Immunoblasts can be numerous. Vascular proliferation is also common. Sarcoid granulomas may be seen. Nonbirefringent crystalline structures throughout parenchyma can be seen after gold therapy.
- IHC stain: CD10(+), BCL6 (+), BCL2(-)GCs, CD138+ plasma cells in the interfollicular areas, and EBER+ in some cases.
- Ancillary studies: no monoclonal IgH rearrangement. Elevated serum RF and anticyclic citrullinated peptide antibodies.

Major Differential Diagnoses

- CD: Morphologically can be very similar; clinical history is essential for differential diagnosis.
- Syphilitic lymphadenitis: Besides follicular hyperplasia and plasmacytosis, vasculitis and perivasculitis are also common. Warthin–Starry special stain or PCR study is helpful to identify spirochetes/*Treponema pallidum*.
- Plasmacytoma (sheets of monoclonal plasma cell with light chain restriction).

Prognosis

Follow-up is needed as these patients are at increased risk of lymphomas and leukemias including, but not limited to, DLBCL (some were EBV positive), classic HL, and large granular lymphocytic leukemia

Treatment

Treat the underlying rheumatoid arthritis.

Sarcoid Lymphadenopathy

Introduction

Sarcoidosis is an inflammatory disorder that primarily affects lung and lymph tissues and is manifested with single or multisystemic granulomatous changes. It commonly affects females at any age (especially middle age, 20–40 years), with the highest prevalence among Black Americans and people with Scandinavian ethnicity.

Pathogenesis

Unknown, both innate and adaptive immune responses are contributable to the onset and progression of the disease. It is an antigen-triggered immune process that could be mediated by antigen-presenting T cells through the major histocompatibility complex II, and the disease is most representative of unresolved immunological paradox (PMID: 30955519).

Diagnosis

- Morphology: The nodal architecture is partially or totally replaced by well-demarcated noncaseating epithelioid granulomas associated with giant cells, and by immunoglobulin deposits with a variety of inclusion bodies, such as Schaumann, asteroid, and Hamazaki-Wesenburg.
- IHC: The lymphocytes surrounding the granulomas are predominantly CD4+ T cells with fewer CD8+ T cells. Special stains for microorganisms are negative, including acid-fast bacteria (AFB), Grocott's methenamine silver stain (GMS), Periodic acid-Schiff stain, etc.
- Ancillary studies: PCR study shows no evidence of T-cell receptor gene rearrangement. Laboratory tests show elevated ESR, angiotensin converting enzyme, hypercalcemia, and CBC study may show cytopenias.

Major Differential Diagnosis

- *Mycobacterium tuberculosis*: mostly necrotizing granuloma, AFB+
- Atypical mycobacteria: AFB+ granuloma
- Fungal lymphadenitis: GMS positive granuloma
- Leprosy: AFB+ mycobacteria, PCR study (sensitivity of 87–100%) for confirmation (PMID: 32229279), on physical exam there will be hypopigmented or erythematous skin patches

Treatment

Systemic corticosteroids are the first line of treatment. Other treatment options (second-line include: methotrexate, azathioprine, leflunomide, and mycophenolate and the third-line drugs (infliximab and adalimumab) are selected for failure of second-line therapy or drug cytotoxicity.

Promising Clinical Studies

Efficacy and Safety of Intravenous Efzofitimod in Patients with Pulmonary Sarcoidosis (NCT 05415137).

Caveats

Lungs and mediastinal/hilar lymph nodes are the most common affected organs. Other commonly involved organs are the skin, liver, eyes, and heart.

HIV-Associated Lymphadenopathy

Introduction

Generalized lymphadenopathy is often seen in the acute phase of HIV but can persist in a subset of patients. Most commonly in the head-and-neck region with superficial adenopathy, more likely to be reactive.

Pathogenesis

Lymphotrophic virus that causes remodeling of lymph nodes, manifesting as lymphadenopathy in three phases.

Diagnosis

- Biopsy not always indicated, consider for enlarging generalized lymphadenopathy or a single site of enlarged nodes.
- Morphology:
  - Stage I: explosive follicular hyperplasia with large GCs
  - Stage II: germinal-center involution and lymphocyte depletion
  - Stage III: vascular proliferation with abundant plasma cells
- Ancillary studies: CD4

Major Differential Diagnosis

- Infection (viral, bacterial, fungal, toxoplasma, and mycobacterial, e.g., tuberculosis or *Mycobacterium avium* complex). EBV and cytomegalovirus infections are the two most common viral infections among patients with AIDS or who are HIV positive. Infectious mononucleosis can resemble stage-I HIV lymphadenopathy.
- Lymphoma, HIV-related (e.g., classical HL, EBV+ DLBCL, Burkitt lymphoma).
- CD.
- Immune reconstitution inflammatory syndrome if recent initiation of highly active antiretroviral therapy, combination antiretroviral therapy (cART).
- Kaposi sarcoma (associated with HHV8 infection).
- Composite lymphoma(s).

Prognosis

Disease stage-related, compliance with HAART therapy-related. Low CD4 count and high viral titers often have a negative impact on prognosis. Low CD4 count among patients with HIV correlates with increased lymphadenopathy. Decreasing lymphadenopathy can be seen with severe lymphocyte depletion and associated with increased risk of transformation to AIDS.

Treatment

Treat underlying HIV with HAART. If coexistence of lymphoma, then chemoregiments should be added accordingly (PMID: 33325733).

IgG4-Related Lymphadenopathy

Now classified as "tumour-like with B-cell predominance" in the *WHO Classification of Tumors* [1, 7, 8].

Introduction

Fibro-inflammatory disorder predominantly seen in extranodal sites (pancreas, salivary and lacrimal glands, and retroperitoneum), and may frequently involve lymph nodes. Clinical manifestations are heterogeneous but usually asymptomatic. The lesions consist of a storiform fibrosis with IgG4-rich plasma-cell inflammatory infiltrate.

Pathogenesis

Likely to be an autoimmune disease. IgG4 production, although a hallmark of this condition, is not thought to be pathogenic but secondary to the increased production of cytokines in the effected lymph nodes.

Diagnosis

It follows the 2020 revised comprehensive diagnostic criteria for IgG4-related disease (PMID: 33274670).

- Morphology: increased IgG4 plasma cells and IgG4/IgG ratio, associated with different backgrounds. Histologically, can be divided into five subtypes:
  - I: multicentric Castleman's-like disease
  - II: follicular hyperplasia with plasmacytosis
  - III: interfollicular expansion with lollipop appearance in some follicles and mature plasma, plasmablasts, immunoblasts, and eosinophils
  - IV: PTGC-like
  - V: inflammatory pseudotumor-like (storiform collagen fibers with plasma cells and lymphocyte infiltration)
- Serum-IgG4 levels are elevated among ⅔ of patients but is neither sensitive nor specific for diagnosis.
- Ancillary studies: CBC with differential, CMP, amylase, lipase, IgG subclasses, IgE, serum protein electrophoresis, serum C3/C4, HgB, hemoglobin A1C, CT, and/or PET/CT.

Major Differential Diagnosis

MCD and for follicular hyperplasiam, see above.

Prognosis

A relapse is common; it is reported as increased risk of malignancy, specifically pancreatic cancer, and lymphoma; e.g., MALT lymphomaIgG4-related disorder is not uncommonly associated with RDD.

Treatment

Initial therapy for patients with symptomatic or progressive disease is typically with glucocorticoids. An additional immunosuppressive or biologic regimen, such as rituximab, can be added. Next-line therapy is steroid-sparing agents, including azathioprine or mycophenolate

Board Questions

1. A 44-year man with painless right-cervical lymphadenopathy and several skin nodules that have slowly grown for the past 7 months. Lymph-node biopsy revealed RDD. Which of the following mutations can be more frequently detected on this lesion?

   A. *MAP2K1*
   B. *BTK* C481S
   C. *BRAF* V600E
   D. *FLT3*-ITD
   E. *JAK2* V617F

Answer: A. Mutations are often involved in MAPK pathology in a subset of patients diagnosed with RDD. *BRAF* V600E has occasionally been reported in RDD. *FLT3* and *JAK2* mutations are more associated with an acute myeloid leukemia and a myeloproliferative neoplasm, respectively.

2. A 45-year-old woman presented with palpable bilateral–cervical lymphadenopathy with no other associated symptoms. Laboratory examination was unremarkable, including normal CBC, CMP, ESR, C-reactive protein, lactate dehydrogenase, serum–protein electrophoresis with immunofixation, and urinalysis. HIV serology was negative. PET–CT showed disease localized to his cervical region without any other nodal or

extranodal involvement. An excisional biopsy of enlarged right-cervical lymph node was compatible with hyaline-vascular CD (HHV8 and EBV by IHC were negative). What is the best treatment option for this patient?

A. Siltuximab
B. Rituximab
C. Lenalidomide, bortezomib, and dexamethasone
D. Complete surgical resection
E. Clinical trial

Answer: D. complete surgical resection based on evidence based consensus and expert guidelines such as the NCCN CD guidelines [9].

References

1. WHO. Classification of tumours. 5th ed. https://tumourclassification.iarc.who.int/chaptercontent/63
2. Masaru K, Motoori T, Asano S, et al. Histological diversity of reactive and atypical proliferative lymph node lesions in systemic lupus erythematosus patients. Pathol Res Pract. 2007;203(6):423–31. PMID: 175405097.
3. Kojima M, Matsuda H, Iijima M, et al. Reactive hyperplasia with giant follicles in lymph node lesions from systemic lupus erythematosus patients: report of three cases. Apmis. 2005;113(7–8):558–63. PMID: 16086828.
4. Dispenzieri A, Fajgenbaum DC. Overview of Castleman disease. Blood. 2020;135(16):1353–64. PMID: 32106302.
5. Abramson JS. Diagnosis and management of Castleman disease. J Natl Compr Canc Netw. 2019;17(11.5):1417–9. PMID: 31766018.
6. Oussama A, Jacobsen C, Picarsic J, et al. Consensus recommendations for the diagnosis and clinical management of Rosai-Dorfman-Destombes disease. Blood. 2018;131(26):2877–90. PMID: 297204852.
7. Vikram D, Zen Y, Chan JKC, et al. Consensus statement on the pathology of IgG4-related disease. Mod Pathol. 2012;25(9):1181–92. PMID: 22596100.
8. Hisanori U, Okazaki K, Kawa D. The 2020 revised comprehensive diagnostic (RCD) criteria for IgG4-RD. Modern Rheumatol. 2021;31(3):529–33. PMID: 332746709.
9. Zelenetz A, Gordon L, Abramson J, et al. JNCCN Clinical Practice Guidelines in Oncology. Castleman disease. National Comprehensive Cancer Network. Available at https://www.nccn.org/professionals/physician_gls/pdf/castleman.pdf. Version 1. 2024.

Hypersplenism and Hyposplenism

49

Franco C. Garcia
and Jennifer Eatrides

The spleen is a well-capsulated small vascular organ located in the upper quadrant of the abdomen measuring 11.0 × 5.0 × 7.0 cm and weighing 70–200 g in a normal adult. It contains both white pulp and red pulp. The white pulp is a secondary lymphoid organ which is composed predominantly of B cells and some T cells and functions similar to a lymph node. The red pulp filters 150 ml of blood per minute via an extensive sinusoidal system lined by macrophages which remove antibody-bound substances, bacteria, foreign material, and damaged red blood cells. The two major functions of the spleen are to store blood and eliminate aged or defective cells. It is also an important secondary immune organ. Disorders of the spleen can have a significant impact on the health of individuals affected by them, leading to anemia, thrombocytopenia, and increased risk of infections. The spleen has hematopoietic potential between the second and sixth months of fetal life,

F. C. Garcia
Department of Satellite and Community Oncology, H. Lee Moffitt Cancer Center and Research Institute, Tampa, FL, USA

J. Eatrides (✉)
Department of Satellite and Community Oncology, H. Lee Moffitt Cancer Center and Research Institute, Tampa, FL, USA

Department of Oncologic Sciences, Morsani College of Medicine, University of South Florida, Tampa, FL, USA
e-mail: Jennifer.Eatrides@moffitt.org

L. Sokol, L. Zhang (eds.), *Non-Neoplastic Hematologic Disorders*,
https://doi.org/10.1007/978-3-031-62373-8_49

but this activity is abolished after bone marrow can perform this function. It is important to note that splenomegaly can be associated with either hypersplenism or hyposplenism. Many of the conditions that cause splenomegaly can cause a functional hyposplenism. Accordingly, the examination and differential are similar for both conditions.

Hypersplenism

Introduction

Hypersplenism is a condition resulting in augmented splenic function and can occur in the setting of splenomegaly (enlarged spleen with a size >11 cm in craniocaudal length, or weights >400 g), but these two parameters do not always coexist. The overactive spleen filters blood cells more efficiently, resulting in extensive splenic sequestration of mature blood cells and leading to an increased destruction of red blood cells, white blood cells, and platelets. In a healthy individual, the spleen will contain roughly $\frac{1}{3}$ of the body's red blood cells and platelets within the red pulp. In the setting of hypersplenism, this proportion can substantially increase, resulting in anemia, thrombocytopenia, and even leukopenia.

Pathogenesis

Hypersplenism can be caused by a variety of factors. It is often a complication of underlying disease, most commonly portal hypertension, but can also occur in the settings of infiltrative disorders, neoplastic disorders, and autoimmune disorders.

Diagnosis

- History and physical exam to assess spleen size and tenderness.
- Complete blood count with differential: typically shows cytopenias.

- Comprehensive metabolic panel to evaluate for liver dysfunction.
- Examination for vitamin deficiencies to rule out other causes of cytopenias.
- Peripheral smear review for circulating abnormal cells.
- Rheumatologic panel if an autoimmune disorder is suspected.
- Disease-specific infection panel.
- Imaging: abdominal ultrasound, computed tomography (CT), or magnetic resonance imaging (MRI) may show enlarged spleen. Nuclear medicine liver/spleen scan to detect colloid shift less commonly used now that CT and MRI are widely available. Positron emission tomography/CT should be guided by initial examination and suspected etiologies.
- Genetic testing in which clinical picture fits infiltrative metabolic disorders (including lipid storage disorders, see dedicated chapter).

Major Differential Diagnosis

Differential diagnosis considers potential causes of cytopenias and splenomegaly, including possible malignancy, underlying splenic infiltrative disorders, and lymphoproliferative disorders, see Table 49.1.

Prognosis

Prognosis is related to the underlying cause which varies widely. The risk of rupture is high among patients with significant splenomegaly.

Treatment

No treatment is needed for asymptomatic splenomegaly. Avoidance of injury or trauma is used to protect from the rupture of an enlarged spleen. Treatment should focus on managing the

Table 49.1 Causes of hypersplenism

Conditions affecting the liver	Cirrhosis Portal hypertension Heart failure (congestive hepatopathy) Venous thrombosis (portal or hepatic)
Infiltrative disorders	Amyloidosis Gaucher disease and other lysosomal Storage diseases Rosai–Dorfman disease (rarely) Sarcoidosis
Hematologic disorders causing splenic sequestration	Sickle cell anemia Thalassemia Hemoglobin SC disease Hemolytic anemias
Autoimmune disorders	Systemic lupus erythematosis Rheumatoid arthritis
Infectious	Infectious mononucleosis Hepatitis Malaria Tuberculosis
Malignancy	Myeloproliferative neoplasms (CML, PMF) MDS/MPN (e.g. CMML) Lymphoma Leukemia (e.g., hairy-cell leukemia) Metastatic carcinoma
Vascular lesions	Hemangiomas
Medications	Oxaliplatin Immunosuppressants
Others	Cysts Trauma induced hematoma

CML chronic myeloid leukemia, *CMML* chronic myelomonocytic leukemia, *PMF* primary myelofibrosis, *SC* sickle-C disease

underlying disease or condition causing the spleen to become overactive, as well as on supportive treatment for cytopenias. In some cases, medications may be prescribed to reduce the activity of the spleen, or blood transfusions may be necessary to replace the destroyed blood cells. When the etiology of hypersplenism is irreversible and the patient has clinically significant cytopenias, such as in the case of liver cirrhosis, a partial splenic embolization or splenectomy can be considered to improve cytopenias. Partial splenic embolization is thought to have similar results in terms of cytopenias, but with fewer complications [1].

Promising Clinical Studies

Studies are ongoing for specific causes of hypersplenism, such as myelofibrosis. Momelotinib (activin-A receptor-type 1 and JAK1/JAK2 inhibitor) showed superior clinical benefit over danazol as well as a 25% reduction in spleen size, recently approved for intermediate/high risk myelofibrosis [2].

Studies with thermal ablation techniques using microwaves or focused ultrasound are of interest.

Caveats

Overall, hypersplenism is managed supportively in case of symptoms secondary to splenomegaly or cytopenias. However, it is important to evaluate for disorders that can be targeted with a specific treatment.

Hyposplenism

Introduction

A condition in which the spleen functions poorly or is absent. This can lead to an increased risk of infections, venous thromboembolism, and certain types of cancer.

Pathogenesis

Hyposplenism refers to reduced splenic function, either secondary to its anatomical absence or physiological capability. The spleen is an important organ of the immune system and plays a vital role in fighting infections, filtering blood, and producing blood cells. When the spleen is not functioning properly, it can lead to a variety of complications, including an increased risk of infections as well as thromboembolism.

The mechanism of hyposplenism can vary depending on the underlying cause. It can be congenital (genetic mutations leading to abnormal or absent development of the spleen), surgical, or acquired. Functional asplenia or hyposplenism can occur in conditions leading to infiltration of the spleen or infarction of the spleen. Myeloproliferative and lymphoproliferative disorders can lead to splenic infiltration and functional asplenia. Decreased blood flow to the spleen secondary to thrombosis of the major vessels can lead to atrophy of the spleen.

Diagnosis

There are no clear guidelines for the evaluation of hyposplenism. The following can be considered depending on clinical presentation [3]. As many patients with hyposplenism may have splenomegaly, peripheral smear is important for identifying functional hyposplenism.

- History and physical examination.
- Complete blood count with differential shows thrombocytosis among the majority of patients after splenectomy.
- Peripheral blood smear demonstrating Howell–Jolly bodies (nuclear remnants in red blood cells typically removed by splenic macrophages) indicates functional asplenia. Nucleated red blood cells may also be seen in hyposplenia, as these are not removed from circulation.
- Imaging studies may be helpful to identify infarct, abscess, or infiltrative disease and should be based on clinical presentation: abdominal ultrasound, CT scan, or MRI of the abdomen [4]. Not sensitive to detect low-level hypofunction.
- IgM memory B cells detectable with flow cytometry.
- Pitted red blood cell count: not widely available and high observer variability.
- Additional laboratory tests: hemoglobin electrophoresis, viral studies, and antiphospholipid syndrome.

Major Differential Diagnosis

It is important to identify the etiology that could lead to hyposplenism, see Table 49.2 for potential causes of hyposplenism.

Prognosis

Prognosis depends on the clinical scenario causing hyposplenism.

Table 49.2 Common causes of hyposplenism

Category	Disease
Congenital aplenia	Hypoparathyroidism syndrome Isolated congenital hyposplenia Ivemark's syndrome Premature birth Other congenital or familial syndromes Stormorken's syndrome, etc.
Infectious disease	HIV/AIDS
Autoimmune disorder	Hashimoto's thyroiditis Rheumatoid arthritis Sjögren's disease Systemic lupus erythematosus
Hematologic disorder (functional hyposplenism)	Sickle cell disease Thalassemia Lymphoma Leukemia Bone marrow transplantation (chronic graft-vs-host disease) Myeloproliferative neoplasms Mastocytosis
Iatrogenic	Splenectomy or partial splenectomy, splenic irradiation
Thrombotic events	Splenic arterial or venous thrombosis Celiac artery thrombosis
Gastrointestinal disorders	Celiac disease Inflammatory bowel disease Whipple's disease
Others	Amyloidosis Sarcoidosis

Treatment

Treatment for hyposplenism typically involves managing the underlying cause of the condition and taking steps to reduce the risk of infections and other complications. This may include vaccinations to protect against certain infections, such as pneumococcal disease and meningococcal disease, and antibiotics to prevent bacterial infections. Vaccinations should occur at least 2 weeks before splenectomy but preferably 12 weeks before (detailed schedule per Table 49.3). The use of prophylactic antibiotics is based on infection history, age, and other comorbidities, such as immunodeficiencies. When daily prophylactic antibiotics are indicated, the preferred regimens are penicillin V, 250 mg twice daily or amoxicillin, 500 mg twice daily with alternative options being cephalexin, 250 mg twice daily or azithromycin, and 250 mg daily.

Table 49.3 Suggested vaccination schedule according to CDC guidelines for patients with asplenia [5]

Vaccine	Schedule
Pneumococcal conjugate vaccine (PCV20 or PCV15)	1 dose of PCV 20 or 1 dose of PCV 15 follow by a dose of the 23-valent pneumococcal polysaccharide vaccine (PPSV23) 1 year later
COVID-19	Schedule and boosters pending brand used
Pneumococcal polysaccharide vaccine (PPSV23)	Administered at least 8 weeks after dose of PCV15 or at 1 year, no booster required. Not needed if PCV20 is used
Meningococcal serotype B (MenB)	2 doses of MenB-4C at least 1 month apart or 3 doses of MenB-FHbp at 0, 1–2, and 6 months. Booster every 2–3 years
Meningococcal conjugate vaccine (MenACWY)	Administered as a two-dose series, with the second dose given 8–12 weeks after first dose. If the patient has already received 1 or more doses of MenACWY, they should receive a booster dose every 5 years
Haemophilus influenzae type b (Hib) vaccine	Administered as a three-dose series, with the second dose given 1–2 months after the first dose, and the third dose given 6 months after the first dose
Influenza vaccine	Administered annually, ideally before flu season

Promising Clinical Studies

Hyposplenism poses its own unique set of difficulties for patients; thus, clinical trials are designed to mitigate common complications, specifically, the risk for infections. The ongoing, large phase-3 French study SPLEMENGO (NCT04166656) seeks to evaluate the immunological response and tolerance of several vaccination schedules with Bexsero and Trumenba against meningococcal infections for patients with asplenia. These vaccines differ according to biochemical composition. Meningococcal-recombinant proteins are compared to conjugate vaccines, made of a capsular polysaccharide and a conjugate. This study aims to elucidate whether reinforcement-vaccination strategies are of benefit for asplenic patients with suboptimal response to a conjugate vaccine.

Caveats

Major concerns are infectious complications related to lack of splenic function.

The absence of Howell–Jolly bodies after splenectomy suggests the presence of accessory spleen.

Board Questions

1. A 22-year-old female college volleyball player presents with a 48-h history of fevers, night sweats, and sore throat. Laboratory tests show mild lymphocytosis with some atypical lymphocytes but a differential within normal limits. Of note, she does report that her roommate may have had a similar illness recently. On physical examination, spleen can be palpated below the left coastal margin, otherwise no other abnormalities are noted. Which is the most appropriate course of management?

   A. Obtain positron emission tomography CT scan
   B. Order spleen MRI
   C. Order peripheral blood flow cytometry
   D. Recommend refraining from sports requiring physical contact for 8 weeks

Answer: D

Explanation: The constitution of symptoms is those of infectious mononucleosis. Given the history of close contact with roommates with a similar illness, a malignant hematological process like lymphoma is less likely. Atypical lymphocytes can be seen on peripheral blood smear of patients with mononucleosis infection. Typical management would be supportive care and avoidance of physical contact sports because of risk of splenic rupture.

2. An 18-year-old male presents to an outpatient hematologic clinic with a history of recurrent respiratory infections as a child, as well as chronic history of intermittent thrombocytosis. Laboratory tests for mild thrombocytosis are otherwise within normal limits. On peripheral blood smear stained with Wright–Giemsa stain, small purple inclusions are seen in red blood cells. What condition could account for all this patient's clinical and laboratory findings?

   A. Asplenia
   B. Common variable immunodeficiency
   C. Chediak–Higashi syndrome
   D. Hereditary spherocytosis

   Answer: A

Explanation: The description of the peripheral blood-smear finding refers to Howell–Jolly bodies, which are small basophilic (purple) nuclear DNA remnants found in red blood cells when there is splenic dysfunction and/or absence. Thrombocytosis can be seen among patients with asplenia, given the lack of the spleen to perform its normal function of removing platelets as they age. Asplenia additionally predisposes patients to encapsulated bacterial infections. Given all these findings, asplenia best fits the said clinical picture.

References

1. Huang Y, Ren D, Gao F, et al. An updated meta-analysis of patial splenic embolization versus splenectomy in treatment of hypersplenism due to cirrhosis. Minim Invasive Ther Allied Techno. 2022;31(5):664–75.
2. Verstovsek S, Gerds AT, Vannucchi AM, et al. Momelotinib versus danazol in symptomatic patients with anemia and myelofibrosis (momentum): results from an international, double-blink, randomized controlled, phase 3 study. Lancet. 2023;401(10373):269–80.
3. Lenti MV, Luee S, Carsetti R, et al. Asplenia and spleen hypofunction. Nat Reve Dis Primers. 2022:8–71.
4. Thipphavong S, Duigenan S, Schindera ST, et al. Nonneoplastic, benign, and malignant splenic diseases: cross-sectional imaging findings and rare disease entities. AMR Am J Roentgenol. 2014;203(2):315–22.
5. William BM, Corazza GR. Hyposplenism: a comprehensive review. Part I: Basic concepts and causes. Hematology. 2007;12(10):1–13. Centers for Disease Control and Prevention. Vaccination of adults with aplenia. Centers for Disease Control and Prevention. 2016. Retrieved April 12, 2023 from https://www.cdc.gov/vaccines/adults/rec-vac/health-conditions/asplenia.html

Common Infections in Patients with Hematologic Neoplasms and Hematopoietic Stem Cell Transplant

50

Oluwatobi Ozoya, Jennifer Eatrides, Ling Zhang, Ana Paula Velez, and Ramon Sandin

Introduction

Infections are common among individuals with hematologic malignancies undergoing therapy and can result in significant morbidity and mortality. The precise incidence of infectious diseases varies depending on the type of hematologic malignancy, stage of disease, type of chemotherapy, kind of trans-

O. Ozoya (✉) · L. Zhang · R. Sandin
Department of Hematopathology, H. Lee Moffitt Cancer Center and Research Institute, Tampa, FL, USA
e-mail: Oluwatobi.Ozoya@moffitt.org

J. Eatrides
Department of Malignant Hematology, H. Lee Moffitt Cancer Center and Research Institute, Tampa, FL, USA

A. P. Velez
Department of Infectious Diseases, H. Lee Moffitt Cancer Center and Research Institute, Tampa, FL, USA

L. Sokol, L. Zhang (eds.), *Non-Neoplastic Hematologic Disorders*,
https://doi.org/10.1007/978-3-031-62373-8_50

plant, length of neutropenia, complications from transplant, including graft-vs-host disease, antimicrobials, previous infections, and immune status. The complex mechanisms driving susceptibility to infections depend on numerous factors [1, 2]. For example, patients who have undergone hematopoietic stem cell transplant (HSCT), especially allogeneic transplants, receive high dosages of immunosuppressants and are highly susceptible to various infections. The type of infection depends on the patient's level of immune deficiency, exposure to pathogens, duration of therapy after transplantation, and sociodemographic factors.

This chapter aims to provide an overview of the pathophysiology, clinical manifestations, and management modalities of common infections in patients with hematologic neoplasms undergoing therapy.

Pathogenesis

Microorganisms

Infections with bacteria, viruses, parasites, and fungi potentially weaken hematopoietic cell function and hemostatic factors in circulation and tissue, thereby suppressing marrow or lymphatic system function [3]. Each has a distinct pathogenesis to be considered when managing infections in this high-risk patient group. SARS-CoV-2 (COVID-19) viral infection provides a classic example of the complex interaction between the immune system and homeostatic factors [4]. The virus infects endothelial cells, causing inflammation and clotting, which blocks blood vessels, causing hypoxia and further tissue damage. The virus also triggers cytokine release, leading to further inflammation and endothelial dysfunction. These mechanisms contribute to significant morbidity and mortality among patients with hematologic malignancies [4].

Underlying Malignancy

Clonal expansion of malignant hematopoietic precursor cells in the bone marrow and mature lymphoid cells interferes with production of normal blood cells and lymphoid cells, causing weakness, cytopenia, and increased susceptibility to infection.

Cytoreduction and Immunotherapy

The mechanisms of immune suppression with chemotherapy are multifaceted and include depletion of white blood cells, inhibition of immune-cell proliferation and activation, damage to bone marrow, and alteration of microbiota. High-dose chemotherapy predisposes to significant immune suppression, with a marked reduction in T-cell function that persists for several months after treatment.

Biologic agents are also used in hematologic malignancies to target pathways that control cellular proliferation and immune or inflammatory responses. These agents target a network of tissue-T-helper cells, cytotoxic CD8+ T cells, and B cells, sometimes resulting in impaired long-term immunologic memory by suppressed CD4+ and CD8+ memory T cells. The therapies may, therefore, affect responses to acute-infection exposures as well as control of latent or chronic infections.

Certain nonchemotherapeutic agents (e.g., methotrexate and mycophenolate mofetil), antiviral or antibiotics (e.g., ganciclovir, valganciclovir, trimethoprim-sulfamethoxazole, and intravenous vancomycin), and occasional H2 blockers are also potentially myelosuppressive.

Normal Flora

Proliferation of natural commensals in the body in the presence of severe immunosuppression is another important mechanism of infection. Common commensals that are potentially fatal include

Staphylococcus epidermidis, methicillin-resistant *Staphylococcus aureus* (MRSA), streptococcus pneumoniae, *Clostridium difficile*, *Neisseria meningitidis*, *Escherichia coli*, viridans streptococci, coagulase-negative staphylococci, *Enterococcus* spp., and *Candida* spp. [5, 6]. Furthermore, severe mucositis and/or enteritis resulting from chemotherapy facilitates local invasion by the pathogen, usually enteric gram negatives and anaerobes with potential translocation to the bloodstream. Moreover, bacteria from the skin can also access the blood from long-term central lines used for treatment.

Pathogens from Donor Cells

Infections can be introduced by reactivation of pathogens from donor or recipient B cells. Commonly occurring organisms include Epstein–Barr virus, hepatitis-B virus, varicella zoster virus, and cytomegalovirus among high-risk patients with immunocompromised status. Therefore, it is important to carefully monitor the immune function in cancer patients undergoing chemotherapy and develop effective strategies to mitigate the associated risk factors.

Diagnosis

The goal of diagnosing infectious diseases in high-risk patients is to achieve prompt diagnosis and rapid treatment. We recommend early involvement of infectious-disease specialists in these often-complicated cases with broad infectious differential. Prophylactic measures are ideal and preferred rather than waiting to confirm an actual pathogen; however, there are challenges to prophylaxis, such as breakthrough multidrug-resistant organisms. Achieving a delicate balance across numerous factors such as dosage, timing, duration of prophylaxis, therapy, and clinical response remain a challenge. Table 50.1 highlights the clinical presentation, appropriate laboratory tests, and treatment.

Table 50.1 Common infectious disorders in patients undergoing High-dose chemotherapy pre- and post-HSCT

Organism	Sources or vector	Clinical presentation	Laboratory tests	Hematologic changes	Treatment
Bacteria					
Gram-positive bacteria including *Staphylococcus aureus*, and other coagulase-negative staphylococci, and *Streptococcus* spp.	Central venous lines, oral mucosa, GI and respiratory tract commensals in the nares, and skin flora	Sepsis syndrome, neutropenic fever, bacteremia Vascular catheter-associated cellulitis (*Staphylococcus epidermidis*), pneumonia	Gram stains and culture of blood, secretions, or tissue. Chromogenic media or PCR for MRSA	Typical leukocytosis may be absent in immunosuppressed patients	Sensitive antibiotics: vancomycin, oxacillin, nafcillin, cefazolin, daptomycin per susceptibility

Table 50.1 (continued)

Organism	Sources or vector	Clinical presentation	Laboratory tests	Hematologic changes	Treatment
Enteric gram-negative rods, pseudomonas, Stenotrophomonas, Acinetobacter, among other nosocomial pathogens	GI, GU, respiratory tract, and nosocomial pathogens from contaminated surfaces, water, hospital equipment, and healthcare personnel	Sepsis syndrome, neutropenic fever, bacteremia, enteritis, diarrhea, pneumonia, urinary tract infection, and bacteremia D	Gram stain and culture of the blood, stool culture, *E. coli* Shiga-like toxin by EIA. Gastrointestinal panel by PCR	Typical leukocytosis may be absent in immunosuppressed patients	Cephalosporins, beta-lactamase inhibitors, carbapenems, quinolones, aminoglycosides per susceptibilities
Clostridium. difficile	Exposure to contaminated surfaces, water, hospital equipment, and healthcare personnel, prolonged antibiotics use	Sepsis syndrome, neutropenic fever, abdominal pain, *C. difficile*–associated diarrhea (CDAD) and colitis, abdominal pain	Toxin-B gene by PCR (preferred initial test)	Leukocytosis may be absent from immunosuppressed patients	Oral vancomycin, fidaxomicin, and metronidazole (alternative therapy)

Mycobacterium TB and non-TB *Mycobacterium* spp.	Reactivation or new exposure (TB *Mycobacterium*), contaminated water supplies (non-TB *Mycobacterium*)	Cough, B-symptoms (fever, weight loss), and several types of pulmonary infiltrates Usually, 100+ day post-HSCT	Acid-fast bacillus culture, special stains (ZN, AFB) MTB by IHC	Anemia leukocytosis, thrombocytopenia, and myelofibrosis but these findings may be absent in immunosuppressed patients	Combination therapy with rifampicin, isoniazid, pyrazinamide for TB *Mycobacterium* infections
Fungi					
Candida spp. and other non-*Candida* yeast spp. (cryptococcus, *Saccharomyces*, *Malassezia*, *Geotrichum*, *Rhodotorula*, among others)	Endogenous, exogenous, environmental, or healthcare personnel	Sepsis, neutropenic fever, esophagitis, erythematous papular skin lesions, hepatosplenic candidiasis	Blood cultures, (1,3)-beta-D-glucan for invasive/disseminated fungal infections *Candida* species by PCR	Peripheral cytopenias, granuloma formation in bone marrow or tissue	Fluconazole, voriconazole, Posaconazole, isavuconazonium, amphotericin B, depending on species and susceptibilities

(continued)

Table 50.1 (continued)

Organism	Sources or vector	Clinical presentation	Laboratory tests	Hematologic changes	Treatment
Aspergillus, fusarium, scedosporium, Mucorales spp.	Inhalation or traumatic inoculation of conidia from vegetation, dust, hospital construction areas	Neutropenic fever, sinusitis, cough, pleuritic pain, cavitary, or nodular pneumonia on imaging, erythematous papular lesions for disseminated mold infection, large eschar surrounded by erythema in traumatic skin inoculation	*Aspergillus* galactomannan antigen by EIA on serum or bronchoscopy PCR tests can be negative, but the diagnosis is presumed by radiological findings in immunosuppressed host	Neutropenia	Voriconazole, Posaconazole, isavuconazonium, amphotericin B, depending on species and susceptibility
Parasites					
Cryptosporidium spp.	Multiple transmission routes exist but person-to-person contact is more common	Diarrhea Less commonly, cholecystitis, cholangitis, hepatitis, and pancreatitis	PCR, ELISA or Special staining (modified acid-fast stain, fluorescent stains) of biopsy specimens		Antidiarrheal medications. Nitazoxanide is less effective for immunocompromised patients

Toxoplasma gondii	Exposure to cat feces and undercooked meat	Disseminated toxoplasmosis (often acute respiratory failure with diffuse infiltrates on imaging)	Real-time PCR targeting a 529-bp genomic fragment has a higher sensitivity Serology and conventional *T. gondii* PCR, targeting the B1 gene is limited	Cytopenias, Leukocytosis. In severe disease, disseminated intravascular coagulation, hemophagocytic lymphohistiocytosis (HLH), granuloma	Treatment with pyrimethamine and sulfadiazine plus folinic acid Prophylaxis with trimethoprim-sulfamethoxazole is more efficacious than pentamidine for prophylaxis
Strongyloides stercoralis	Skin exposed to contaminated soil	Disseminated strongyloidiasis (acute respiratory distress syndrome) Persistent diarrhea (>14 days)	Strongyloides antibody, IgG by ELISA, serum (positive results in patients from endemic areas may not be true active infection) Ova and parasite examination of urine or body fluid	Eosinophilia	Ivermectin

(continued)

Table 50.1 (continued)

Organism	Sources or vector	Clinical presentation	Laboratory tests	Hematologic changes	Treatment
Virus					
HSV	HSV-seropositive patients not on antiviral prophylaxis often have HSV reactivation	Mucositis (oral cavity, oropharynx, and esophagus), encephalitis	Secretions and tissue for HSV1/HSV2 by PCR Immunohistochemistry. HSV meningitis/encephalitis panel by PCR		Treatment and prophylaxis with acyclovir, valacyclovir, famciclovir. The doses vary for treatment vs prophylaxis
CMV	CMV-seropositive patients not on antiviral prophylaxis often have viral reactivation	Pneumonia, colitis	CMV by quantitative NAAT, on plasma or qualitative PCR on saliva		Prophylactic or pre-emptive anti-CMV regimen: ganciclovir, valganciclovir, foscarnet, letermovir, and maribavir. Treatment with ganciclovir, valganciclovir, foscarnet, and maribavir
HCV	Needle-sharing, contaminated medical equipment	Hepatic sinusoidal syndrome Early cirrhosis	PCR, FibroSure test, and ultrasound-based elastography		Sofosbuvir–velpatasivir Glecaprevir–pibrentasvir

HBV	Reactivation post-engraftment in HBsAg-negative patients from occult HBV infection	Acute hepatitis	HBV core Ab IgM, HBV surface Ag, HBV DNA by PCR		Entecavir, tenofovir, lamivudine
EBV	Reactivation from donor or recipient B cells	IM-type acute illness with or without malignant B-cell transformation, PTLD (can present as fever, nodal or extranodal LPD in diverse organs)	CT/PET, Biopsy, immunohistochemical panel including EBV–LMP, flow cytometry, in situ hybridization. EBV DNA by qPCR in PB	IM, chronic EBV infection, lymphomas, aggressive NK-cell leukemia, ENNKL, PTLD-associated lymphoid proliferation	Reduce immunosuppression, EBV-specific cytotoxic T cells, rituximab. Less effective antiviral agents include ganciclovir and acyclovir
Respiratory viruses*	Respiratory droplets inhalation	Sinusitis, pneumonia	Respiratory virus mini panel by PCR		Prevention with influenza-inactivated vaccine immunization. Treatment with neuraminidase inhibitors (zanamivir, oseltamivir), baloxavir marboxil

(continued)

Table 50.1 (continued)

Organism	Sources or vector	Clinical presentation	Laboratory tests	Hematologic changes	Treatment
VZV	Reactivation-seropositive patients. Contact exposure to contagious patient or following live VZV vaccination	Chicken pox, shingles, encephalitis, hepatis, pneumonia	VZV by PCR on blood, CSF, tissue and vesicle fluid, ocular fluid	–	Avoid exposure to potentially contagious individuals Consider vaccine prophylaxis with recombinant zoster vaccine vs antivirals (acyclovir, famciclovir, valacyclovir) in transplant patients and with some chemotherapy regimens VariZIG to seropositive pretransplant, T cell–depleted allograft, high-dose glucocorticoid therapy. Postexposure valacyclovir

HHV-6	Reactivation	Encephalitis, bone marrow suppression, and delayed platelet engraftment, rashes, encephalitis, pneumonia, and hepatitis	PCR from blood or CSF	–	Prophylaxis not recommended
Parvovirus B-19	Respiratory secretions or blood products	Profound anemia a/w post-HSCT	Serology, PCR, IHC, intracellular virus inclusion identified in early stage erythroblasts	Red blood cell aplasia, bone marrow suppression	Reduce immunosuppression, IVIG, supportive transfusions
BK polyomavirus	Respiratory secretions, contact with infected urine/feces, blood transfusion or donor organ, reactivation	Hemorrhagic cystitis*, nephritis	PCR in blood, and urine, decoy cells, tissue biopsy	–	Reduce immunosuppression, supportive care, IVIG. Cidofovir

(continued)

Table 50.1 (continued)

Organism	Sources or vector	Clinical presentation	Laboratory tests	Hematologic changes	Treatment
Adenovirus (More common in children than adults)	Respiratory secretions, fecal–oral, blood products, or direct contact	Hemorrhagic cystitis*, URT infection, conjunctivitis, pneumonitis (severe), hepatitis, enteritis, hemorrhagic colitis, nephritis	PCR, antigen detection	–	Supportive care, consider cidofovir
Enteric viral pathogens (coxsackie A, rotavirus, echovirus, norovirus)	Fecal–oral route	Mouth ulcers, gastroenteritis, enteritis with prolonged and significant diarrhea, pericarditis	PCR, antigen detection	Predisposing factor: lymphopenia	Supportive care

HIV	Homosexual behavior, drug use, exposure to HIV-contaminated blood products or body fluid, vertical (fetal-maternal) infection	Flu-like, B-symptoms, generalized lymphadenopathy, rash	PCR, ELISA	HIV-related lymphoproliferative disorders/lymphoma	ART
COVID-19	Respiratory pathway	Flu-like symptoms	PCR, antibody tests	Atypical lymphocytes	Prophylactic vaccination Nirmatrelvir+ritonavir if no contraindications or medication interactions Remdesivir based on severity

(continued)

Table 50.1 (continued)

Organism	Sources or vector	Clinical presentation	Laboratory tests	Hematologic changes	Treatment
HTLV 1/2	Endemic HTLV1/2 exposure	Carriers usually asymptomatic	PCR, antibody tests	ATLL	No treatment if not developed ATLL
HHV-8	HIV or immunosuppressed individual	Symptoms and signs upon type of disease	IHC, PCR	Kaposi sarcoma, Castleman disease, HHV8-associated lymphoproliferative disorder	Limited role for antivirals Treatment of HIV rituximab +/– chemotherapy

*Respiratory viruses: including respiratory syncytial virus, influenza, parainfluenza, and adenovirus, and toxicity to the bladder mucosa from the conditioning regimen used pretransplant (cyclophosphamide, ifosfamide, busulfan, and total body irradiation), or BK polyomavirus and adenovirus occurred post-transplant

Ab Antibody, *ART* Anti-retroviral therapy, *ATLL* adult T-cell lymphoma/leukemia, *a/w* associated with, *CDAD Clostridium difficile*-associated diarrhea, *CMV* cytomegalovirus, *CSF* cerebrospinal fluid, *CT* computed tomography, *CTV* cytomegalovirus, *EBV* Epstein–Barr Virus, *EIA* enzyme-linked immunoassay, *ELISA* Enzyme-Linked ImmunoSorbent Assay, *ENNKL* Extranodal Natural-killer cell lymphoma, GI gastrointestinal, *GvHD* graft-vs-host disease, *HBsAg* hepatitis-B surface antigen, *HBV* Hepatitis B, *HCV* Hepatitis C, *HHV* human herpes virus, *HSCT* hematopoietic stem cell transplant, *HSV* Herpes simplex virus, *HTLV* Human T-lymphotropic virus, *IgG* immunoglobulin, *IHC* immunohistochemistry, *IM* infectious mononucleosis, *IVIG* Intravenous immunoglobin, *LMP* latent membrane protein, *LPD* lymphoproliferative disorder, *MRSA* methicillin-resistant *Staphylococcus aureus*, *MTB Mycobacterium tuberculosis*, *NAAT* Nucleic Acid Amplification, *NK* natural-killer, *PB* peripheral Blood, *PCR* polymerase chain reaction, *PET* positron-emission tomography, *PTLD* post-transplant lymphoproliferative disease, *qPCR* quantitative PCR, *TB* Tuberculosis, *URT* upper respiratory tract, *VariZIG* varicella zoster immune globulin, *VZV* varicella zoster virus, *ZN* Ziehl-Neelsen

Differential Diagnosis

A syndromic approach to infectious workup is preferred because of certain similarities in clinical manifestations across different organisms and medications. These syndromes can be localized to organs or have systemic manifestations. Noninfectious causes, such as direct toxicity or side effects from chemotherapeutic and nonchemotherapeutic medications, must be considered. For example, diarrhea can be caused by direct toxicity, viral, parasitic, or bacterial pathogens. Some diseases that could clinically, or histologically mimic infectious diseases should be excluded (Table 50.2). Disease-specific ancillary tests should be ordered in addition to microbiological tests.

Table 50.2 Common mimickers of infectious diseases

Infectious type	Resembling diseases	Additional tests
Bacteremia/sepsis with leukemoid reaction	Myeloid neoplasms	Bone marrow biopsy, cytogenetics, FISH, and NGS
Mycobacteria	Benign histiocytic proliferation or histiocytoma	Tissue biopsy with AFB stain
Parvovirus B19	Aplastic anemia, pure red blood cell aplasia	Bone marrow biopsy
HTLV1/2 carrier	Adult T-cell leukemia/ Lymphoma	Flow cytometry, tissue-specific PCR for HTLV1/2
IM (EBV infection)	EBV+ DLBCL	Flow cytometry, FISH panel for MYC rearrangement
Toxoplasma gondii involving CNS	CNS lymphoma, GBM	Biopsy for flow cytometry, IHC, and genetic studies
Viral infection with lymphadenopathy (e.g., HIV, EBV, COVID-19)	Lymphoma	Lymph node biopsy

AFB Acid fast bacilli, *CNS* central nervous system, *DLBCL* diffuse large B-cell lymphoma, *EBV* Epstein–Barr virus, *FISH* florescent in situ hybridization, *GBM* Glioblastoma multiforme, *HTLV* Human T-lymphotropic virus, *IHC* immunohistochemistry, *IM* infectious mononucleosis, *ITP* immune mediated thrombocytopenia, *NA* not applicable, *NGS* next-generation sequencing, *PCR* polymerase chain reaction, *PE* pulmonary embolism

Prognosis

Infectious-disease severity and prognosis among patients with hematologic neoplasms and HSCTs depend upon early diagnosis, patients' immune status, expected immune recovery, and prompt and effective treatment. Localized infectious disease can be more easily eradicated with better outcome, while systemic or disseminated infectious disease shows worse outcome and requires critical care and close monitoring. Administering colony-stimulating factors and certain cytokines during engraftment has been shown to enhance immunity and outcomes.

Treatment

The therapy for infections in patients undergoing HSCT covers pre-emptive, prophylactic, and post-confirmed infection. Pre-emptive therapy is a dynamic approach that requires serial measurement of blood levels of the organism following transplant and treating those who develop detectable disease where applicable [7]. Prophylactic therapy involves commencing therapy for the organism based on established risk profile without an identifiable organism. Toxicity from prolonged administration is a potential downfall of prolonged prophylactic therapy. The consensus of most appropriate approach has not been reached; therefore, the decision to give prophylactic or pre-emptive therapy is personalized, considering the risk profile of each patient, in particular for those high-risk patients.

There are clinical situations where organisms may not be identified despite the presence of clinical features; these situations warrant being cognizant of direct toxicity from chemotherapeutic agents and mitigating these effects. We consider in these cases whether underlying disease may be contributing to symptoms suggestive of infection.

Infection control using strict hand-hygiene practices and contact-droplet airborne precautions is critical to prevent transmission when managing these high-risk patient groups. It may be prudent to delay transplant until resolution of symptoms in the symptomatic patient provided relapse or progression of disease is not imminent. Physical distancing should be employed with individuals suspected of having community-acquired respiratory viral infection. Chlorhexidine bathing for all HSCT recipients is recommended. Passive and active immunizations should be considered because of lost immunity following transplant. More detailed information regarding organism-directed prophylaxis and vaccinations after HSCT is discussed elsewhere [8].

Promising Clinical Studies

Preventive and prompt treatment for infections following HSCT is not always effective and can have toxic side effects. Successful infection control requires the regeneration of T cells. Therefore, T-cell immunotherapy has been studied as a substitute or complement to pharmacotherapy. Research has shown that introducing donor-derived T cells aimed at specific viruses guided by monitoring viral DNA can re-establish immunity and protect against viral infections [9, 10]. Many of these initial studies are not FDA-approved, yet they provide hope for the potential of T-cell immunotherapy to enhance pathogen-specific immunity. Vaccines against many respiratory viruses are under investigation with good premise; however, few are clinically available.

Board Questions

1. The following are important viruses commonly associated with infection in HSCT recipients except:

   a. Cytomegalovirus
   b. Epstein–Barr virus
   c. Human herpes virus 6
   d. Hepatitis-B virus
   e. HIV

Correct answer: e

Explanation: All the viruses above are commonly associated with infection in HSCT recipients except HIV. HIV is usually associated with high-risk sexual behavior or drug use, not after HSCT.

2. The most common fungal pathogen in patients undergoing HSCT is:

    a. *Candida* pre-engraftment, *Aspergillus* post-engraftment
    b. *Candida* post-engraftment, *Aspergillus* post-engraftment
    c. *Candida* post-engraftment, *Aspergillus* pre-engraftment
    d. *Candida* pre-engraftment, *Aspergillus* pre-engraftment

Correct answer: a

Explanation: Before the advent of routine antifungal prophylaxis, *Candida* spp. accounted for most fungal infections in the pre-engraftment HSCT patients, followed by *Aspergillus* spp. *Aspergillus* is also the most common fungal species infecting HSCT recipients, occurring most commonly in post allogeneic HSCT recipients who have severe graft-vs-host disease while on immunosuppressive therapy, including steroids.

References

1. Rothman KJ. Causes. Am J Epidemiol. 1995;141(2):90–5. https://doi.org/10.1093/oxfordjournals.aje.a117417.
2. Wingard JR, Hsu J, Hiemenz JW. Hematopoietic stem cell transplantation: an overview of infection risks and epidemiology. Infect Dis Clin North Am. 2010;24(2):257–72. https://doi.org/10.1016/j.idc.2010.01.010.
3. Hu B, Huang S, Yin L. The cytokine storm and COVID-19. J Med Virol. 2021;93(1):250–6. https://doi.org/10.1002/jmv.26232.
4. Bikdeli B, Madhavan MV, Jimenez D, et al. COVID-19 and thrombotic or thromboembolic disease: implications for prevention, antithrombotic therapy, and follow-up: JACC state-of-the-art review. J Am Coll Cardiol. 2020;75(23):2950–73. https://doi.org/10.1016/j.jacc.2020.04.031.
5. Nathan S, Ustun C. Complications of Stem Cell Transplantation that Affect Infections in Stem Cell Transplant Recipients, with Analogies to Patients with Hematologic Malignancies. Infect Dis Clin North Am.

2019;33(2):331–59. https://doi.org/10.1016/j.idc.2019.01.002. Epub 2019 Mar 30. PMID: 30940464.
6. Misch EA, Andes DR.Bacterial Infections in the Stem Cell Transplant Recipient and Hematologic Malignancy Patient. Infect Dis Clin North Am. 2019;33(2):399–445. https://doi.org/10.1016/j.idc.2019.02.011. PMID: 31005135.
7. Dukkipati SS, Velez AP, Yacoub AT, Greene J. Prophylaxis for infections following allogeneic hematopoietic stem cell transplantation. Infect Dis Clini Pract. 2015;23(1):7–12.
8. Tomblyn M, Chiller T, Einsele H, et al. Guidelines for preventing infectious complications among hematopoietic cell transplantation recipients: a global perspective. Biol Blood Marrow Transp. 2009;15(10):1143–238.
9. Leen AM, Bollard CM, Mendizabal AM, et al. Multicenter study of banked third-party virus-specific T cells to treat severe viral infections after hematopoietic stem cell transplantation. Blood. 2013;121(26):5113–23. https://doi.org/10.1182/blood-2013-02-486324.
10. Tzannou I, Papadopoulou A, Naik S, et al. Off-the-shelf virus-specific T cells to treat BK virus, human herpesvirus 6, cytomegalovirus, Epstein-Barr virus, and adenovirus infections after allogeneic hematopoietic stem-cell transplantation. J Clin Oncol. 2017;35(31):3547–57. https://doi.org/10.1200/JCO.2017.73.0655.

Microorganism-Induced Benign Hematologic Conditions

51

Jennifer Eatrides and Guy Handley

Many infections present with hematologic manifestations, prompting consultation with a hematologist. Hematologic abnormalities may be correctable by treating the underlying infection and often require a multidisciplinary approach with infectious-disease consultation. We will focus on a brief review of selected infections and their benign hematologic manifestations in this chapter. We summarize these selected infections, as well as several others (HIV, cytomegalovirus, brucellosis, and leishmaniasis) in Table 51.1. Infections commonly present in or associated with hematologic malignancies and post-transplantation will be discussed in a separate Chap. 50.

J. Eatrides (✉)
H. Lee Moffitt Cancer Center and Research Institute, Tampa, FL, USA

Department of Oncologic Sciences, Morsani College of Medicine, University of South Florida, Tampa, FL, USA
e-mail: jennifer.eatrides@moffitt.org

G. Handley
H. Lee Moffitt Cancer Center and Research Institute, Tampa, FL, USA

Department of Medicine, Division of Infectious Disease and International Medicine, Morsani College of Medicine, University of South Florida, Tampa, FL, USA

L. Sokol, L. Zhang (eds.), *Non-Neoplastic Hematologic Disorders*,
https://doi.org/10.1007/978-3-031-62373-8_51

Table 51.1 Microorganisms with benign hematologic manifestations and differential diagnosis

Microorganism	Benign hematologic manifestations	Differential diagnosis	Key points in examination	Treatment
Parvovirus [1]	PRCA Transient aplastic crisis HLH*	DBA Thymoma-associated PRCA Autoimmune or malignancy-associated PRCA (caused by T-cell proliferation or T-cell LGL) Aplastic anemia Hypoplastic MDS	Reticulocyte count inappropriately low in setting of severe anemia Serology or parvovirus PCR to confirm diagnosis (depending on immune status) BMBx considered in unclear cases	Reduce immunosuppression IVIG in refractory cases
EBV [2]	Pancytopenia Aplastic anemia Thrombocytopenia Lymphocytosis Lymphadenopathy HLH*	Viral infections: CMV, HIV, viral hepatitis HL and NHL	Monospot (IM) Serology based on phase of illness Evaluation for LPD including tissue biopsy +/− BMBx based on clinical picture with EBER in situ hybridization	IM: supportive care EBV-related PTLD: Reduce immunosuppression Rituximab in select populations

HHV8 [3]	MCD HLH*	Reactive lymphadenopathy Idiopathic MCD KS, PEL Lymphoma Solid tumor HIV lymphadenitis Autoimmune disorder Sarcoidosis	CBC, CMP, HIV, ESR, CRP Tissue biopsy/IHC for HHV8 LANA-1 for diagnosis	ART if concurrent HIV Rituximab in MCD Various cytotoxic chemotherapy regimens for refractory disease Unclear role of antivirals
HCV [4]	Mixed cryoglobulinemia Aplastic anemia Thrombocytopenia	Viral infections: EBV, CMV, HIV, HBV Lymphoproliferative disorders Autoimmune disease (rheumatoid arthritis, Sjögren's syndrome) Other causes of vasculitis (ANCA, infection-related, drug-induced, etc.)	Cryoglobulins (>5 mg/dL; cryocrit >0.5–1% for diagnosis), SPEP/IFE Histopathology for leukocytoclastic vasculitis BMBx may be considered in examination for aplasia, cytopenias	Direct antiviral therapy (ex glecaprevir–pibretasvir or sofosbuvir–velpatasvir) Immunologic Phenomena: high-dose steroids +/– Rituximab Cyclophosphamide in refractory cases

(continued)

Table 51.1 (continued)

Microorganism	Benign hematologic manifestations	Differential diagnosis	Key points in examination	Treatment
HIV [5]	Aplastic anemia ITP Neutropenia Lymphopenia Lymphadenopathy	Viral infections: EBV, CMV, viral hepatitis HL and NHL Myeloproliferative disorders	Fourth generation combined antigen/antibody immunoassay Quantitative viral load PCR CD4+ T-cell count BMBx may be considered in examination for aplasia	Initiation of ART Consider IVIG, dexamethasone for refractory ITP
CMV (acute infection) [6]	Hemolytic anemia Pancytopenia HLH*	Viral infections: EBV, HIV, viral hepatitis Lymphoma	Serology PCR for DNA pp65 antigen	Acute infection: supportive care Antivirals only for select populations with CMV disease from reactivation or high risk (eg, HCT)
Babesia [7]	Hemolytic anemia DIC Splenic rupture	Noninfectious causes of hemolytic anemia Other tick-borne illnesses: borreliosis, ehrlichiosis anaplasmosis or rickettsial infections *Plasmodium* species	Peripheral smear with *Maltese cross* PCR to confirm Serology (does not require treatment in isolation)	Atovaquone + azithromycin Alternative: Clindamycin + primaquine Asymptomatic: no treatment required

Plasmodium species/ Malaria [8]	Hemolytic anemia Thrombocytopenia Splenomegaly Microvascular sequestration	Noninfectious causes of hemolytic anemia Other arboviral illnesses Typhoid fever, leptospirosis, viral hepatitis	Thick and thin smear for parasites (ring, trophozoite, and schizont forms may provide species) Assays for *Plasmodium* lactate dehydrogenase or PfHRP2 (*P. falciparum* only) PCR	Severe: IV artesunate (initial) IV quinine (alternative) Uncomplicated: artemether–lumefantrine Other second-line agents (Castro et al, PMID: 37847222)
Brucella [9]	Pancytopenia Hepatosplenomegaly Lymphadenopathy HLH*	Viral infections: HIV, EBV, CMV Lymphoproliferative disorders Tuberculosis Malaria, typhoid	Gram stain and culture (variable sensitivity; bone marrow culture highest yield) Serology (variable sensitivity) PCR Imaging based on clinical picture Histopathology with noncaseating granulomas	Doxycycline + aminoglycoside or rifampin based on extent and site of disease

(continued)

Table 51.1 (continued)

Microorganism	Benign hematologic manifestations	Differential diagnosis	Key points in examination	Treatment
Leishmania (Visceral) [10]	Pancytopenia Hepatosplenomegaly HLH*	Viral infections: HIV, EBV, CMV, viral hepatitis Brucella Tuberculosis Leukemia malnutrition	Histopathology shows amastigote (may require bone marrow biopsy) PCR Culture Serology Test for HIV coinfection	Liposomal amphotericin B Alternatives: stibogluconate + paromomycin miltefosine *Depends on immunocompetence, endemic area, and availability

*In cases where HLH diagnosed in context of above infections, treatment of underlying cause is primary treatment with consideration to add steroids (dexamethasone) and/or etoposide per HLH-2004 protocol based on severity and clinical context

+In general, examination for cytopenias includes CBC with differential and peripheral smear, and may include examination for hemolysis with LDH, haptoglobin, reticulocyte count, and direct Coombs test

ANCA antineutrophilic cytoplasmic antibody, *ART* antiretroviral therapy, *BMBx* bone marrow biopsy, *CBC* complete blood count, *CMP* complete metabolic panel, *CMV* cytomegalovirus, *CRP* C-reactive protein, *DBA* Diamond Blackfan anemia, *DFA* direct fluorescent antibody, *DIC* disseminated intravascular coagulation, *EBER* Epstein–Barr virus encoded small RNAs, *HBV* hepatitis B virus, *HCT* hematopoietic cell transplant, *HIV* human immunodeficiency virus, *HL* Hodgkin's lymphoma, *HLH* hemophagocytic lymphohistiocytosis, *IFE* immunofixation, *IM* infectious mononucleosis, *IPF* immature platelet fraction, *ITP* immune thrombocytopenic purpura, *IVIG* intravenous immunoglobulin, *KS* Kaposi sarcoma, *LANA-1* latency-associated nuclear antigen-1, *LDH* lactate dehydrogenase, *LGL* large granular lymphocytic leukemia, *LPD* lymphoproliferative disorder, *MCD* multicentric Castleman disease, *MDS* myelodysplastic syndrome, *NHL* non-Hodgkin's lymphoma, *PCR* polymerase chain reaction, *PEL* primary effusion lymphoma, *PRCA* pure red cell aplasia, *PTLD* post-transplant lymphoproliferative disorder, *SPEP* serum protein electrophoresis, *VEGF* vascular endothelial growth factor

Human Parvovirus B19 (B19V)

Introduction

Human parvovirus B19 (B19V) is a single-stranded DNA virus with a wide range of clinical presentations depending on patient's net state of immunosuppression. It causes a mild febrile illness, typically in childhood, with a characteristic *slapped-cheek* rash (fifth disease or erythema infectiosum). However, B19V may also cause severe illness in patients with underlying chronic hemolytic disorders, or it may present with a pure red blood cell (RBC) aplasia (PRCA) in immunocompromised patients.

Pathogenesis

B19V infects erythroid progenitors through the surface-P antigen. Increased RBC destruction or decreased RBC production predisposes to a transient aplastic crisis, characterized by severe anemia, absent reticulocytosis, and viral inclusions in early erythroblasts with PRCA in the patient's bone marrow (PMID: 27337440).

Diagnosis

- Serology is the recommended test for immunocompetent patients.
- B19V nucleic acid amplification testing/polymerase chain reaction (PCR) is less sensitive as viremia may resolve before symptom onset but can help immunocompromised patients or those with hemolytic disorders.
- Immunohistochemical staining on bone-marrow samples.

Prognosis

Disease course is typically self-limited in immunocompetent patients, but immunocompromised patients may have complications or relapses.

Treatment

Management depends on manifestations of infection, but for PRCA and aplastic crisis, supportive treatment with transfusions is required until aplasia resolves along with reduction of immunosuppression. There is no specific antiviral therapy, but intravenous (IV) immunoglobulin can be considered for immunocompromised patients with persistent infection.

Promising Clinical Studies

There are no active clinical trials for treating B19V. Areas of interest have been with B19V human immunoglobulin-G monoclonal antibodies and B19V-tailored nano-systems.

Caveats

- Patients whose RBCs do not express P antigen are resistant to B19V.

Epstein–Barr Virus (EBV)

Introduction

Epstein–Barr virus (EBV) infection occurs at any age. Most cases are asymptomatic, but clinical infection could result in cytopenias, hemolytic or aplastic anemia, reactive lymphocytosis, lymphadenopathy, and hepatosplenomegaly. Rarely, chronic active infection persists, but, for most, symptoms resolve, and the virus establishes lifelong latency. EBV gene products may be involved in oncogenesis or other lymphoproliferative processes after primary infection, particularly in the setting of immunosuppression state (PMID 2952635).

Pathogenesis

EBV infects oropharyngeal epithelial cells and undergoes lytic replication and then spreads to resting memory B cells to establish a lifelong latent infection with potential reactivation. It can infect and reactivate in any organ system with variable, potentially life-threatening, manifestations. Asymptomatic DNAemia is common but can be associated with lymphoproliferative disorders and overt malignancy. In addition, EBV can also cause the following nonmalignant disorders:

- Lymphomatoid granulomatosis: Clonal EBV-infected B cells that cause B symptoms and can involve the lungs, kidneys, skin, liver, and central nervous system and progress into EBV+ diffuse large B-cell lymphoma.

- X-linked lymphoproliferative disease: selective immunodeficiency to EBV caused by mutation in *SH2D1A* or *XIAP* gene.
- Post-transplant lymphoproliferative disorders.
- Hemophagocytic lymphohistiocytosis (HLH): both with primary infection and in the setting of subsequent EBV-associated lymphoproliferative disorders.

Diagnosis

- Monospot/heterophile antibody test in case of classic infectious mononucleosis (IM)
- EBV-specific serology for viral capsid antigen and nuclear antigen 1 if concerned for IM.
- EBV–PCR

- Immunohistochemical staining for EBV-latent-membrane protein or in situ hybridization using EBV-encoded RNA probe (EBER) of tissue.

Prognosis

Prognosis ranges widely based on the presence, severity, and duration of immunosuppression. Most recover without sequelae, whereas immunocompromised patients can have life-threatening and even refractory symptoms and/or disease from EBV infection or malignant progression.

Treatment

Disease course is typically self-limited with no treatment indicated. In general, antivirals have not shown a benefit. Steroids may be used in the instance of critical airway obstruction from lymphadenopathy or severe hemolytic anemia. In EBV-associated lymphoproliferative disorders, reduction in immunosuppression should be pursued. Rituximab has a role in treating EBV in select patients with CD20+ lymphoproliferative processes. Routine screening for DNAemia is not recommended except for those at high risk for EBV-associated lymphoproliferative processes.

Promising Clinical Studies

- Vaccine trials: viral vaccine targeting gp350/220 and a phase 1 study evaluating mRNA-EBV vaccine (NCT05831111)
- EBV-specific cytotoxic T lymphocytes (NCT03266653)
- Chimeric antigen receptor T-cell therapy/tabelecleucel in EBV-associated disease (NCT04554914)

Caveats

- Because of the significant delay from time of infection to symptoms, serology from viral capsid antigen and EBV nuclear antigen 1 is required to differentiate acute from past infection.
- The monospot/heterophile antibody test may have false positives with neoplastic or rheumatologic conditions and should primarily be used in classic presentations of IM.
- There are data for pre-emptive rituximab for EBV–DNAemia in select patient populations at high risk of lymphoproliferative disorders.

Human Herpes Virus 8 (HHV8)

Introduction

Human herpes virus 8 (HHV8) is endemic but with high geographic variability causing several neoplasms, including Kaposi sarcoma (KS), primary effusion lymphoma, and multicentric Castleman disease (MCD). This section will address nonmalignant MCD, but it is important to evaluate for concurrent KS, PEL, and other neoplasms in such patients.

Pathogenesis

HHV8+ MCD typically presents with lymphadenopathy and *B symptoms*, including fevers, night sweats, and unintentional weight loss. Patients may also have cytopenias, skin rash, hepatosplenomegaly, as well as organ dysfunction.

Diagnosis

- Immunohistochemical staining for LANA-1 on tissue biopsy is the gold standard for HHV8+ MCD.
- HHV8 PCR may be helpful but is nonspecific and not always present.

Prognosis

Prognosis of HHV8+ MCD is poor without treatment, and up to 20% of patients may go on to develop lymphoma, but this prognosis has improved substantially with the use of rituximab.

Treatment

- Antiretroviral therapy for all HHV8+ MCD patients who have HIV.
- Rituximab with or without chemotherapy for HHV8+ MCD depending on the severity.
- Chemotherapy with etoposide with progressive organ dysfunction or life-threatening disease and pegylated liposomal doxorubicin if there is concurrent KS.

Promising Clinical Studies

- NCT06052618 will evaluate pacritinib, a JAK2/FLT3 inhibitor, but is not yet open.

Caveats

- HIV should be checked in all patients with diagnosis of HHV8-associated disorder.
- The management differs significantly in HHV8-negative MCD.
- Rituximab monotherapy may exacerbate or lead to KS in HHV8+ MCD.

Hepatitis C Virus (HCV)

Introduction

Hepatitis C virus (HCV) invades hepatocytes but can present with hematologic manifestations. Most infections are asymptomatic, but symptoms may include fever, abdominal pain, and jaundice with associated elevated liver-function tests.

Pathogenesis

After acute infection, a minority of patients clear the infection, while most others develop chronic HCV, which can cause cirrhosis and hepatocellular carcinoma. Hematologic manifestations range from benign cytopenias to lymphoproliferative disorders and overt lymphoma. Thrombocytopenia occurs via immune-mediated mechanisms, including antiplatelet antibodies and non-immune mechanisms, including hypersplenism, bone marrow suppression, and decreased thrombopoietin production by the liver. HCV may trigger aplastic anemia, PRCA, and autoimmune hemolytic anemia. Mixed cryoglobulinemia can be seen in patients with HCV and presents as an inflammatory syndrome with vasculitis symptoms (purpura, neuropathy, renal involvement, and arthralgias) that are attributed to immune-complex deposition in capillaries and arterioles, but most patients with cryoglobulins do not have vasculitis (PMID: 11439948).

Diagnosis

- HCV serology and quantitative viral load PCR.
- Lactate dehydrogenase, haptoglobin, direct antiglobulin test, reticulocyte count in patients with anemia to evaluate for autoimmune-mediated hemolysis.
- Cryoglobulins should be tested in patients with vasculitis symptoms.

Prognosis

Prognosis varies. Direct antiviral therapy is mostly curative and may correct hematologic abnormalities. Autoimmune cytopenias respond to treatments used for patients without HCV but with some increased risk of complications, such as thrombosis risk with splenectomy. Prognosis for cryoglobulinemia varies with extent, and worse outcomes are associated with lung, gastrointestinal tract, kidney involvement, and age greater than 65 years (PMID: 26622988).

Treatment

Management involves treating the underlying virus and potential immunosuppressive therapy. Direct antiviral therapy has largely replaced prior treatment regimens with cure rates of 98%, but regimens are specific to genotype. Cytopenias and cryoglobulinemia may be treated with steroids with or without rituximab, as well as with cyclosporine or cyclophosphamide in refractory patients.

Promising Clinical Studies

- NCT05168475 will evaluate biologics in patients with refractory non-antineutrophilic cytoplasmic antibody vasculitis.

Caveats

- Cryoglobulin testing must be collected in prewarmed tubes (37 °C) without anticoagulants.
- Patients treated and cured of hepatitis C with direct antivirals can become re-infected. A long-run laboratory monitoring is needed.

Intraerythrocytic Parasites

Babesia *Species*

Introduction

Babesia are protozoan intraerythrocytic parasites. Most infections are asymptomatic or have mild constitutional symptoms, but for some, particularly immunocompromised patients, it can present with fevers, hemolytic anemia, malaise, respiratory distress, and organ dysfunction which can be severe or life-threatening. While typically transmitted by tick vectors (*Ixodes scapularis*, commonly called deer ticks or blacklegged ticks), infection may occur through blood transfusion or organ transplant (PMID: 22716978).

Pathogenesis

Sporozoites delivered by the tick use glycosaminoglycans and sialoglycoproteins to invade erythrocytes and mature into trophozoites and then merozoites, which rupture host erythrocytes and invade other erythrocytes.

Diagnosis

- Microscopy/peripheral smear demonstrating pleomorphic ring forms of trophozoites or *Maltese cross* inclusions.
- PCR (helpful in setting of low parasitemia)

Prognosis

Prognosis varies. Risk factors for severe babesiosis include asplenia, immunosuppression, and age greater than 50 years. Complications include acute respiratory distress syndrome, disseminated intravascular coagulation, organ failure, or splenic rupture.

Treatment

Asymptomatic patients do not require antimicrobial therapy. Ambulatory patients with mild-to-moderate symptoms should receive 7–10 days of oral atovaquone and azithromycin. Hospitalized patients with severe disease should receive atovaquone and azithromycin as well; however, up to 6 weeks with

2 weeks of resolution of parasitemia may be required for some immunocompromised patients. Clindamycin and quinine were previously preferred for severe disease but is now an alternative regimen. Exchange transfusion can be considered with high-grade parasitemia (>10% of patients) or severe hemolytic anemia and/or with severe pulmonary, hepatic, or renal failure based on limited data (PMID: 33252652).

Promising Clinical Studies: Caveats

- Consider babesiosis in patients with other *Ixodes* tick-borne infections, including Lyme disease and human granulocytic ehrlichiosis.
- Patients with babesiosis are excluded from donating blood for a period because of risk of transmission in transfusions.

Plasmodium *Species*

Introduction

Five distinct *Plasmodium* species that cause malaria in humans include *P. falciparum, P. vivax*, *P. malariae*, *P. ovale*, and *P. knowlesi* with transmission through the *Anopheles* mosquito vector. Most infection is from *P. falciparum*, which carries the highest mortality, and from *P. vivax*, ranging from a mild flu-like illness, often with cyclic fever, to multi-organ failure, coma, and death.

Pathogenesis

Sporozoites enter via mosquito bites and infect hepatocytes via the lymphatic system where they form many merozoites which are released into circulation. Gametocytes are taken up by a mosquito to renew the cycle. *P. vivax* and *P. ovale* develop dormant hypnozoite forms within the liver. *P. falciparum* may infect erythrocytes and reticulocytes. Hematologic abnormalities can include thrombocytopenia (potentially with an autoimmune component), impaired platelet adhesion, anemia (including a severe hemolytic anemia), intravascular coagulation (though rarely disseminated intravascular coagulation), and splenomegaly (PMID: 28770814).

Diagnosis

- Microscopic examination of thick and thin smears of stained blood films remains the gold standard and is important for determining parasitemia.
- Assays for pan-species lactate dehydrogenase enzyme or *P. falciparum* histidine-rich protein can provide rapid diagnosis.

Prognosis

Prognosis varies widely by strain, geographic region, access to treatment, and severity. Criteria for severe *P. falciparum* malaria include clinical and laboratory criteria, including hemoglobin less than 7 g/dL in adults, hypoglycemia less than 40 mg/dL, acidosis with lactate greater than 5 mmol/L, creatinine greater than 3 mg/dL, or parasitemia greater than 10% among others, and is a true medical emergency. Protective factors among hosts include sickle-cell trait, blood group O, and certain thalassemias, while sickle-cell disease, blood group B, HIV, and asplenia increase risk of severe malaria.

Treatment

Severe malaria requires treatment with IV artesunate, while less-effective quinine is an alternative. Serial parasite-density monitoring every 6–12 h should be performed to ensure clearance. As of 2023, artemether–lumefantrine is now recommended for all adult patients with uncomplicated malaria, even in pregnancy (PMID: 37847222). Resistant strains to nearly all agents are emerging, including artemisinin-resistant strains. Adjunct therapies, including exchange transfusion and steroids, have been trialed but have not shown efficacy.

Promising Clinical Trials

- Antimicrobial agents targeting blood schizonts are under development.
- Over ten vaccine trials are currently recruiting patients.

Caveats

- The absence of the Duffy glycoprotein on RBCs can be protective against *P. vivax*.

Glucose-6-phosphate dehydrogenase deficiency may protect against severe malaria but increases risks of hemolytic anemia with primaquine treatment, and activity should be confirmed before using with *P. vivax* and *P. ovale*.

Board Questions

1. You are consulted on a 23-year-old patient who has had persistently high fevers, cytopenias, splenomegaly, and a ferritin level of 50,000 ng/mL. What are your considerations for potential triggers for this inflammatory syndrome?

    a. EBV
    b. Brucellosis
    c. Leishmania
    d. Hodgkin's lymphoma
    e. All of the above

    Correct answer: e

    Explanation: The patient described has symptoms suspicious for HLH, and this should be considered in patients with markedly elevated ferritin. HLH is an inflammatory syndrome that can be triggered by various infections, autoimmune disease, or underlying malignancy.

2. A 45-year-old with no significant medical history presents with fevers, confusion, nausea, vomiting, and diarrhea after returning from a 3-week vacation in Sub-Saharan Africa. He is

jaundiced, obtunded, and laboratory tests reveal a hemoglobin of 6 g/dL and a creatinine of 3.7 mg/dL. A peripheral smear obtained in the emergency department shows ring forms in approximately 15% of cells, and you are consulted by the emergency department after they were alerted by the laboratory. Which of the following is the most important next step?

a. Initiation of IV artesunate
b. Initiation of po atovaquone and IV azithromycin
c. Exchange transfusion
d. High-dose IV corticosteroids

Correct answer: a

Explanation: This patient is presenting with malaria, likely *P. falciparum*, with several criteria for severe infection, including hemoglobin of <7 g/dL, creatinine <3 mg/dL, parasitemia >10%, and cerebral dysfunction. IV artesunate is superior to other agents and should be initiated without delay. Mortality in cerebral malaria approaches 20% even when treated. Exchange transfusion has not shown a benefit and is not recommended. Atovaquone and azithromycin is therapy for babesiosis; however, such a severe presentation is unlikely in an otherwise immunocompetent host.

References

1. Landry M. Parvovirus B19. Microbiol Spectr. 2016;4(3):1–13. PMID: 27337440.
2. Thorley-Lawson D. EBV Persistence – introducing the virus. Curr Top Microbiol Immunol. 2015;390:151–209. PMID: 26424647.
3. Carbone A, et al. Castleman disease. Nat Rev Dis Primers. 2021;7(84):1–18. PMID: 34824298.
4. Kedia S, et al. Benign and Malignant hematological manifestations of chronic hepatitis C virus infection. Int J Prev Med. 2014;5(suppl 3):S179–92. PMID: 26622988.
5. Vishnu P, et al. Haematological manifestations of human immune deficiency virus infection. Br J Haematol. 2015;171(5):695–709. PMID: 26452169.

6. Boeckh M. Complications, diagnosis, management, and prevention of CMV infections: current and future. Hematology Am Soc Hematol Educ Program. 2011:305–9. PMID: 22160050.
7. Krause P, et al. Clinical Practice Guidelines by the Infectious Diseases Society of America (IDSA): 2020 guidelines on diagnosis and management of babesiosis. Clin Infect Dis. 2021;72(2):e49–64. PMID: 33252652.
8. Phillips, et al. Malaria. Nat Rev Dis Primers. 2017;3(17050):1–24. PMID: 28770814.
9. Pappas G, et al. Brucellosis. N Engl J Med. 2005;352(22):2325–36. PMID: 15930423.
10. Shiferaw, et al. Hematological profiles of visceral leishmaniasis patients before and after treatment of anti-leishmanial drugs at University of Gondar Hospital; Leishmania Research and Treatment Center Northwest, Ethiopia. BMC Infect Dis. 2021;21(1):1005. PMID: 34565339

Index

L. Sokol, L. Zhang (eds.), *Non-Neoplastic Hematologic Disorders*, https://doi.org/10.1007/978-3-031-62373-8

B

GPSR Compliance

The European Union's (EU) General Product Safety Regulation (GPSR) is a set of rules that requires consumer products to be safe and our obligations to ensure this.

If you have any concerns about our products, you can contact us on ProductSafety@springernature.com

In case Publisher is established outside the EU, the EU authorized representative is:

Springer Nature Customer Service Center GmbH
Europaplatz 3
69115 Heidelberg, Germany

Batch number: 10732632

Printed by Printforce, the Netherlands